MW01517433

European Committee for Hyperbaric Medicine
ECHM

THE ECHM COLLECTION
Volume I

Consensus Conferences and Workshops 1994 – 1999

European Committee for Hyperbaric Medicine
ECHM

THE ECHM COLLECTION
Volume I

Consensus Conferences and Workshops 1994 – 1999

Editors
A. Marroni, D Mathieu, F. Wattel

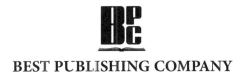

BEST PUBLISHING COMPANY

Copyright © 2005, by Best Publishing Company

International Standard Book Number: 1-930536-25-9

Library of Congress: 2004097985

Published by
Best Publishing Company
Post Office Box 30100
Flagstaff, AZ 86003-0100

www.bestpub.com

TABLE OF CONTENTS

Section I - Part 2 1-143
The 2nd European Consensus Conference on Hyperbaric Medicine

CONTENTS

CONTENTS

CONTENTS

Foreword

A. Marroni, D. Mathieu, F. Wattel

WHY THIS BOOK?

The European Committee for Hyperbaric Medicine has, during the last decade, become a common referral for state-of-the-art hyperbaric medicine practice and guidelines in Europe as well as internationally, with special reference to the European scene. The action of the ECHM, since its inception, has been characterized by a pragmatic and direct approach to the many problems connected to the development and acceptance of hyperbaric medicine in a multifaceted, multilingual, and extremely variegated reality, such as the European one.

This has been done thanks to the enthusiastic action—and devotion—of a small group of dedicated individuals who represented the best of hyperbaric medicine in many European countries and were the clinical and/or academic reference persons in their respective countries, either acting as single recognized specialists or representatives of national scientific societies.

The production of the ECHM during this period has been indeed remarkable, with 4 European Consensus Conferences, 3 Thematic Workshops, 2 ECHM Reports and a fifth European Consensus Conference planned for the year 2001.

Although all of the Consensus Conferences, Workshops and Reports are published, this did not happen in an orderly and standardized manner: most of the publications have been made in the form of Conference Proceedings, some of which were printed in only limited quantity and essentially distributed to the attendants and to some selected Academic, Scientific and Public Administration Institutions.

One Consensus Conference, the third one on Acute Musculo-skeletal Trauma, was partially published by Best Publishing Company, together with the proceedings of the Joint International Meeting of the International Congress of Hyperbaric Medicine, the European Underwater and Baromedical Society and the European Committee for Hyperbaric Medicine, which was held in Milano, Italy, in 1996.

The first Workshop, on Wound Healing, Safety and Cost-effectiveness, which was held in Belgrade in 1998 and printed locally, was then internationally published and distributed again by Best Publishing Company.

This started a productive relationship between the ECHM and Best, and particularly with its President Jim Joiner, who accepted to help and support the mission and the action of the ECHM by the regular publication of its key documents.

This volume is intended to be the first one of a series, hence the name "ECHM Collection", and covers the action of the ECHM since its inception until 1999. The multifaceted production of the ECHM will be, this way, more readily available to the international scientific community.

Other documents of the ECHM, such as the proceedings of the Workshop on New Indications of Hyperbaric Oxygen Therapy, held in Malta in 2000 and those of the Fifth ECHM Consensus Conference on Hyperbaric Oxygen Therapy in the treatment of Radio-induced Lesions in Normal Tissues, Lisbon, Portugal, October 19-20th, 2001, will be published with the next volumes of this ECHM Collection.

We, as the Editors, are glad to acknowledge Jim Joiner and Best Publishing Company for the essential support to this initiative and to the mission of the European Committee for Hyperbaric Medicine.

Alessandro Marroni, Daniel Mathieu, Francis Wattel

INTRODUCTION

The European Committee for Hyperbaric Medicine

History, Mission, and Achievements of the European Committee for Hyperbaric Medicine

A. Marroni, D. Mathieu, F. Wattel

I—HISTORY

- The first proposition to found the Committee was made in Milano in February 1989 during an informal and friendly discussion between some distinguished gentlemen involved in diving and hyperbaric medicine.
- The first meeting of the promoting members was held in Lille at the Hyperbaric Medical Center of the Intensive Care Department of the Calmette Hospital in November 1989 in order to state the scope and goals of the Committee, nominate the executive board and the members of the Committee, plan the next actions.

The promoting members were Dirk BAKKER, Jordi DESOLA, Alessandro MARRONI, Daniel MATHIEU, Giorgio ORIANI, Paolo PELAIA, Jörg SCHMUTZ, Francis WATTEL, Jörg WENDLING.

The promoting members decided to act as the executive board of the committee and, by unanimous decision, Professor Francis WATTEL was elected President of the Executive Board of the ECHM, and Professor Alessandro MARRONI was elected Secretary.

The executive board decided that all the presidents of the European Undersea and Baromedical Society and of the European National Underwater and Hyperbaric Medical Societies should be invited to be ex-officio members of the committee. For the European countries where there is no organized Hyperbaric Medicine Scientific Body, the leading authorities in Hyperbaric Medicine should be invited to be members of the committee. All the western and eastern European countries, included Turkey, Iceland, Cyprus and Malta should be represented in the committee. Dr Lee J. GREENBAUM, in his quality of executive director of the Undersea and Hyperbaric Medical Society (UHMS, USA), and Dr Frederick CRAMER, in his quality of secretary of the Foundation for the International Congress on Hyperbaric Medicine (ICHM), will also be members of the committee.

- The first plenary meeting of the ECHM was held in Amsterdam in August 1990, where the immediate tasks for the committee were defined as follows:
  - To officially constitute the committee
  - To enlarge its representativeness to all or most of the European countries
  - To pursue the definition of European Standards for Hyperbaric Medicine and official contacts with EEC Health Authorities

- Following to this, the Committee was officially constituted and its bylaws legally registered on 19 February 1991, in Milano, Italy, with Act REP15RAC3 of Notary Public Andrea Fezzara, registered in Codogno, Milano at number 75 series number 1, on 24 January 1991 and validated with State Seal of the Italian Government, protocol N 4/91 RA, on 29 January 1991, according to the European Convention of The Haye, of 5 October 1961.

- Official letters of invitation to become a member of the Committee were then sent to those European Scientists and Organizations, involved in Hyperbaric Medicine, who had not yet been formally invited.

- Every year, Plenary Meeting of the ECHM was called during the annual meeting of the European Underwater and Baromedical Society while ECHM Executive Committee meetings were hold twice times a year.

II—SCOPE AND GOALS OF THE ECHM

II.1. The scope and goals of the Committee are defined as follows :

- Studying and defining common indications for hyperbaric therapy, research and therapy protocols, common standards for therapeutic and technical procedures, equipment and personnel, cost-benefit and cost-effectiveness criteria

- Acting as a representative body with the European Health Authorities.

- Promoting further cooperation among existing scientific organizations involved in the field of Diving and Hyperbaric Medicine.

- An effective cooperation between ECHM and numerous scientific medical or technical organizations was promoted and organized particularly with the European Underwater and Baromedical Society (EUBS), the Underwater and Hyperbaric Medical Society (UHMS), the Foundation for the International Congress on Hyperbaric Medicine (ICHM), the Medical Subcommittee on the European Diving Technical Committee (EDTC), DAN EUROPE and International DAN, the Medical Committee of CMAS, the Japanese Society for Hyperbaric Medicine, etc. and an official presentation of the ECHM was done to the General Direction for Health and Safety and General Direction for Science, Research and Development, European Community, Brussels.

- But the most important action of the Committee was to define European standards for Hyperbaric Medicine Practice regarding indications, patient care and quality assurance, equipment and quality control, personnel and training policies, and research.

II.2. Planning the action

II.2.1. The initial draft document on which the committee has worked was a synthesis of the current international indications for HBOT.

Then, it was decided to elaborate a draft document named *European Standards for Hyperbaric Medicine* and composed of the following sections :

   I. Indications. Section Editors F. Wattel, D.J. Bakker
  II. Patient Management. Protocols. Section Editors G. Oriani, J. Wendling
 III. Safe and efficient use of hyperbaric chambers and medical equipment under hyperbaric conditions. Section Editors P. Pelaia, I. Mekjavic
 IV. Personnel and training policies. Section Editors J. Desola, J-L. Ducassé
  V. Research. Section Editors J. Schmutz, M. Lamy

Regarding the HBOT indications (Section I), the ECHM elaborated a preliminary list of indications already accepted, under investigations, or controversial in the different European countries (Committee meetings in Ancona, Italy in Nov./Dec. 1991 and in Toulouse, France in May 1992).

The accepted indications included decompression sickness, acute gas embolism, carbon monoxide poisoning and smoke inhalation, cyanide poisoning, Clostridium myonecrosis, necrotizing fasciitis, refractory osteomyelitis, sudden deafness, acute post-anoxic encephalopathy, mandibular osteoradionecrosis, hemorrhagic radiation cystitis, compromised skin graft and flaps, diabetic foot lesions, crush and compartment syndromes, reimplantations, arterial insufficiency ulcer or delayed wound healing, acute and chronic vascular insufficiency.

The group of investigated indications contained hydrogen sulfide poisoning, carbon tetrachloride poisoning, brain, pulmonary, liver abscesses, mycosis, head and spinal cord injuries, soft tissue radiation damage (cutaneous, subcutaneous, enteritis, proctitis, myelitis), burns, stroke.

Controversies concerned fetal hypoxia due to maternal vascular insufficiency, multiple sclerosis, blood loss.

II.2.2. In order to allow the validation of the proposed European Standards for Hyperbaric Medicine and to obtain the most complete agreement by the medical community, the ECHM decided to organize the First European Consensus Conference on Hyperbaric Medicine.

More than 350 specialists from 21 different countries participated at the conference that was held in September 1994 at the Medical university of Lille, France. An international jury : E.M. CAMPORESI, New York (USA), A. GASPARETTO, Roma (Italy), M. GOULON, Paris (France), L.J. GREENBAUM, Bethesda (USA), E.P. KINDWALL, Milwaukee (USA), M. LAMY, Liège (Belgium), D. LINNARSSON, Stockholm (Sweden), JM. MANTZ, Strasbourg (France), C. PERRET, Lausanne (Switzerland), President of the jury, P. PIETROPAOLI, Ancona (Italy), H. TAKAHASHI, Nagoya (Japan), C. VOISIN, Lille (France), with the support of a panel of 62 conference experts and rapporteurs was called to formulate recommendations that could answer to the 6 following questions after each one of them has been discussed and debated during monothematic workshop.

- Which treatment for decompression illness ?
- Which acute indications for hyperbaric oxygen therapy ?
- Which chronic diseases need adjunctive hyperbaric oxygen therapy ?
- Which design and safety requirements for chambers and medical equipment for hyperbaric use ?
- Which initial training and which continuing education for clinical hyperbaric medicine ?
- Which research to expect and plane for the next five years period ?

To reach a consensus between European hyperbarists on these questions and facilitate the work of the jury, the Scientific Committee of the Conference (D.J. BAKKER, A. MARRONI, D. MATHIEU, G. ORIANI) had elaborated instructions for jury members and rapporteurs. Recommendations of the jury were done and accepted at the end of the conference and proceedings published in 1995.

II.2.3. *Continuing the action*

The scope of the Lille Conference was to establish an agreement on the situation of Hyperbaric Medicine in Europe with regards to the different characteristics of a medical discipline: field of indications, material design, operational rules, procedures and safety requirements, training of dedicated personnel, research and development. It was an initial assessment, based on a minimal consensus and completed by numerous proposals of action regarding the field of hyperbaric and diving medicine and leading to the ECHM restructure.

- Face to the heterogeneous nature of the different conditions grouped under the definition "Decompression Illness," and regarding the recent significant development of recreational diving which, notwithstanding the stringent safety rules and procedures, is accompanied by the occurrence of decompression accidents, the ECHM Committee decided to organize the 2nd European Consensus Conference in Marseille, on May 1996 devoted to "The treatment of decompression accidents in recreational diving" in order to obtain a more precise evaluation and recommendations. The goal was reached and the expert reports and recommendations of the International Jury (P. PELAIA, Trieste (Italy), President, D. BAKKER, Amsterdam (Netherlands), P. CARLI, Paris (France), D. ELLIOTT, London (United Kingdom), B. GRANDJEAN, Ajaccio (France), B. LAMY, Liège (Belgium), JM. MELIET, Toulon (France), G. ORIANI, Milano (Italy), M. SARRIAS, Barcelona (Spain), PH. UNGER, Geneve (Switzerland), U. VAN LAAK, Kiel (Germany) were published in January 1997.

- The hyperbaric field is presently in active motion and significant critical debates are occurring within practitioners themselves. But regarding with the HBOT indications, especially when HBO constitutes an important adjunctive part of a complex treatment including at first surgical procedures or requiring a multidisciplinary approach, it is necessary to pursue the concerned specialists and obtain their faithful support for prescribing HBOT with the best condition for the patient. It is the reason why the ECHM Committee decided that the International Jury of the 3th European Consensus Conference devoted to the role of HBOT in acute musculoskeletal trauma (International Joint Meeting Milano, September 1996) would be only set up with orthopedist, traumatologists, intensivists and other specialists non involved in hyperbaric medicine : PG. MARCHETTI, Bologna (Italy), President of the jury, A. BRIENZA, Bari (Italy), A. DUQUENNOY, Lille (France), D.LINNARSSON, Stockholm (Sweden), F. MALERBA, Milano (Italy), R. MARTI, Amsterdam (The Netherlands), C. MARTIN, Marseille (France), R. VILADOT, Barcelona (Spain).

- The 4th European Consensus Conference devoted to hyperbaric oxygen in the treatment of foot lesions in diabetic patients was hold in London, December, 1998, with the support of the British Hyperbaric Association. A.J.M. BOULTON, London (United Kingdom), President of the jury was assisted by G. CATHELINEAU, Paris (France), E. CHANTELAU, Dusseldorf (Germany), E. FAGLIA, Milano (Italy), DINIS DA GAMA, Lisboa (Portugal), ALBERTO DE LEIVA, Barcelona (Spain), F. MALERBA, Bologna (Italy), J. ROSS, Aberdeen (United Kingdom), P. PRIOLLET (France), S. THOM (USA). Most of them were involved in the medical, vascular or surgical treatment of the disease and their recommendations spread in the European Diabetic Medical Community.

- European Workshops have been done to prepare panel discussion and guidelines: wound healing, safety, cost-effectiveness of HBOT (Beograd, May, 1998), New-Methods of fire fighting in hyperbaric chambers—theory and life tests (Lübeck, 1999). The next one will be joint to the EUBS meeting (Malta, September, 2000) and devoted to the new indications for HBOT.

- The 5th European Consensus Conference will be devoted to HBOT radionecrosis, to be held in Lisboa, October 19-20th, 2001.

III - ECHM STRUCTURE AND REGULATIONS

III.1. The general business meeting of the members of the ECHM, called in Milano, on September 7th 1996, during the International Joint Meeting on Hyperbaric and Underwater Medicine, has unanimously approved the proposed variations to the ECHM bylaws and the regulations, as presented by the ECHM Executive Committee (meetings of 11-14 May 1995 and 9-12 May 1996).

The European Committee for Hyperbaric Medicine should be enlarged to represent all the European Countries and the Non European Mediterranean Countries.

The ECHM regulations were therefore updated as follows :

1. The members of the European Committee for Hyperbaric Medicine (ECHM) are individuals who are either members in their capacity of the current Presidents of the Diving and Hyperbaric Medicine Scientific Societies existing in the represented countries and/or invited individuals particularly experienced and active in the baromedical field in their countries.

2. The ECHM is governed by the ECHM Board of Representatives (BR), which is formed by individuals who are members in their capacity of the current Presidents of the Diving and Hyperbaric Medicine Scientific Societies existing in the represented countries.

3. The founding members of the ECHM are permanent members of the ECHM Board of Representatives. Any decision of the BR must be approved by at least two thirds of the professionally active founding members.

4. Those individuals who are serving as the Immediate Past and the Past Presidents of the Diving and Hyperbaric Medicine Societies existing in the

represented countries, invited distinguished baromedical scientists and clinician nominated and elected by majority vote of the ECHM Executive Board or Board of Directors, and the Past Presidents of the ECHM are members of the ECHM and form the ECHM College of Advisors.

5. The ECHM Board of Directors, upon nomination by the ECHM members, elects the ECHM Executive Board (EB), which is composed of 9–12 members who will serve for a 4 year term, renewed by 1/2 every 2 years, without limit to re-election. The minimum number of the ECHM Countries represented in the EB should be at least 1/2 + 1 of the number of the EB members. The first interim members of the ECHM Executive Board are the current ECHM Executive Committee members, for a period of two years and with the task to implement the present variations to the ECHM regulations, to prepare voting regulations and procedures and to call the next ECHM general business meeting and elections.

6. The President of the ECHM is nominated by the members of the ECHM and elected/ratified by the BR. The President serves for a two year term and can be re-elected for one further term only.

7. The President of the ECHM is the Chairman of the Executive Board.

8. All invited members of the ECHM are nominated by the ECHM members, approved by the ECHM Board of Representatives and invited by the ECHM Executive Board in the person of its Chairman and President of the ECHM.

9. The Executive Board periodically calls for nominations of the new ECHM officers and members, as appropriate.

10. The Executive Board nominates :
    a) Consensus Conference Bureau with the scope to indicate to the ECHM EB the themes for future Consensus Conferences, to indicate the most adequate individuals to serve as the Scientific Committee Members of the Consensus Conferences, and to define the best possible dates. The first members of the Consensus Conference Bureau were A. Marroni, D. Mathieu, F. Wattel.
    b) Finance Bureau, with the mission of defining modalities and procedures to find financial support to the action of the ECHM. The first members of the Finances Bureau were G. Oriani and J. Schmutz.

11. The following ECHM Sub-Committees are instituted :
    a) Research Sub-Committee : this is composed of 9–12 members, nominated by the ECHM members and elected/ratified by the Committee Board. The members of the Research Sub-Committee serve for a 3 year term, and can be re-elected for one further term only. The Sub-Committee is renewed by 1/3 every 3 years.
        1) The Research Sub-Committee of the ECHM will be divided into an Ethics Section and a Research Section. The two sections will be formed of different individuals and will work separately for the

scientific and ethical evaluation of European research projects in baromedical sciences.

2) The Chairman of the Sub-Committee is elected within the Sub-Committee by its members. First members of the Sub-Committee were : Bakker, Frey, Linnarsson, Lamy, Mathieu, Niinikoski, Pelaia, Perret, Ross, Tempe, Wendling.

b) Technical and Training Sub-Committee : composed of 9–12 members, nominated by ECHM members and elected/ratified by the Committee Board. The members of the Technical and Training Sub-Committee serve for a 3 year term, and can be re-elected for one further term only. The Sub-Committee is renewed by 1/3 every 3 years. The Chairman of the Sub-Committee is elected within the Sub-Committee by its members. First members of the Sub-Committee were : Desola, Wendling, Elliott, Wattel, Pelaia, Lind. The interim members will prepare an action plan for the Sub-Committee to be approved by the ECHM EB and BR. It is in particularly stressed that the Technical and Training Sub-Committee will liaise with the European Diving Technology Committee (EDTC), according to the recommendations of the 1st European Consensus Conference on Hyperbaric Medicine of the ECHM.

III.2. The general business meeting of the members of the ECHM called in Malta, on September 15th 2000, has unanimously approved the proposed variations of the ECHM by laws and the new regulations as presented by the ECHM Executive Committee (meetings of 20 May 1999 - Lübeck and 30 August 1999 - Haifa).

III.2.1. It is confirmed that the ECHM is structured around 3 bodies :

- The ECHM Board of Representatives (BR) formed by all the current President of the Diving and Hyperbaric Medicine Scientific Society (ies) existing in the European Countries. The ECHM BR is the governing body of the ECHM.

- The ECHM College of Advisors formed by the immediate past and past presidents of these societies, invited distinguished baromedical scientists and clinicians, nominated and elected by a majority vote of the ECHM EB or BD, and the past presidents of the ECHM.

- The ECHM Executive Board formed by 9–12 members coming from at least 1/2 + 1 European countries. The ECHM EB is elected by the ECHM Board of Representatives and is in charge of the everyday business.

III.2.2. ECHM is represented by its President who is elected by the BR. Other specific offices are Vice President in charge of international affairs, General Secretary and Treasurer.

III.2.3. ECHM is working through permanent and ad-hoc subcommittees.

- Permanent subcommittees are :
  - Workshop and Consensus Conference Bureau:
    Scope: Topics, Scientific Committee and Jury member selection,
    localisation and date, local organiser, publication.
    Actual members: F. Wattel, A. Marroni, D. Mathieu
  - Finance Bureau:
    Scope: Modality and procedure to find financial support
    Actual member: J. Schmutz
  - Research Sub Committee:
    Scope: to establish guidelines in order to improve the level of
    fundamental/clinical research in Hyperbaric Medicine, to propose
    and to implement multicentric studies
    Actual members: the COST B 14 action by its working groups
    B and C serves as Research Subcommittee
  - Education and Training Subcommittee:
    Scope : to establish recommendation and guidelines for training and
    continuous education of both medical and non medical persons
    involved in Hyperbaric Medicine activity(ies)
    Actual members: J. Desola, J. Wendling, P. Pelaia
    (suppl: P. Longobardi)

IV—PRESENT REALISATIONS AND ONGOING ACTIONS OF THE ECHM

At the moment 4 relevant actions have been conducted.

1. The definition of European standards for HBOT indications
2. ECHM recommendations for safety in multiplace medical
   hyperbaric chambers
3. Propositions for personnel education and training policies to be used by the
   European College of Baromedicine (ECBM), created in 1999 with the support
   of the university of Malta, with the following general principles for application
   common syllabus, common faculty, regional organization for theory
   teaching, Practical training in agreed centers, Agreement and mutual
   recognition of final examination, common graduation.
4. Creation of a research network by inclusion of HBOT evaluation in the
   COST B 14 program of the European Union.

As, due to the collaboration established with Best Publishing Company, the
proceedings of the Consensus Conferences and workshops, the safety recommendations
for the practice of HBOT and the education program are published "in extenso"
hereafter, only a digest of the ECHM recommendations about the accepted indications
for HBOT are done in this introductory chapter.

IV.1. ECHM Indications for HBOT

Many diseases or syndromes have as a major component a cellular O_2 insufficiency usually locally and HBOT represents a technically well-developed approach designed to enhance O_2 supply. The ECHM has developed, using the methodology of consensus conferences and reports of expert workshops, an ongoing approach to define indications for HBOT that may be periodically revised.

1. Methodology

Medical practice is changing and the change, which involves using the medical literature more effectively in guiding medical practice is profound enough that it can appropriately be called a paradigm shift. To get rid of the blame being "a therapy in search of disease" (1) and define accepted indications hyperbaric oxygen therapy (HBOT) has to prove its effectiveness in comparison with alternative therapeutic procedures, as well as to be technically feasible and safe, with a minimum of possible adverse effects. It is now accepted that virtually no drug—and hyperbaric oxygen must be considered as a drug—can enter clinical practice without a demonstration of its efficacy in clinical trials.

- One of the possibilities to give an opinion on the effectiveness of HBOT therapy and to help clinicians in treating the patients is to consider the best available evidence from experimental and clinical studies that have been reported in the literature on the subject, using the procedure of the Evidence-Base Medicine (EBM), a new approach to teaching the practice medicine by application of formal rules of evidence evaluating the clinical literature (2). The approach and tools used by EBM have been well described. They include the use of prospective, randomized, double blind controlled clinical trials to answer specific questions, the use of measures rather than their assessments as the primary end points of clinical trials, the collation of results through the Cochrane collaboration, and meta-analysis of multiple clinical trials to resolve variations in results. However at the moment, inevitably, as in numerous fields of medicine, only a very small proportion of all the issues involved in the cure of patients with HBOT have been assessed in this way.
  - Each therapeutic procedure has its own requirements. Clinicians should remember the following facts :
    - clinical decision making is usually based on the balance of evidence rather than the level of evidence that would be required to establish proof beyond all reasonable doubt.
    - An absence of evidence of benefit does not equal evidence of absence of benefit. That is until an adequate study has been performed, the verdict on usefulness of a procedure or treatment should remain open.
    - There is a hierarchy of evidence and that just because multiple large clinical trials have not been performed, it does not mean that there isn't reasonable evidence to support a clinical decision.

- Analysis of the medical literature demonstrate just how few of procedures commonly used are supported by the highest level of evidence. It is the reason why the scientific committee of the ECHM decided to define HBOT indications by using the methodology of the consensus conference.

- An International Jury assisted by experts and rapporteurs is called to formulate recommendations that could answer to the questions chosen by the Scientific Committee Members of the Consensus Conferences, and with regard to the theme of the conference. To facilitate the work of the jury, instructions have been elaborated. It was proposed that the jury members note and grade relevant arguments and recommendations made by each expert or rapporteur, using the same scale than in Consensus Conference in other medical disciplines to assess the weight of their recommendations :
  a. Recommendation based on at least 2 concordant, large, double-blind, controlled randomized studies with no or only weak methodological bias.
  b. Recommendation based on double-blind controlled, randomized studies but with methodological bias, or concerning only small sample, or only a single study.
  c. Recommendation based only on uncontrolled studies : (historic control group, cohort study, ...).

As large scale double blind controlled studies are often lacking in HBOT medicine, it was suggested that facts, arguments, and recommendations would be divided into three groups (Basic Studies: animal studies with control group, human studies and clinical trials) and graded as follows :

4. strong evidence of beneficial action (equivalent to A in the previously exposed classification),
3. evidence of beneficial action (equivalent to B),
2. weak evidence of beneficial action (equivalent to C),
1. no evidence of beneficial action, case report only, methodological or interpretation bias preclude any conclusion.

- So HBOT evaluation, conducted from assessment of reported experimental and clinical data according to available medical evidence, using recommendations of experts Committee and conclusions of consensus conference juries leads to recognize the usefulness of HBOT with regard to the weight of recommendation as well :
  - type 1 recommendation (1R) : HBOT is strongly recommended because it is recognized that HBOT positively affects the prognosis for survival. This implies that the patient is transferred to the nearest hyperbaric facility as soon as possible.
  - type 2 recommendation (2R) : HBOT is recommended because it is recognized that HBOT constitutes an important part of the treatment of that given disease which, even if it may not influence the prognosis for patient's survival, it is nevertheless important for the prevention of serious disorders. This implies that the transfer to a hyperbaric facility is made, unless this represents a danger to the patient's life.
  - type 3 recommendation (3R) : HBOT is optional because HBOT is

regarded as a additional treatment modality which can improve
clinical results.

In other situations, where sufficient evidence in favour of HBOT is not available,
it is necessary to start evaluation procedures based on multicentric studies and on
clearly defined protocols, as approved by a suitable ethical committee. Only after the
completion of such studies, will it be possible to accept a new indication.

IV.2. Acute indications for HBOT

2.1. General

- Hyperbaric facilities accepting emergency indications in potentially Intensive
  Care requiring patients should be hospital based and located in or close to the
  hospital Intensive or Emergency Care Department.
- Technical competence and personnel skills at the hyperbaric facility must be
  adequate. The patient's condition must not interfere with the decision to
  accept an indication for HBOT. The chamber must be equipped for
  any eventuality.
- Hyperbaric oxygen Therapy must be seen as a part of a therapeutic
  continuum, without any interruption of the chain of treatment. It cannot be
  considered as an isolated treatment modality.

2.2. Diving decompression accident and air embolism (DCS and AE)

The need for recompression to decrease bubble size and elimination of N_2 from
the inspired gas to enhance movement of N_2 molecules from tissue to blood and hence
to alveolar gas sets HBOT as the general treatment of choice for both DCS and
AE. However, a large number of questions remain unanswered. Some are very basic
whereas others are of simple, practical significance to the patient with DCS or AE. Areas
of fundamental science include elucidation of predisposing factors, mechanisms of
bubble formation and movement. Areas of applied science include strategies for
education and prevention; continuing development and evaluation of adjunctive
therapies, especially when chambers are not available; optimization of chamber regimes
for treatment; and methods for assessing organ function.

2.3. Decompression accidents in recreational diving

Decompression accidents are true medical emergencies that must benefit from
treatment in specialized centers as soon as possible. The victims of a decompression
accident should be immediately directed from the site of the diving accident to the
closest specialized center (type 1 R).

- Initial recompression modality
  - Minor decompression accidents (pain only) should be treated with oxygen
    recompression tables at 18 meters depth maximum (type 1 R)
  - Regarding more serious decompression accidents (neurological and
    vestibular accidents), there are presently two acceptable protocols, as

neither one has been proven better by any scientifically valid study to date : oxygen recompression tables at 2.8 ATA (with possible extension) or hyperoxygenated breathing mixtures at 4.0 ATA.

- The choice between the two may depend on personal experience and on local logistics. However, under no circumstance the un-availability of one of the two accepted modalities should delay the treatment (type 1 R).
- The following optional treatment modalities may also be considered (type 3 R) :
- compression to 6 ATA in case of cerebral arterial gas embolism, with the condition that this compression is performed using hyperoxygenated mixtures and not compressed air and that the delay to treatment is not more than a few hours.
- saturation treatment tables in case of persistent symptoms.
- Finally, in water recompression should never be undertaken as the initial recompression modality for a decompression accident (type 1 R).

- Fluid treatment
- On site : oral hydration is recommended only if the patient is conscious (type 1 R). Contra-indications to oral re-hydration are stringent and include : any consciousness abnormality, nausea and vomiting, suspected lesions of the gastro-intestinal tract. Oral hydration should be done with plain water, possibly with the addition of electrolytes but with no gas, adapted to the patient's thirst and acceptance.

- Venous re-hydration should be preferred if a physician is present, using preferably Ringer Lactate as the infusion fluid.
- At the hospital, intravenous rehydration is recommended while controlling the routine physiological parameters : urinary output, hemodynamics, CVP, Standard laboratory tests.

- Drug treatment
- Normobaric oxygen is strongly recommended (type 1 R). The administration of normobaric oxygen allows for the treatment of hypoxemia and favours the elimination of inert gas bubbles. Oxygen should be administrated with an oronasal mask with reservoir bag, at a minimal flow rate of 15 l/min, or with CPAP mask circuit, using either a free flow regulator or a demand valve, in such a way to obtain a FiO_2 close to 1. In case of respiratory distress, shock or coma, the patient should be intubated and ventilated with a $FiO_2 = 1$ and setting the ventilator to avoid pressure and volume trauma. Normobaric oxygen should be continued until hyperbaric recompression is started (with a maximum of 6 hours when the FiO_2 is 1).

- Any necessary drug for the support treatment of an intensive care patient (adequate first aid kit) is recommended (type 2 R). The role of specific drugs at this early stage remains unresolved and suitable for further studies, so the use of aspirin is optional.

- Treatment protocol for persistent symptoms after the initial recompression. There are no scientifically valid data to allow for a recommended approach to this issue.

- Results
  - Oxygen first aid and hyperbaric treatment in clinical outcome of 202 DCS cases of the DAN Europe 1989-1993 diving accident database objective total recovery in 176 cases (87.13 %) and incomplete or negative in 26 cases (12.87 %). Comparing the group of injured divers who receive oxygen first aid (119) with those who did not (82) the negative results were only 5 (4.2 %) in the first group and 25 (30 %) in the second non-treated group. Difference between the two groups is statistically significant (3).

2.4. Gas embolism (AE)

Its origin is mainly iatrogenic and it may happen in surgical setting (neurosurgery, cardiac surgery, laparoscopy as well as in medical setting (central venous catheterisation, pleural and pulmonary endoscopy or biopsy, hemodialysis...). Whatever the symptomatology of air embolism may be morbidity and mortality of AE remain high. All patients (AGE or VGE) with neurological abnormalities should receive recompression treatment; HBOT is strongly recommended. The minimal treatment pressure must not be lower than 3 ATA (type 1 R). The outcome after recompression treatment of AE is good in both animals studies and clinical series (4) with immediate recompression treatment being most effective (5).

2.5. Carbon monoxide (CO) intoxication

- 2.5.1. CO poisoning is actually the first cause of accidental poisoning in Europe and north America. This intoxication remains frequent, severe and overlooked. In addition to hypoxemic hypoxia (effect on oxygen transport) CO poisoning induces a histotoxic hypoxia (CO binding to myoglobin and to cytochromes). This process is self-worsening, in good agreement with the clinical presentation and experience (heart damage, pulmonary edema, late neurological sequelae, CO intoxication during pregnancy). Hyperbaric oxygen is well recognized as the treatment of choice due to its effects on accelerated dissociation of CO hemoproteins and its role in preventing reoxygenation injury (6, 7), even if some controversy remains concerning the treatment of poisoning of minor importance and if different HBOT profiles should be compared to determine optional treatment for a given set of conditions.

- 2.5.2. Recommendations
  - Carbon monoxide intoxications must be treated with normobaric oxygen as a first aid treatment (type 1 R).
  - Carbon monoxide intoxications presenting with consciousness alterations, clinical neurological, cardiac, respiratory or physiological signs must be treated with Hyperbaric Oxygen Therapy, whatever the carboxyhemoglobin value may be (type 1 R).

- Pregnant women must be treated with Hyperbaric Oxygen Therapy, whatever the clinical situation and the carboxyhemoglobin value may be (type 1 R).
- In minor carbon monoxide intoxication, there is a choice between normobaric oxygen therapy for at least 12 hours and HBOT. Until the results of randomized studies are available, HBOT remains optional (type 3 R).

- 2.5.3. Results
  - In a series of 774 patients managed with HBOT according to these recommendations, results at 1 year objective only 4.4 % of patients suffer from persistent manifestations and only 1.6 % have major functional impairment (motor or sensory impairment, hypertonia) by comparison with report of 10 % or more of immediate gross neurological sequelae and more than 30 % of delayed personality deterioration and memory disturbance when patients received inadequate therapy (any oxygen in the emergency treatment, delayed therapy with or without HBOT) (8).

2.6. Clostridial myonecrosis (gas gangrene) and anaerobic or mixed bacterial necrotizing soft tissue infections (NSTI)

- 2.6.1. For the onset of gas gangrene two conditions are necessary : the presence of clostridial spores, and an area of lowered oxidation-reduction potential caused by circulatory failure in a local area or by extensive soft tissue damage and necrotic muscle tissue, an area with a low pO_2 where clostridial spores can flourish into the vegetative form.

The clostridial bacteria surround themselves with toxins. Local host defense mechanisms are abolished when the toxin concentration is sufficiently high, and then begins the ever-increasing tissue destruction and further clostridial growth.

The progressive nature of gas gangrene depends on the continuous production of alpha toxin by Clostridia. Unless toxin production and bacterial multiplication are stopped, the patient will die.

The local condition of the wound is far more important than the presence of Clostridia and can be considered as the clinically deciding factor for the onset of gas gangrene.

- Regarding the clinical presentation 3 remarks may be focused :
  1) patients who are at risk for infection in general (e.g., patients with predisposing factors such as ischemia, diabetes mellitus, lowered resistance, foreign bodies etc; patients with underlying systemic diseases; elderly people; debilitated patients with gastrointestinal, biliary, or genitourinary tract infection ; drug addicts, etc.) are also more vulnerable to gas gangrene.
  2) The local picture of gas gangrene is not like that other pyogenic infection. Signs and symptoms depict an overwhelming process.

3) Extreme severity of the disease is characterized by a toxic psychosis, caused by the direct influence of circulating alpha toxin on the central nervous system, a jaundice partly caused by hemolysis by alpha toxin and partly by hepatic insufficiency, an acute renal failure due to the hemolytic uremic-syndrome and septic shock.

- The present treatment for gas gangrene includes surgery, antibiotics, general resuscitative and ancillary measures and hyperbaric oxygen (type 1 R).
  The action of hyperbaric oxygen on Clostridia and other anaerobes is based on the formation of oxygen free radicals in the absence of free radical degrading enzymes such as superoxide dismutases, and peroxidases. A tissue pO_2 over 250 mmHg can be reached with 100% oxygen breathing at 3 ATA when the patient is at 3 ATA and breathing 100% oxygen, virtually all dangerous alpha toxin has disappeared after 30 min. Moreover HBOT interacts with antimicrobial agents and reinforces a specific immune response (phagocytic killing, adherence of leukocytes to the vascular endothelium) (9).

- It is very important that hyperbaric oxygen therapy starts as early as possible, because the best treatment results are achieved in the earliest possible stage of the infection : Early hyperbaric oxygen is life-saving, limb- and tissue-saving, and clarifies the demarcation between dead and still-living tissue within 24–30h. The recommended treatment profile is 3 ATA pure oxygen for 90 minutes (multiplace chamber), 3 times in the 1st 24 hours and then twice delay for the next 4–5 days. A control of the treatment should be done by using transcutaneous and intramuscular PO_2 measurements before, during, and after the HBOT sessions.

- Before hyperbaric oxygen therapy became available, the treatment of gas gangrene was almost entirely surgical. The main objective was to excise or amputate as soon as and as generously as possible so as to remove all diseased tissue. Mortality remained between 20 and 55 %. Moreover, patients who lived were often disabled and subjected to long-lasting physical and psychological rehabilitation programs. The incidence of demolitive and seriously disabling amputations is over 60 % (10).

- Animal experiments and clinical data show that combination of hyperbaric oxygen, local debridement, and antibiotics led to less mortality and morbidity than any of these treatment modalities alone. The incidence of demolitive amputation is reduced to less than 15 % and overall mortality to less than 20 % (11).

- 2.6.2. Anaerobic or mixed bacterial necrotizing soft tissue infection (NSTI).
  - Mechanistically HBOT should be helpful in all NSTI. The rationale for using adjunctive HBOT and the mechanisms have been outlined extensively by Mader (12). However, if antibiotic and surgical treatment are generally effective in a type of necrotizing infection, then adjunctive

HBOT probably is not cost effective. But when the morbidity and/or mortality of a particular infection is high, then adjunctive HBOT may be life-saving as well as cost-effective (13) : Mortality in NSTI is also related to the size of the infectious process (14). Adjunctive HBOT is strongly recommended for compromised hosts with crepitant anaerobic cellulitis and necrotizing fasciitis, including Fournier's disease and cervical necrotizing fasciitis. Patients with non-clostridial myonecrosis have also an extreme morbidity and mortality risk. These patients should receive adjunctive HBOT. These recommendations (type 1 R) are supported by in vivo and in vitro studies and clinical observations (12, 15-18).

2.7. Acute soft tissue ischemia and acute musculoskeletal trauma

- 2.7.1. HBOT therapy has to be considered as an adjunctive treatment modality. Optimal surgery and resuscitation have to be done before or simultaneously.

There is experimental and clinical evidence supporting that HBOT acts to correct post-traumatic tissue edema and delayed bone healing (19). There is some experimental evidence showing a positive effect of HBOT in preventing reperfusion injury, but there is not sufficient clinical evidence. However, no study showed a detrimental effect of HBOT in increasing the oxydative stress, in injured tissue (20). In prevention of post-traumatic superimposed infections, the procedure of choice is surgery (repeated if necessary), but HBOT can be recommended as an adjunctive treatment to enhance antibiotic efficacy, to improve tissue oxygenation and prevent surinfection.

- 2.7.2. Recommendations of the international jury of the 3rd ECHM Consensus Conference devoted to the role of HBOT in acute musculo-skeletal trauma (Milano, September 1996) have confirmed and given details in accordance with the Lille Conference recommendations.
  - In limb crush trauma and reperfusion post-traumatic syndromes, adjunctive HBOT is recommended (Type 2 R) because in case of severe tissue damage, with dubious vitality, there is experimental and clinical evidence that HBOT improves tissue salvage and clinical outcome (21). In cases of open fractures with extensive soft tissue and/or vascular damage (corresponding with type III/B/C of Gustillo's classification) adjunctive HBOT is recommended (Type 2 R). In less severe cases, HBOT adjunctive to surgery can be used in compromised hosts (Type 3 R).
  - In compromised skin grafts and myo-cutaneous flaps, HBOT is recommended (Type 2 R). It cannot be overemphasized that patient selection and the timing of HBOT treatment are the keys to a successful outcome for most conditions in plastic surgery. Although HBOT research has become more scientific and less anecdotal, there is still a need for further experimental and prospective clinical studies to more accurately define and confirm the specific role of HBOT in this field (22).

- In the re-implantation of traumatically amputated limbs, HBOT is optional (Type 3 R) as in post-vascular surgery reperfusion syndromes.
- In every case the measurement of transcutaneous oxygen pressure under hyperbaric oxygen is needed as an index for the definition of the HBOT indication and follow-up (Type 2 R).

The cost of the adjunctive HBOT will be at least compensated by the decrease in morbidity in these patients (e.g. lower amputation rate).

2.8. Burns

- Encouraging theoretical and experimental evidence as well as clinical results exist for the adjunctive use of HBOT in the acute phase of selected critical thermal burns. However well-controlled clinical studies are lacking and considerable controversy still exists in the burn surgeon community. Broad-based justification for the use of adjunctive HBOT in burns depends on favourable results from well-controlled prospective and randomized clinical trials in burn with HBOT capabilities to which patients are taken within a few hours of injury (23).

At the moment, HBOT is strongly recommended when the burn is associated with carbon monoxide intoxication and smoke inhalation injury, (Type 1 R). In the absence of a carbon monoxide intoxication, HBOT is optional when burns exceed 20 % of body surface, are of 2nd degree or more, or involve critical body parts (face, hands, feet, and perineum), consist of circumferential burns of the extremities or are electrical burns (type 3 R). If burned areas are less than 20 % of body surface, HBOT therapy is not advised.

2.9. Post-anoxic encephalopathy—traumatic brain injury

- Utilization of adjunctive HBOT in post anoxic encephalopathy remains controversial. The potential benefit (24) must be balanced against its potential toxicity. Even if HBOT was classified as optional (type 3 R) with regard to cerebral anoxia, it may be used under clinical research trial, associated with other therapeutic procedures. HBOT modalities (recompression level, duration, delay, number of sessions) must be precisely defined and prospective randomized controlled studies are needed (25).

2.10. Hearing disorders (sudden vascular deafness, objective tinnitus)

- Utilization of HBOT remains to be objectively evaluated. Clinical reports are very numerous, in favour of efficacy of HBOT according to electrophysiological evaluation, but HBOT is often associated with other treatment measures such as hemodilution, and the respective efficacy of the two treatment modalities is not known at the moment. HBOT may be classified as optional (Type 3 R) before having results of conducted prospective trials.

2.11. New frontiers

- In the future, HBOT may constitute an adjunctive therapy to antibiotics and drainage in particular forms of aeroanaerobic intracranial abscesses, aero-anaerobic lung abscesses, empyema and mediastinitis, intra-abdominal sepsis and peritonitis. Shoke, acute coronary insufficiency and myocardial infarction may also constitute a possible indication. If first and anecdotal reports indicate a beneficial action, multicentric randomized prospective and well controlled studies are needed before concluding to recommend HBOT as well as further clinical researches may include well-controlled human trials of HBOT as a preventive approach in post surgical wound infection.

3. Chronic indications for HBOT

- 3.1. Defective wound healing and osteoradionecrosis
  - 3.1.1. Defective wound healing (DWH) is a major health problem, with corresponding financial implications. Basic research strongly supports the potential for HBOT and clinical studies encourage inclusion of HBOT in the management of DWH although controlled, randomized studies are still limited. Oxygen deficiency caused by impaired O_2 delivery is the most common cause of DWH. Wounds fail to heal and become infected when sufficiently hypoxic. DWH is commonly associated with: diabetes, peripheral venous stasis, arterial insufficiency, decubitus pressure, irradiation of tissue, collagen vascular diseases, pulmonary disease, malnutrition, and sickle cell disease. Contributing factors in these diseases include: inadequate blood supply (insufficient oxygenation and nutrient delivery); repeated physical trauma; persistent infection; inadequate inflammatory and/or immunologic responses, and interference with healing by prescribed drugs such a steroids, immunosuppressive agents, and antimetabolites. Additional factors include general debility, malnutrition, and chronic diseases (such as malignancy, anemia, chronic renal failure, possible AIDS).

    Blood flow in normal tissues and the process of vascular regeneration are both sensitive to local PO_2 Measuring oxygen tension in wounded tissue so that HBOT can be properly evaluated and determining the upperlimit beyond which further increases in oxygen tension are harmful have been experimentally assessed while concomitant exploration of the micro-circulation using laser doppler velocymetry and videomicroscopy have helped to understand the role of O_2 in healing process face to the hetero geneity of the local microcirculatory bed. If HBOT augments PO_2 but simultaneously reduces local perfusion, the net effects on inflammatory cell accumulation, nutrient supply, metabolite clearance, and ultimately wound healing require attention.

    At the biochemical level, the key ingredient to successful wound healing (synthesis and deposition of collagen) is O_2 dependent. If collagen is not adequately hydroxylated because of insufficient O_2, it is degraded rather than deposited for wound healing and the result can be DWH. Animal skin grafting studies indicate a beneficial role of HBOT on graft survival across a variety of grafting approaches and species (26). In clinical practice, transcutaneous oxygen pressure measurements and intramuscular oxygen pressure measurements at the wound level have been shown to reflect oxygen delivery to tissues and constitute, a very useful and reliable test to predict efficacy of HBOT and to follow evolution, when measurement are done under pure hyperbaric oxygenation (27).

- 3.1.2. In chronic critical leg ischemia with arteriosclerotic ulcer and in diabetic foot lesions, clinical trials have demonstrated the benefit of adjunctive HBOT to surgical debridements and wound dressings, which induces a reduction in the amputation rate statistically significant by comparison with the non HBOT treated group (28).
  - So, in arteriosclerotic patients the use of HBOT is recommended in case of a chronic critical ischemia, if transcutaneous oxygen pressure readings under hyperbaric conditions (2.5 ATA, 100 % oxygen) are higher than 50 mmHg (type 2 R).
  - Diabetic foot lesions
    - The three conditions adversely affecting the outcome and length of treatment are persistent soft tissue infection, critical limb ischaemia, and osteomyelitis. "The Jury of the London Conference is aware of the lack of studies in animal models and humans specifically addressing the above points in diabetes. However, there is evidence of the efficacy of HBOT in animal and human studies in radiotherapy-induced hypoxia. There is evidence from animal studies in non-diabetic models of the efficacy of HBOT in osteomyelitis and soft tissue infections, however evidence from diabetic models remains to be presented. This is Level 1 evidence."

    - Patients with diabetic foot problems warrant treatment by foot care teams with careful evaluation of metabolic, neuropathic, and vascular factors. Potential candidates for HBOT may include those with Wagner grade three to five lesions treated unsuccessfully by standard methods when amputation seems a possibility. There is some evidence from a number of trials, each of which suffers from methodological problems, to support the use of HBOT in ischaemic limb-threatening problems in diabetic patients. This is Level 2 evidence. A result of the meeting is the recognition of urgent need for a collaborative international trial for the application of HBOT in diabetic foot lesions. Pre-treatment evaluation should include an assessment of the probability of its success which might include $TcPO_2$ & O_2 challenge at pressure and assessment of peripheral circulation by invasive/non-invasive methods.

    - "There is evidence that the multidisciplinary team approach reduces the incidence of recurrent ulcerations and amputations. This is Level 3 evidence. If HBOT is to be used in the diabetic foot, it should always be in the multidisciplinary team setting. Data suggest that the cost of HBOT is equivalent to other new treatments in the diabetic foot and may be cost effective."

- In diabetic patients, the use of HBOT is recommended in the presence of a chronic critical ischemia as defined by the European Consensus Conference on Critical ischemia, if transcutaneous oxygen pressure readings under hyperbaric conditions (2.5 ATA, 100 % oxygen) are higher than 100 mmHg (type 2 R, Lille conference).

- 3.1.3. A specific focus of HBOT is osteoradionecrosis where it has been shown to be efficacious as part of comprehensive management, including surgery, antibiotics, and general care such as nutritional support and local wound toilet (30). Cost-effectiveness is well documented for HBOT in osteoradionecrosis (29). So, HBOT is strongly recommended in osteoradionecrosis (type 1 R). The most frequently adopted treatment protocol implies 20 HBOT sessions pre-surgery and 10 sessions post-surgery. HBOT is strongly recommended as a preventive treatment for dental extraction in irradiated or osteonecrotic bone (type 1 R). The most frequently adopted treatment protocol implies 20 HBOT sessions pre-extraction and 10 sessions post-extraction.

  HBOT is also strongly recommended in soft tissue radionecrosis such as radionecrotic cystitis (type 1 R), except in radionecrotic lesions of the intestine where HBOT has to be considered only as optional (type 3 R). HBOT is optional in spinal cord radionecrosis (type 3 R).

- 3.2. Refractory chronic osteomyelitis
  Several early clinical reports describe the benefit of adjunctive HBOT to patients with refractory osteomyelitis. In vitro and in vivo studies have been designed to quantify and define the value of HBOT. A PO2 of 40 mmHg or more seems necessary for clinical healing of infected bone in experimental settings. Success rates between 70–85 % have been reported when treated with adjunctive HBOT (30). So HBOT is recommended in chronic refractory osteomyelitis defined as osteomyelitic lesions persisting more than six weeks after adequate antibiotic treatment and at least one surgery (type 2 R). In cranial (except the mandible) and sternal osteomyelitis, HBOT should be started simultaneously with antibiotics and surgical treatment (type 2 R).

- 3.3. New frontiers concern peripheral arteriopathies (early stages), drepanocytosis, perineal ulcerations and fistula in Crohn disease, dermatological diseases as epidermolysis bullosa, Hansen's disease, pyoderma gangrenosum, cerebral palsy. At the moment, HBOT is not recommended and remains to be evaluated.

REFERENCES

1. Gabb G, Robin ED (1987) - hyperbaric oxygen : a therapy in search of diseases. Chest 92 : 1074-1082.
2. Gyatt G and the Evidence Based Medicine working group (1992) - Evidence based medicine. A new approach to teaching the practice of medicine. JAMA, 268 : 2420-2425.
3. Marroni A (1996) - The Divers Alert Network in Europe : risk evaluation and problem management in a European recreational divers population. In : Oriani G, Marroni A, Wattel F (eds) Handbook on hyperbaric medicine. Springer verlag, Milano, Italy, pp.265-267.
4. Dutka AJ (1991). Air or gas embolism - In : camporesi EM, Barker AC (eds) hyperbaric oxygen therapy : a critical review. Undersea and Hyperbaric Medical Society, Bethesda, MA, USA, pp.1-10.
5. Moon RE (1996) Gas embolism - In : Oriani G, Marroni A, Wattel F (eds) Handbook on hyperbaric medicine. Springer Verlag, Milano, Italy, pp.229-248.
6. Thom S (1993) - Leukocytes in carbon monoxide mediated brain oxidative injury - Toxicol Appl Pharmacol, 123 : 234-247.
7. Thom S (1993) - Functional inhibition of leukocyte B2 integrins by hyperbaric oxygen in carbon monoxide mediated brain injury in rats - Toxicol Appl Pharmacol, 123 : 248-256.
8. Mathieu D, Wattel F, Neviere R, and Mathieu-Nolf M (1996) - Carbon monoxide poisoning : mechanism, clinical presentation and management. In : Oriani G, Marroni A, Wattel F (eds) Handbook on hyperbaric medicine. Springer Verlag, Milano, Italy, pp.281-296.
9. Park MK, Muhvich KH, Myers RAM and Mazella L (1994) - Effects of hyperbaric oxygen infectious diseases : basic mechanisms. In : Kindwall EP (ed) Hyperbaric medicine practice. Best Publishing Company, Flagstaff, AZ, USA, pp.141-172.
10. Hart GB, Strauss MB (1990) - Gas gangrene - clostridial myonecrosis - a review. J of hyperbaric Med. 5 : 125-144.
11. Bakker D.J. , Van der kleij AJ (1996) Clostridial myonecrosis. In : Oriani G, Marroni A, Wattel F (eds) Handbook on hyperbaric medicine. Springer Verlag, Milano, Italy, pp.362-385.
12. Mader JT (1988) Mixed anaerobic and aerobic soft tissue infections. In : Davis JC, Hunt TK (eds). Problem wound : the role of oxygen, Elsevier, New-York, USA, pp.153-172.
13. Marroni A, Oriani G; Wattel F, (1996) Cost-benefit and cost efficiency evaluation of hyperbaric oxygen therapy. In : Oriani G, Marroni A, Wattel F (eds) Handbook on hyperbaric medicine. Springer Verlag, Milano, Italy, pp.879-886.
14. Wattel F, Mathieu D, Neviere R (1996) - Les indications de l'oxygÈnothÈrapie hyperbare - organisation d'une unitÈ de traitement. Formation des personnels. Bull. Acad. Nat. Med. 180 : 949-964.
15. Wattel F, Ohresser Ph, Mathieu D, Durand-Gasselin J, Vanalbada T (1986)—Perineal gangrene—clinical presentation and management. J. Hyperbare Med., I : 215-221.
16. Mathieu D, Neviere R, Chagnon JL, Wattel F (1995) - Cervical necrotizing fasciitis - clinical manifestations and management. Clin. Infect. Dis. 21 : 51-56.
17. Bakker D.J. , Van der Kleij AJ (1996) - Soft tissue infection excluding clostridial myonecrosis : diagnosis and treatment. In : G. Oriani, A. Marroni, F. Wattel (eds), Handbook on hyperbaric medicine, Springer Verlag, Milano, Italy, pp. 343-361.
18. Riseman JA, Zamboni WA, Curtis A (1990) - Hyperbaric oxygen therapy for necrotizing fasciitis reduces mortality and the need for debridements. Surgery 108 : 847-850.
19. Niniikoski J., Hunt T.K (1996) - Oxygen and healing wounds : tissue-bone repair enhancement. In: G. Oriani, A. Marroni, F. Wattel (eds), Handbook on hyperbaric medicine, Springer Verlag, Milano, Italy, pp. 485-507.
20. Zamboni WA (1994) - The microcirculation and ischemia-reperfusion : basic mechanisms of hyperbaric oxygen. In : Kindwall EP (ed) Hyperbaric medicine practice. Best Publishing Company, Flagstaff, AZ, USA, pp.551-564.
21. Bouachour G, Cronier P. (1996) - Hyperbaric oxygen in crush injuries. In: G. Oriani, A. Marroni, F. Wattel (eds), Handbook on hyperbaric medicine, Springer Verlag, Milano, Italy, pp. 428-442.
22. Zamboni WA (1996) - Applications of hyperbaric oxygen therapy in plastic surgery. In: G. Oriani, A. Marroni, F. Wattel (eds), Handbook on hyperbaric medicine, Springer Verlag, Milano, Italy, pp. 443-483.
23. Lind F (1996) HBOT therapy in burns and smoke inhalation injury. In: G. Oriani, A. Marroni, F. Wattel (eds), Handbook on hyperbaric medicine, Springer Verlag, Milano, Italy, pp. 509-520.
24. Wattel F, Mathieu D (1998) - Hyperbaric oxygen in the treatment of post-hanging cerebral anoxia. In : Gullo A (ed) APICE 12, Springer Verlag, Milano, Italy, pp. 459-473.
25. Ducasse JL, Cathala B (1996) - Brain injuries and HBOT. In: G. Oriani, A. Marroni, F. Wattel (eds), Handbook on hyperbaric medicine, Springer Verlag, Milano, Italy, pp. 404-408.
26. Nemiroff PM, Merwin GE, Brant T, Cassisi NJ (1985) - Effects of hyperbaric oxygen and irradiation on experimental skin flaps in rats, Otolaryngol Head Neck Surg, 93 : 485-491.
27. Mathieu D, Neviere R, Wattel F (1996) - Transcutaneous oxymetry in hyperbaric medicine. In: G. Oriani, A. Marroni, F. Wattel (eds), Handbook on hyperbaric medicine, Springer Verlag, Milano, Italy, pp. 686-698.
28. Van Merkesteyn JPR, Bakker D.J. , Kooijman R (1996). Radionecrosis - In: G. Oriani, A. Marroni, F. Wattel (eds), Handbook on hyperbaric medicine, Springer Verlag, Milano, Italy, pp. 387-401.
29. Marx RE - Radiation injury to tissue (1994). In : Kindwall EP (ed) Hyperbaric medicine practice. Best Publishing Company, Flagstaff, AZ, USA, pp. 448-503.
30. Britt M, Calhoun J. Mader JT, Mader JP (1994). The use of hyperbaric oxygen in the treatment of osteomyelitis. In : Kindwall EP (ed) Hyperbaric medicine practice. Best Publishing Company, Flagstaff, AZ, USA, pp.419-427.

SECTION I – PART 1

The 1st European Consensus
Conference on Hyperbaric Medicine

The 1st European Consensus Conference on

Hyperbaric Medicine

Section I – Part 1

September 19-24, 1994—Lille, France

CONTENTS

REPORTS AND RECOMMENDATIONS

EXPERTS

ALLEMA J.H., Amsterdam
(The Nederlands)
ALTASALO K., Turku (Finland)
BAKKER D., Amsterdam
(The Nederlands)
BARGIARELLI J.P., Marseille (France)
BENNETT P.B., Durham (USA)
BERGMANN E., Marseille (France)
BOUACHOUR G., Angers (France)
BRUBBAK A., Trondheim (Norway)
CALI-CORLEO R., St-Julians (Malta)
CATHALA B., Toulouse (France)
CAVENEL Ph., Toulon (France)
CHAGNON J.L., Lille (France)
CIMSIT M., Istanbul (Turkey)
COGET J.M., Lille (France)
DAUMANN R., Bordeaux (France)
DELAUZE H.G., Marseille (France)
DESOLA J., Barcelona (Spain)
DUCASSE J-L., Toulouse (France)
ELLIOTT D., Haslemere (UK)
ESTEVE-FRAYSSE M.J.,
Toulouse (France)
FAGLIA E., Milano (Italy)
FONTAINE P., Lille (France)
GIUFFRIDA G.F., Milano (Italy)
GRANDJEAN B., Ajaccio (France)
GREENBAUM L.J., Bethesda (USA)
HAMABE I., Kobe-Shi (Japan)
HAMILTON-FARREL M.R.,
London (UK)
HAMPSON N.B., Seattle (USA)
JAMES P.B., Dundee, Scotland (UK)
JOANNY P., Marseille (France)
LARENG L., Toulouse (France)

LE PECHON J.C., Paris (France)
LIND F., Stockholm (Sweden)
LINNARSSON D., Stockholm (Suède)
LONGONI C., Zingonia, Bergamo (Italy)
MACCHI J.P., Marseille (France)
MAGNI R., Milano (Italy)
MARC-VERGNES J.P., Toulouse (France)
MARRONI A., Ancona (Italy)
MATHIEU D., Lille (France)
MELIET J.L., Marseille (France)
MIANI G., Milano (Italy)
MYERS R.A.M., Baltimore (USA)
NEVIERE R., Lille (France)
NIINIKOSKI J., Turku (Finland)
ORIANI G., Milano (Italy)
ORNHAGEN H., Horsfjerden (Sweden)
PELAIA P., Roma (Italy)
PERRINS D.J.D, Abingdon (UK)
POISOT D., Bordeaux (France)
RAPHAEL J.C., Garches (France)
ROCCO M., Roma (Italy)
SAINTY J.M., Marseille (France)
SCHMUTZ J., Bâle (Switzerland)
TEMPE J.D., Strasbourg (France)
THOM S., Philadelphia (USA)
VAN DER KLEIJ A.J., Amsterdam
(The Nederlands)
VAN LAAK U., Kiel (Germany)
VAN MERKEYSTEN J.Ph.R., Leiden
(The Nederlands)
VERIN Ph., Bordeaux (France)
VEZZANI G., Fidenze (Italy)
WENDLING J., Bienne (Switzerland)
ZANNINI D., Genova (Italy)

ORGANISED BY
The European Committee for Hyperbaric Medicine

SPONSORED BY

- Société de Physiologie et de Médecine Subaquatiques et
  Hyperbares de Langue Française
- European Underwater and Baromedical Society
- Undersea and Hyperbaric Medical Society
- International Congress of Hyperbaric Medicine
- Société de Réanimation de Langue Française
- DAN Europe and Internation DAN
- Societa italiana di Medicina Subacquea e Iperbarica
- Societa italiana di Anestesia Analgesia Rianimazione e Terapia Intensiva
- British Isles Group of Hyperbaric Therapists
- Geselschaft für Tauch und Uberdruckmedizin
- Nederlandse Vereniging voor Duikgeneeskunde
- Société Suisse de Médecine Subaquatique et Hyperbare
- Comite Coordinador de Centros de Medicina Hiperbarica (Espagne)
- Japanese Society for Hyperbaric Medicine

The scope of the First European Consensus Conference on Hyperbaric Medicine was to establish an agreement on the situation of Hyperbaric Medicine in Europe with regard to the different characteristics of a medical discipline: field of indications, material design, operational rules, procedures and safety requirements, training of dedicated personnel, research and development.

More than 350 specialists from 21 different countries participated at this conference. An international jury, assisted by a panel of 62 experts and rapporteurs was called to formulate recommendations that could answer to the 6 following questions, after each one of them has been discussed and debated during monothematic workshop.

1. Which treatment for decompression illness ?
2. Which acute indications for hyperbaric oxygen therapy ?
3. Which chronic diseases need adjunctive hyperbaric oxygen therapy ?
4. Which design and safety requirements for chambers and medical equipment for hyperbaric use ?
5. Which initial training and which continuing education for clinical hyperbaric medicine ?
6. Which research to expect and plan for the next five years period ?

To reach a consensus between European Hyperbarists on these questions and facilitate the work of the jury, the Scientific Committee of the Conference (D.J. Bakker, A. Marroni, D. Mathieu, G. Oriani) had elaborated instructions for jury members and rapporteurs.

It was proposed that each workshop would be attended by 2 jury members who noted and graded relevant arguments and recommendations made in the introductory report and by each expert. It was suggested that the same scale than in consensus conference in other medical disciplines would be used to assess the weight of their recommendations:

A: Recommendation based on at least 2 concordant, large, double-blind, controlled randomized studies with no or only weak methodological bias.

B: Recommendation based on double-blind controlled, randomized studies but with methodological bias, or concerning only small sample, or only a single study.

C: Recommendation based only on uncontrolled studies: (historic control group, cohort study, ...)

As large scale double-blind controlled, randomized studies are often lacking in HBO Medicine, it was suggested that facts, arguments and recommendations presented at the conference would be divided in three groups and graded as follows:

Basic studies (Tissular, cellular, or subcellular level)

4. strong evidence of beneficial action
3. evidence of beneficial action
2. weak evidence of beneficial action
1. no evidence of beneficial action or methodological or interpretation bias preclude any conclusion

Animal studies with control group

4. strong evidence of beneficial action
3. evidence of beneficial action
2. weak evidence of beneficial action
1. no evidence of beneficial action or methodological or interpretation bias preclude any conclusion

Human studies

4. strong evidence of beneficial action
   (equivalent to A in the previously exposed classification)
3. evidence of beneficial action
   (equivalent to B in the previously exposed classification)
2. weak evidence of beneficial action
   (equivalent to C in the previously exposed classification)
1. no evidence of beneficial action (Case report only) or methodological or interpretation bias preclude any conclusion

In particular, the Scientific Committee suggested that the following points were noted and graded during the workshop.

Workshop 1. Decompression illness

Question: Which treatment for decompression illness?

- Classification: pertinence, accuracy, usefulness
- Evaluation of recompression tables: air, oxygen/nitrogen, oxygen/helium

- Adjunctive medical treatment
- Treatment to be applied in case of incomplete resolution.

Workshop 2. Acute hyperbaric oxygen therapy indications

Question: Which acute indications for HBO?

Workshop 3. Chronic hyperbaric oxygen therapy indications

Question: Which chronic diseases need adjunctive HBO?

For each indication, studies had to be divided in basic, animal, and clinical studies and graded as previously exposed.

Prior to the consensus conference, the ECHM had elaborated a preliminary list of indications: already accepted, under investigation, or controversial in the different European countries, during committee meetings at the 3rd European Conference on Hyperbaric Medicine in Nov/Dec 1991 in Ancona, Italy and in Toulouse, France in May 1992.

The accepted indications included:

- decompression sickness
- acute gas embolism
- carbon monoxide poisoning and smoke inhalation
- cyanide poisoning
- Clostridium myonecrosis
- necrotizing fasciitis
- refractory osteomyelitis
- sudden deafness
- acute post anoxic encephalopathy
- mandibular osteoradionecrosis
- hemorragic radiation cystitis
- compromised skin grafts and flaps
- diabetic foot lesions
- crush and compartment syndromes
- reimplantation
- arterial insufficiency ulcer or delayed wound healing
- acute and chronic vascular insufficiency

The group of investigated indications contained:

- hydrogen sulfide poisoning
- carbon tetrachloride poisoning
- brain, pulmonary, liver abscesses
- mycosis
- head injury
- spinal cord injury
- osteoradionecrosis (other bone localizations)

- soft tissue radiation damage (cutaneous, subcutaneous, enteritis and proctitis, myelitis)
- burns
- stroke

Controversies concerned:

- fetal hypoxia due to maternal vascular insufficiency
- multiple sclerosis, blood loss

The purpose of these two workshops was to validate (with or without modifications) this approach and with regard for the accepted indications, to give a particular attention to the character strongly recommended (or mandatory) recommended or optional of the indication.

Workshop 4. Material, equipment, safety

Questions:

- Which design and safety requirements for chamber and medical equipment for hyperbaric care?
- What was minimal requirements in chamber design, medical equipment, and safety device for treating a critical care patient with HBO?
- What was minimal requirements in chamber design, medical equipment, and safety device for treating a patient with chronic illness?
- Could we still accept the use of pure oxygen hyperbaric chamber?
- What safety regulations had to obtain an agreement throughout Europe?
- What methodology had to be followed to evaluate medical equipment to be brought inside HBO chamber? (interest of a cooperation network between HBO centers?)

Workshop 5. Personnel education and training policies

Questions:

- Which initial formation and training had to follow personnel involved in HBO?
- Which categories of personal work in an HBO center?
  For each of them:
    Initial formation:
      - minimal educational level required
      - syllabus and length of formation
      - final examination content
      - need for an official approval
    Permanent training:
      - content and minimal time per year
      - validation

Workshop 6. Patient evaluation, quality assessment and research guidelines in hyperbaric therapy

Questions:

- What research for hyperbaric medicine in the next 5 years?
- Did the actual research effectively support clinical use of HBO?
- What had to be the directions of future research?
  (Basic studies, animal experimentation, and clinical studies)
- What had to be its means?
  (methodologic improvement, controlled studies, center cooperation,...)

The President of the Conference would like to thank all the participants of this meeting for their responsibility and the hard work done. Two days were needed to elaborate a consensus from expert and rapporteur presentations and jury deliberation.

The papers published in this proceeding book are grouped by question and presented in the original language (French or English); each subject includes a preliminary report, the expert presentations and synthesis. The jury recommendations have been approved in plenary session.

This first meeting would initiate further consensus conferences that the European Committee for Hyperbaric Medicine will promote.

D. MATHIEU, MD   F. WATTEL, MD
General Secretary of the Conference   President of ECHM
                                        President of the Conference

DECOMPRESSION ILLNESS
What We Do Know, What We Don't Know
—Introductory Report

Alf O. Brubakk, Dept Biomedical Engineering, University of Trondheim, Norway

INTRODUCTION

Decompression has generally been regarded as safe as long as it does not lead to clinical symptoms requiring treatment. Traditionally, the symptoms following decompression (dysbarism) has been distinguished according to where the main symptoms occur:

Table 1
Classification of decompression disorders (dysbarism)

Decompression sickness

Type I (mild)	Type II (serious)
- Muscles and/or joints (bends, niggles)	- Spinal
- Skin	- Cerebral
- Lymph	- Vestibular
- Malaise/Fatigue ?	- Cardiopulmonary (Chokes)

Arterial gas embolism

Barotrauma

This classification implies that the different categories are well defined disease entities and that there is reasonable agreement between doctors about the classification. Both the study of Smith et al. (1) and a study by Kemper et al. (2) demonstrate that there is considerable uncertainty between experts about classification. For instance, cerebral DCS can in many cases not be distinguished from arterial gas embolism or vestibular barotrauma. Furthermore, several studies have shown that symptoms only from joints are quite rare, they are usually accompanied by central nervous symptoms (3,4). Extreme fatigue can be classified as a harmless sign or be a sign of subclinical pulmonary embolism (5). Francis et al. (6) therefore suggested the term decompression illness to include both decompression sickness and arterial gas embolism.They furthermore suggested that the disease should not classified as Type I and type II, but instead described according to clinical symptoms and their development. Using this classification scheme, a high degree of concordance between different doctors was reached (7).

For discussing the more general problem related to the effect of decompression, several other definitions may be used:

Table 2
Possible definitions of decompression disorders

1. "Acute clinical symptoms requiring treatment in individuals who have been exposed to a reduction in environmental pressure."

2. "Acute clinical symptoms in individuals who have been exposed to a reduction in environmental pressure."

3. "Organic and/or functional decrements in individuals who have been exposed to a reduction in environmental pressure."

4. "Vascular gas bubbles without reported clinical symptoms in individuals exposed to a reduction in environmental pressure."

The first definition is the one traditionally used and is incidentally the one used to evaluate the effectiveness of decompression procedures. This is probably quite accurate if serious symptoms occur. If, however, the symptoms are less marked, a considerable under-reporting of symptoms may happen (see below) and the second definition may prove to give a more accurate description. The third definition includes both acute and chronic changes related to decompression. These may be related to acute clinical symptoms or develop subclinically. A recent consensus conference determined that such changes, even in individuals with few or no reported symptoms, have been found in the bones, central nervous system and the lungs (8).

The last definition is similar to the so-called "silent bubbles" described by Behnke (9). Most will probably not regard this as DCI. However, the fact that such bubbles are present during most decompressions is similar to the situation in many infectious diseases with detectable pathological flora and little or no symptoms. The question still remains if these bubbles can have an effect on the organism.

There is probably little argument that severe violation of decompression procedures will lead to serious symptoms and that this is caused by widespread gas bubble formation in many different organs. However, decompression illness requiring treatment is a rare disease. In commercial diving, the incidence of treated DCI is probably below 0.1% (10). In sport-divers, the incidence is probably considerably below this. However, these general numbers hide the fact that some types of dives, even in commercial operations, have a much higher incidence of DCI. Figure 1 shows an example of this. These data is taken from a commercial air diving operation in Norway, where all incidents happened on the deeper and longer dives. This is the same results that was seen in the study by Shields and Lee (11), where the majority of the incidents happened in the more stressful dives, as defined by a high pt, where p is the maximal depth of the dive in bar and t is the duration of the dive. However, other studies show a different picture, as is demonstrated in Figure 2. Here we see the relationship between depth and duration of the dive for professional divers treated for decompression illness in Norway in the time period 1978-92 (Risberg, personal communication, 1994). As can be seen, a large number of the incidents happened on short, shallow dives.

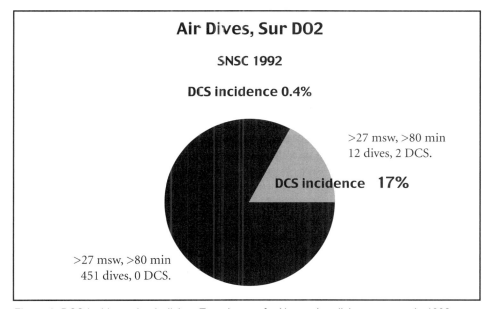

Figure 1. DCS incidence in air diving. Experience of a Norwegian diving company in 1992.

Even if decompression illness is quite rare, a large percentage of divers have been treated. In a survey among divers in an off-shore diving company in 1985, 38% of the divers with 1–9 years experience and 62% of those with 10–24 years of experience had been treated for decompression sickness (12). A recent survey of a large population of Norwegian divers, showed that 3% of the sport divers and 28% of the experienced professional divers had been treated (13).

IS DECOMPRESSION ILLNESS A DISEASE?

According to Webster (14) a disease is "a condition of an organ, part, structure or system of the body in which there is incorrect function resulting from the effect of

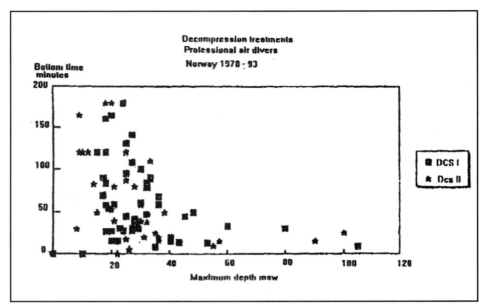

Figure 2. Decompression treatments of professional divers at the Norwegian Navy Hyperbaric Chamber, 1978-93 (Riseberg 1994, personal communication).

heredity, infection, diet, or environment. A disease is a serious, active, prolonged, and deep-rooted condition."

In contrast to this: "A disorder is usually a physical or mental derangement, frequently a slight or transitory one."

I think there is probably no disagreement when we say that DCI is potentially a disease if it is not treated properly, I will also claim that it can be a disorder if proper action is taken. The aim of all our effort must be to keep DCI as a disorder. In order to do this we need a much more extensive knowledge of the decompression process and its effect on the body.

PROPHYLAXIS

Everybody involved in problems related to decompression would probably agree that the primary cause of DCI is separation of gas in the body. Furthermore, it is also well established that this gas separation is determined by the degree of gas supersaturation in different tissues.

However, there is still many factors about this that are very poorly understood. The same decompression stress will produce quite a different amount of gas in two different individuals as can be demonstrated in Figure 3. Furthermore, differences in work load, temperature, and blood flow, may have a significant effect upon decompression outcome (15). This can be seen in Figure 4, where the Doppler scores from two group of divers are depicted. The Doppler score from the group of individuals performing a dry dive in a chamber is significantly less than that from a group of divers working in the water in hot-water suits during the bottom time.

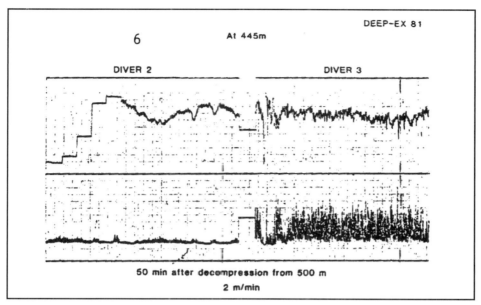

Figure 3. Ultrasonic recordings from the femoral vein of two divers performing an ascending excursion from 500-445 msw during a heliox saturation dive. Top curve shows velocity of blood flow, bottom curve intensity of the reflected signal. The high intensity peaks in the right recording (diver 3) are gas bubbles.

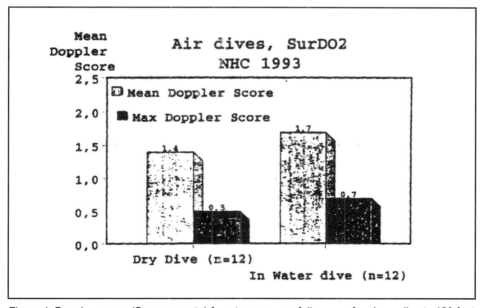

Figure 4. Doppler scores (Spencer scale) from two groups of divers performing a dive to 120 feet for 60 minutes. One group of divers was sitting in the chamber at ambient temperature during the bottom period (dry dive), the other performed an in-water dive in hot-water suits while performing light work. Decompression using surface decompression was performed in the dry for both groups.

The best prophylaxis is properly performed decompressions. One of the major problems is that we have a very limited knowledge about how to do this. We still are still in the position that was pointed out by Behnke in 1951 (9).

"The problem of bringing a diver or caisson worker out of a compressed-air atmosphere has not been solved although there now has accumulate a mass of empirical data which have led to reasonably safe procedures."

The main reason for our uncertainty is that we have to rely on reported clinical symptoms to evaluate our procedures. As is described below, there are many reasons why this may not be adequate. Another approach is to try to use some objective means of determining how effective decompression is, like for instance the formation of gas (16,17).

THE DECOMPRESSION PROCESS

Already in 1715, van Musschenbroek (18) described that he believed that the main problem in decompression was that the bubbles blocked the vessels and interfered with the blood supply, which was particularly damaging to the brain.

A very significant factor in decompression is the fact that since the introduction of ultrasound, it has been demonstrated that gas bubbles will probably be formed in the vasculature during all decompressions (19). Several studies have documented that there is a relationship between the occurrence of many bubbles and the risk for clinical symptoms requiring treatment. Tissue bubbles are probably also formed during the majority of decompressions (20). Due to the fact that even very severe violations of the decompression procedures will not always lead to clinical symptoms, this means that the sites where bubbles are formed must have considerable resistance to the effects of these bubbles.

The most predominant theory about the growth of bubbles is that bubbles grow from preformed nuclei, as the resistance of "pure solutions" to supersaturation and gas phase development is considerable (21). The fact that bubbles seem to be detected at all supersaturations, makes it likely that the nuclei are composed of small (approx. 1 micron) stable gas bubbles (22). The speed of growth of these bubbles is significantly influenced by the size of the nuclei. If gas bubbles are present before the dive, the growth can be explosive as is demonstrated in Figure 5. In this experiment, gas was inadvertently infused into an animal (Murat 3) at altitude prior to a dive to 22.5 msw for 40 minutes. After the dive, this led to an explosive bubble formation and death. Note that no bubbles could be detected in the pulmonary artery shortly after air infusion. The response of another animal (Murat 2) without prior bubbles can be seen for comparison.

CLINICAL DIAGNOSIS AND REPORTING

"The major symptoms and signs of decompression sickness are pain (bends), asphyxia (chokes) and paralysis. Minor effects are rash and fatigue. The parts of the body chiefly involved are the extremities (bends), cardiorespiratory system (chokes) and the spinal cord"(9).

Even today, there is probably little to add to this description of Behnke in 1951, with the possible exception that we believe today that the brain may be more frequently and that extreme fatigue may be a more serious sign than previously thought (5).

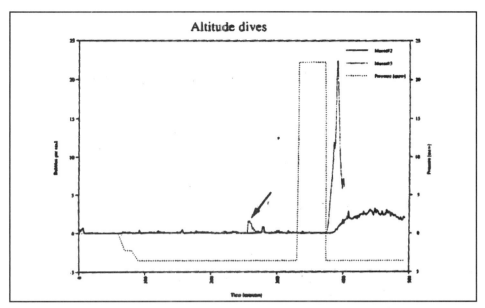

Figure 5. Ultrasonically detected gas bubbles in the pulmonary in two pigs performing an altitude dive. In one pig (Murat 3) a small amount of gas was inadvertently infused at the arrow. Data supplied by O. Eftedal.

Table 3 shows an overview of symptoms of decompression sickness in several studies over a time period of 90 years.

Even given the possibility that there may be differences in reporting, there are remarkable differences in the symptomatology. Of particular interest is to note that pain is only present in about half of the cases in the amateur divers. Furthermore, that serious injuries of the spine and symptoms from the lungs are quite common in the amateur divers. This might fit in with the observation that 17% of the amateurs had experienced extreme fatigue. This sign has been described as a sign of subclinical pulmonary embolism (5). According to Lehner et al. (27), shallow and long or deep and short dives have a high incidence of chokes. The latter dives also have a high incidence of central nervous DCI. The main difference between these dives are the tissues that will be supersaturated. Thus, the change in symptomatology might indicate a different diving practice and that the decompression procedures are not adequate for the more stressful dives.

There has for many years been anecdotal evidence that clinical symptoms of DCI is underreported to a considerable degree. We have recently asked a large group of Norwegian divers about this (13). Nineteen percent of the sports divers, 50% of the professional air divers and 63% of the saturation divers reported that they had symptoms that had not been treated, a majority of these symptoms were related to the CNS. Interestingly enough, there was a statistical relationship between this and later minor central nervous symptoms.

TABLE 3
Incidence of symptoms in DCI

	Caisson workers	US Navy	Prof. Divers		Amateurs	Amateur Prof.
	Keays 1909(23)	Behnke 1947(9)	Rivera 1964(24)	Kidd 1969(25)	DAN 1993(26)	Kelleher 1994(4)
n	3.692	159	935		1.249	225
	%	%	%	%	%	%
Pain	89	72	92	70	57	67
Rash		14	15		4	5
Paralysis	0.9	0.6	6		6	
Fatigue			1		17	13
Visual dist.		5	7		6	4
Chokes/ Dyspnoea	1.6	4	2		9	8

RELATIONSHIP BETWEEN VASCULAR BUBBLES AND DCI

There is little reason to doubt that the localized pain in a joint is caused by local gas formation. This has been elegantly demonstrated by Webb (28), who showed that gas could be seen in periarticular and perivascular tissue spaces, and that there was a correlation between the occurrence of gas and pain. Ferris and Engels further demonstrated that strain and muscular activity were correlated with pain at the site where the strain had been applied (29). One further observations would tend to support this, namely the fact that local compression can in many cases remove the pain. Ferris and Engels claim that the pain can be eliminated by eliminating arterial inflow.

Given the fact that vascular gas bubbles is quite common, the above seems to indicate that if the diver complains of pain in a joint, he is most likely suffering from two different disease entities, namely tissue gas in and around the joint and vascular gas in the pulmonary circulation.

It has often been claimed that gas bubbles as can be detected in the pulmonary artery is a poor predictor of DCI. The main reason for this is that gas bubbles has been detected without clinical signs of DCI (30). There seems, however, to be agreement that the risk of DCI increases with increasing number of bubbles. In my own experience, after carefully having monitored many hundreds of air dives and numerous saturation dives, I have never seen an individual without pulmonary artery gas bubbles who had clinical symptoms. The same observation was made by Davies (31), who claims that clinical symptoms were never observed when gas bubbles could not be detected in the muscles of the thigh. Nishi (32) points out that for air dives, decompression illness was always accompanied by bubbles if all monitoring sites are considered.

Published data seem to support this. In Table 4, an overview of several studies have been made.

One interesting observation is the considerable differences in DCI incidence in the different studies. In all groups with bubbles, the incidence is considerably above what is considered acceptable. It can be very difficult in many cases to distinguish between an occasional bubble and no bubbles using the Doppler method (35). Thus it is possible that the few individuals with DCI and no observed gas bubbles actually had a few bubbles that were not detected.

We performed a study where we compared the incidence of gas bubbles in two surface decompression procedures (36). One was the USN standard surface decompression table using oxygen, the other a new table developed by the Institute of Environmental Medicine (IFEM), University of Pennsylvania. The DCI cases were all skin rashes, except one case of knee pain. The divers were monitored postdive using Doppler equipment, the results were graded according to the Kisman-Masurel scale.

This study only considers few subjects, but seem to indicate that a bubble grade in excess of 2 increases the risk of DCI. When evaluating this, it must be kept in mind that the grading system used is non-linear and probably close to logarithmic (Eftedal and Brubakk, unpublished).

The data shown above indicate that even few bubbles in the pulmonary artery increases the risk of having clinical symptoms.

An interesting set of data from recent animal experiments support the assumption that bubbles in the pulmonary artery is a good indicator of decompression stress. In pigs, the circulation to one limb was reduced during decompression. The consequence of this is a considerable increase in supersaturation in this leg as compared to the other, with very few bubbles transported to the pulmonary artery. In the pulmonary

TABLE 4
AIR dives, precordial bubbles at rest

		Bubble grade	
		0	I-IV
Nishi 1993(33)	n	1265	331
	DCI incidence (%)	0.6	8
Spencer& Johansen 1974(33)	n	110	64
	DCI inc.(%)	1.0	22
Nashimoto& Gotho 1977(34)	n	64	88
	DCI inc (%)	0	19

TABLE 5
Comparison of bubble grades after surface decompression (KM scale)

Depth (feet)/ Duration (min)	n	USN Max bubble grade	DCI inc %	n	IFEM Max bubble grade	DCI inc %
80/70	10	2.2	10	12	1.4	0
110/40	10	2.0	10	10	1.7	10+
100/50	10	1.9	0	16	1.7	0
120/40	13	2.2	7.7	30	1.2	0
Mean (all dives)	43	2.4	7.5	68	1.5	1.5

+ One individual with transitory and spontaneously resolved shoulder pain.

artery, a considerable increase in gas bubbles could be seen when circulation was restored, as is demonstrated in Figure 6. Furthermore, changes in the skin, a symptom often related to serious pulmonary decompression illness (chokes), could only be seen in the leg where the circulation had been restrained, as is demonstrated in Figure 7.

ARE "BENDS" A RED HERRING ?

Skin rash, muscle pain and other minor symptoms are regarded as non-serious symptoms of DCI and a decompression procedure is usually considered adequate if only such symptoms occur in a small percentage of cases. Generally, standard treatment procedures will adequately eliminate these symptoms. The question remains, however, to which extent gas bubbles are also formed simultaneously at other sites and if the treatment procedures are just as effective in eliminating these. This is a question that at the present time can not be adequately answered, but there seems to be no doubt that the lungs are involved in all cases of DCI, and probably also in all decompressions regardless of symptomatology. It is well documented from older literature that severe central nervous decompression symptoms frequently have been accompanied by symptoms from the lungs (24,27).

EFFECT OF BUBBLES

In vitro studies have demonstrated that gas bubbles have an effect upon both formed elements and biochemical processes in the body. Using gas bubbles in vitro,

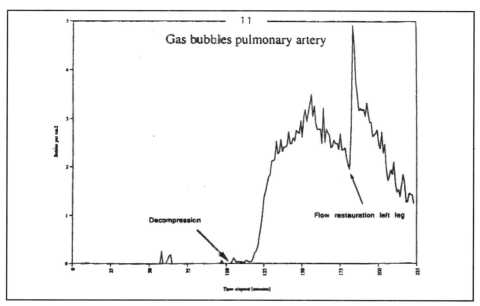

Figure 6. Ultrasonically detected gas bubbles in the pulmonary artery in one pig performing a dive to 5 bar for 45 minutes, 2 minutes decompression. During and after decompression flow was reduced by approximately 80% to the left leg. Note the increase in bubbles at restoration of flow to this leg. Data supplied by O. Eftedal.

Thorsen et al. (38), showed that gas bubbles lead to aggregation of thrombocytes. Furthermore, the degree of aggregation does not seem to be dependent upon the gas content of the bubble, but only on its surface properties (39). In vivo, it has been demonstrated that the activation of thrombocytes occur during the bottom phase of a saturation dive (40). As is shown in Figure 8, thrombocyte aggregation can also be seen following exposure to hypoxia. Thus, in-vivo, thrombocyte aggregation caused by decompression and gas bubbles will be added on to the effects or other environmental factors.

Ward et al. (41) demonstrated that gas bubbles could activate complement in-vitro. Using a different technique, Bergh et al. (42) was able to verify this. During this study, it was also shown that the response was similar regardless of the content of the bubble, indicating that it was the surface of the bubble that was of importance for activation (Figure 9). However, Ward et al. also showed that individuals could be divided into sensitive and non-sensitive individuals according to the degree of activation of complement and that clinical symptoms of decompression illness was related to the degree of activation (43). In a recent study on air divers, Hjelde et al. has not been able to verify this (44). However, interestingly enough, those individuals who had a low level of C5a before the dive produced many gas bubbles, as is shown in Figure 10. Furthermore, a single air dive seemed to reduce the level of C5a. This seems to indicate that diving and gas bubbles may activate C5a receptors as well as C5a. If this is the case, this raises the possibility of ways to treat the effect of gas bubbles on the organism.

Activation of C5a has also been demonstrated by Stevens et al. (45) in divers up to 14 hours after they had been treated for DCI.

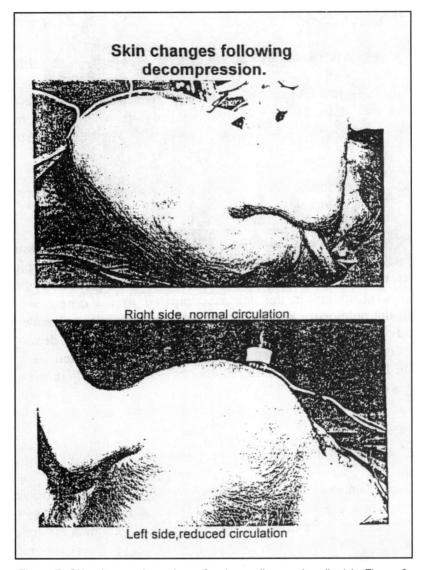

Figure 7. Skin changes in a pig performing a dive as described in Figure 6.
Pictures taken about 40 minutes after decompression. Pictures by S. Koteng.

Complement activation is an interesting and plausible model for how intravascular gas bubbles effect the organism. As can be seen from Figure 11 (46), complement activation will lead to activation of neutrophils and the formation of multiple membrane attack complexes (MAC) that will lead to destruction of nucleated cells. This process leads to adhesion of leukocytes to the endothelial layer and eventually to its transport through the endothelium. That decompression lead to activation of neutrophils can be demonstrated by comparing the activation of neutrophils at surface, after pressure exposure and during decompression. While no activation occur when leucocytes are studied at pressure (Bjerkvik, personal communication, 1994),

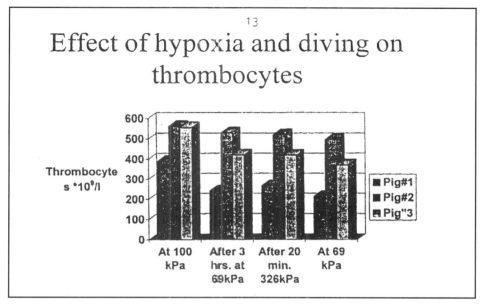

Figure 8. Number of thrombocytes in three pigs performing an altitude dive.

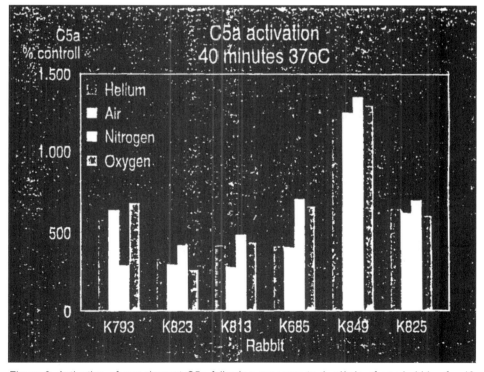

Figure 9. Activation of complement C5a following exposure to 1 ml/min of gas bubbles for 40 minutes. The bubbles contained helium, air, nitrogen and oxygen respectively. Data by A. Hjlede.

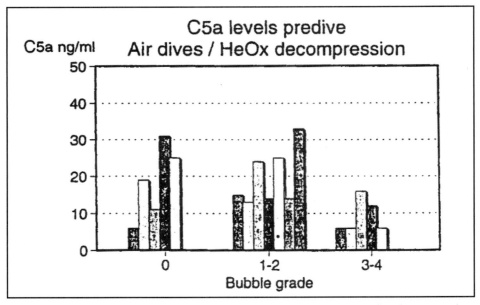

Figure 10. C5a levels predive in divers performing an air dive followed by heliox decompression. Each bar represents one diver, the bubbles are graded according to the Spencer scale. Data from (44).

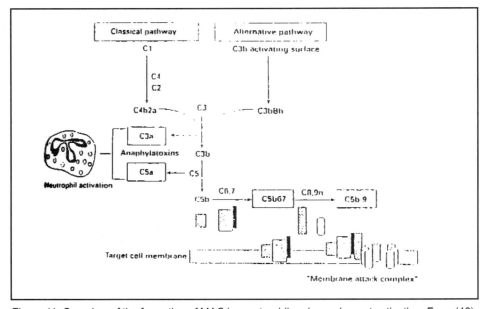

Figure 11. Overview of the formation of MAC by neutrophil and complement activation. From (46).

considerable activation is seen during decompression (47), Figure 12. In the skin, C5a will lead to erythema and edema and promote infiltration of inflammatory cells (48). This is a picture that is very similar to what can be actually observed in the skin of pigs undergoing decompression, as can be seen in Figure 13. Another important effect of C5a is that it leads to vasoconstriction and a reduction in flow (49). If circulation of blood is reduced in a leg during decompression, this leads to a reduction in gas elimination and considerable bubble formation. After circulation is restored, flow to the affected leg does not show the expected reaction, where ischemia normally is followed by a considerable overshoot of flow (Figure 14). Both vascular bubbles and C5a activation may contribute to this.

The changes seen in the lungs in pigs after decompression are similar to what could be expected after complement activation. This is demonstrated in the pig, where considerable leukocyte invasion is seen in the lungs from a pig that had been exposed to a considerable amount of bubbles (Grade III-IV KM scale) for about 100 minutes after decompression (Figure 15). Complement activation seems to be the main mechanism for acute lung injury (50). The changes in lung function seen in divers, with a reduction in carbon monoxide diffusion capacity and reduction in compliance (51), would support the hypothesis that inflammatory processes in the lungs is a result of the decompression process. The reduction in diffusion capacity is quite rapid and follows the development of bubbles as can be seen from Figure 16 (52). Neutrophil activation leads to the production of oxygen radicals (53), thus it is reasonable that exposure to increased oxygen tensions would lead to similar changes and that actually increased oxygen tension and bubbles may have additive effects. This could have implications for treatment of DCI.

Based on the above, the lungs must be considered a primary target organ for gas bubbles, and is probably exposed to gas bubbles to a larger or smaller degree in all decompressions. Generally, the main focus on the lungs has been on its role as a filter, where the bubbles are eliminated before they can be transmitted to the arterial side, where their potential for damage is greater. However, if the gas load on the lungs is large, the filtering capabilities of the lungs will be exceeded and gas will enter the arterial circulation (54). Furthermore, if an open foramen ovale is present, as it is in about 25-30% of the younger population (55), gas bubbles will be transmitted to the arterial side at much lower pressures. Figure 17 shows an example of this in the pig. These data clearly show that, at least in the pig, an increase in pulmonary artery pressure of only about 30% is sufficient to facilitate arterialization of venous gas bubbles. In addition to this, bubbles will increase the shunt fraction of the lungs considerably (56), causing a reduction of arterial oxygen tension. An increase in inspired oxygen tension will have the same effect, where an increase from 21 to 100 to 200 kPa in the inspired gas will increase shunt fraction from 7 to 21 to 45% respectively (56) (Figure 18).

CENTRAL NERVOUS SYSTEM

Central nervous changes in DCI are probably caused by several mechanisms. In severe DCI, both vascular bubbles and in-vivo bubble formation probably plays a role (57). A large percentage of divers probably are exposed to bubbles in the cerebral circulation regularly. For instance, in deep saturation diving, it has been shown that gas bubbles are present in the carotid artery in nearly all divers performing excursions (58). The possible effects of these gas bubbles are of importance.

Exposure to vascular bubbles do not seem to have a serious effect upon the spinal cord (59). In this group of 10 amateur and 10 professional divers, five of whom had suffered from DCI, no changes could be seen. In the brain, changes in the endothelial layer of the ventricles could be detected in a group of divers (60). This is probably not an effect of intravascular gas bubbles in the brain, but may be related to circulatory changes that may cause changes in venous pressure, e.g., pulmonary embolism. It is thus of interest to note that the changes were more marked in air divers than in saturation divers, maybe due to the fact that air divers are subjected to more severe decompressions with higher amounts of pulmonary gas. Another possible explanation is that this damage is caused by gas bubbles in the spinal fluid, such bubbles will probably primarily adhere to the lining of the ventricles. Chrysanteou et al. have shown that animals exposed to decompression will show breakage of the blood-brain-barrier (61). Broman et al. has demonstrated that even very short contact between gas bubbles and endothelium (1–2 minutes) will lead to such breakage (62). Furthermore, studies in rabbits indicate that such contact leads to endothelial damage and progressive reduction on cerebral blood flow and function (63).

In Figure 19, an overview of the possible effect of gas bubbles in the vessels is seen.

TREATMENT OF DCI

Many different treatment protocols are in use, while the USN6 is probably the one used most extensively. Experience till now seems to indicate that this is adequate in the majority of cases where treatment is initiated immediately following the insult. Usually, there is considerable delay in initiating treatment, and many of the secondary effects described above may play a role. For instance, Kelleher has recently shown that initial treatment is only effective in about 66% of the cases (4). Usually, the treatment protocol is determined by the severity of the clinical symptoms. Studies have demonstrated, however, that none of the proposed protocols are superior to Table USN 6A (64). However, the severity of symptoms is not the only variable worth considering. As the different tissues has a different rate of uptake and elimination of gas, the majority of the gas bubbles may have a different location in long dives than in short dives and thus, treatment protocols may have to be different. Heliox dives may differ from air dives, due to the differences in partition coefficients of helium and nitrogen in different tissues. Furthermore, as the treatment procedure always contains a decompression part, further gas may be picked up during this phase. Finally, as mentioned above, increased oxygen tensions may increase the shunt fraction in the lung and also decrease the rate of gas elimination (Flook et al., unpublished, 1994).

The use of different gas mixes, particularly helium as the breathing gas, is controversial. Some clinical data seem to indicate that helium is of benefit. Experimentally, air bubbles in tissue disappear more quickly from the spinal cord at 1 ATA if heliox is used instead of pure oxygen (65). However, at a pressure of 2.8 bar, the reverse is true (66). Our own data, showing an increased shunt in the lung as well as a reduction of gas elimination at increased oxygen tensions, would indicate that there is actually little benefit in using high oxygen tensions and that lower tensions may be of advantage.

Over the years, many attempts have been done to improve treatment of decompression by introducing drugs. Generally, this have had little success, mainly because our understanding of the way in which gas interacts with the body is not known.

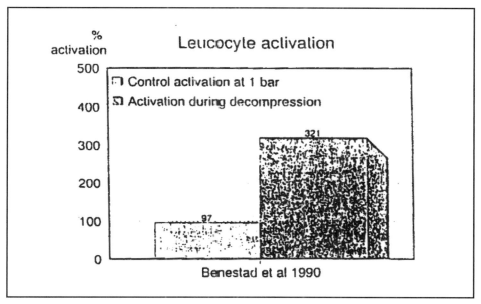

Figure 12. Activation of leucocytes during decompression. Data from (47).

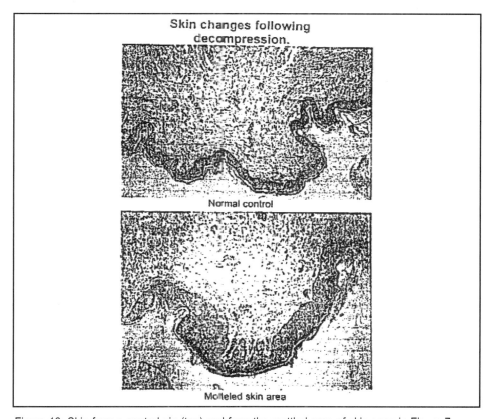

Figure 13. Skin from a control pig (top) and from the mottled area of skin seen in Figure 7.

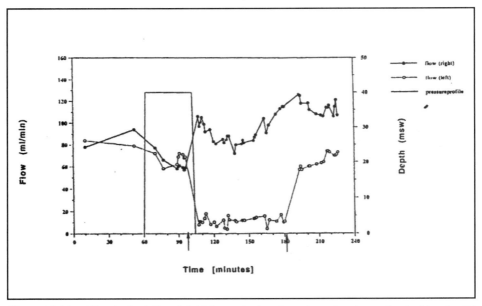

Figure 14. Blood flow in the left and right femoral artery in a pig performing a dive to 5 bar for 45 minutes. Flow is restricted to the left leg as indicated by the arrows.

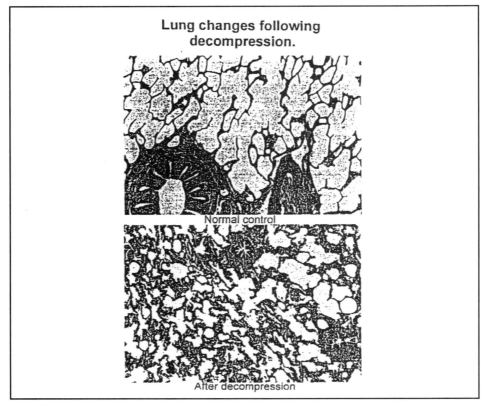

Figure 15. Lung changes in the pig following exposure of approx. grade III bubbles (Spencer scale) for 100 minutes (bottom panel).

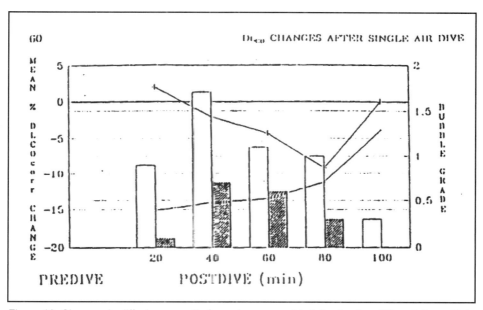

Figure 16. Changes in diffusion capacity for carbon monoxide following two different dives. Note that the changes in diffusion capacity closely follows the changes in bubble grade (Spencer scale). From (52).

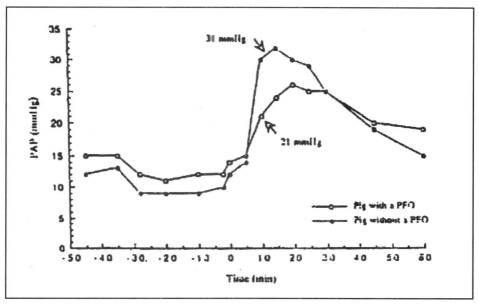

Figure 17. Pulmonary artery pressure in two pigs (one with and one without an open foramen ovale) following decompression. The increase in pressure is caused by gas bubbles. Breakthrough of gas to the arterial side is indicated by the arrows. Data from A. Vik.

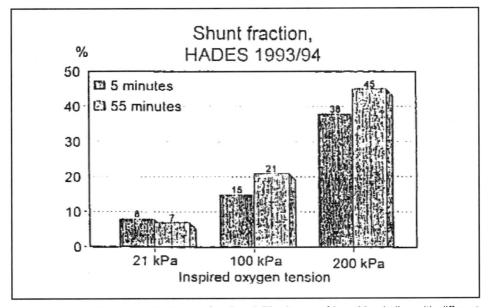

Figure 18. Shunt fraction in the lungs after 5 and 55 minutes of breathing heliox with different oxygen tensions during a nitrox dive to 3 bar. Data from (56).

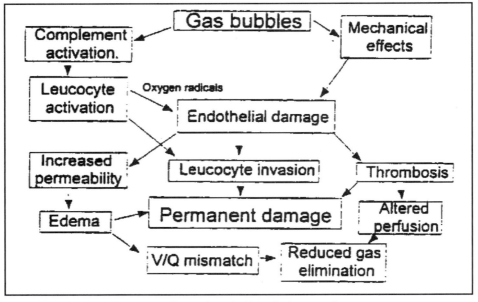

Figure 19. Overview of possible effects of gas bubbles in the vessels.

There are, however, some interesting possibilities that have only been insufficiently been tested. One is the use of fluorocarbons, substances that have a much higher solubility for nitrogen than has plasma. In a study in rats, Lutz and Herrmann (67) were able to substantially reduce the mortality of rats undergoing rapid decompression from 8 ATA if a fluorocarbon was infused after decompression.

If complement activation and in particular its effect on the leukocyte-endothelium adhesion plays an important role in DCI, then drugs that can interfere with this is of considerable interest.

CONCLUSIONS

This review has focused upon several factors that may be of importance for evaluating decompression illness. It has deliberately been aimed at describing the changes caused by gas bubbles in the vessels, as this is the only feature that has been demonstrated to be present in most if not all decompressions used today. If we want to reduce the incidence of decompression illness, there are two possible ways to go. One is to develop decompression procedures that reduces the amount of gas to the lowest possible amount. This will require studies on gas elimination and uptake under various conditions and an increased understanding of the individual factors that may influence bubble formation. Among these are for example differences in surface tension. The other is to understand how gas bubbles effect the body. This will enable us to specifically treat the biochemical effect of gas on the body, not only its mechanical effect.

We also need to know more precisely the relationship between minor clinical symptoms and signs and the changes in the body. In order to do this we will have to improve the reporting system as well as improving the medical follow up of all divers.

ACKNOWLEDGMENTS

The help and participation of researchers and students of the "Trondheim" group is gratefully acknowledged. Without their enthusiastic support and hard work this study would not have been possible. The economic support of Phillips Petroleum Norway (the HADES program), Statoil, Hydro, Saga (The FUDT/OMEGA program), the Norwegian Oil Directorate, Health and Safety Executive, UK, British Gas, University of Trondheim, and SINTEF UNIMED is gratefully acknowledged.

REFERENCES

1.   Smith DJ, Francis TJR, Pethybridge RJ, Wright JM, Sykes JJW. Concordance: A problem with the current classification of diving disorders. Undersea Biomed Res 1992;19(suppl): 40.
2.   Kemper GB, Stegman BJ and Pilmanis AA. Inconsistent classification and treatment of Type I / Type II decompression sickness. Aviat Space Environ Med 1992; 63: 386.
3.   Denoble P, Vann RD, Dear GdeL. Describing decompression illness in recreational divers. Undersea & Hyperbaric Medicine 1993;20(suppl):18.
4.   Kelleher PC, Francis TJR. INM diving accident database analysis of 225 cases of decompression illness. INM Report No. R93048, Institute of Naval Medicine, Alverstoke 1994.
5.   Hallenbech JM, Elliott DH, Bove AA. Decompression sickness studies in the dog. In Lambertsen CJ (ed). Underwater Physiology V, Fed Am Soc Exp Biol, Bethesda 1975: pp.
6.   Francis TJR, Smith DJ, Sykes JJW. The prevention and management of dicing accidents. INM Report No. R93002, Institute of Naval Medicine, Alverstoke, 1993.
7.   Smith DJ, Francis TJR, Tehybridge RJ, Wright JM, Sykes JJW. An evaluation of the classification of decompression disorders. Undersea & Hyperbaric Medicine 1993;20(suppl):17.
8.   Hope A, Elliott DH, Halsey M (eds). Long term health effects of diving. NUTEC, Bergen 1994 (In press).
9.   Behnke AR. Decompression sickness following exposure to high pressures. In: Fulton JF. Decompression sickness. WB Saunders Company, London 1951: pp 53-89.
10.   Imbert JP. Decompression safety. In:Subtech 93, Kluwer Academic Publishers 1993: pp 293-249.
11.   Shields TG, Duff PM, Lee WB, Wilcock SE. Decompression sickness from commercial offshore air-diving operations on the UK continental shelf during 1982-1986. OT O-89-029. Robert Gordons Institute of Technology, Aberdeen 1989.
12.   Brubakk AO, Fyllingen J. Occupational health service for diving ships. In: Schrier LM (ed). Proc XII EUBS, Rotterdam 1986:149-158.
13.   Brubakk AO, Bolstad G, Jacobsen. Helseeffekter av luftdykking. SINTEF Report STF23 A93053, Trondheim 1993.
14.   Webster's Encyclopedic unabridged Dictionary of the English Language. Gramercy Books, New York 1989.
15.   Vann RD. Exercise and circulation in the formation and growth of bubbles. In Brubakk AO, Hemingsen BB, Sundnes G.(eds), Supersaturation and bubble formation in fluids and organisms. Tapir Publishers Trondheim 1989: pp 235-258.
16.   Daniels S, Bowser-Riley F, Vlachonikolis IG. The relationship between gas bubbles and symptoms of decompression sickness. In: In Brubakk AO, Hemingsen BB, Sundnes G.(eds), Supersaturation and bubble formation in fluids and organisms. Tapir Publishers Trondheim 1989:pp 387-399.
17.   Flook V, Brubakk AO. Designing bubble-free profiles - Impossible? Underwater technology 199319: 23-29.
18.   Van Musschenbroek P. De aeris presentia in humoribus animalibus. Lugd Bat, S Luchtmans 1715.
19.   Eckenhoff RG, Olstad CS, Carrod G. Human dose-response relationship for decompression and endogenous bubble formation. J Appl Physiol 1990;69:914-918.
20.   Daniels S. Bubble formation in animals during decompression. In: Brubakk AO, Kanwisher J, Sundnes G (eds). Diving in animals and man. Tapir Publishers, Trondheim 1986:pp 229-264.
21.   Hemingsen EA. Nucleation of bubbles in vitro and in vivo In Brubakk AO, Kanwisher J, Sundnes G (eds). Diving in animals and man. Tapir Publishers, Trondheim 1986:pp 43-59.
22.   Yount DE. Growth of bubbles from nuclei. In Brubakk AO, Kanwisher J, Sundnes G (eds). Diving in animals and man. Tapir Publishers, Trondheim 1986:pp 131-164.
23.   Keays FL. Compressed air illness with a report of 3.692 cases. Publ Cornell Univ med Coll Depth Med 1909;2:1-55.
24.   Rivera JC. Decompression sickness among divers; an analysis of 935 cases. Milit Med 1964;129: 314-334.
25.   Kidd DJ, Elliott DH. Decompression disorders in divers. In Bennett PB, Elliott DH (eds). The Physiology and Medicine of Diving. 2nd ed, Bailliere Tindall, London 1969:pp 471-495.
26.   Elliott D, Moon RE. Manifestations of the decompression disorders. In Bennett PB, Elliott DH (eds). The Physiology and Medicine of Diving, 4th ed. WB Saunders Company, London 1993:pp 481-505.
27.   Lanphier EH, Lehner CE. Animal models in decompression. in Lin YC, Shida KK (eds). Man in the sea 1990:pp 273-295.
28.   Webb JP, Engel GL, Romano J, Ryder HW, Stevens CD, Blankenhorn MA, Ferris EB. The mechanism of pain in aviators bends. J Clin Invest 1944;23:034-935.
29.   Ferris EB, Engel GE. The clinical nature of high altitude decompression sickness. In: Fulton JF. Decompression sickness. WB Saunders Company, London 1951: pp 4-52.
30.   Nishi RY. Doppler evaluation of decompression tables. In Lin YC, Shida KK (eds). Man in the sea. Best Publishing Company San Pedro 1990:pp 297-316.
31.   Davies JM. Studies on bubble formation after decompression. PhD thesis, Dept of Pharmacology, University of Oxford 1983.
32.   Nishi RY. Doppler and ultrasonic bubble detection In Bennett PB, Elliott DH (eds). The physiology and medicine of diving. 4th ed, WB Saunders Company London 1993:pp 433-453.
33.   Spencer MP, Johanson DC. Investigation of new principles for human decompression schedules using the Doppler ultrasonic blood bubble detector. Tech Report , Inst. Environ Med and Physiol, Seattle 1974.

34. Nashimoto I, Gotoh Y, Relationship between precordial Doppler ultrasound records and decompression sickness. In Shilling CW, Beckett MW (eds) Underwater Physiology VI. Undersea Medical Society, Bethesda 1978:pp 497-501.

35. Sawatzky KD, Nishi RY. Assessment of inter-rater agreement on the grading of intravascular bubble signals. Undersea Biomed Res 1991; 18: 373-396.

36. Brooks S, Brubakk AO, Eftedal O, Flook V, Holmes C, Hjelle J, Risberg J, Vik A. Decompression from air dives using surface decompression. SINTEF Report SINTEF23 F93013. SINTEF Trondheim 1993.

37. Behnke AR, Shaw LA. The use of oxygen in the treatment of compressed air illness. Nav med Bull 1937; 35: 61-73.

38. Thorsen T, Brubakk A, Yvstedal T, Farstad M, Holmsen H. A method for production of N2 microbubbles in platelet-rich plasma in an aggregometer-like apparatus, and effect of platelet density in vitro. Undersea Biomed Res 1986;13:271-288.

39. Thorsen T, Klausen H, Lie RT, Holmsen H. Bubble-induced, aggregation of platelets: effects of gas species, proteins and decompression. Undersea & Hyperbaric Med 1993;20:101-120.

40. Klausen H, Hjelle JO, Flood PR, Holmsen H. Activation of blood platelets in man during deep saturation diving- a morphological approach. European J Clin Invest. In press 1994.

41. Ward CA, Koheil A, McCullough D, Johnson WR, Fraser WD. Activation of complement at plasma-air or serum air interface of rabbits. J Appl Physiol 1986;60:1651-1658.

42. Bergh K, Hjelde A, Iversen O-J, Brubakk AO. Variability over time of complement activation induced by air bubbles in human and rabbit sera. J Appl Physiol 1993, 74:1811-1815

43. Ward CA, McCullough D, Fraser WD. Relation between complement activation and susceptibility to decompression sickness. J Appl Physiol 1987;62:1160-1166.

44. Hjelde A, Brubakk AO, Bergh K, Iversen O-J. Complement activation in divers following repeated air/heliox dives and its possible relevance to decompression sickness. Submitted J Appl Physiol 1994.

45. Stevens DM, Gartner SL, Pearson RR. Complement activation during saturation diving. Undersea & Hyperbaric Med 1993;20:279-288.

46. Kilgore KS, Friedrichs GS, Homeister IW, Lucchesi BR. The complement system in myocardial ischemia/ reperfusion injury. Cardiovascular Res 1994;28:437-444.

47. Benestad HB, Hersleth IB, Hardersen H, Malvær OI. Functional capacity of neutrophil granulocytes in deep-sea divers. Scand J Clin Lab Invest 1990;50:9-18.

48. Swerlick RA, Yancey KB, Lawlwy TJ. A direct in vivo comparison of the inflammatory properties of human C5a and C5a des arg in human skin. J Immunol 1988;140:2376-2381.

49. Martin SE, Chenoweth DE, Engler RL, Roth DM, Longhurst JC. C5a decreased regional coronary blood flow and myocardial function in pigs; implications for a granulocyte mechanism. Circ Res 1988;63:483-491.

50. Ward RA, Till GO, Kunkel R et al. Evidence for the role of hydroxyl radical in complement and neutrophil-dependent tissue injury. J Clin Invest 1983;72:789-801.

51. Thorsen E. Segadal K, Kambestad B, Gulsvik A. Divers' lung function: small airways disease. Brit J Industr Med 1990;47:519-523.

52. Dujic Z, Eterovic D, Denoble P, Krstacic G, Tocilj J, Gosovic S. Effect of single air dive on pulmonary diffusing capacity in professional divers. J Appl Physiol 1993;74:55-61.

53. Rivkind AI, Siegel JH, Littleton M, De Gaetano A, Mamatov T, Laghi F, Soklosa JC. Neutrophil oxidative burst activation and the pattern of respiratory physiologic abnormalities in the fulminant post-traumatic adult respiratory distress syndrome. Circulatory Shock 1991;33:48-62.

54. Vik A, Brubakk AO, Hennessy, Jenssen BM, Ekker M, Slørdahl SA. Venous air embolism in swine: transport of gas bubbles through the pulmonary circulation. J Appl Physiol 1990;69:237-244.

55. Hagen PT, Scholz DG, Edwards WD. Incidence and size of patent foramen ovale during the first 10 decades of life: an autopsy study of 965 normal hearts. Mayo Clin Proc 1984;59:17-20.

56. Flook V, Koteng S, Holmen IM, Ustad A-L, Brubakk AO. The differential effects of oxygen and bubbles on lung function. Undersea & Hyperbaric Medicine 1994 In press.

57. Francis TJR, Gorman DF. Pathogenesis of the decompression disorders. In: Bennett PB, Elliott DH (eds). The physiology and medicine of diving, 4th ed. WB Saunders Company, London 1993:pp454-480.

58. Brubakk AO, Peterson R, Grip A, Holand B, Onarheim J, Segadal K, Kunkle TD, Tønjum S. Gas bubbles in the circulation in divers after ascending excursions from 300 to 250 msw. J Appl Physiol 1086;60:45-51.

59. Mørk S, Morild I, Eidsvik S, Nyland H, Brubakk AO, Giertsen JC. Does diving really damage the spinal cord? A neuropathological study of 20 professional and amateur divers. Undersea Biomed Res 1992;19(suppl):111.

60. Morild I, Mørk SJ. A neuropathologic study of the ependymoventricular surface in divers brains. Undersea & Hyperbaric Medicine 1994;21:43-51.

61. Chrysanteou C., Springer M, Lipschitz S. Blood- brain and blood-lung barrier alterations by dysbaric exposure. Undersea Biomed Res 1977;4:111-116.

62. Broman T, Branemark PI, Johansson B, Stenwall O. Intravital and post-mortem studies on air embolism damage of the blood-brain-barrier. Acta Neur Scand 1966;42:146-152

63. Helps SC, Parsons DW, Reilly PL, Gorman DF. The effect of gas emboli on rabbit cerebral blood flow. Stroke 1990;21:94-99.

64. Leitch DR, Green RD. Additional pressurization for treating nonresponding cases of serious air decompression sickness. Aviat Space Environ Med 1985;56:1139-1143.

65. Hyldegård O, Møller M, Madsen J. Effect of He-O2, O2 and N2-O2 breathing on injected bubbles in spinal white matter. Undersea Biomed Res 1991;18:361-371.

66. Hyldegård O, Madsen J, Kerem D, Melamed Y. Effect of combined recompression and air, heliox or oxygen breathing on air bubbles in rat spinal white matter. In: Eidsmo Reinertsen R, Brubakk AO, Bolstad G (eds). Proc XIX EUBS, Trondheim1993:pp 292-296.

67. Lutz J, Herrman G. Perfluorochemicals as a treatment of decompression sickness in rats. Pflugers Archiv 1984;401:174-177.

DECOMPRESSION ILLNESS
—Final Report

A. Marroni, MD, President, DAN Europe

The following paper resumes the conclusions and the recommendations made by the invited international experts and the following productive discussion with the many specialists in the field convened in Lille from all Europe as well as from many countries outside Europe.

DEFINITION, PHYSIOPATHOLOGY AND EPIDEMIOLOGY

Decompression Illness is a complex condition which can appear with a wide variety of signs and symptoms. The classification criteria adopted so far—i.e., Type I or Type II Decompression Sickness and Arterial Gas Embolism—are generic and presume that the underlying diagnosis criteria are of common and uniform knowledge. Indeed a great variation and a significant level of disagreement has been observed between different experienced specialists called to define the same cases of decompression disorders using the traditional classification. A descriptive form of classification, using the common term "Decompression Illness," followed by a description of the clinical signs and symptoms and of their onset and development characteristics, is both more universally understandable and simpler to explain and to adopt, and it showed a much higher degree of concordance between the specialists who were asked to define the same cases of decompression disorders using this kind of classification criteria.

Any organic or functional decrements in individuals who have been exposed to a reduction in environmental pressure must be considered as a Decompression Illness case and treated as such until the contrary is proven. This applies to acute, sub-acute and chronic changes related to decompression and may be related to acute clinical symptoms or to situations which may develop sub-clinically and deceptively. It is in fact generally accepted that sub-clinical forms of Decompression Illness, with little or no reported symptoms may cause changes in the bones, the central nervous system and in the lungs.

Generally speaking, a disorder is a physical derangement, frequently slight and transitory in nature; a disease is instead a condition of an organ, part, structure or system of the body in which there is incorrect function resulting from the effect of heredity, diet, or environment. A disease is a serious, active, prolonged, and deep-rooted condition (Webster). Decompression Illness should be considered a disorder due to a physical primary cause that can transform into a disease if adequate and timely action is not undertaken to abort or to minimize the patho-physiological effects of bubbles on the body tissues.

The primary physical cause of Decompression Illness is the separation of gas in the body tissues, due to inadequate decompression and determining an excessive degree of gas supersaturation in the body tissues. Inadequately rapid speed of ascent after an exposure to increased environmental pressure, as much as the omission of the prescribed decompression stops, are the origin and the cause of gas separation in body tissues. The best prevention of Decompression Illness is therefore achieved by calculating and observing appropriate ascent and decompression procedures.

Unfortunately the current knowledge as to which ascent or decompression procedures are the most appropriate is largely empirical and not yet reliable. The incidence of "unexplainable" cases of DCI is very significant and about 50% of the recreational diving DCI cases reported by DAN internationally are apparently "undeserved."

In fact the role of other contributing factors of DCI, such as a Patent Foramen Ovale, the wide variation in individual susceptibility to DCI, the role of Complement activation in the presence of gas bubbles and the relationship between gas bubbles, blood cells, the capillary endothelial lining and DCI, are still undefined and obscure.

It is apparent that DCI can manifest itself with minor and very subtle changes, likely to be ignored or denied if an adequate information is not provided to individual divers as well as to diving training organizations and to the examining non-specialized physicians and there is growing evidence that under-reported, under-estimated, and under-treated signs and symptoms of DCI can result in permanent organic or functional damage.

Although the presence of doppler-detectable gas bubbles in the blood is not always predictive of clinically evident DCI, it has been observed during many field and experimental human studies that no individual without detectable pulmonary artery and venous bubbles developed signs and symptoms of DCI. On the contrary, there is growing experimental and clinical evidence that asymptomatic "silent" bubbles present in the body tissues can cause cellular and biological reactions and the release of potentially damaging biochemical substances in the blood.

Epidemiologically, there is universal consensus among the diving medicine international community, that the incidence of DCI is generally very low and that there is no gender-related significant difference. There is equally uniform consensus on the fact that neurological manifestations of DCI are by far the most common form of the condition among recreational divers. Universal data, based of wide epidemiological information, are unfortunately still lacking.

Many yet unknown aspects of DCI are currently the object of ongoing international studies, such as the relationship between gas separation and DCI Injury, the relationship between clinical symptoms and the severity of the disease, the relationship between initial clinical onset, treatment results and permanent sequelae, the reason for the large variation in individual susceptibility to DCI, the life time of gas bubbles, and the real incidence of DCI.

THE TREATMENT OF DCI

DCI is generally considered a benign condition, if adequate treatment is promptly started, with a success rate in excess of 80–90%.

There is universal consensus that 100% oxygen should be administered immediately as the single most important first aid treatment of any DCI case related to surface-oriented diving, and that rehydration is a very valuable adjunct during field first aid of such DCI cases.

Hyperbaric treatment should be started with the shortest possible delay from surfacing or from the onset of the first DCI signs and symptoms. Hyperbaric Treatment tables using 100% oxygen at environmental pressures not exceeding 2.8 bars, with various depth/time profiles, showed to assure very good results in more than 80% of the treated cases. There is no significant evidence that any other therapeutical scheme may provide better results and be therefore preferable as the hyperbaric treatment of first choice for DCI related to surface-oriented diving.

It is accepted by many specialists in Europe that the use of high pressure (generally 4 bars maximum) treatment tables using a gas mixture of 50% helium and 50% oxygen may prove highly effective and provide good results in the cases that do not quickly and satisfactorily respond to the standard low pressure hyperbaric oxygen treatment tables.

Although conclusive scientific evidence suggesting the use of any pharmacological treatment other than oxygen is missing, the administration of adjunctive fluid therapy is considered very important and generally recommended by the diving-hyperbaric medicine specialists in Europe, whereas the role of other drugs, such as steroids and anticoagulants, although widely used without any apparent adverse effect, is still controversial.

The continuation of hyperbaric oxygen therapy, combined with a specific rehabilitation protocol in neurological cases, when the initial DCI treatment tables are not totally successful, is considered essential by the European Hyperbaric Specialists, and there is growing scientific evidence that it significantly contributes to achieving an eventually better functional recovery.

FINAL RECOMMENDATIONS

In conclusion the recommendations originating from the Workshop on Decompression Illness of the 1st European Conference on Hyperbaric Medicine, held in Lille, France, on September 19–21, 1994, are the following:

1. DCI is best classified descriptively.
2. On-site Oxygen First Aid and fluid therapy are strongly recommended.
3. Therapeutic Recompression in a hyperbaric chamber must be started as soon as possible.
4. Low Pressure Oxygen Treatment Tables are the tables of first choice for the treatment of DCI related to surface-oriented diving.
5. High pressure (4 bars) Helium-Oxygen Treatment Tables are recommended in selected cases.
6. Deep, not surface-oriented, mixed gas and saturation diving may require special treatment protocols.
7. Adjunctive Fluid Therapy is generally useful and recommended, while the use of other drugs, such as steroids or anticoagulants, although widely adopted without any apparent adverse effect, is controversial and considered optional.
8. The continuation of a combined Hyperbaric Oxygen and Rehabilitation Treatment Protocol is recommended until clinical stabilization or no further amelioration is achieved.

NOTES

HBO INDICATIONS FOR EMERGENCY AND RESUSCITATION PURPOSES
—Introductory Report

Jean Louis Ducassé, MD, Purpan University Hospital (F 31059 Toulouse)

This report on HBO indications in emergency and resuscitation wards first considers the indications usually found in the literature (gas embolism, acute carbon monoxide poisoning, anaerobic infectious), raising a number of specific issues for experts. It then goes on to consider other indications that are found less often in the literature (brain anoxia, burns, crush injury, sudden deafness). For reasons pertaining to the organisation of the Consensus Conference, we shall not deal with diving accidents which are naturally emergencies but which will be dealt with in Workshop 1 of the conference.

ACUTE GAS EMBOLISM (AGE)

Air embolism is the consequence of accidental penetration of air or gas in the vascular system. The degree of severity of such accidents is essentially determined by the extent of cerebral damage. The increased frequency of such accidents observed in recent years is proportional to the reinstatement of the vascular approach in medicine both for therapeutic and diagnostic purposes, making endogenous air embolism due to diving or high altitude flight accidents more secondary. Recent developments in endoscopic surgery techniques such as CO_2 pneumoperitoneum do not appear to have increased the frequency of AGE occurrence (6, 7, 12). Twenty years after its introduction in medical practice, hyperbaric oxygen treatment (HBO) has yet to be submitted to a randomized study under controlled conditions which would enable its impact on the treatment of AGE to be defined with certainty (13).
There are, however, specific grounds for its use (4):

- physical grounds based on Boyle-Mariotte's law according to which the reduction in the volume of a gas bubble is directly proportional to pressure increase. However, more than the volume of the bubble, it is its size that impedes normal circulation of blood. In the case of a spherical bubble, the reduction of the diameter is proportional, not to the pressure increase itself but rather to the latter's cubic root. Hence, at 4 ATA, a 75 % reduction in volume is achieved, whereas the diameter is decreased only by 40 %.
- physico-chemical grounds based on denitrogenation. In pure oxygen, whereby the input of inert gases is eliminated, a partial pressure gradient for nitrogen in the blood-alveolar air direction is established. Then as the blood is denitrogenated, a bubble-blood-alveolar air gradient is created which appears to be sufficient, in the case of air embolism, to bring about total denitrogenation. However, it should be observed that tissue denitrogenation is a function of tissue period. The decrease in local blood rates found in cases of AGE increases the period.

- pathophysiological grounds, AGE achieves a double association—ischemia/hypoxia and cerebral oedema/intracranial hypertension—on which HBO is active due to the passage from an anaerobic cerebral energy metabolism to an aerobic metabolism (76) and by reducing intracranial pressure.

In combination with symptomatic resuscitation techniques, HBO is proposed in cases of AGE with cerebral or coronary symptomatology (2, 3). It is also common to recommend that this treatment be applied as early as possible and, in all cases, before the 6th hour (15). Some observations do, however, point to its efficacy even after significant periods (1, 5, 16).

The choice of a therapeutic scheme may be either in favor of an initial recompression at 6 ATA in air, followed by a therapeutic step at 2.8 ATA, of cisc directly at 2.8 ATA in pure oxygen as shown by experimental work on dogs performed by Leitch et al. (8, 9, 10). There has been no human study showing the superiority of one scheme over another (14).

It would appear that no other measure, apart from symptomatic resuscitation, need be associated with the HBO session. Experimental work on cats done by McDermott et al. has shown the superiority of a 2.8 ATA session for 130 minutes over the absence of treatment, as well as its superiority over the same treatment associated with a lidocaine perfusion. The analysis was performed by recording the evoked somesthetic potentials (11).

ANAEROBIC INFECTIONS

Because of their discrepancies, these pathologies may be classified into three large categories, according to the extent of lesion, with a distinction being made between (18).

- muscle necrosis, essentially characteristic Clostridial myonecrosis typically associated with major, generalised, toxic-infectious signs.
- progressive bacterial gangrene or cellulitis which are local infectious of the skin and of the sub-cutaneous tissue with few or no general signs.
- necrotizing fasciitis, i.e., sub-cutaneous tissue infectious that rapidly spread to the fascia and to the skin by thrombosis of sub-cutaneous vessels, often accompanied by major general signs. The general principle behind the treatment of such infectious is based on the association of surgery, antibiotic administration, and hyperbaric oxygen treatment. However, it should be recognized that no prospective, randomized survey has yet assessed the value of HBO in the various clinical states.

CLOSTRIDIAL MYONECROSIS

Clostridial myonecrosis is an invasive infectious of the muscular mass characterized by toxemia, extensive oedema, significant tissue destruction, and a certain degree of gas production. The germs responsible are encapsulated, Gram positive aerobic bacilli belonging to the Clostridium family. Among the twenty or so toxins of Clostridium perfringens, one alpha toxin, lecithinase C, prevails. It is responsible of hemolysis and tissue destruction. An oxygen pressure greater than 250 mm Hg is necessary to inhibit its production (24, 26, 34), i.e., an exposure to 3 ATA.

Some less recent experimental works (22, 27) have shown the efficacy of the association of HBO, antibiotics, and surgery, but do not specify the exact impact of HBO, antibiotics, and surgery. Recently, Stevens et al., working on experimental model of infectious by Clostridium perfringens in the mouse, found that clindamycine has a superior effect to penicillin, metronidazole, and HBO, and that its action is not potentiated by supplementing it with H_3O (39). Similarly, Hirm et al. recently showed that supplementing surgery with HBO reduces the morbidity of experimentally produced multi-microbial gas gangrene, but does not reduce its mortality (29).

In clinical practice, the initial approach consisted in performing surgical debridement and administrating antibiotics. The rate of survival varied from 30 (20) to 86 % (17). In 1963, Brummelkamp et al. added HBO to the treatment scheme and reported that the survival rate for selected patients was 95 % (19). Since then, many publications have confirmed the relevance of this triple association (23, 25, 28, 40, 41). However, the significant difference in the mortalities reported (from 5 to 31 %) may be due to a bias introduced in the selection of patients by the difference in speed of diagnostic, the interval between the diagnostic and surgery (and its nature), on the one hand, and administration of antibiotics and HBO on the other. Although a clinical consensus on the association of surgery, antibiotics and HBO appears to have been reached, there is no agreement on when HBO should be administered. Some teams recommend HBO before surgery whereas for others surgery is most urgent (21).

The usual HBO pattern is 3 ATA for 90 minutes, three times in the first 24 hours and twice a day for the next 4 or 5 days.

NECROTIZING FASCIITIS

This includes Meleney's ulcer (35) and Fournier's syndrome (21). It is characterized by an initial necrosis of the superficial and deep fascia, followed by extension towards the neighbouring tissues. The preferred location of Fournier's syndrome is in the scrotal, vulvar (38), and/or perianal regions (31). The germs involved are anaerobic (Bacteroides fragilis, Peptostreptococcus, etc.), but also aerobic (enterobacteria, Staphylococci, Streptococci, etc.).

Mortality for these disorders is generally high (12.5 to 48%), depending on the speed of diagnosis and treatment, the patient's medical background, and the treatment scheme.

Several investigations have emphasized the importance of associating surgery, antibiotics and HBO (30, 33, 36, 37, 41, 42). Others do no mention HBO (38).

ANAEROBIC CELLULITIS

This raises the issues of definition, classification and treatment. Should anaerobic cellulitis be treated and how? (1)

ACUTE CARBON MONOXIDE POISONING

Once a diagnosis is established, sometimes in rather special conditions (52, 53), treating patients suffering from acute carbon monoxide (CO) poisoning raises the issue of whether HBO is indicated. Prospective, randomized studies (46, 64) have attempted to identify the respective roles of H_3O and normobaric oxygen (NBO) in the treatment of these acute cases of poisoning. Furthermore, the daily experience of emergency and resuscitation wards has given rise to a number of practical treatment schemes (49, 63).

Carbon monoxide does not bind only to haemoglobin but also to cytochromes, in particular the a3 cytochrome of the mitochondrial respiratory chain. Carbon monoxide's action on the mitochondrial respiratory chain is to inhibit the enzyme responsible for oxidation of the a3 cytochrome. CO poisoning therefore brings about a blockage of electron transportation in the respiratory chain. However, in the event of CO poisoning, the respiratory chain is capable of moderating its sensitivity to CO. The time lag for this reaction to operate depends on each individual's own enzymatic system capable of altering the membranous electron flow in the respiratory chain. Its activation, however, partly depends on the individual's metabolic state. Some known factors that affect this reaction are metabolic acidosis, calcium, alcohol, and HBO. Acidosis and alcohol rate are thought to operate against the activation of the enzymatic system, and therefore lead to greater toxicity. Conversely, magnesium is thought to inhibit the intracellular flow of Ca^{++} and this could contribute to a significant reduction in CO binding.

Using HBO in the carbon monoxide poisoning indication was first reported in 1960 (67). Its relevance at the time was connected with studies on the elimination of CO in the blood (59, 62). Using 18 volunteers, Peterson and Stewart (62) showed that inhalation of 500 ppm of CO for 2.3 hr led to a carboxyhemoglobin (HbCO) rate of 25% and that inhalation of oxygen at a rate of 10 liters/min. under atmospheric pressure achieved the elimination half-life at approximately the ninetieth minute. This value falls to 23 minutes in the case of exposure at 3 times atmospheric pressure. Alongside the acceleration of the elimination half-life of HbCO, HBO inhalation at 3 ATA reduces the CO-cytochrome a3 (44) compound and restores the respiratory chain's functional mode. Similarly, Thom showed that HBO administered to a rat (3 ATA, 45 minutes) inhibits the cerebral lipoperoxidation induced by CO (69).

Very few clinical studies under controlled conditions have investigated the respective impact of NBO and HBO in the treatment of CO poisoning in non-comatose patients. From an important study performed on a limited number of patients that were not unconscious upon admission (46), it appears that HBO is more effective than NBO as regards clinical progress, electroencephalograms, and cerebral vasomotricity. Conversely, in a study performed on 629 adults (64), HBO did not prove to be useful for treating carbon monoxide poisoning in the absence of initial disorders of consciousness. Furthermore, the authors conclude that in the case of severe consciousness disorders, performing one or two HBO sessions does not achieve significant differences as regards progress. However, this work raised a number of reservations concerning methodology (45). Alongside the results of these studies, teams have varying practical approaches ranging from no use of HBO to treat poisoning (50) to routine HBO treatment for all types of poisoning (56) and a series of intermediate approaches (54, 58). Depending on the medical teams, HBO pressures vary from 2 to 3 ATA, and its duration from 45 to 90 minutes. Similarly, there is no standard practice as regards the optimal point in time at which HBO is administered (48, 66, 68).

One important factor concerning the cerebral prognosis of CO poisoning is the existence of initial hyperglycemia, which appears to act negatively (61) and should be considered for clinical and experimental protocols (60).

In 1994, it appears to be widely accepted that:

- the decision to administer NBO or HBO must not be based on the rate of CO or HbCO in the blood (57). Concerning clinical practice, early clinical signs are unspecified (43) and are furthermore modifies by normobaric oxygen administration prior to admission.
- pregnancy requires urgent HBO treatment. The prospective multicenter study performed by Koren et al. (51) indeed establishes that HBO must be applied at an early stage in pregnant women to decrease the risks connected with fetal hypoxia and to improve fetal prognosis.
- the risk of a delayed syndrome occurring is such that criteria for discharging patients who have suffered cerebral hypoxia due to acute CO poisoning must be carefully defined (47). A formal rate of HbCO is not in itself sufficient evidence and it would seem necessary to perform neuropsychological tests to avoid a delayed syndrome (55 65).

Among the open issues that arise from the divergence in the controlled studies and methodological criticisms, the following should be considered:
- Criteria for selection and protocols for treatment of severe carbon monoxide poisoning: what issues do they raise?
- How many hyperbaric oxygen treatment sessions should be performed for treating acute carbon monoxide poisoning?

OTHER HBO INDICATIONS IN EMERGENCY AND RESUSCITATION WARDS

Many pathologies found in emergency and resuscitation situations have been treated by HBO and the results thereof published (71, 72, 73). We cannot report on them all here. The Organization Committee of the Consensus Conference has chosen a number of indications that appear to be relevant to hyperbaric medicine.

BRAIN ANOXIA

The action of HBO on anoxic encephalopathy is based on the correction of an energy deficit involving a modification of the cerebral energetic metabolism (76, 78). HBO also has a cerebral anti-oedematous effect and enable the ischemic circulatory disorders to be partially corrected (79) and to improve cerebral hemo-rheology by increasing the deformability of red blood cells under HBO (83).

The only randomized work on HBO and anoxic encephalopathy is an experimental study performed on cats (80). Following a heart arrest lasting 5 minutes, the animals in the group treated with HBO (2.5 hr, 1.5 ATA, O_2 100%) showed speedier recovery on the EEG and more rapid improvement in the lactate rate of the CSF than the animals in the control group. The first clinical case dates back to September 8, 1951, when a one hour session at 3 ATA was successfully applied to a man aged 51 who 6 hours earlier had suffered per-op cardiac arrest (81). Other clinical works (77, 82, 84, 85) have confirmed the relevance of this treatment on cerebral hypoxia. However, no randomized clinical studies have been performed and the question of whether cerebral hypoxia should be treated with HBO[4] can be legitimately raised.

BURNS

The basis for applying HBO is vasoconstriction which decreases peripheral oedema during the oedematous post-burn stage, and the decrease of plasma extravasation (89). A number of teams have treated patients with repeated HBO sessions. Results involving more than 1100 patients are good (88). Cianci et al. (86, 87) also find a significant decrease in the length of time burns patients (19 to 50 % of body surface burned) are hospitalized and a reduction in unit patient cost by $31,600. This practice almost solely concerns North America and the question is worth considering in Europe— should hyperbaric oxygen treatment be used for treating burns?

CRUSH INJURY

Theoretically, HBO at 2 to 3 ATA is an important supplementary treatment for serious trauma of the limbs because it acts against tissue hypoxia, reduces post-traumatic oedema, accelerates healing and contributes to the prevention of infections (92). However, the following question deserves attention does HBO reduce reperfusion lesions in acute ischemia and cases of crush injury?

In clinical terms, various situations have been reported (91), in which the effect of HBO as complementary treatment is not negligible. Randomized studies in controlled conditions concerning its exact relevance in the treatment scheme have not been yet published. Research teams are working on evaluating its efficacy by means of transcutaneous oxygen pressure measurements (90).

SUDDEN DEAFNESS

The pathogenesis of sudden deafness is not thoroughly known and there are several hypotheses. A partial drop in the oxygen pressure in the internal ear of animals has been reported and HBO was found to be the best available treatment for restoring the hypoxia (95). Several European and Japanese teams (93, 94, 96, 97, 98) have reported highly satisfactory results. Three controlled studies have been published (93, 94, 98) involving more than 200 patients; they emphasize the best results obtained when HBO is included in the treatment scheme. However, the diversity of these clinical states and moreover the importance of the time lag involved before the treatment is begun has raised the question of HBO's position in emergency treatment of sudden deafness.

The development of hyperbaric medicine in Europe undoubtedly requires the intensification of means than enable intensive care techniques to be associated with hyperbaric treatment. Indeed, out of the 12 indications recognized by the Undersea and Hyperbaric Medicine Society and accepted by the major US insurance companies for compensation purposes, 7 relate to emergency and resuscitation situations.

Other prospective, randomized studies in controlled conditions have been published in recent years, some of which are contradictory (70, 75). They raise the issue of the difficulties involved in performing such investigations with the required methodological stringency. However for hyperbaric medicine to become more widespread, conducting controlled studies is necessary, otherwise, in the future, we shall continue to refer to hyperbaric oxygen treatment as an old technique still lacking proper validation (74).

REFERENCES

Acute gas embolism

1. Armon C; Deschamps C; Adkinson C; Fealey RD; Orszulak-TA Hyperbaric treatment of cerebral air embolism sustained during an open-heart surgical procedure. Mayo Clin Proc 1991; 66: 565-571.
2. Catron PW; Dutka AJ; Biondi DM; Flynn ET; Hallenbeck JM Cerebral air embolism treated by pressure and hyperbaric oxygen. Neurology. 1991 ; 41: 314-315.
3. Davis FM; Glover PW; Maycock E. Hyperbaric oxygen for cerebral arterial air embolism occurring during caesarean section. Anaesth Intensive Care. 1990; 13 : 403-405.
4. Ducassé JL, Cathala B. L'oxygène hyperbare dans le traitement de l'embolie gazeuse cérébrale. Rev Méd Toulouse, 1983;1:179-185.
5. Dunbar EM; Fox R; Watson B; Akrill F Successful late treatment of venous air embolism with hyperbaric oxygen. Postgrad Med J. 1990 ; 66 : 469-470
6. Etches RC. Hyperbaric oxygen and C02 embolism Can J Anaesth; 1990; 37:270-27 1.
7. Larson GM, Vitale GC, Casey J et al. Multipractice analysis of laparoscopic cholecystectomy in 1983 patients. Am J Surg; 1992; 163:221-226.
8. Leitch DR, Greenbaum LJJ, Hallenbeck JM. Cerebral arterial air embolism: I. Is there benefit in beginning HBO treatment at 6 bar? Undersea Biomed Res. 1984; 11: 22 1-235.
9. Leitch DR, Greenbaum LJJ, Hallenbeck JM. Cerebral arterial air embolism: II Effect of pressure and time on cortical evoked potential recovery. Undersea Biomed Res. 1984; 11: 237-248.
10. Leitch DR, Greenbaum LJJ, Hallenbeck IM. Cerebral arterial air embolism: III. Cerebral blood flow after decompression from various pressure treatments Undersea Biomed Res. 1984 11:237-248.
11. McDermott JJ; Dutka AJ; Evans DE; Flynn ET. Treatment of experimental cerebral air embolism with lidocaine and hyperbaric oxygen. Undersea Biomed Res. 1990; 17 : 525-534.
12. McGrath BJ, Zimmerman JE, Williams JF. Carbon dioxide embolism treated with hyperbaric oxygen. Caiz J Anaesth 1989; 36 : 586-589.
13. Orebaugh SL.Venous air embolism: clinical and experimental considerations. Crit. Care Med. 1992 ; 20: 1169-1177.
14. Peirce EC. : Cerebral gas embolism (arterial) with special reference to iatrogenic accidents, HBO Review, 1980; 1, 161-184.
15. Watiel F., Gosselin B., Chopin C. : Les embolies gazeuses et leur traitement par l'O.H.B. Lille Méd. 1975, 20, 9 1-95.
16. Weissman A; Peretz BA; Michaelson M; Paldi E. Air embolism following intra-uterine hypertonic saline instillation : treatment in a high-pressure chamber, a case report. Eur J Obstet GynecolReprodBiol. 1989; 33 : 27 1-274.

Anaerobic infections

17. Altemeier W.A., Fullen W.D. Prevention and treatment of gas gangrene JAMA 1971 ; 217: 806-813.
18. Bakker D.J. Pure and mixed aerobic and anaerobic soft tissue infectious. HBO rev. 1985 : 665-96.
19. Brummelkamp W.D., Hogendijk J., Boerema I. Treatment of anaerobic infectious (Clostridial myositis) by drenching the tissues with oxygen under high pressure. Surgery 1961; 49: 299-301.
20. Darke S.G., King A.M., Slack W.K. Gas gangrene and related infectious : classification, clinical features and aetiology, management and mortality. A report of 88 cases. Br J Surg 1977 64: 104-112.
21. De Jong Z., Anaya Y., Pontonnier F., Ducassé JL., Izard P., Bloom E., Rougé D. Evolution et traitement de huit malades atteints d'une gangrène périnéo-scrotale de Fournier. Ami. Urol.; 26: 364-367; 1992.
22. Demello F.J., Haglin J.J., Hitchcock C.R. Comparat ve study on experimental Clostridium perfringens infection in dogs treated with antibiotics, surgery and hyperbaric oxygen Surgery 1973 ; 73 : 936-941.
23. Desola J; Escola E; Moreno E; Murioz MA; Sanchez U; Murillo F. Tratamiento combinado de la gangrena gaseosa con oxigenoterapia hiperbarica, cirugia y antibioticos. Estudio colaborativo multicentrico nacional. Med Clin Barc. 1990 ; 94: 641-650.
24. Gottlieb S.F. Effects of hyperbaric oxygen on micro-organisms. Ann Rev. Microbiol. 1971 ;25:111-152.
25. Heimbach R.D. Gas gangrene : review and update . HBO Rev. 1980; 1: 41-46.
26. Hill G.B., Osterhout S. Experimental effects of hyperbaric oxygen on selected Clostidial species. I. In vitro studies. J Infect Dis 1972; 125: 17-25.
27. Hill G.B., Osterhout S. Experimental effects of hyperbaric oxygen on selected Clostridial species. II. In vivo studies in mice. J Infect Dis 1972; 125 : 26-35.
28. Hirn-M; Niinikoski-J. Hyperbaric oxygen in the treatment of Clostridial gas gangrene. Ann Chir Gynaecol. 1988; 77: 37-40.
29. Hirn-M; Niinikoski-J.; Lehtonen O.P. Effect of hyperbaric oxygen and surgery on experimental multimicrobial gas gangrene. Eur Surg Res. 1993 ; 25 265-269.
30. Him-M; Niinikoski-J. Management of perineal necrotizing fasciitis (Fournier's gangrene). Ann Chir Gynaecol. 1989; 78 : 277-8 1.
31. Iorianni P.; Oliver G.C. Synergistic soft tissue infectious of the perineum. Dis Color Rectum. 1992; 35 : 640-644.

32.   Ketterl R; Beckurts T; Kovacs J; Stubinger B; Hipp R; Claudi B. Gas-gangrene following arthroscopic surgery. Arthroscopy. 1989; 5 : 79-83.
33.   Lucca M; Unger HD; Devenny AM. Treatment of Fournier's gangrene with adjunctive hyperbaric oxygen therapy. Am-J-Emerg-Med. 1990; 8 : 385-387.
34.   Mader J.T. Phagocyting killing and hyperbaric oxygen : antibacterials mechanisms. HBO rev. 1983 ; 2, 37-54
35.   Meleney FL Hemolytic streptococcus gangrene. Arch Surg 1924; 9 : 3 17-364.
36.   Paty R. ; Smith A.D. Gangrene and Fournier's gangrene. Urol. Clin. North. Am. 1992: 19 149-162.
37.   Riseman J.A., Zamboni W.A., Curtis A., Graham D.R., Konrad H.R. Ross D.S. Hyperbaric oxygen therapy for necrotizing fasciitis reduces mortality and the need for debridements. Surgery 1990; 108: 847-850.
38.   Stephenson H., Dotters D.J., Katz V., Droegemueller W. Necrotizing fasciitis of the vulva. Am J Obsret Gynecol 1992; 166: 1324-1327.
39.   Stevens D.L., Bryant A.E., Adams K., Mader J.T. Evaluation of therapy with hyperbaric oxygen for experimental infection with Clostridium perfringens. J Jnfect Dis 1993; 17 : 231- 237.
40.   Trivedi D.R.; Raut V.V. Role of hyperbaric oxygen therapy in the rapid control of gas gangrene infection and its toxaemia. J Postgrad. Med. 1990; 36: 13-15.
41.   Topper S.M. ; Piaga B.R. ; Burner W.L. Necrotizing myonecrosis and polymicrobial sepsis. The role of adjunctive hyperbaric oxygen. Orthop Rev. 1990; 19: 895-900.
42.   Wattel F., Ohresser Ph., Mathieu D. Perineal gangrene. J Hyperbaric Med 1986, 1: 215-221.

Carbon monoxide poisoning

43.   Barret L., Danel V., Faure J. Carbon monoxide poisoning : a diagnosis frequently overlooked. Clin Toxicol 1985; 23 : 309-3 13.
44.   Brown SD, Piantadosi CA. Reversal of carbon monoxide-cytochrome c oxidase binding by hyperbaric oxygen in vivo. Adv-Exp-Med-Biol. 1989; 248: 747-754.
45.   Brown SD, Piantadosi CA, Hyperbaric oxygen for CO poisoning. Lancet, 1989, 2, 1032.
46.   Ducassé J.L., Izard P., Celsis P., Leclercq C., Marc-Vergnes JP, Catala B. Moderate carbon monoxide poisoning : hyperbaric or normobaric oxygenation? Human randomized study with tomographic cerebral blood flow measurement. In : Hyperbaric Medicine Proceedings. Bakker & Schmutz Eds, Basel, 1990, pp 289-297.
47.   Ducassé J.L. Neurologic sequelae from CO poisoning. In Proceedings of "The realm of Hyperbaric Therapy" EM Camporesi, G Vezzani, A Pizzola Editors, Parma, 1992, pp 192-201.
48.   Gibson AJ; Davis FM; Ewer T; McGeoch G Delayed hyperbaric oxygen therapy for carbon monoxide intoxication—two case reports. N-Z-Med-J. 1991 104: 64-65.
49.   Ilano AL; Raffin TA Management of carbon monoxide poisoning. Chesr. 1990; 97: 165- 169.
50.   Jardin F. L'oxygènothérapie hyperbare au cours des intoxications oxycarbonnées. Une thérapeutique théoriquement justifiée mais pratiquement discutable. Presse Méd., 1985, 14, 283.
51.   Koren O; Sharav T; Pastuszak A; Garrettson LK; Hill K; Samson I; Rorem M; King A; Dolgin JE A multicenter, prospective study of fetal outcome following accidental carbon monoxide poisoning in pregnancy. Reprod-Toxicol. 1991:5 . 397-403.
52.   Hampson NB; Norkool DM Carbon monoxide poisoning in children riding in the back of pickup trucks. JAMA. 1992; 267 : 538-540.
53.   Hampson NB; Kramer CC, Dunford RG, Norkool DM Carbon monoxide poisoning from indoor burning of charcoal briquets. JAMA. 1994; 271: 52-53.
54.   Mathieu D., Nolf M., Durocher A. Wattel F. Acute carbon monoxide poisoning. Risk of late sequelea and treatment by hyperbaric oxygen. Clin. Toxicol., 1985, 23, 3 15-324.
55.   Messier LD; Myers RA. A neuropsychological screening battery for emergency assessment of carbon-monoxide-poisoned patients. J Clin Psychol. 1991 :47 . 675 -684.
56.   Micheels J., Colignon M., Lamy M. Les intoxications à l'oxyde de carbone (CO) et l'oxygénothérapie hyperbare (OHB). Méd. et Hvg., 1989, 47, 3607-36 10.
57.   Myers-RA; Britten-JS. Are arterial blood gases of value in treatment decisions for carbon monoxide poisoning ? Crit Care Med. 1989; 17: 139-142.
58.   Myers R.A.M., Snyder S.K., Linberg S., Cowley R.A. Value of hyperbaric oxygen in suspected carbon monoxide poisoning. JAMA, 1981, 246, 2478-2480.
59.   Pace N., Stajman E., Waiker EL. Acceleration of carbon monoxide elimination in man by high pressure oxygen. Science, 1950, 111, 652-654.
60.   Penney DO. Acute carbon monoxide poisoning in an animal model : the effects of altered glucose on morbidity and mortality. Toxicology; 1993 ; 80 : 85- 101.
61.   Penney DO. Hyperglycemia exacerbates brain damage in acute severe carbon monoxide poisoning. Med Hypotheses; 1988; 27 : 241-249.
62.   Peterson J.E., Stewart R.D., Absorption and elimination of carbon monoxide by inactive young men. Arch. Environ. Health., 1970, 21, 165-171.
63.   Piantadosi CA. Carbon monoxide intoxication. In : Vincent JL, ed. Update in Intensive care and emergency medicine. New York, NY : Springer-Verlag; 1990; 10 : 460-471.
64.   Raphaël J.C., Elkharrat D., Jars-guincestre M.C. Trial of normobaric and hyperbaric oxygen for acute carbon monoxide intoxication. Lancet, 1989, 2, 414-418.
65.   Samuels AH; Vamos MJ; Taikato MR Carbon monoxide, amnesia and hyperbaric oxygen therapy. Aust-N-Z-J-Psychiatry. 1992; 26 : 316-319.

66. Sloan EP; Murphy DO; Har R; Cooper MA; Turnbull T; Barreca RS; Ellerson B. Complications and protocol considerations in carbon monoxide-poisoned patients who require hyperbaric oxygen therapy: report from a ten-year experience. Ann Emerg Med. 1989; 14: 629-634.
67. Smith GI, Sharp GR. Treatment of carbon monoxide poisoning with oxygen under pressure; Lancet, 1960, 1, 905-906.
68. Thom SR; Keim LW. Carbon monoxide poisoning: a review epidemiology, pathophysiology, clinical findings, and treatment options including hyperbaric oxygen therapy. J-Toxicol-Clin-Toxicol. 1989; 27: 141-156.
69. Thom SR. Functional inhibition of leukocyte b2 integrins by hyperbaric oxygen in carbon monoxide-medited brain injury in rats. Toxicol Appl Pharmacol; 1993; 123 : 248-256 .

Other HBO indications in emergency and resuscitation wards

70. Anderson-DC; Bottini-AG; Jagiella-WM; Westphal-B; Ford-S; Rockswold-GL; Loewenson-RB A pilot study of hyperbaric oxygen in the treatment of human stroke. Stroke. 1991 Sep: 22(9): 1137-42.
71. Bouachour O., Gouello JP., Aiquier Ph. L'oxygénothérapie hyperbare : les indications en urgence Rev Prat 1994; 246: 2 1-26.
72. Davis JC. Hyperbaric oxygen therapy. Intensive Care Med. 1989: 4 : 55-57.
73. Mathieu D., Poisot D., Wattel F. Oxygénothérapie hyperbare en réanimation. Réan Soins intens Méd Urg, 1986; 2 : 71-83.
74. Raphaël JC. L'oxygénothérapie hyperbare : une technologie ancienne en mal d'évaluation. Rev Prat 1994; 246 : 7.
75. Rockswold-GL; Ford-SE; Anderson-DC; Bergman-TA; Sherman-RE Results of a prospective randomized trial for treatment of severely brain-injured patients with hyperbaric oxygen. J-Neurosurg. 1992 Jun; 76(6): 929-34 .

Brain anoxia

76. Ducassé JL: Oxygène hyperbare et cerveau: Action de l'OHB sur l'hémodynamique et le métabolisme cérébral. In Ohresser Ph, Bergmann E.: L'oxygénothéapie hyperbare. Masson Ed., Paris, 1991.
77. Ducassé JL, Genestal M, Hugot B, Marc-Vergnes JP Boé M, Cathala B, Lareng L: Effets de l'oxygénothérapie hyperbare sur les différences artério-veineuses cérébrales dans les comas anoxiques. Med. Sub. Hyp., 1, 103-110, 1982.
78. Ducassé JL, Marc-Vergnes SP, Cathala B, Genestal M, Lareng L: Early cerebral prognosis of anoxic encephalopathy using brain energy metabolism. Crit. Care Med., 12, 897-900, 1984.
79. Ducassé J.L., Catala B, Marc-vergnes J.F. Experimental research on cerebral metabolic changes during an hyperbaric oxygen session. Undersea Biomed Research, 1990, 17:139-140.
80. Kapp JP, Phillips M, Markov A, Smith FR: Hyperbaric oxygen after circulatory arrest: Modification of postischemic encephalopathy. Neurosurgery, 1,496-499, 1982.
81. Koch A,Vermeulen-Cranch DME: The use of hyperbaric oxygen following cardiac arrest. Brit J Anaesth, 34, 738-740, 1952.
82. Lareng L, Cathala B, Ducassé JL: L'oxygénothérapie hyperbare dans les comas après arrêt circulatoire récupéré: appréciation de son efficacité par l'étude du métabolisme énergétique cérébral. Bull.Acad.Nat.Med., 165,461-470,1981.
83. Mathieu D, Coget J, Vinckier L, Saulnier F, Durocher A, Wattel F: Filtrabilité éythrocytaire et oxygénothérapie hyperbare. Med.Sub.Hyp., 3, 100-104, 1984.
84. Mathieu D, Wattel F, Gosselin B, Chopin C, Durocher A : Hyperbaric oxygen in the treatrnent of posthanging cerebral anoxia J Hyperbaric Med, 1987, 2 63 67.
85. Whalen RE, Heyman A, Saltzman H: The protective effect of hyperbaric oxygenation in cerebral anoxia Arch Neurol, 14 15-20, 1966.

Burns

86. Cianci-P; Williams-C; Lueders-H; Lee-H; Shapiro-R; Sexton-J; Sato-R Adjunctive hyperbaric oxygen in the treatment of thermal burns An economic analysis -Burn-Care-Rehabil. 1990 Mar-Apr, 11(2)140-3.
87. Cianci-P, Lueders-HW, Lee-H. Shapiro-RL, Sexton-J Williams-C, Sato-R Adjunctive hyperbaric oxygen therapy reduces length of hospitalization in thermal bums -Burn-Care-Rehabil. 1989 Sep-Oct; 10(5): 432-5.
88. Grossman AR , Grossman AJ. Update on hyperbaric oxygen and treatment of burns. HBO rev; 1982; 3: 5 1-62.
89. Nylander G., Nordstram H., Eriksson E., Effects of hyperbaric oxygen on oedema formation after a scald burn. Burns, 1984, 10: 193-196.

Crush injury

90. Mathieu D. Wattel F.E. et al. Post traumatic limb ischemia. Prediction of final outcome by transcutaneous oxygen measurements in hyperbaric oxygen. J.Trauma,1 990; 20: 307-314.
91. Strauss MB. Role of hyperbaric oxygen therapy in acute ischemias and crush injuries. HBO Rev., 1981,2: 87-106.
92. Strauss MB, Hart GB. Crush injury and the role of hyperbaric oxygen. Topics in Emergency Med., 1984,6 : 9-24.

Sudden deafness

93.   Dauman R, Cros AM, Poisot D Treatment of sudden deafness first results of a comparative study. J Otolaryngol 1985; 14 : 49-56..

94.   Goto F., Fujita T., Kitani Y. Hyperbaric oxygen and stellete ganglion blocks for idiopathic sudden hearing bss. Acta Otolaryngol 1979; 88 : 335-342.

95.   Lamm H., Lamm K. The effect of hyperbaric oxygen on the inner ear. In : Kindwall EP (Ed) Proceedings of the 8th international congress of hyperbaric medicine. San Pedro, p 35..

96.   Lamm H., Klimpel L. Hyperbare Sauerstofftherapie bei Innenohr und Vestibularisstörungen. HNO; 1971; 19: 363-369.

97.   Orhesser Ph., Jean C., Alessandrini G. Traitement par l'oxygène hyperbare de la surdité brusque: étude sur 160 cas. Med Aéro Spat Med Sub Hyp. 1980; 19: 58-60.

98.   Pilgramm M., Lamm H., Schumann K. Zur hyperbaren Sauerstofftherapie beim Hörsturz. Laryngol Rhinol Otol. 1985; 64: 351-354..

ACUTE INDICATIONS OF HBO THERAPY
Final Report

G. Oriani, MD
Anesthesia - Intensive Care and Hyperbaric Service
Istituto Ortopedico Galeazzi - Milano

INTRODUCTION

The purpose of this final report was to clearly indicate the pathologies that have to be considered as acute indications for hyperbaric oxygen therapy.

Introduction of the subject firstly needed to precisely define the maining of acute indications and criteria used for utilization of HBO in therapeutical protocols.

First of all, acute indications for HBO therapy concern pathologies in which HBO therapy can be considered of primary importance in saving the life of the patient, because therapy is able to restore one or more compromised vital functions. Patients relevant to these emergency indications are most often critically ill patients, in unsteady state.

Acute indications of HBO also include pathological situations for which a fast application of the therapy may result in saving a body segment (for example to avoid amputation for traumatic limb ischemia), or because a timely and urgent application of the therapy may preserve a function or save organ (for example in sudden deafness). In these situations, HBO therapy can be considered an important part of the therapy in preventing serious disability but not primary life saving.

Criteria used for the introduction of HBO therapy in therapeutical protocols are relevant to the same rules that those applied in other medical fields, by using a graded scale to assess the weight of recommendations, with regard to basic studies, animal studies with control group, and human studies. Three lines of evidence have been used to justify HBO therapy in clinical practice: strong evidence of beneficial action, evidence of beneficial action, weak evidence of beneficial action, versus no evidence of beneficial action.

Moreover, classification previously suggested by the European Committee for Hyperbaric Medicine (ECHM Scientific Board Meeting, Toulouse, France, May 1992) must be used as an initial step for discussion to facilitate elaboration of proposals. HBO indications were divided in three groups: already accepted, under investigation or controversial indications, and, with respect to the acute indications, a particular attention for the right place of HBO regarding patient recovery was done. So characterization of acute HBO indications such as strongly recommended, recommended or optional appears of primary importance face to the possible applicative method of the therapy, that may be performed as the sole treatment, or be included in a multi-disciplinary therapeutic approach.

At least, it would be of major interest to precisely define for each indication, an application scheme: O_2 pressure, periods of treatment, duration and frequency of hyperbaric cycles, etc.

During the workshop, the following pathologies were considered that represent acute indications of HBO previously proposed by the ECHM.

- Carbon monoxide intoxication
- Arterial gas embolism
- Gas gangrene
- Serious mixed infections of soft tissue including diabetic gangrene
- Crush injuries and compartment syndrome
- Burns, burns with smoke inhalation
- Post-anoxic encephalopathy
- Sudden deafness
- Serious vascular visual pathologies

CARBON MONOXIDE INTOXICATION

It is a serious intoxication that causes immediate and subsequent consequences to the nervous cardiocirculatory system. The immediate damage is connected with the relation between the porphyrinic groups (haemoglobin, myoglobin, cytocrome) and the carbon monoxide and so, related to the incapacity to bring oxygen to the tissues and to the cytocrome inhibition. The minor damage is the consequence of a post-anoxic syndrome, and it appears in a time period of few days till 40 days from the poisoning. The most damaged organs are the brain (with the appearance of psychical disturbances of different intensity) and the heart (with alterations of kinesis and structural alterations of the myocardial fibre). The clinical evidence of a favourable outcome determined by the hyperbaric oxygen therapy has been proved by many authors in about 30 year application. The last evidence is represented by Thom's study (39). Two further evidences have been reported in this session: epidemiological data by Hampson (19) and a French randomized controlled study concerning minor forms of carbon monoxide poisoning (28).

It has been recalled that normobaric oxygen must be used as soon as the patient is reserved and till HBO session.

Many evidences have been reported that HBO efficacy is maximal if the period between CO poisoning and HBO is less than 6 hours (18,26,27,31).

Indications for HBO have to be based on clinical presentation: coma and conscience impairment, neurological, psychological, cardiological abnormalities whatever carboxy-hemoglobin level may be. Pregnant women must also undergo HBO whatever their clinical state.

The hyperbaric therapy for CO poisoning has to be considered strongly recommended and urgent. It must be used for the best in a 6 hour period, in a protocol using normobaric oxygen as a first aid measure and followed by a neurological, cardiological, and behavioural follow up. In case of HBO indication, pressure to be used and the number of HBO session (one or two) are actually not firmly established, but the protocol most frequently used is 2.5 ATA during 90 minutes and repetition of HBO session is currently done by many centers in case of persistent critical abnormalities.

ARTERIAL GAS EMBOLISM (AGE)

Causes of arterial gas embolism are diverse. In underwater hyperbaric practice, AGE may be caused by a pulmonary over-inflation and/or by ignored patent foramen ovale. In the clinical practice, AGE may be caused by surgical operations (cardio-, neuro-, thoracic surgery), during haemodialysis or by central venous catheter. What is important is not the nature of the gas present in the circulatory system but its quantity. HBO works by two ways: hydrostatic pressure for recompression and so for reduction of the gas bubble volume, and hyperoxygenation for tissue hypoxia and local metabolic acidosis correction.

Works on animals (10,24) as well as data collected in humans (34) have proved the benefit of the therapeutical recompression.

The clinical experience on serious ill patients has shown that use of pressure up to 6 ATA, rather than use of pure oxygen under lower pressure, results in the same favourable outcome, thus reducing the risks connected with illness of the patient.

Treatment must include a single recompression with a maximum pressure compatible with the respiratory gas used (3 ATA for oxygen and 6 ATA for mixture). Following treatments may be used but only to correct local perfusion damages (to consider like reperfusion damage).

The HBO in arterial gas embolism must be considered strongly recommended and urgent. It must be applied, together with an intensive care protocol to support the cardiocirculatory system and alveolocapillary exchanges.

GAS GANGRENE

The Clostridium myonecrosis (gas gangrene) is a rapid infection, caused by an anaerobic bacteria (Clostridium genier). The Clostridium-induced alterations are either direct or mediated by an alpha-exotoxin which produces tissue necrosis, hemolysis and specific neurological disturbances.

Clostridium needs low oxygen pressure to grow. Necrotic process leads to further tissue destruction and to lower local perfusion. These conditions are very favorable either for the bacterial reproduction or for specific toxin production. Hyperbaric oxygen is lethal for anaerobic micro-organisms and stops alpha-toxin production completely when tissue PO_2 is > 250 mmHg.

Favourable evidence was demonstrated years ago (3,12). In 1988, Bakker had proposed a soft tissue infection classification and a pluridisciplinary approach based on surgery (local debridement)—antibiotics and early HBO (5), associated to general resuscitative and ancillary measures.

It is very important that HBO therapy start as early as possible, because the best treatment results are achieved in the earliest possible stage of the infection (21). The advantages of early hyperbaric oxygen treatment are that:

- it is life-saving because less heroic surgery needs to be performed in very ill patients, and the cessation of alpha-toxin production is rapid.
- it is limb and tissue-saving because no major amputations or excisions are done in advance, and, when demarcation becomes clear, far less tissue appears to be lost than initially thought.
- it clarifies the demarcation, so that there is a clear distinction between dead and still-living tissue within 24–30 hours (4).

Since then, many authors had reported same evidence: the lowest morbidity and mortality are achieved with initial conservatrice surgery and rapid initiation of HBO therapy. By now, there is no doubt about the role of hyperbaric oxygen in this pathology (13,22,37,41).

HBO therapy in gas gangrene must be considered as highly recommended, urgent, and should start quickly, for the best within 12–18 hours from the clinical manifestation, never as an isolated therapy but associated with surgery (fasciotomy) and antibiotics. The most often recommended treatment profile consist of oxygen at 3.0 ATA pressure for 90 minutes, three times in the first 24 hours and then twice per day for the next four to five days. Decision of termination of treatment depends on the patient's response to HBO therapy.

COMPARTMENT SYNDROME

Causes of compartmental syndrome are multiple: traumatic, vascular, dismetabolic. After severe trauma, local circulation is compromised. The decrease in blood flow may be either functional or anatomical, but results always in local hypoxia, where infection or necrosis may appear. After an ischemic injury, revascularisation may induce reperfusion damage in the so called ischemic-reperfusion injury.

The ischemic reperfusion injury is a complex pathological entity in which the tissue damage paradoxically becomes more severe after the obtained vascular reperfusion. The endothelial cell swelling, the release of intracellular enzymes and proteins and the increased microvascular permeability to protein, are all factors that lead to the development of muscle edema which, together with concomitant vasomotor changes, may compromise tissue perfusion. This is particularly evident in the muscles enclosed within a fascial sheath where the increase in internal pressure quickly reaches a level where compressive tissue necrosis and concomitant neuropathy appears (compartment syndrome). The key event initiating local reperfusion injury appears to be the release of oxygen derived free radicals (FRO) within muscle tissue, with production of Xanthine oxidase-derived superoxide anions.

The HBO therapy, in this compartment syndrome, allows the increase of tissue oxygen pressure, the reduction of vasogenic edema, the demarcation between live and dead tissue and finally the resolution of this "Paradox effect" on FRO production.

Initially the use of HBO in this field was controversial, due to hypothesis that HBO could exacerbate ischaemia-reperfusion injury by adding extra oxygen to the system and increasing free radical production. The experimental studies of Zamboni on a rat ischemic axial skin flap survival demonstrated a significant improvement of skin flap survival after HBO administration during reperfusion in spite of 8 hours of global ischemia (44).

	Progressive Bacterial Gangrene	Necrotizing Fasciitis	Diabetic gangrene
Surgery	debridement and Graft	debridement and Drainage	debridement and vascular surgery
Antibiotics	Facultative	Always	Always
HBO	Immunodepressed and lucking patient	Always	Always

Recently Thom, studying an animal model of brain reperfusion injury, has demonstrated the HBO effect in inhibiting neutrophil adherence and the deleterious cascade of events that follow reperfusion (38).

Another important effect of HBO is on the rhabdomyolysis of reperfused muscle. The myoglobin released into the circulation may precipitate in the renal tubules and cause renal tubular necrosis; this is particularly likely in the presence of a metabolic acidosis and deshydratation. A more rapid decrease of the creatinphosphokinase values has been reported during HBO therapy (33).

Our own 10 year clinical experience of 181 compartmental syndrome, with excellent results (restitutio ad integrum = 80 %) and the other reported studies as a recent randomized prospective clinical trial by Bouachour (7) lead to consider that **HBO therapy for this syndrome (either traumatic or vascular) is recommended and urgent, preferably within 4 to 6 hours of the injury. It has to be included in a multi-disciplinary protocol, which includes vascular and bone reconstruction.** The most often used protocol consists of two sessions a day at 2.4/2.5 ATA pure oxygen during 3–5 days.

The measurements of transcutaneous oxygen pressure is an useful index for the definition of HBO indication and follow up (8,25).

SOFT TISSUE MIXED INFECTIONS

A local tissular hypoxia inhibit PMN microbicidal activity. Thus, a local infection may appear and develop. This, associated with toxic catabolism product accumulation, do reduce the oxy-reduction potential that allows the development of an anaerobic sur-infection. This category includes the crepitant and anaerobic cellulitis, progressive bacterial gangrene, necrotizing fasciitis, non Clostridial myonecrosis, and Fournier Syndrome. Patient evaluation is extremely important in all these cases. HBO is useful in all the necrotizing infections, but the patient basic health situation may influence the evolution. The clinical benefit of the hyperbaric oxygen has been demonstrated by Bakker (2). Allema (1) has presented the dutch positive experience. Riseman (35) has reported in a comparative study, that adjunctive HBO therapy had significantly improved the evolution of this pathology. Zamboni (45) has presented a report about the HBO efficacy in the Streptococcus beta-hemolitic necrotizing fasciitis, and the HBO Italian SIAARTI study group had collected 130 cases who had undergone HBO with positive result (36). All these authors, and many others publications do agree to enclose surgery, antibiotics, and HBO therapy in a one and only therapeutic protocol.

Diabetic gangrene requires a particular attention; on the one hand, diabetes is a complex metabolic pathology, often complicated by a reduced peripheral perfusion and sensibility caused by a neurovasculopathy. This explain why diabetic patients get more easily peripheral infections and septic process. On the other hand, the diabetic gangrene is the most important reason for amputation in diabetics. International literature agrees with the enormous rate of amputations in diabetics. HBO therapy in the last years has become a specific therapy because of its effect on mixed bacterial flora, its demarcation action of the infected area, and the reparation support of the surrounding tissue. In 1987, Baroni and Oriani (6) have demonstrated the usefulness of the HBO therapy for the diabetic gangrene. Many authors have determined the advantage of a special protocol that includes patient metabolic control, frequent debridement, antibiotics, and HBO therapy (17,29,42).

In our previous randomized work, we demonstrated a statistically significant difference either in the final result or in the average length of hospital stay (6).

TcPO$_2$ measurements are useful for selecting patient for HBO and to follow evolution. They have to be repeated (cf. infra workshop 3).

HBO therapy in mixed soft tissue infections is recommended and urgent, specially in diabetic gangrene. TcPO$_2$ measurements should be included in the management of these patients.

BURNS WITH SMOKE INHALATION

Burn injury not only damages the skin, but when of sufficient size, affects all the body systems, in direct relation to its extent. It induces a progressive ischemia with continuing tissue damage beyond the initial thermal trauma. Edema and stasis result from a combination of histamine-mediated and oxygen free radical mediated damage to endothelial cells, leading to an increase in microvascular permeability.

A burn-induced inflammatory response mediated by activation, production, and release of endogenous mediators (serotonin, bradykinin, prostaglandins, leukotrienes) may contribute to organ system injuries with the subsequent development of MOF (Multiple Organ Failure).

This pathology is extremely serious when burned surface is extended or when the burn level is deep. Burns are frequently associated with respiratory damage and circulatory failure.

There are many reasons for using HBO in this pathology:

- The presence of carbon monoxide poisoning or the inhalation of smoke considerably worsens the prognosis, and HBO has been proved to be determinant in this regard, both in the acute stage and in preventing further damage.
- Using a New Zealand white rabbit model system, Yamaguchi et al. (43) studied the effects of HBO on various combinations of smoke inhalation and cutaneous burn injuries. Results indicate that the use of HBO reduced the severity of pulmonary edema. This may occur by vasoconstriction of capillaries because elevated O$_2$ pressure is thought to restrict the permeability of the endothelium to fluids.
- Thom showed that HBO inhibits neutrophil adherence and occurrence of lipidic peroxidation connected to it. This lipidic peroxidation is one of the critical factors in lung damage after burn, so it is certainly wise to reduce it (40).
- One of the major features of serious burns is the fast and impressive loss of blood and plasma following an extensive burn. Both Hart (20), in a controlled and randomized trial on 16 patients, Cianci (11), and other researchers have shown that the plasma loss is reduced by 35 % in the first 24 hours, in the group treated with HBO, compared with the control group.

HBO has been definitively proposed as an adjunct for acute burns. The vast majority of animal experiments and clinical studies of the past two decades have demonstrated the beneficial effect of HBO in thermal burns.

When treating burns, HBO should be not used in case of limited or modest injuries unless the patient is immunodepressed.

In the case of serious burns, **HBO should be considered as highly recommended and urgent if there is also CO or smoke poisoning; in this case, it should be given as quickly as possible, several times a day, together with a specially dedicated intensive therapy.** Therefore, it is essential that the hyperbaric centre, taking in charge these patients, is located inside an Intensive Care Department (23).

HBO is to be considered recommended and to be used as fast as possible in burns, in cases where the surface involved exceeds 20 % of the body, with deep injuries, when circulation in the extremities is impaired or if due to electrocution.

POST-ANOXIC ENCEPHALOPATHY

This term is used to designed brain damage resulting from a global cerebral injury, whatever its origin. For example, it may result from a circulary arrest such as during ventricular fibrillation or asystole, or from a cervical compression impeding cerebral blood flow, such as in hanging.

The use of HBO in post-anoxic encephalopathies is based on the increased oxygen supply to the cells, with a reduction of the energy debt and modification of the glucose metabolism (directing it towards an oxidation-type metabolism and thus causing a reduction in lactate formation) (15). Secondly, the vascular constriction induced by HBO leads to a reduction of cerebral blood flow and then to a reduction of the intracranial blood volume and intracranial pressure (14). Thirdly, as any anoxic condition, the hypoxia induced by the brain ischemia decreases the flexibility of erythrocytes and increases the blood viscosity.

HBO improves erythrocytes flexibility and improves blood viscosity, restoring a proper flow. So, HBO effects in post anoxic encephalopathy, even if limited merely to the treatment time, may be of interest because it improves local oxygenation by diffusion, limits the ischemic damage and decreases the intracranial pressure.

However, there are many disagreements, both concerning pressures to use and time to treat. Post anoxic encephalopathy is a very important question, where further controlled research have to be wait for providing greater certainty.

However, prescription of HBO for post-anoxic encephalopathy is to be considered optional. In any case, it must be used as quickly as possible, less than 6 hours after the accident, at moderate pressure, and must be included within an intensive reanimation program.

SUDDEN DEAFNESS

Sudden deafness is a symptom that results from various causes such as trauma, viral infection, noise... It is well known that cochlear activity requires for this system to be constantly supplied with oxygen.

It has been shown that a very loud noise and/or a very high wave of pressure (rifle shot) can cause an hypoxic crisis at the cochlear level and this hypoxic crisis can, via a self-supporting mechanism, causes functional ischemic damage.

Many studies have shown that the performance of the auditory system can be improved after intense application of oxygen, as if the injured cochlear cells had a possibility of improvement (9).

In the protocol used in France, HBO is considered a useful adjunct in a multi-disciplinary treatment, which includes also haemodilution and use of vasoactive drugs (16). In a previous work, we have shown that a extremely prompt treatment with HBO, within the first 24–36 hours, lead to a very significant reduction of the functional injury and, above all, to the reappearance of the standard waves and peaks on the evoked potentials (32). If the delay between injury and treatment is too long, the positive outcome becomes drastically reduced, up to the point that, in a non-acute stage, our practice is only to treat patients with persistent cochlear ear discharges.

However, since controlled studies are lacking, **the prescription of HBO for sudden deafness should be considered recommended and urgent. HBO has to begin quickly and to be associated with other measures such as haemodilution and vasoactive drugs.**

VASCULAR VISUAL PATHOLOGY

Effects on visual function and ophtalmological benefits of HBO have been recently assessed (30,32). HBO therapy has been used in retinal arterial thrombosis, in association with other measures (vasodilators, thrombolytics), and has been shown effective if performed urgently, as soon as possible, in patients who can still tell the difference between light and dark.

It has also been used in retinal venous thrombosis for its effect on vasogenic edema. Results are also dependent on the delay between thrombosis occurrence and HBO.

HBO has to be considered as optional in acute ocular vascular pathologies (retinal artery occlusion, retinal venous occlusion). In these cases, it must be given as quickly as possible and combined with other pharmacological treatments.

REFERENCES

1. Allema JK., Van der Kleij AJ., Bakker DJ. Should we treat soft tissue infections with hyperbaric oxygen therapy? And How? Proc. of the 1st European Consensus Conference on Hyperbaric Medicine, Lille 1994;1:102-107.

2. Bakker DJ. The use of hyperbaric oxygen in the treatment of certain infectious diseases, especially gas gangrene and acute dermal gangrene. Drukkerij Veenman BV., Wageningen University of Amsterdam 1984;74-90.

3. Bakker DJ. Pure and mixed aerobic and anaerobic soft tissue infections. HBO review 1985;6:65-96.

4. Bakker DJ. Clostridium myonecrosis in problem wounds : the role of oxygen. J.C. Davis and T.K. Hunt edit., 1 vol, Elsevier, N6Y, 1988 : 153-172.

5. Bakker DJ., Kox C. Classification and therapy of necrotizing soft tissue infections: The role of surgery, antibiotics and hyperbaric oxygen. In : Current problems in general surgery 1988;5(4):489-500.

6. Baroni G., Porro T., Faglia E., Pizzi G., Mastropasqua A., Oriani G., Pedesini G., Favales F. Hyperbaric oxygen in diabetic gangrene treatment. Diabetes Care 1987;10:81-86.

7. Bouachour G., Cronier P., Gouello J.P., Toulemonde J.L., Tahla A., Alquier Ph. Results of a randomized prospective clinical trial of hyperbaric oxygen therapy versus placebo in crush injuries: HBO improves wound healing and reduces the need for surgery. Proc. of the XXth EUBS annual meeting, Istanbul 1994, 1: 172.

8. Bouachour G., Gouello J.P., Perrotin F., Alquier Ph. Usefulness of transcutaneous oxygen monitoring in hyperbaric oxygen in patients with crush injuries. Results of a randomized prospective study. Proc. of the XXth EUBS annual meeting, Istanbul 1994, 1: 393.

9. Cavallazzi GM., Oriani G., Zurlo T., Montino O., Michael M., Prendini P., Sacchi C., Ronzio A. HBO and the physiopathology of the auditory function. Proceedings of XIX European Undersea Medical Society 1993; 1: 54-62.

10. Catron PW., Dutka AJ., Biondi DM, Flynn ET., Hallenbeck JM. Cerebral air embolism treated by pressure and hyperbaric oxygen. Neurology 1991;41:314-315.

11. Cianci P., Sato R. Adjunctive hyperbaric oxygen therapy in the treatment of thermal burns : a review. Burns 1994;20(1):5-14.

12. Demello FJ., Haglin JJ., Hitchcox CR. Comparative study on experimental Clostridium perfrigens infection in dogs treated with antibiotics, surgery and hyperbaric oxygen. Surgery 1973;73:936-941.

13. Desola J., Escola E., Moreno E., Munoz MA. Sanchez U., Murillo F. Tratamiento combinado de la Gangrena gaseosa con oxigenoterapia hiperbarica, cirugia y antibioticos. Estudio collaborativo multicentrico nacional. Med Clin Barc 1990;94;641-650.

14. Ducassé JL., Marc-Vergnes JP., Cathala B., Genestal M., Lareng L. Early cerebral prognosis of anoxic encephalopathy using brain energy metabolism. Crit Care Med 1984;12:897-900.

15. Ducassé JL.Oxygène Hyperbare et cerveau: action de l' OHB sur l'hémodynamique et le métabolisme cérébral. In: Ohresser Ph. Bergmann E. Médecine hyperbare Masson Ed 1991:53-60.

16. Esteve Fraysse MJ., Fraysse B. Attitude actuelle face à une surdité brusque. Proc. of the 1st European Consensus Conference on Hyperbaric Medicine, Lille 1994;1: 137-142.

17. Faglia E., Baroni G., Favales F., Ballerio G. Traitement de la gangrène diabétique par l'oxygénothèrapie hyperbare. Journées annuelles Diabetol. Hot. Dieu 1987:209-216.

18. Goulon M., Barois A., Rapin M , Nouilhat E. Grobuis S., Labrousse J. Intoxication oxycarbonée et anoxie aigue par inhalation de gaz de charbon et d'hydrocarbures. Ann. Med. Int. (Paris), 1969, 120: 335-439 - English translation: J. Hyperbaric Med., 1986, 1: 23.47.

19. Hampson NB., Dunford RG., Kramer CC., Norkool DM. Selection criteria utilized for hyperbaric oxygen treatment of acute carbon monoxide poisoning: Results of a North American survey. Undersea Hyperbaric Med 1994; 21 (Suppl).

20. Hart G., Strauss M., Lennon P., Whitcraft D. Treatment of smoke inhalation by hyperbaric oxygen. J Emerg Med 1985;3:211.

21. Heimbach R.D. Gas gangrene : review and update. HBO Rev., 1980, 1: 41-61.

22. Hirn M., Niinikoski J., Lehtonen OP. Effects of Hyperbaric oxygen and Surgery on experimental multimicrobial gas gangrene. Eur Surg Res 1993;25:265-269

23. Lind F. Rationale for the use of HBO in thermal burns. Proc. of the 1st European Consensus Conference on Hyperbaric Medicine, Lille 1994;1:118-130.

24. McDermott JJ., Dutka AJ., Evans DE., Flynn ET. Treatment of experimental cerebral air embolism with lidocaine and hyperbaric oxygen. Undersea Biomed Res 1990;17:525-534.

25. Mathieu D., Wattel F., Bouachour G., Billard V., Defoin J.F. Post traumatic limb ischemia. Prediction of final outcome by transcutaneous oxygen measurements in hyperbaric oxygen. J. Trauma, 1990, 20 : 307-314.

26. Mathieu D., Wattel F., Neviere R., Mathieu-Nolf M. Carbon Monoxide poisoning. Acta Anaesthesiologica Italica 1992;43(2):167-176.

27. Myers RAM., Messier LD. Development of a neuropsychological screening battery for assessment of Carbon Monoxide patients. Journal of Clinical Psychology 1991;47(5):675-684.

28. Neviere R., Mathieu D., Mathieu-Nolf M., Durak C., Tempe JP., Bouachour G., Sainty JM., Grandjean B., Wattel F. Intoxication par le Monoxide de Carbone. Résultats intermédiaires d'une étude randomisée comparant l'efficacité d'une séance d'OHB à 12 heures d'ONB dans les intoxications non comateuses. Proc. of the 1st European Consensus Conference on Hyperbaric Medicine, Lille, 1994, 1.

29. Oriani G., Meazza D., Favales F., Pizzi GL., Aldeghi A., Faglia E. Hyperbaric oxygen therapy in Diabetic Gangrene. J Hyperbaric Medicine 1990; 5(3) : 171-175.

30. Oriani G., Magni R., Musini A., Meazza D., Brancato R. A new electrophysiological test to assess opthalmological benefits of hyperbaric oxygen treatment. J Hyperbaric Med 1990;5(4):231-237.

31. Oriani G., Sala G., Meazza D., Sacchi C., Ronzio A., Campagnoli P., Montino O. Post-interval syndrome: incidence after HBO therapy. Acta anaesthesiologica Italica 1992;43 (3):462-469.

32. Oriani G., Magni R., Zurlo T. Hyperbaric Oxygen activity on visual and auditory function. III International Course on Anesthesia and Intensive care - Alimini- 1994;1: 145-155.

33. Oriani G., Miani S. Ischemia reperfusion injury: indications and role of hyperbaric oxygen therapy. Proc. of the 1st European Consensus Conference on Hyperbaric Medicine, Lille 1994;1: 131-136.

34. Peirce EC. Cerebral gas embolism (arterial) with special reference to iatrogenic accidents. HBO review 1980;1:161-184.

35. Riseman JA., Zamboni WA., Curtis A., Graham DR., Konrad HR., Ross DS. Hyperbaric Oxygen Therapy for necrotizing fasciitis reduces mortality and the need for debridements. Surg 1990;108:847-850.

36. SIIARTI Study Group. Recommendations for HBO application Ed. Mandragola - Italian Society of Anesthesia and Intensive Care, 1994.

37. Stevens DL., Bryant AE., Adams K., Mader JT. Evaluation of therapy with hyperbaric Oxygen for experimental infection with Clostridium perfrigens. J Infect Dis 1993;17:231-237.

38. Thom SR. Xanthine dehydrogenase conversion to oxidase and lipid peroxidation in brain after CO poisoning. J Applied Physiology 1992;73:1584.

39. Thom SR., Taber RL., Mendiguren I. Delayed neuropsychiatric sequelae following CO poisoning and the role of treatment with 100% O2 or hyperbaric Oxygen - A prospective,randomized clinical study. Undersea biomed Res 1992;19(Suppl):47.

40. Thom SR. Leukocytes in carbon monoxide-mediated brain oxidative injury. Toxicol Appl Pharmacol 1993a;123:234-247.

41. Topper SM., Plaga BR., Burner WL. Necrotizing Myonecrosis and polymicrobial sepsis. The role of adjunctive hyperbaric oxygen. Orthop Rev 1993;19:895-900.

42. Wattel F., Mathieu D., Coget JM., Billard V. Hyperbaric oxygen in chronic vascular wound management. Angiology 1990;41:59-65.

43. Yamaguchi KT., Taira MT., Stewart RJ, Roshdieh BB., Mason SW., Dabbasi NI. and Naito MS. Thermal and inhalation injury: Effects of fluid administration and hyperbaric oxygen. J Hyperbaric Medicine 1990; 5(2):103-109.

44. Zamboni WA., Roth AC., Russell RC., Graham B., Suchy H., Kucan JO. Morphological analysis of the microcirculation during reperfusion of ischaemic skeletal muscle and effect of hyperbaric oxygen. Plast reconstr Surg 1993;91:1110-1123.

45. Zamboni, Kindwall E. Flesh-eating bacteria can be zapped by HBO Pressure, 1994 ; 23-4 : 1-7.

CHRONIC HYPERBARIC OXYGEN THERAPY INDICATIONS
Hyperbaric Oxygenation and Healing Disorders
—Introductory Report

Juha Niinikoski, Department of Surgery, University of Turku, Turku, Finland

INTRODUCTION

The use of hyperbaric oxygenation in chronic indications is strongly based on its application as a therapeutic adjunct in the management of repair tissues which exist in chronic oxygen deficiency and where the local oxygen tension is far below optimal for healing.

The injury which incites the repair also injures local blood vessels. Injured vessels thrombose while nearby vessels dilate thrombocytes and leukocytes stick to the endothelium and soon white cells migrate through the vessel walls into the wounded tissue. Within a few hours the injured area becomes infiltrated with rapidly metabolizing leukocytes and macrophages that will later be replaced by highly metabolic fibroblasts. Consequently, the nutritional and metabolic need of the repair process is greatest at the very time when the local circulation is least able to satisfy it. Since the requirements of inflammation and repair overwhelm the capacity of nutritional supply the wound soon faces a local "energy crisis" (Hunt et al., 1972).

WOUND OXYGEN ENVIRONMENT

The wound architecture is partly controlled by the energy needs of the wound cells. New wound capillaries are stimulated to migrate towards the hypoxic and acidotic area at the wound edge. Cells in the van of the advancing wound edge produce lactate, growth factors, and chemotactic stimuli that diffuse back towards the developing microvasculature. The growth of new vessels needs stromal support. On the other hand, the fibroblasts which supply stromal support require nutrients to make collagen, fibronectin, and proteoglycans. Thus, in the wound milieu a delicate interaction exists between the inflammatory cells, new vessels, and fibroblasts (Hunt and Halliday, 1980, Niinikoski et al., 1991).

Reparative cells must necessarily migrate into the wound space. Migration usually occurs along concentration gradients, and steep concentration gradients are found in wounded and healing tissue. Gradients of oxygen, carbon dioxide, pH, lactate, and glucose have been measured and others undoubtedly exist. Measurements of oxygen tension gradients demonstrate that PO_2, which is of the order of 60–90 mmHg over the most distal capillary at the wound edge, decreases to near zero at the zone of macrophages and the central dead space (Silver, 1969, 1980; Niinikoski et al., 1972). In the area of dividing fibroblasts, which is almost confined to the leading capillary zone, the PO_2 is in the region of 30–80 mmHg.

Almost no cell division can be found where the oxygen tension is consistently below 20 mmHg. According to Silver (1980), maximum synthetic and collagen cross-linking activity takes place in a zone in which the PO_2 is 20–60 mmHg and where the oxygen diffusion gradients are much less steep than those at the wound edge.

EFFECTS OF INCREASED OXYGEN TENSIONS ON WOUND HEALING

The discovery that oxygen is a pivotal nutritional ingredient of healing has stressed the importance of efficient oxygen supply to the repair tissue. Reports from several laboratories have indicated that in many types of wounds increased oxygen tensions enhance healing and, conversely, reduction in available oxygen inhibits repair (Lundgren and Zederfeldt, 1969; Niinikoski, 1969; Silver, 1971; Stephens and Hunt, 1971; Hunt and Pai, 1972).

Niinikoski (1969) showed that the tensile strength of incisional wounds in rats increases as ambient oxygen concentrations increase from 18 to 70 volume per cent. When 70 % oxygen was administered, the tensile strength was 35 % above the control level in 10 day wounds. Systemic hypoxia suppressed the healing rate, and the optimal conditions were passed when the oxygen treatment was extended to 100 per cent oxygen at 1 ATA pressure. Parallel observations in subcutaneous cellulose sponge implants demonstrated that the favourable effect of oxygen resulted from enhanced accumulation of collagen, augmented cross-linking of collagen, and increased synthetic activity of wound cells, as indicated by a rise in their RNA/DNA ratio. These findings were confirmed by several investigators who showed that the oxygen effects apply to healing of ear chambers and wire mesh cylinders in rabbits and that not only wound strength and collagen deposition but also angiogenesis and epithelialization are enhanced by moderate systemic hyperoxia.

Collagen synthesis is crucially dependent on the availability of molecular oxygen. Oxygen is incorporated into the peptide chain to form hydroxyprolyl and hydroxylysyl residues. Hutton et al. (1967) found a close correlation between the rate of proline hydroxylation and oxygen concentration over the range of 0.51–14.9 volume per cent of oxygen by using a partially purified chick embryo hydroxylase. The K_m value for oxygen was 2.6 volume per cent, equalling a PO_2 of about 20 mmHg. These results were confirmed by Myllylä et al. (1977) and more recently challenged by de Jong and Kremp (1984) who suggest a higher figure. Partly because hydroxylation of proline is one of the terminal steps of collagen synthesis, its rate tends to limit the rate of collagen synthesis under most physiological conditions. This also means that the synthesis of collagen will be limited by the oxygen tension in any fibroblast which exist in an environment in which PO_2 is less than about 50 mmHg.

The rate of collagen accumulation in healing wounds is a function of arterial PO_2 over a certain physiological range (Hunt and Pai, 1972). Niinikoski (1980) showed that the accumulation of collagen is definitely impaired at a mean oxygen tension of approximately 20 mmHg. This value accords with observations made with ultramicro oxygen electrodes in rabbit ear chambers in which the minimal PO_2 in the area of newly formed collagen fibers is of the order of 20–30 mmHg (Silver, 1980). The ear chamber studies have also shown, however, that oxygen tensions in healing tissues are heterogeneous. Even in normal physiological circumstances, areas of oxygen tensions in the limiting range are found.

Chvapil et al. (1968) reported that cross-linking of collagen in chick embryo skin slices increased almost linearly when oxygen concentration in the incubation gas was elevated from 20 to 95 volume per cent. Lysyr oxidase, which catalyses some of the important covalent bonds which cross-link collagen peptides, also uses molecular oxygen as a substrate. The critical or limiting range of oxygen tension is in the same range as in the case of prolyl hydroxylase.

HYPERBARIC OXYGEN AND WOUND HEALING

The greatest benefit of hyperbaric oxygenation in wound healing may be achieved in situations in which the nutritive flow and oxygen supply to the repair tissue are markedly compromised, as for instance by local injury or infection, but in which the regional blood supply is intact. In uncomplicated surgical incision wounds possessing adequate nutritive flow, the optimal oxygen tension for healing is probably passed when the oxygen treatment is extended to hyperbaric conditions. This is supported by the finding that the rate of gain in the tensile strength of incision wounds is significantly lower in rats treated intermittently with hyperbaric oxygen at 2 ATA than in rats breathing air. Hyperbarically oxygenated normal wounds contain less collagen hydroxyproline as well as less DNA and RNA than control wounds (Niinikoski, 1969).

The healing of open wounds involves contraction and epithelization, processes of little significance in the healing of incisional wounds. In a study of rats, long-term intermittent hyperbaric oxygenation at 2 ATA had no effect on the healing rate of open wounds in which the circulation was left intact. When wound edges were devascularized, however, hyperbaric oxygen enhanced the rate of wound closure in the final stages of healing, thus counteracting the delay caused by disturbed blood supply (Kivisaari and Niinikoski, 1975).

HYPERBARIC OXYGENATION IN PROBLEM WOUNDS

Ulcers Due to Arterial Insufficiency

Many of the peripheral vascular diseases are accompanied by ulceration of the skin of the legs or even gangrene. Ledingham et al. (1963) obtained satisfactory results with hyperbaric oxygenation at 2 ATA in ulcers typical of thromboangiitis obliterans. In arteriosclerosis the response was less satisfactory until prolonged courses of treatment were instituted. Hart and Strauss (1979) used hyperbaric oxygen at 2 ATA to treat 16 patients with arteriosclerotic ulcers, which were refractory to conventional treatments. In 75 per cent of cases the ulcers healed completely. Perrins and Barr (1986) described their results in 50 geriatric patients with arteriosclerotic ulcers treated with hyperbaric oxygen at 1.5-3 ATA alone. Healing was achieved in 52 per cent and improvement in 20 per cent. Amputation was avoided in 65 per cent of patients. The authors concluded that: 1) Many patients with ulcers due to peripheral vascular disease that have resisted treatment by other means can be healed by prolonged courses of hyperbaric oxygen therapy. 2) The response is dose-dependent. Some ulcers respond to 1.5 ATA, while others require up to 3 ATA. Some fail to respond to treatment for a total of two hours per day, others heal with less than one hour a day. 3) The period required for healing can be reduced considerably if the ulcer base is prepared with a course of hyperbaric oxygen therapy before split skin grafting.

In the treatment of ulcers due to peripheral arterial occlusive disease it is stressed that a prerequisite for complete and permanent healing is an effective arterial reconstruction bypassing major dominating obstructions in large- and middle-sized arteries.

Venous Stasis Ulcers

Slack et al. (1966) reported on hyperbaric oxygen therapy of 17 patients with varicose ulcers of the extremities. They used hyperbaric oxygen at 2.5 ATA once a day in a monoplace chamber until maximum benefit was achieved. Five of the patients healed completely, six showed marked improvement, and another four slight improvement. Perrins and Barr (1986) treated 12 patients with hyperbaric oxygen at 1.5–3 ATA and there was healing in 50 per cent. In another six patients treated with hyperbaric oxygen and split skin grafts there was 100 per cent healing.

Creutzig et al. (1985; cf. Fischer et al., 1988) measured oxygen pressure fields in leg ulcers of 11 patients with chronic venous insufficiency. They found low PO_2 values with microcirculatory disturbance of the ulcer tissue. After a compression bandage had been applied to the legs, the tissue oxygen tension of the ulcers increased markedly, probably as the result of diminished venous stasis. These ulcers healed without any other special treatment or hyperbaric oxygen therapy.

Diabetic Ulcers

Diabetes is one of the common causes of nonhealing in ulcers. Before considering hyperbaric oxygen therapy in diabetic ulcers one has to consider whether tissue oxygen in the ulcer area can be augmented by hyperbaric oxygenation. The response of ulcer tissue PO_2 to hyperbaric oxygen depends upon the degree and level of obstruction in the vasculature. If there is adequate large vessel function and the occlusive process is in the microcirculation, oxygen inhalation may be able to normalize wound oxygen tension to enhance leukocyte bacterial killing of microorganisms and to increase the rate of fibroblast collagen production to support capillary angiogenesis (cf. Niinikoski et al., 1991). If large vessel obstruction is amenable to revascularization surgery to perfuse large- and medium-sized vessels, oxygen hyperbaric treatment may be of value in achieving healing of foot wounds. However, oxygen has its limits. Even hyperbaric oxygen will fail to achieve significant elevation of wound PO_2 in peripheral tissue that is barely viable (Davis et al., 1988).

A decision as to whether hyperbaric oxygen will be a useful adjuvant to surgery, antibiotics, and metabolic control in the diabetic foot should start with peripheral vascular evaluation. Palpation and Doppler evaluation of pedal pulses, ankle pressure determination, and angiography may determine the level of occlusive disease. When results are borderline or significant questions remain, transcutaneous oxygen measurements over the skin adjacent to the ulcer and outside any zone of inflammation may help to determine whether oxygen, even at hyperbaric pressures, can be delivered to relatively ischemic tissues of the foot (Emhoff and Myers, 1984). Perrins and Barr (1986) treated 24 patients with diabetic ulcers using hyperbaric oxygen therapy. Sixty-seven per cent of the ulcers healed and in 18 per cent of cases amputation was avoided.

Decubitus Ulcers

Decubitus ulcers are caused by pressure on the skin, which interferes with circulation on the point of contact. Prolonged immobilization in one position may lead to this within a few hours. These ulcers are usually located over bony prominences such as the sacrum and the heel. Seiler and Stähelin (1984) measured transcutaneous oxygen tension in tissues under pressure. Pressure of 15 kPa was found to lead to anoxia and a pressure sore in two hours.

Fischer (1969) treated 26 patients with pressure sores using topical hyperbaric oxygen at 1.03 ATA. An improvement in almost all the cases was found within six hours of treatment. A pinkish color developed and the inflammatory reaction subsided. This was followed by granulation and epithelization. Topical hyperbaric oxygenation suppressed bacterial growth and stimulated granulation tissue before plastic surgical repair. Measurements with ultramicro oxygen electrodes showed that topically applied oxygen can penetrate in a depth of about 300 micrometers from the surface of open moist granulating wounds (Silver, personal communication).

Post-Traumatic Ischemic Lesions

Severe trauma to soft and hard tissues can produce damage to large vessels and also injure microcirculation. Vascular reconstructive surgery can deal effectively with large vessel trauma, but the vicious cycle of ischemia, hypoxia, and edema may be resistant to vascular repair techniques.

Strauss et al. (1983) demonstrated a significant reduction in compartment pressure and muscle necrosis in hyperbaric oxygen-treated experimental compartment syndrome in dogs. Nylander et al. (1985) used a rat limb model of ischemia to demonstrate a significant and lasting reduction in postischemic edema of muscles of hyperbaric oxygen-treated animals. Both of these reports recommended hyperbaric oxygenation as an adjuvant to fasciotomy, vascular repair, fracture stabilization, and debridement.

The protocol recommended by Strauss (1981) in crush injuries is 90 minutes of 100 per cent oxygen inhalation at 2 ATA every eight hours for two days, every 12 hours for the next two days, and once a day for the next two days. If hyperbaric oxygen is needed to promote healthy granulation tissue or control infection, it is continued once or twice daily during osseous and soft tissue reconstruction.

Mathieu and coworkers (1990) from Ulle suggested that transcutaneous oxygen measurements at 2.5 ATA oxygen are a valuable, noninvasive adjunctive method for prediction of the final outcome of major vascular trauma of the limbs.

Radiation-Induced Soft Tissue Wounds

Hyperbaric oxygen therapy has been used successfully in cases of soft tissue radiation necrosis to achieve healing or to prepare a healthy receptor bed for myocutaneous flaps (Davis et al., 1983). While hyperbaric oxygen provides capillary angiogenesis in previously irradiated, partially ischemic, hypoxic tissue, debridement of all necrotic tissue must be performed. Reconstruction or primary healing can then proceed in well-vascularized tissue. Usually, more than 20 hyperbaric oxygen treatment sessions are needed.

Pyoderma Gangrenosum

Intermittent correction of soft tissue wound hypoxia has been a useful adjuvant to debridement and soft tissue grafting in patients with pyoderma gangrenosum (Davis et al., 1987; Cardwell et al., 1988; Wasserteil et al., 1992). The etiology of pyoderma gangrenosum remains obscure, and treatment with corticosteroids and local wound care remains empirical. Eighty per cent of cases are reported to have associated collagen vascular disorders, notably ulcerative colitis and rheumatoid arthritis. Those with inflammatory bowel disease may experience resolution of pyoderma after appropriate bowel surgery. The remaining 20 per cent have no associated disorders. With the apparent common features of small vessel obliteration and infection in these wounds, skin grafting has been considered futile and is not recommended without preparation with preoperative hyperbaric oxygen.

HYPERBARIC OXYGENATION AS AN AID TO SURVIVAL OF SKIN FLAPS AND FREE SKIN GRAFTS

Perrins (1966) used hyperbaric oxygenation as an adjunctive treatment in skin flaps with a disturbed circulation. During the first exposure to hyperbaric oxygenation at 3 ATA ischemic skin flaps came to life and turned vivid pink. Treatment was usually continued intermittently over the next week and ultimately, the flap often healed without scarring. In 1970 Pernns and coworkers carried out a controlled study in patients undergoing split skin grafting. After surgery, the patients were treated either conventionally or by exposure to 100 per cent oxygen at 2 ATA for two hours twice daily for three days. The better results were obtained in the treated group of 24 patients where 92 per cent of the surface area of the graft survived compared to 63 per cent in the controls. Complete take occurred in 64 per cent of the treated patients but in only 17 per cent of the controls.

Experimental evidence of the beneficial effect of hyperbaric oxygen therapy in ischemic skin flaps and grafts has been obtained by several research groups (McFarlane and Wermuth, 1966; Champion et al., 1967; Wald et al., 1968; Niinikoski, 1970 and 1974; Nemiroff et al., 1985). Measurements of tissue gas tensions in ischemic tubed pedicle skin flaps and free composite grafts in rats by means of an implanted Silastic tonometer indicated that exposure of the animals to hyperbaric oxygen at 2 ATA elevated significantly tissue oxygen tensions in both flaps and composite grafts (Niinikoski 1974). The beneficial effect of hyperbaric oxygen on tissue PO_2 was over within 30 minutes after return to a normal atmosphere and no reserve of oxygen was created. Since the oxygen consumption of skin is only 0.33 ml per 100 g of tissue per minute, the requirements of a flap must be low. It has been postulated that the skin can survive for several hours in hypoxic condition, and that intermittent correction can significantly prolong this period (Perrinns, 1967).

HYPERBARIC OXYGENATION AND BONE HEALING

Several reports suggest that the supply of oxygen is a fundamental and, to a great extent, limiting factor in the healing of fractures and recovery from osteomyelitis.

Basset and Herrmann (1961) showed that variations in oxygen supply can alter the type of tissue that differentiates in a culture of multipotent mesenchymal cells. In their studies, hyperoxia caused a differentiation to osseous tissue whereas hypoxia resulted in cartilage formation.

Makley and his associates (1967) found that fracture healing in air at 0.5 atmosphere pressure was markedly reduced in unacclimatized animals. Studies by Penttinen and his associates (1971) indicated that acute tissue hypoxia retards the regeneration of bone by reducing both the synthesis of the collagenous matrix and mineralization.

Hyperbaric oxygenation has been found to stimulate the healing of fractures. Coulson and his colleagues (1966) observed that fractured femurs of rats treated daily under hyperbaric oxygen had a greater uptake of radioactive calcium and a higher breaking strength than the control rats at atmospheric pressure. Yablon and Cruess (1968) demonstrated by autoradiography with tritiated thymidine that all phases of fracture repair were accelerated under the influence of hyperbaric oxygen. On the other hand, when the daily duration of hyperbaric treatment was extended from four to six hours per day at 2 atmospheres of oxygen, breaking strength was reduced as described by Wray and Rogers (1968).

Experiments in fractured rat tibias showed that the growth of callus tissues accelerated by intermittent treatment under hyperbaric oxygen (Niinikoski et al., 1970; Penttinen et al., 1972a and b). Exposure to hyperbaric oxygen at 2.5 ATA for two hours twice daily resulted in enhanced accumulation of minerals and accelerated formation of collagen and other proteins in callus tissues as compared with atmospheric controls. However, no significant differences were noted either in the mechanical strength of the fractures or in the RNA/DNA-ratio of callus cells. This suggest that hyperbaric oxygen does not accelerate the sequence of bone healing in normal animals although a callus luxurians with a larger amount of regenerating tissue does develop.

HYPERBARIC OXYGENATION IN REFRACTORY OSTEOMYELITIS

Clinically, hyperbaric oxygen therapy has been successfully applied in the treatment of supportive pseudoarthrosis and osteomyelitis when conventional methods, such as intensive antibiotic therapy, curettage drainage of sinuses, and removal of foreign material, were ineffective. Slack and associates (1965) found that hyperbaric oxygenation can favorably influence the course of a persistent sinus in chronic osteomyelitis and given sufficient exposure, most lesions will heal, at least temporarily.

Measurements of bone tissue gases in animals have shown that by increasing the respiratory oxygen concentration, one can indeed raise the oxygen tension of regenerating tissue both in infected and uninfected bone (Niinikoski and Hunt, 1972; Kivisaari and Niinikoski, 1975). Using a rabbit model of *Staphylococcus aureus* osteomyelitis, Mader et al. (1978) demonstrated that hyperbaric oxygen alone could eradicate bone infection. Searching for the mechanism of action by using the same osteomyelitis model, Mader et al. (1980) demonstrated hypoxia of mean PO_2 of 21 mmHg in infected bone compared to 45 mmHg in normal bone. Breathing of pure oxygen at 2 ATA raised oxygen tension in osteomyelitic bone to a mean of 104 mmHg and in normal bone to 321 mmHg. In the same study, they found impaired leukocyte killing of *S. aureus* at the hypoxic oxygen tension of osteomyelitic bone and significantly improved killing at oxygen tensions of normal bone or tensions achieved by hyperbaric oxygen in osteomyelitic bone.

At present, data obtained from experimental and clinical studies are adequate to support the following:

1. infected bone is hypoxic,
2. hyperbaric oxygen can elevate PO_2 in infected bone proportional to vascularity,
3. hypoxia impairs leukocyte bacterial killing,
4. hypoxia impairs fibroblastic collagen production to support angiogenesis,
5. in controlled studies in animal models, hyperbaric oxygen alone can eradicate *S. aureus* in infected bone (Davis and Heckman, 1988).

In a clinical situation where the local circulation is so badly impaired that even 100 per cent oxygen breathing at 3 ATA cannot bring significant amounts of oxygen into the infected tissue, no response at all can be expected. In addition to hyperbaric oxygen therapy, treatment of refractory osteomyelitis should include thorough surgical debridement, parenteral antibiotics, as well as autogenous bone grafts and/or soft tissue grafts.

HYPERBARIC OXYGEN IN MAXILLOFACIAL OSTEOMYELITIS AND OSTEORADIONECROSIS

Clinical applications of hyperbaric oxygen in maxillofacial surgery are useful in conditions such as osteomyelitis and osteoradionecrosis, where tissue hypoxia is present. Hyperbaric oxygen is not used as the sole treatment for osteomyelitis and osteoradionecrosis, but as adjunctive therapy in conjunction with general supportive care, antibiotic therapy based on bacterial cultures and sensitivity testing, meticulous local wound care, and surgical intervention.

The pathophysiology of maxillofacial osteomyelitis and osteoradionecrosis involves ischemic bone and tissue hypoxia. Bone infection persists and osteogenesis is retarded until vascular proliferation is induced. Hyperbaric oxygen therapy improves vascularity and stimulates osteogenesis in these conditions (Mainous, 1977; Marx and Johnson, 1988).

In the treatment of established osteoradionecrosis, hyperbaric oxygen is able to identify the need and the degree of maxillofacial surgery required to completely resolve the disease and then rehabilitate resulting tissue defects (Marx, 1983). In osteoradionecrosis prevention, hyperbaric oxygen has been shown to provide a wide safety margin when irradiated tissue is wounded, thus preventing the clinical manifestation of a nonhealing wound with exposed bone (Marx et al., 1985). In refractory osteomyelitis and sclerosing osteomyelitis of the jaws, the addition of hyperbaric oxygen to standard treatment regimens increases the rate of remission or resolution (Van Merkenstyn et al., 1984).

The clinical application of hyperbaric oxygen in cancer-related deformities of the jaws has been dramatic. Although the initial use of hyperbaric oxygen for this purpose was solely in the post surgical phase, the data now clearly indicate that the use of presurgical hyperbaric oxygen leads to far superior results. The University of Miami Protocol for elective maxillofacial reconstruction in irradiated tissue is as follows:

1. Twenty sessions of hyperbaric oxygen at 2.4 ATA pure oxygen for 90 minutes each session,
2. reconstructive surgery, and
3. ten postsurgical sessions at 2.4 ATA pure oxygen for 90 minutes each session. The postsurgical hyperbaric oxygen exposures are not intended to further revascularize the tissue bed, but rather to oxygenate and stimulate revascularization in what amounts to a free graft within a large tissue dead space (Marx and Johnson, 1988).

According to Marx and Johnson (1988) the greatest challenges in the effective application of hyperbaric oxygen in maxillofacial surgery are as follows:

1. Identifying patients who can respond to hyperbaric oxygen without jaw resection,
2. knowing when to intervene with surgery,
3. determining what degree of surgical intervention is required,
4. providing total functional and cosmetic reconstruction to all those who require jaw resection,
5. coordinating hyperbaric oxygen with surgery to resolve—not merely arrest—osteoradionecrosis without later recurrences, and
6. keeping hyperbaric oxygen exposures and costs to a minimum.

CONCLUSION

Hyperbaric oxygenation is an important therapeutic adjunct in the management of wounds and bone lesions, which exist in chronic oxygen deficiency and where the local oxygen tension is below optimal for healing. Hyperbaric oxygen therapy seems to produce no apparent benefit to the repair of normal, uncomplicated wounds. However, in the treatment of hypoxic and ischemic wounds the value of hyperbaric oxygenation is established.

The greatest benefit of hyperbaric oxygen therapy is achieved in situations where the nutritive flow and oxygen supply to the repair tissue are compromised by local injury or infection, but in which the regional vascular network, a prerequisite for oxygen to reach tissues is intact or only partially damaged. On the other hand, hyperbaric oxygen seems to possess significant angiogenic potential in tissues suffering from chronic lack of oxygen due to defective vasculature.

In healing wounds the synthesis of collagen by fibroblasts is crucially dependent on the availability of molecular oxygen as is the ability of endothelial cells to form new vessels. The main function of polymorphonuclear leukocytes in the repair tissue is to resist infection. An important mechanism by which white cells selectively kill bacteria uses oxygen. Thus, any treatment that augments the local oxygen supply or helps to avoid hypoperfusion of the repair tissue tends to increase the rate of healing and decrease the susceptibility to infection.

REFERENCES

1. Basset AC, Herrmann I. Influence of oxygen concentration and mechanical factors on differentiation of connective tissue in vitro. Nature 190:460, 1961.
2. Cardwell RJ, Taha AM, Venu P. Hyperbaric oxygen therapy in pyoderma gangrenosum. J Hyperbaric Med 3:73, 1988.
3. Champion WM, McSherry CK, Goulion D. Effect of hyperbaric oxygen on the survival of pedicled skin flaps. J Surg Res 7:583, 1967.
4. Chvapil M, Hurych J, Ehrlichova E. The influence of various oxygen tensions upon proline hydroxylation and the metabolism of collagenous and non-collagenous proteins in skin slices. Z Physiol chem 349:211, 1968.
5. Oouison DB, Ferguson AS, Diehi RC. Effect of hyperbaric oxygen on the healing femur of the rat. Surg Forum 17:449, 1966.
6. Davis JC, Buckley CJ, Barr PO. Compromised soft tissue wounds: correction of wound hypoxia. in: Davis JC, Hunt TK (Eds.), Problem Wounds. The Role of Oxygen. Eisevier Science Publishing, New York, pp. 143-152, 1988.
7. Davis JC, Heckman JD. Refractory Osteomyelitis. In: Davis JC, Hunt TK (Eds.), Problem Wounds. The Role of Oxygen. Elsevier Science Publishing, New York. pp. 125-142, 1988.
8. Davis JC, Landeen JM, Levine RA. Pyoderma gangrenosum: Skin grafting after preparation with hyperbaric oxygen. Plast Reconstr Surg 79:200. 1987.
9. De Jong L, Kemp A. Stoichiometry and kinetics of the prolyl 4-hydroxylase partial reaction. Biochem Biophys Acta 787:105, 1984.
10. Fischer BH. Topical hyperbaric oxygen treatment of pressure sores and skin ulcers. Lancet :405, 1969.
11. Fischer B, Jain KK, Braun E et al. Handbook of Hyperbaric Oxygen Therapy. Springer Verlag, Berlin, p. 106, 1988.
12. Hart GB, Strauss MB. Responses of ischaemic ulcerative conditions to OHP. In: Smith G (Ed.), Hyperbaric medicine. Aberdeen University Press, Aberdeen, pp. 312-314, 1979.
13. Hunt TK, Halliday B. Inflammation in wounds: from 'laudable pus' to primary repair and beyond. In: Hunt TK (Ed.), Wound Healing and Wound Infection: Theory and Surgical Practice, Appleton-Century-Crofts, New York, pp. 281-293, 1980.
14. Hunt TK, Niinikoski J, Zederfeldt B. Role of oxygen in repair processes. Acta Chir Scand 138:109, 1972.
15. Hunt TK, Pai MP. The effect of varying ambient oxygen tensions on wound metabolism and collagen synthesis. Surg Gynecol Obstet 135:561, 1972.
16. Hutton JJ, Tappel AL, Udenfriend S. Cofactor and substrate requirements of collagen proline hydroxylase. Arch Biochem 118231, 1967.
17. Kivisaari J, Niinikoski J. Effect of hyperbaric oxygenation and prolonged hypoxia on healing of open wounds. Acta Chir Scand 141:14, 1975.
18. Ledingham IMcA. Some clinical and experimental applications of high pressure oxygen. Proc R Soc Med 56:999, 1963.
19. Lundgren CEJ, Zederfeidt B. Influence of low oxygen pressure on wound healing. Acta Chir Scand 135:555, 1969.
20. Mader JT, Brown GL, Guckian JC et al. A mechanism for the amelioration by hyperbaric oxygen of experimental staphylococcal osteomyelitis in rabbits. J Infect Dis 142:915, 1980.
21. Mader JT, Guckian JC, Glass DL et al. Therapy with hyperbaric oxygen for experimental osteomyelitis due to Staphylococcus aureus in rabbits. J Infect Dis 138:312, 1978.
22. Mainous EG. Hyperbaric oxygen in maxillofacial osteomyelitis, osteoradionecrosis and osteogenesis enhancement. In: Davis JC. Hunt TK (Eds.), Hyperbaric Oxygen Therapy. Undersea Medical Society, Bethesda, Maryland, pp. 191-203, 1977.
23. Makley JT, Heiple KG, Chase SW et al. The effect of reduced barometric pressure on fracture healing in rats. J Bone Joint Surg 49A:903, 1967.
24. Marx RE. A new concept in the treatment of osteoradionecrosis. J Oral Maxillofac Surg 41:351, 1983.
25. Marx RE, Johnson RP. Problem wounds in oral and maxillofacial surgery: The role of hyperbaric oxygen. In: Davis JC, Hunt TK (Eds.), Problem Wounds. The Role of Oxygen. Elsevier Science Publishing, New York, pp. 65-123, 1988.
26. Marx RE, Johnson RP, Kline SN. Prevention of osteoradionecrosis: A randomized prospective clinical trial of hyperbaric oxygen versus penicillin. J Am Dent Assoc 111:49, 1985. Mathieu D, Wattel F, Bouachour G et al.
27. Mathieu D, Wattel F, Bouachour G et al. Post-traumatic limb schemia: Prediction of final outcome by transcutaneous oxygen measurements in hyperbaric oxygen. J Trauma 30:307, 1990.
28. McFarlane RM, Wermuth RE. The use of hyperbaric oxygen to prevent necrosis in experimental pedicle flaps and composite skin grafts. Plast Reconstr Surg 37:422, 1966.
29. Myllylä R, Tuderman L, Kivirikko KI. Mechanism of the prolyl hydroxylase reaction. 2. Kinetic analysis of the reaction sequence. Eur J Biochem 80:349, 1977.
30. Nemiroff PM. Merwin GE, Brant T et al. Effects of hyperbaric oxygen and irradation on experimental skin flaps in rats. Otolaryngol Head Neck Surg 93:485, 1985.
31. Niinikoski J. Effect of oxygen supply on wound healing and formation of experimental granulation tissue. Acta Physiol Scand 334(Suppl.):i, 1969.
31. Niinikoski J. Viability of ischemic skin in hyperbaric oxygen. Acta Chir Scand 136:567, 1970.

32.   Niinikoski J. Viability of ischemic skin flaps in hyperbaric oxygen. In: Trapp WG, Banister EW, Davison AJ, Trapp PA (Eds.), 5th International Hyperbaric Congress Proceedings, Simon Fraser University, Bumaby, B.C., Canada, pp. 244-252, 1974.

34.   Niinikoski J. The effect of blood and oxygen supply on the biochemistry of repair. In: Hunt TK (Ed.), Wound Healing and Wound Infection: Theory and Surgical Practice, Appleton-Century-Crofts, New York, pp. 56-71. 1980.

35.   Niinikoski J, Gottrup F, Hunt TK. The role of oxygen in wound repair. In: Janssen H, Rooman R, Robertson JIS (Eds.), Wound Healing, Wrightson Biomedical Publishing, pp. 165-174, 1991.

36.   Niinikoski J, Hunt TK Oxygen tensions in healing bone. Surg Gynecol Obstet 134:746, 1972.

37.   Niinikoski J, Hunt TK, Dunphy JE. Oxygen supply in healing tissue. Am J Surg 123:247. 1972.

38.   Niinikoski J. Penttinen R, Kulonen E. Effect of hyperbaric oxygenation on fracture healing in the rat. Calcif Tissue Res 4(Suppl.):1 15, 1970.

39.   Nylander G, Lewis D, Nordström H et al. Reduction of postischemic edema with hyperbaric oxygen. Plast Reconstr Surg 76:596, 1985.

40.   Penttinen R, Niinikoski J, Kulonen E. Hyperbaric oxygenation and fracture healing. A biochemical study with rats. Acta Chir Scand 138:39, 1 972a

41.   Penttinen R, Niinikoski J, Rantanen J et al. Effects of hyperbaric oxygenation and reduced barometric pressure on the nucleid acid contents of healing fractures. A biochemical study with rats. Acts Chir Scand 138-269, 1972b.

42.   Penttinen R, Rantarien J, Kulonen E. Effect of reduced air pressure on fracture healing. ISR J Med Sci 7:444, 1971.

43.   Perrins DJD. Hyperbaric oxygenation of ischemic skin flaps and pedicles. In: Brown IW, Cox BG (Eds.). Proceedings of the 3rd international congress on hyperbaric medicine. Duke University Press, Durham NC, pp. 613-620, 1966.

44.   Perrins DJD. Influence of hyperbaric oxygen on the survival of split skin grafts. Lancet i:868, 1967.

45.   Perrins DJD. The influence of hyperbaric oxygen on the survival of split skin grafts. In: Wada J, Iwa T (Eds.), Proceedings of the Fourth International Congress on Hyperbaric Medicine. Bailliére Tindall & Casseli, London, pp. 369-376, 1970.

46.   Perrins DJD, Barr PO. Hyperbaric oxygenation and wound healing. In: Schmutz J (Ed.). Proceedings of the 1st Swiss symposium on hyperbaric medicine. Foundation for Hyperbaric Medicine, Basal, pp. 119-132, 1986.

47.   Seiler WO, Stähelin HB. Dekubitus. Neue Forschungsmethode in der Dekubituspathogenese. Hospitalis 6:319, 1984.

48.   Silver IA. The measurement of oxygen tension in healing tissue. Progr Resp Res 3:124, 1969.

49.   Silver IA. Wound healing and cellular microenvironment. Final technical report. US Army Contract No. DMA 37-70-2328, 1971.

50.   Silver IA. The physiology of wound healing In: Hunt TK (Ed.), Wound Healing and Wound Infection: Theory and Surgical Practice, Appleton-Century-Crofts, New York, pp. 11-31, 1980.

51.   Slack WK, Thomas DA, Deiode LRJ. Hyperbaric oxygen in treatment of trauma, ischemic disease of limbs and varicose ulcerations. In: Brown IW, Cox B (Eds.), Proceedings of the 3rd international congress on hyperbaric medicine. Duke University Press, Durham NC, pp. 621-624, 1966.

52.   Slack WK, Thomas DA, Perrins DJD. Hyperbaric oxygenation in chronic osteomyelitis. Lancet :1093, 1965.

53.   Stephens FO, Hunt TK. Effect of changes in inspired oxygen and carbon dioxide tensions on wound tensile strength. Ann Surg 173:515, 1971.

54.   Strauss MB. Role of hyperbaric oxygen therapy in acute ischemias and crush injuries—An orthopedic perspective. HBO Review 2:87, 1981.

55.   Strauss MB, Hargens AR, Gershuni DH et al. Reduction of skeletal muscle necrosis using intermittent hyperbaric oxygen in a model compartment syndrome J Bone Joint Surg 65A:656.1983.

56.   Wald HI, Georgiade NG, Angelillo J et al. Effect of intensive hyperbaric oxygen therapy on the survival of experimental skin flaps in rats. Surg Forum 9:497, 1968.

57.   van Merkenstyn JPR, Bakker DJ, Van Der Waal I, et al. Hyperbaric oxygen treatment of chronic osteomyelitis of the jaws. Int J Oral Surg 13:386, 1984.

58.   Wray JB, Rogers LS. Effect of hyperbaric oxygenation upon fracture healing in the rat. J Surg Res 8:373, 1968.

59.   Wasserteil, Bruce S, Sessoms SL et al. Pyoderma gangrenosum treated with hyperbaric oxygen therapy. Internet J Dermatol 31:594, 1992.

60.   Yablon IG, Cruess RL. The effect of hyperbaric oxygen on fracture healing in rats. J Trauma 8:186, 1968.

NOTES

CHRONIC HYPERBARIC OXYGEN THERAPY INDICATIONS
—Final Report

D.J. Bakker MD PhD, J. Niinikoski MD PhD

INTRODUCTION

In his introductory report, Niinikoski stated that the use of hyperbaric oxygen in chronic indications is strongly based on its application as a therapeutic adjunct in the stimulation of tissue repair. This goes especially for those tissues in which the local oxygen tension is far below optimal for normal healing to take place; that is tissues with a chronic oxygen deficiency.

Even in "normal" oxygenated tissues the nutritional and metabolic needs of the repair processes are greatest at the time when local circulation is the least able to provide these requirements (22).

PO_2 measurements of oxygen tension gradients demonstrate that a PO_2 of 60-90 mm Hg exists over the most distal capillary at the wound edge, decreasing to 30-80 mm Hg in the area of dividing fibroblasts and further decreasing to near zero in the zone of macrophages and the central dead space (53,56).

Virtually no cell division is found in areas where the oxygen tension is below 20 mm Hg.

Maximum synthesis and cross-linking of collagen takes place at a tissue PO_2 of 20–60 mm Hg (55). Thus, tissue repair depends on the availability of molecular oxygen and an efficient oxygen supply.

In many types of wounds increased oxygen tensions enhance healing and, on the other hand, reduction in available oxygen inhibits repair (21,28).

Even in normal physiological circumstances, oxygen tensions in healing tissues are found to be heterogenous and sometimes suboptimal for normal healing.

THE USE OF HYPERBARIC OXYGEN IN WOUND HEALING

The greatest benefit of hyperbaric oxygen is achieved in situations where the nutritive flow and oxygen supply to the tissues is compromised by local injury and/or infection, but in which the local and regional vascular network, a prerequisite for oxygen delivery to the tissues, is intact or only partly damaged.

On the other hand, hyperbaric oxygen possesses significant angiogenic potential in tissues suffering from chronic lack of oxygen due to a defective vasculature (27,37,38).

Hyperbaric oxygen gives no apparent benefit in the repair of normal, uncomplicated wounds. In normal surgical incision wounds with an adequate nutritive flow, optimal oxygen tension for healing is even passed under hyperbaric conditions. This is shown by the finding that the rate of gain in tensile strength of incision wounds is significantly lower in rats treated intermittently with hyperbaric oxygen at 2 ATA than in rats breathing air. Hyperbarically oxygenated normal wounds contain less collagen-hydroxyproline as well as less DNA and RNA than control wounds (50).

Long term intermittent hyperbaric oxygenation at 2 ATA had no effect on the healing of open experimental wounds in rats with an intact circulation. However, the rate of closure was enhanced with hyperbaric oxygen, when the wound edges were devascularized (25).

CONCLUSIONS

1. The value of hyperbaric oxygenation in the treatment of hypoxic and ischemic wounds is well established.
2. Augmentation of the local oxygen supply also decreases the susceptibility to infection by stimulation of the oxygen dependent white cell (polymorphonuclear leucocytes) killing mechanism (32).
3. It is not so much the etiology of the wound that forms an indication for adjunctive hyperbaric oxygenation, but the existing tissue hypoxia, on the condition that hyperbaric oxygen is shown to be able to correct this tissue hypoxia.

CHRONIC INDICATIONS

The European Committee had a preliminary list of indications: Already accepted; Under investigation or Controversial in the different European countries. This was decided upon during Committee meetings during the 3rd. European Conference on Hyperbaric Medicine in Nov/Dec 1991 in Ancona, Italy and in Toulouse, France in May 1992.

The accepted chronic indications included:

- chronic vascular insufficiency
- arterial insufficiency ulcer or delayed wound healing
- diabetic foot lesions
- compromised skin grafts and flaps
- hemorrhagic radiation cystitis
- mandibular osteoradionecrosis
- refractory osteomyelitis

The group of investigated chronic indications contained among others:

- soft tissue radiation damage
- osteoradionecrosis (other than mandibular)

Multiple sclerosis remained highly controversial.

During the Consensus Meeting in Lille, France, 1994, the following indications were discussed and under investigation in the "chronic" group.

1. CHRONIC ISCHEMIC ULCERS DUE TO
   a. arterial insufficiency
   b. venous insufficiency
   c. diabetic vascular insufficiency

    d. decubitus
    e. post-traumatic
    f. post-radiation
    g. pyoderma gangrenosum

2. RADIATION TISSUE DAMAGE
    a. mandibular osteoradionecrosis
    b. cystitis
    c. proctitis
    d. laryngeal necrosis
    e. xerostomia
    f. enteritis
    g. myelitis
    h. preventive hyperbaric oxygenation before surgery in irradiated tissues

3. CHRONIC REFRACTORY OSTEOMYELITIS
    a. maxillo-facial osteomyelitis
    b. chron. refractory osteomyelitis in other locations

4. HBO AS AN AID TO SURVIVAL OF SKIN FLAPS AND
   FREE SKIN GRAFTS

5. BONE HEALING

CHRONIC ISCHEMIC ULCERS

Arterial insufficiency

A prerequisite for complete and permanent healing is an effective arterial reconstruction (including endarterectomy, bypass-surgery incl. femoro-pedal bypasses if possible, and endovascular procedures by the intervention radiologist).

Uncontrolled, open studies show a beneficial effect of hyperbaric oxygenation in arteriosclerotic ulcers, which are refractory to conventional treatments. Amputation could be delayed or became unnecessary. Controlled prospective studies however, are lacking and have to be performed.

Hyperbaric oxygen treatment is recommended in these ulcers when:

- arterial reconstruction is impossible
- seriously delayed wound healing despite arterial reconstruction
- ulcer $PO_2 \geq 100$ mmHg at 2 ATA 100 % O_2 breathing
- toe pressure ≥ 30 mmHg and ankle pressure ≥ 55 mmHg (41,42)

Diabetic ulcers

Many uncontrolled studies have been published showing beneficial effects and healing in ulcers refractory to conventional treatment without hyperbaric oxygen. One controlled prospective study has been published[11,58].

Before considering hyperbaric oxygen therapy one has to investigate whether tissue oxygen in the ulcer area is too low for healing and can be raised by hyperbaric oxygen.

In case of adequate large vessel function and occlusion in the microcirculation, oxygen inhalation is able to normalize wound oxygen tension.

Furthermore white blood cell bacterial killing is enhanced, the rate of fibroblast collagen production is increased, and capillary angiogenesis is supported. Hyperbaric oxygen is an useful adjuvant to surgery, antibiotics, and metabolic control.

With hyperbaric oxygen there is an increased deformability of erythrocytes with improvement of the circulation, while in diabetics a decreased deformability of erythrocytes has been shown (41,26).

Adjunctive hyperbaric oxygenation for diabetic ulcers is recommended when

- arterial reconstruction is impossible or no healing or delayed healing takes place after reconstruction
- $TcpO_2$ ≥200 mmHg at 2.5 ATA 100 % O_2 breathing
- and/or toe pressure ≥30 mmHg and ankle pressure ≥75 mmHg.

A strong recommendation is given to initiate prospective randomized multicenter trials using a uniform classification (Wagner, Wagner-Boulton), the same, above mentioned criteria, and an identical treatment scheme.

Venous ulcers

Uncontrolled studies and anecdotal reports on the possible benefit of hyperbaric oxygen in venous ulcers have been published. No evidence of any beneficial action has been shown. The percentage of healing with and without HBO was the same. Hyperbaric oxygen therapy is optional in delayed wound healing with low tissue PO_2 that can be corrected by hyperbaric oxygen, adjunctive to operative and/or conservative treatment in high risk, immunocompromised patients. Hyperbaric oxygen can be used to prepare the woundbed for skin grafting (62,63,51,54), otherwise not indicated.

Decubital ulcers

Decubitis ulcers are caused by pressure on the skin usually over bony prominences such as the ankle, hip, sacrum etc. Prolonged immobilization in one position may lead to this even within a few hours. Measurements of $TcpO_2$ in tissues under pressure showed that pressures of 15 kPa lead to anoxia and pressure sores in two hours (71).

Only reports on the use of topical oxygen under slightly increased pressures (1,03 ATA) are in the literature (14).

Hyperbaric oxygenation is not recommended in these ulcers; only to prepare the woundbed for flap surgery or skin grafting (see under venous ulcers).

Post-traumatic ischemic lesions

These indications were not further discussed by experts on the Consensus Meeting itself. It is however well known that serious trauma can cause damage to soft and hard tissues and also damage to the macro- and microcirculation. Indicated surgical repair measures as well as vascular reconstructive surgery have to be performed but despite this the vicious circle of ischemia, hypoxia and edema may be resistant to vascular repair techniques. In these selected cases adjunctive hyperbaric oxygenation must be considered and is recommended based on experimental and clinical work outlined in the introductory report by Niinikoski (74,75,57,42).

Radiation ulcers

Will be discussed under Radiation Tissue Damage.

Pyoderma gangrenosum

This subject was not discussed by experts during the Meeting.

Etiology of pyoderma gangrenosum is still obscure. The large majority of cases have associated collagen vascular disorders, ulcerative colitis, rheumatoid arthritis etc. Some patients with ulcerative colitis show healing of their pyoderma after appropriate bowel surgery.

Adjunctive hyperbaric oxygen therapy as intermittent correction of soft tissue wound hypoxia is recommended in selected cases to prepare the wound bed for grafting. Good results have been published (71,8,5,78).

RADIATION TISSUE DAMAGE

The basic pathology of radiation tissue damage is normal tissue cellular kill, and in normal tissue sublethal cellular damage leading to progressive obliterative endarteriitis with resultant tissue ischemia, loss of collagen and fibrosis (35,3).

In irradiated, hypovascular tissue, little oxygen is available and because of the ill-defined and diffuse nature of the boundary between the damaged irradiated and normal tissues, there is a very gradual change in the tissue oxygen gradient. Thus neovascularization is not initiated and damaged fibroblasts at an oxygen tension below 20 mmHg cannot produce collagen. Moreover secondary infections often occur in compromised tissues already having poor healing characteristics, leading to major clinical problems. The mechanism whereby hyperbaric oxygen is able to revascularize irradiated tissues is through creation of steep oxygen gradients that are present naturally in non-compromised, normal wounds. In this way the body recognizes the irradiated area as a "wound" and chemotaxis and biochemical messenger responses proceed as in normal tissue angiogenesis (17,24). Greenwood and Gilchrist demonstrated the effectiveness in reducing the extent of ischemic necrosis of skin flaps created in previously irradiated rats (17).

A controlled study has shown that 100% oxygen at normal atmospheric pressure does not produce angiogenesis in irradiated tissues.

Results were no different than in airbreathing controls (38). So there will be no effect until significant vascular damage has occurred. We do not know, however, at what point postradiation hyperbaric treatment becomes useful, where vascular damage has not yet posed a clinical problem such as ulceration or osteoradionecrosis (24).

An adequate series of hyperbaric treatments raises the tissue PO_2 in irradiated tissues to levels of 75–80% of the PO_2 in non irradiated tissues (37). This level, however, is adequate for tissue healing and it was shown that the new hyperbaric-induced vessels did not involute after cessation of hyperbaric oxygen faster than the normal rate of aging (40).

Hyperbaric oxygen treatment for radiation tissue damage must occur in close coordination with the appropriate specialist and must be part of an overall treatment plan including, debridement, or resection of non-viable tissues, specific antibiotic therapy, soft tissue flap reconstruction, and bone grafting as may be indicated (23).

Mandibular osteoradionecrosis
Recommended and accepted treatment protocol: 2.4 ATA oxygen in a monoplace and 2.8–3.0 ATA oxygen in a multiplace chamber, 90 minutes, once a day, 5–7 days a week.

- 30 sessions HBO followed by evaluation of tissue response.
- When wound healing occurs, 10 or more additional sessions are given. If the lesion does not respond to treatment, surgical debridement is indicated, followed by 10 additional sessions of HBO. Three months after resection of the mandible, reconstruction may be performed without additional HBO (46,48).

Hemorrhagic radiation cystitis
The first case of hyperbaric-oxygen treated radiation cystitis was published in 1986 (70). Weiss et al. used a successful hyperbaric oxygen protocol of 2.0 ATA, 100% oxygen for 2 hours on a daily basis for 60 treatments (79,80). We used a slightly different, also successful, protocol of 2.8-3.0 ATA, 100% oxygen for 90 minutes on a daily basis for 20 treatments (66). Tissue response by cytoscopy is evaluated after 20 treatments. When no residual tumor is present and tissue response is not completely, an additional 10 hyperbaric sessions may be given. In the total number of patients, 54, treated with hyperbaric oxygen between 1989-1993, 80% or 44 patients had complete resolution of symptoms or marked improvement.

Other soft tissue radionecrosis
This includes radionecrosis after radical neck dissections, after laryngectomies, proctitis, and enteritis. Marx recommends the so-called 20/10 protocol; 20 hyperbaric treatments at 2.4 ATA, 100 % oxygen for 90 minutes on a once-a-day basis. A minimum of 20 hyperbaric treatments are given before surgery.
Bouachour published results in the treatment of 8 patients with radiation-induced proctitis with good results (2).
A randomized prospective study in 160 patients requiring soft-tissue flap surgery clearly showed the advantages of a combination of surgery and hyperbaric oxygen. The total wound dehiscence difference was statistically highly significant in favor of the combined treatment protocol (40).
We recommend the 20–30/10 treatment protocol in soft tissue radionecrosis although more experience is needed in the proctitis/enteritis patients. Here hyperbaric oxygen treatment is considered optional.
Laryngeal radionecrosis occurs in 1–7% of cases within 2 years following completion of radiotherapy for laryngeal cancer.
Two series of 8 and 9 patients suffering from severe laryngeal radionecrosis treated with hyperbaric oxygen were published with excellent results in 16 patients (maintaining larynx and a functional voice). In 1 patient laryngectomy was necessary (12,13).
Adjunctive hyperbaric oxygen therapy is recommended for this indication.

Radiation myelitis
Hyperbaric oxygen has shown little effect in the treatment of irradiated neural tissue. HBO was ineffective in improving brain function and of minimal to no use in radiation myelitis of the spinal cord (24).

On the treatment of optic neuropathy with hyperbaric oxygen only anecdotal data and case reports have been published showing some effect (67). We consider hyperbaric oxygen therapy in this indication as optional.

Radiation-induced xerostomia

There are two reports in the literature showing a beneficial effect of hyperbaric oxygen treatment in radiation-induced xerostomia (15,68). Since a multicenter, prospective randomized, placebo-controlled study is underway, results of this have to be awaited before a decision can be made. Until that time HBO will remain optional.

Prophylactic use of hyperbaric oxygen in tooth extraction in the irradiated jaw

Trauma-induced mandibular osteoradionecrosis follows in 89% of tooth extractions in the irradiated jaw. Marx et al. showed in a prospective trial a fast reduction in the incidence of mandibular osteoradionecrosis using the 20/10 hyperbaric oxygen protocol (36). Therefore hyperbaric oxygen treatment for this indication is strongly recommended.

The same goes for prevention of osteoradionecrosis in other locations and for the prevention of soft tissue radionecrosis in irradiated tissues (without previous HBO treatment).

CHRONIC REFRACTORY OSTEOMYELITIS

We will distinguish three different entities in this category:

- chron. refr. osteomyelitis of the jaws
- chron. refr. osteomyelitis in other locations
- acute osteomyelitis of the skull, sternum and/or vertebrae

Chronic refractory osteomyelitis of the jaws

Chronic osteomyelitis of the jaws is a disease found most often in the mandible. It is less frequent in the maxilla due to a difference in vascularisation.

The use of HBO has been advocated in chronic osteomyelitis refractory to surgical and antibiotic therapy (39,43).

Two basic types of mandibular osteomyelitis have to be distinguished:

1. chronic diffuse sclerosing osteomyelitis
2. chronic suppurative osteomyelitis

Chronic diffuse sclerosing osteomyelitis (CDSO)

This disease is characterized by a long history of recurrent pain and swelling without suppuration. Van Merkesteyn et al. found no evidence of an infectious etiology in clinical, radiographic, bacteriologic and histologic studies. The lesion is a reactive hyperplasia of bone due to a chronic tendoperiostitis caused by muscular overuse. This was supported by electromyographic studies. Treatment is based on muscle relaxation therapy and hyperbaric oxygen is not indicated (18,45,47).

Chronic suppurative osteomyelitis

Chronic suppurative osteomyelitis of the mandible is caused in most cases by odontogenic infections, trauma, or surgery. Treatment consists of removal of the source of infection and surgical debridement or decortication in combination with intra-venous antibiotic therapy. I.V. antibiotics should be continued for at least one week and be followed by oral antibiotic therapy for at least two or three weeks. This regimen leads to resolution of the disease in most cases (20,39,43,46).

When refractory to this protocol or in cases with severely compromised vascularization of the mandible or compromised host-defense mechanisms, HBO can be considered as an adjunct to surgical and antibiotic therapy (39,43).

HBO is indicated in chronic (duration more than 3 months) cases refractory to adequate treatment (see above), in cases of concomitant systemic disease compromising the vascularization (osteopetrosis, pycnodysostosis), or in cases of severely compromised immune response (44).

Recommended protocol: 20 sessions 2.8-3.0 ATA 100% O_2 in a multiplace chamber, or 2.4 ATA 100% O_2 in a monoplace chamber for 90 minutes followed by 20 postoperative sessions.

Chronic refractory osteomyelitis in other locations

Slack and associates were the first who found that hyperbaric oxygenation could favorably influence the outcome of chronic osteomyelitis (72).

Refractory osteomyelitis is chronic osteomyelitis which has persisted of recurred after appropriate interventions (failure of surgery to cure and failure of 6 weeks of antibiotics to cure) (76).

Data obtained from experimental and clinical studies support the following:

1. infected bone is hypoxic.
2. hyperbaric oxygen can elevate PO_2 in infected bone proportional to vascularity.
3. hypoxia impairs leucocyte bacterial killing.
4. hypoxia impairs fibroblastic collagen production to support angiogenesis.
5. in controlled studies in animal models, hyperbaric oxygen alone can eradicate S. aureus in infected bone (4,9,29,30,33).
6. aminoglycoside transport across the bacterial wall is oxygen dependent. HBO enhances antibiotic efficacy in a hypoxic environment (31,77).

The Cierny-Mader classification of osteomyelitis can be used as a guide to determine which types of osteomyelitis may be benefitted by adjunctive hyperbaric oxygen.

This classification distinguishes medullary osteomyelitis, superficial osteomyelitis, localized osteomyelitis, and diffuse osteomyelitis. Patients with diffuse osteomyelitis include those who have through-and-through osteomyelitis and who are structurally unstable, either before or after debridement surgery.

These osteomyelitis patients can also be classified as an A (normal host), a B (compromised host) and a C (a host in whom the treatment of the disease is worse than the disease) (6).

We follow the report of the Hyperbaric oxygen therapy Committee of the UHMS and recommend the use of adjunctive hyperbaric oxygen to treat the most difficult stages, localized and especially diffuse osteomyelitis in the B-host. Hyperbaric oxygen is advised in patients with 3 B (a locally or systemically compromised host with a localized osteomyelitis) and 4 B (a locally or systemically compromised host with a diffuse osteomyelitis).

Of course the abovementioned definition of chronic refractory osteomyelitis must also be met and hyperbaric oxygen must be part of an overall therapy scheme of antibiotics, surgery and nutritional support (23).

Malignant external otitis is a special form of chronic osteomyelitis. Three clinical stages can be distinguished.

I: purulent discharge and infected granulation tissue in the floor of the external auditory canal.
II: extension into the soft tissue and bone under the base of the skull with involvement of cranial nerves XI and XII.
III: extracranial extension.

In stage III no survivors have been reported before hyperbaric oxygen was used. Pseudomonas aeruginosa is always cultured in these infections. It is clear from the available literature that hyperbaric oxygen is useful as an adjunct in patients with an advanced disease (stages II and III).

The downhill course in stage III patients reversed promptly when hyperbaric oxygen was added to the treatment regimen. HBO is also indicated in recurrent cases and cases where the process has become refractory to antibiotic treatment (7,10,23,69).

Recommended protocols vary from 2.8-3.0 ATA 100% O_2 for 90 minutes twice a day in a multiplace chamber to 2.0-2.5 ATA 100% O_2 90–120 minutes, twice daily in a monoplace chamber. When the infection is under control the patient may be treated once a day until further healing has occurred.

Acute osteomyelitis in skull, sternum, and/or vertebrae

Hyperbaric oxygen is sometimes used in the treatment of acute osteomyelitis in critical sites such as skull, vertebrae, hand, elbow, or other life- or function-threatening acute cases which have not responded at once to surgery and antibiotics. Although a theoretical benefit of adjunctive hyperbaric oxygen can be constructed in these cases, data are unavailable or too scarce to support a recommendation.

In selected, individual, high-risk cases hyperbaric oxygen, if available, adjunctive to other treatment modalities should not be denied to these patients.

The protocol for chronic osteomyelitis should be used and treatments should be given twice daily.

Extensive practical experience has confirmed the efficacy of adjunctive hyperbaric oxygen in infected, failing or failed sternal wounds. Adjunctive HBO can be recommended for all patients with acute and delayed sternal wound breakdowns and/or infections.

A protocol of 100 % O_2 at 2 ATA for 90 minutes in a monoplace chamber twice daily for three days and once daily thereafter may be used (65).

HYPERBARIC OXYGEN AS AN AID TO SURVIVAL OF SKIN FLAPS AND FREE SKIN GRAFTS

Hyperbaric oxygen therapy is not necessary nor recommended for the support of normal, uncompromised skin grafts or flaps.

However, in cases of preoperative or postoperative irradiated tissues or other cases with a decreased microcirculation or hypoxia, HBO has been extremely useful in preservation of these tissues.

Perrins was the first to use HBO as an adjunctive treatment in skin flaps with a disturbed circulation showing better results in tissue survival in a controlled prospective study (62,63,64). The beneficial effect of hyperbaric oxygen in the treatment of ischemic skin grafts and flaps in animal experiments confirmed the clinical experiences. It was shown, with several methods, that exposure of the animals to hyperbaric oxygen significantly raised tissue oxygen tensions (49,54).

A review of the extensive work that has been done to show the efficacy of HBO on enhancement of the survival of flaps and grafts is recently published. Several authors have shown the cost efficacy and the savings that can be reached by decreasing morbidity, mortality, fewer flaps lost, shorter hospital stay, less surgical re-interventions, less re-hospitalization, etc., with the use of HBO in ischemic flaps (36,49a).

Treatments are given at pressure of 2.0–3.0 ATA and range from 90–120 minutes, dependent on the available HBO facility.

One should start with twice daily treatments which can be diminished to once daily when the graft or flap appears more viable and stable. When grafting in irradiated tissues is required the recommended treatment protocol is the 20/10 protocol of Marx or the 20/20 protocol when 10 postoperative treatments appear to be insufficient (40-49a).

HYPERBARIC OXYGEN IN BONE HEALING

Basset and Hermann showed that hypoxia leads to cartilage formation and hyperoxia leads to osseous tissue formation in a culture of multipotent mesenchymal cells (1).

Further experimental work showed that hypoxia retards bone regeneration and reduced fracture healing (34,59).

Experiments in fractured rat tibias however lead to the conclusion that hyperbaric oxygen does not accelerate the sequence of bone healing in normal animals, although a callus luxurians with a larger amount of regenerating tissue develops (52,60,61).

Strauss and Hart reported their clinical experience with hyperbaric oxygen treatment in fracture healing. They treated 20 patients with 24 long bone fractures and had the best results in the group of patients that were treated with HBO within 20 days of the injury (100% healing versus 75% in the patients where HBO was started 10 or more days post-injury).

They conclude that early application of adjunctive hyperbaric oxygen should be considered in any fracture where there is a significant risk of delayed or non-union (as for example in fractures with a compromised blood supply to the bone fragments) (73).

Although the theoretical benefit of hyperbaric oxygen in fractures at risk for delayed or non-union is shown in animal experiments and supported by limited clinical experiences, there is insufficient evidence as yet to propose a formal recommendation in this indication hyperbaric oxygen treatment here remains optional.

REFERENCES

1. Basset AC, Hermann I. influence of oxygen concentration and mechanical factors on differentiation of connective tissue in vivo. Nature 1961: 190 460.
2. Bouachour GJ, Rongeray J, Ben Bouali A et al. Hyperbaric oxygen in the treatment of radiation-induced proctitis. A report on 8 cases. Undersea Biom Res 1990 ; 17s : 171-172.
3. Bras J, Jonge HKT de, Merkesteyn JPR van. Osteradionecrosis of the mandible : Pathogenesis. Am J Otolaryngol 1990 ; 11 : 244-250.
4. Britt M, Calhoun J, Mader JT et al. The use of hyperbaric oxygen in the treatment of osteomyelitis. In : Kindwall EP (ed). Hyperbaric Medicine Practice. Best Publ Flagstaff, Ar. 1994 : 419-428.
5. Cardwell RJ, Taha AM, Venu P. Hyperbaric oxygen therapy in pyoderma gangrenosum. J Hyp Med 1988 ; 3 : 73.
6. Cierny G, Mader JT, Penninck JJ. A clinical staging system of adult osteomyelitis. Contemp Orthop 1985; 10 : 17-37.
7. Corey JP, Levandowski RA, Panweaker AP. prognostic implication of therapy for necrotizing external otitis. Am J SPOtol 1985 ; 6 : 353-357.
8. Davis JC, Landeen JM, Levine RA. Pyoderma gangrenosum : Skin grafting after preparation with hyperbaric oxygen. Plast Reconstr Surg 1987 ; 79: 200.
9. Davis JC, Heckman JD. Refractory osteomyelitis. In : David JC, Hunt TK (eds). Problem wounds: The role of oxygen. Elsevier Science Publ, New York 1988: 143-152.
10. Davis JC, Gates GA, Lerner C et al. Acjuvant hyperbaric oxygen in malignant external otitis. Arch Otolaryngol 1992 ; 118 : 89-93.
11. Faglia E, Baroni GC, Favales F et al. Traitement de la gangrène diabétique par l'oxygénothérapie hyperbare. Journ Ann Diabetol Hotel Dieu 1987 : 209-216.
12. Feldmeier JJ, Heimbach RD, Davolt DA et al. Hyperbaric oxygen as an adjunctive treatment for severe laryngeal necrosis : A report of nine consecutive cases. Undersea Hyperb Med 1993 ; 20 : 329-335.
13. Fergusson BJ, Hudson WR, Farmer JC. Hyperbaric oxygen therapy for laryngeal radionecrosis. Ann Otol Rhinol Laryngol 1987 ; 96 : 1-6.
14. Fischer BH. Topical hyperbaric oxygen treatment of pressure sores and skin ulcers. Lancet, 1969 ; i : 405.
15. Fontanesi J, Golden EB, Cianci P. Hyperbaric oxygen therapy can reverse radiation-induced xerostomia. J Hyperb Med 1991 ; 6 : 215-221.
16. Greenwood TW, Gilchrist AG. The effect of hyperbaric oxygen on wound healing following ionizing radiation. In: Trapp WC, Banister WE, Davidson AJ et al. (Eds) : Proc. Vth Internat Congr Hyperb Med. Burnaby BC, Canada : Simon Fraser University, 1973 : 253-263.
17. Greenwood TW, Gilchrist AG. Hyperbaric oxygen and wound healing in post-irradiation head and neck surgery. Br J Surg 1973 ; 60 : 394-397.
18. Groot RM, Ongerboer de Visser BW, Merkesteyn JPR van et al. Changes in masseter inhibitory reflex responses in patients with diffuse sclerosing osteomyelitis of the mandible. Or Surg Or Med Or Pathol 1992 ; 74 : 727-732.
19. Guy J, Schatz NJ. Hyperbaric oxygen in the treatment of radiation-induced optic neuropathy. Ophtalm 1986 ; 93: 1083-1088.
20. Hjorting-Hansen E. Decortication in treatment of osteomyelitis of the mandible. Or Surg Or Med Or Pathol 1970 ; 29 : 641-655.
21. Hunt TK, Pai MP. The effect of varying oxygen tensions on wound metabolism and collagen synthesis. Surg Gynecol Obst, 1972 ; 135 : 561.
22. Hunt TK, Niinikoski J, Zederfeldt B. Role of oxygen in repair processes. Act Chir Scand 1972 ; 138 : 109.
23. Hyperbaric Oxygen Therapy. A Committee report. Hyperbaric Oxygen Therapy Committee. Thom SR, chair-man. UHMS Publ nr 30CR (HBO) 1992. Undersea and Hyperbaric Medical Society, Kensington, MD.
24. Kindwall EP. Hyperbaric oxygen effects on radiation necrosis. Clin Plast Surg 1993; 20(3): 473-483.
25. Kivisaari J, Niinikoski J. Effect of hyperbaric oxygenation and prolonged hypoxia on healing of open wounds. Acta Chir Scand, 1975; 141: 14.
26. Kleij van der AJ, Vink H, Bakker DJ et al. Does hyperbaric oxygen alternates nailfold capillary red blood cell velocity ? Proc XVIII Ann Meeting EUBS, Basel, 1992: 51-53.
27. Knighton DR, Silver IA, Hunt TK. Regulation of wound healing angiogenesis: Effect of oxygen and inspired oxygen concentrations. Surg 1981; 90: 262-270.
28. Lundgren CEJ, Zederfeldt B. Influence of low oxygen pressure on wound healing. Acta Chir Scand 1969, 135 : 555.
29. Mader JT, Guckian JC, Glass DL et al. Therapy with hyperbaric oxygen for experimental osteomyelitis due to staphylococcus aureus in rabbits. J Infect Dis 1978; 138: 312-318.
30. Mader JT, Brown GL, Guckian JC et al. A mechanism for the amelioration of hyperbaric oxygen of experimental staphylococcal osteomyelitis in rabbits. J Infect Dis 1980; 142: 915-922.
31. Mader JT, Adams KR, Couch LA et al. Potentiation of tobramycin by hyperbaric oxygen in experimental Pseudomonas aeruginosa osteomyelitis. Presented at the 27th Interscience Conference on antimicrobial agents and chemotherapy 1987.
32. Mader JT. Mixed Anaerobic and Aerobic soft tissue infections. In : Davis JC, Hunt TK (Eds). Problem wounds: The role of oxygen. Elsevier Science Publishing. New York, 1988: 173-186.
33. Mader JT, Adams KR, Wallace WR et al. Hyperbaric oxygen as adjunctive therapy for osteomyelitis. Infect Dix Clin N Am 1990; 4 : 430-433.

34. Makley JT, Heiple KG, Chase SW et al. The effect of reduced barometric pressure on fracture healing in rats. J Bone Joint Surg 1967; 49A: 903.

35. Marx RE. Osteoradionecrosis. Part I: A new concept in its pathophysiology. J Oral Maxillofac Surg 1983; 4: 283-288.

36. Marx RE, Johnson RP, Kline SN. Prevention of radionecrosis. A randomized prospective clinical trial of hyperbaric oxygen versus penicillin. J Am Dent Assoc 1985; 111: 49-54.

37. Marx RE, Johnson RP. Problem wounds in oral and maxillofacial surgery : The role of hyperbaric oxygen. In ; Davis JC, Hunt TK (Eds). Problem wounds: The role of oxygen. Elsevier Science Publishing, New York, 1988: 65-123.

38. Marx RE, Ehlers WJ, Tayapongsak P, Pierce LW. Relationship of oxygen dose to angiogenesis induction in irradiated tissue. Am J Surg, 1990 ; 160: 519-524.

39. Marx RE. Chronic osteomyelitis of the jaws. Surg Clin N Am 1991 ; 3 : 367-381.

40. Marx RE. Radiation injury to tissue. In : Kindwall EP (ed.) Hyperbaric Medicine Practice, 1994, Best Publ Co Flagstaff AZ, 447-504.

41. Mathieu D, Coget JM, Wattel F et al. Filtrabilité érythrocytaire et oxygénothérapie hyperbare. Med Sub Hyp, 1984 ; 3 : 100-104.

42. Mathieu D, Wattel F, Bouachour G et al. Post-traumatic limb ischemia : Prediction of final outcome by transcutaneous oxygen measurements in hyperbaric oxygen. J Trauma, 1990 ; 30-307.

43. Merkesteyn JPR van, Bakker DJ, Waal I van der et al. Hyperbaric oxygen treatment of chronic osteomyelitis of the jaws. Int J Oral Surg 1984 ; 13 : 386-395.

44. Merkesteyn JPR van, Bras J, Vermeeren JIJF et al. Osteomyelitis of the jaws in pycnodysostosis. Int J Or Maxillofac Surg 1987 ; 16 : 615-619.

45. Merkesteyn JPR van, Groot RM, Bras J, Bakker DJ. Diffuse sclerosing osteomyelitis of the mandible : Clinical, radiographic and histopathologic findings in 27 patients. J Or Maxillofac Surg 1988 ; 46 : 825-829.

46. Merkesteyn JPR van, Bakker DJ, Dellemijn HL. The use of hyperbaric oxygen in the treatment of osteomyelitis and osteoradionecrosis of the jaw. In: Bakker DJ, Schmutz J (eds). Proc. 2nd Eur Conf Hyperb Med. Found Hyperb Med, Basel 1990; 70: 414-419.

47. Merkesteyn JPR van, Groot RH, Bras J, Bakker DJ et al. Diffuse sclerosing osteomyelitis of the mandible : A new concept of its etiology. Or Surg Or Med Or Path 1990 ; 70 : 414-419.

48. Merkesteyn JPR van, Bakker DJ. Treatment of radiation damage in the head and neck in 66 patients : Value of hyperbaric oxygen. In : Schmutz J, Wendling J (eds). Proc Joint Meeting on diving and hyperbaric medicine. Basel. Found for Hyp Med, 1992: 156-159.

49. Nemiroff PM, Merwin GE, Brant et al. Effects of hyperbaric oxygen and irradiation on experimental skin flaps in rats. Otolaryngol Head Neck Surg 1985 ; 93 : 485-491.

49a. Nemiroff PM. Hyperbaric oxygen in skin grafts and flaps. In: Kindwall EP (ed). Hyperbaric Medicine Practice. Best Publ Flagstaff, Ar. 1994 : 565-679.

50. Niinikoski J. Effect of oxygen supply on wound healing and formation of experimental granulation tissue. Acta Physiol Scand, 1969; 334 (suppl.): 1.

51. Niinikoski J. Viability of ischemic skin in hyperbaric oxygen. Acta Chir Scand, 1970; 135: 567.

52. Niinikoski J, Penttinen R, Kulonen E. Effect of hyperbaric oxygenation on fracture healing in the rat. Calc Tissue Res 1970 ; 4 (suppl): 115.

53. Niinikoski J, Hunt TK, Dunphy JE. Oxygen supply in healing tissue. Am J Surg 1972;123: 247.

54. Niinikoski J. Viability of ischemic skin flaps in hyperbaric oxygen. In : Trapp WG, Banister EW, Davison AJ, Trapp PA (eds). 5th Internat Hyperb Congr Proc, Simon Fraser University, Burnaby BC, Canada, 1974 : 244-252.

55. Niinikoski J. The effect of blood and oxygen supply on the biochemistry of repari. In : Hunt TK (Ed), Wound healing and wound infection : Theory and surgical practice, Appleton-Century-Crofts, New York, 1980 ; 56-71.

56. Niinikoski J, Gottrup F, Hunt TK. Role of oxygen in wound repair. In : Janssen H, Rooman R, Robertson JIS (eds), Wound healing, Wrightson Biomedical Publishing, 1991 : 165-174.

57. Nylander G, Lewis D, Nordstrom H et al. Reduction of postischemic edema with hyperbaric oxygen. Plast Reconstr Surg, 1985 ; 76 : 596.

58. Oriani G, Meazza D, Favales F et al. Hyperbaric oxygen therapy in diabetic gangrene. J Hyper Med 1990 ; 5(3) : 171-175.

59. Penttinen R, Rantanen J, Kulonen E. Effect of reduced air pressure on fracture healing. Isr J Med Sci 1971 ; 7 : 444.

60. Penttinen R, Niinikoski J, Kulonen E. Hyperbaric oxygenation and fracture healing. A biochemical study with rats. Acta Chir Scand 1972a ; 138 : 39.

61. Pentinnen R, Niinikoski J, Kulonen E. Effects of hyperbaric oxygenation and reduced barometric pressure on the nucleic acid contents of healing fractures. A biochemical study with rats. Acta Chir Scand 1972b ; 138 : 269.

62. Perrins DJD. Hyperbaric oxygenation of ischemic skin flaps and pedicles. In: Brown IW, Cox BG (eds.). Proc 3rd Intern Congr Hyperb Med. Duke University Press, Durham NC, 1966 : 613-620.

63. Perrins DJD. Influence of hyperbaric oxygen on the survival of split skin grafts. Lancet 1967 ; i : 868.

64. Perrins DJD. The influence of hyperbaric oxygen on the survival of split skin grafts. In : Wada J, Iwa T(eds). Proc 4th Internat Congr Hyperb Med. Bailliere, Tindall & Cassell, London 1970 : 369-376.

65. Riddick MF. Sternal wound infections, dehiscence and sternal osteomyelitis: The role of hyperbaric oxygen therapy. In : Kindwall EP (ed). Hyperbaric Medicine Practice. Best Publ Flagstaff, Ar 1994 : 429-446.

66.   Rijkmans BG, Bakker DJ, Dabhoiwala NF et al. Successful treatment of radiation cystitis with hyperbaric oxygen. Eur Urol 1989 ; 16 : 354-356.

67.   Roden D, Bosley TM, Fowble B et al. Delayed radiation injury to the retrobulbar nerves and chiasm. Clinical syndrome and treatment with hyperbaric oxygen. Ophtalm 1990 ; 97 : 346-351.

68.   Roveda SIL, Williamson JA, Goss AN et al. A multi-centre, non-randomized, internally controlled pilot trial : Hyperbaric oxygen therapy for post-irradiation xerostomia in patients with head and neck neoplasia. Undersea Hyperb Med 1993 ; 20 : 24.

69.   Rubin J, Yu VL, Malignant otitis : Insights into pathogenesis, clinical manifestations, diagnosis and therapy. Am J Med 1998 ; 85 : 391-398.

70.   Schoenrock GL, Cianci P. Treatment of radiation cystitis with hyperbaric oxygen. Urol 1986 ; 27 : 271-272.

71.   Seiler WO, Stahelin HB. Dekubitus. Neue Forschungsmethode in der Dekubituspathogenese. Hospitalis, 1984 ; 6 : 319.

72.   Slack WK, Thomas DA, Perrins DJD. Hyperbaric oxygenation in chronic osteomyelitis. Lancet 1965 ; i : 1093-1094.

73.   Strauss MB, Hart GB. Clinical experience with OHB in fracture healing. In: Smith G (ed). Proc 6th Internat Congr Hyperb Med. Aberdeen University Lancet 1979 : 329-332.

74.   Strauss MB. Role of hyperbaric oxygen therapy in acute ischemias and crush injuries. An orthopedic perspective. HBO Review, 1981 ; 2 : 87.

75.   Strauss MB, Hargens AR, Gershuni DH et al. Reduction of skeletal muscle necrosis using intermittent hyperbaric oxygen in a model compartment syndrome J Bone J Surg, 1983 ; 65A : 656.

76.   Strauss MB. Refractory osteomyelitis. Hyperb Med 1987 ; 2 : 147-159.

77.   Verklin RN jr, Mandell GL. Alteration of effectiveness of antibiotics by anaerobiosis. J Lab Clin Med, 1977 ; 89 : 65-71.

78.   Wasserteil V, Bruce S, Sessoms SL et al. Pyoderma gangrenosum treated with hyperbaric oxygen therapy. Int J Dermat 1992 ; 31 : 594.

79.   Weiss JP, Boland FP, Mori H et al. Treatment of radiation-induced cystitis with hyperbaric oxygen. J Urol 1985 ; 134 : 352-354.

80.   Weiss JP, Neville EC. Hyperbaric oxygen : Primary treatment of radiation-induced hemorrhagic cystitis. J Urol 1989 ; 142 : 43-45.

81.   Wyrick WJ, Mader JT, Butler E et al. Hyperbaric oxygen treatment of pyoderma gangrenosum. Arch Dermat 1978 ; 114 : 1232-1233.

NOTES

HYPERBARIC OXYGEN THERAPY: MATERIAL, EQUIPMENT AND SAFETY
—Introductory Report

Dr. Ulrich van Laak, Flottenarzt, Kronshagen, Germany

INTRODUCTION

During the last four decades after Boerema had introduced Hyperbaric Oxygen Therapy (HBO) as a clinical method in the treatment of clostricial myonecrosis, HBO has made a steady progress, however, at a measured pace.

Knowledge about material, equipment and safety regulations as well as training used to be more or less based upon experienced personnel of experimental diving units, air forces and navies in the different countries. When more and more major hospitals in Europe introduced their HBO program as a new supportive clinical method within their departments of anaesthesiology or surgery those standards became extremely important for operational safety guarantee.

In Europe, multiplace double-lock compressed air chambers became the majority whereas monoplace oxygen chambers became more accepted in the U.S.A.

If there was a relatively high standard in clinical HBO medicine the contrary applied for most of the non clinical, usually privately maintained institutions. For instance in Germany ambulant HBO therapy for various, usually chronic disorders became very "en vogue" during the last 5 years after there had been a deep depression following a fatal catastrophe in 1976 (1). Although this catastrophe was only possible because the patients did not get HBO therapy but had only a "therapeutical" pressure exposure all kinds of chambers, regardless whether they had been located in university hospitals or wheresoever, fell into disrepute. In my report I will focus on that historic black day for some minutes.

In Europe we still have to face a lack of well-accepted regulations for clinical and out-patient, ambulant, HBO therapy. Our aim today is to achieve common standards and to find generally accepted answers for the questions

1. What requirements must be met for hyperbaric chambers to allow HBO treatment of patients in stable chronic conditions?
2. What requirements must be met for hyperbaric chambers to allow HBO treatment of patients in critical state?
3. What safety requirements are needed in medical hyperbaric chambers?
4. What safety and user requirements are needed for medical device to allow its use in hyperbaric chambers?

My introductory report is more intended to raise problems rather than to give final answers to these questions. This will be the result of the workshop coming up this afternoon. However, I will proceed with a lessons-learned report on the chamber accident I have already introduced to you, discuss the situation for HBO patients in critical state versus stable chronic condition, and remind you of the basic technical requirements for hyperbaric chambers. Before I conclude with a short preliminary summary I would like to talk about the special requirements for medical devices in hyperbaric chambers.

LESSONS LEARNED—THE CHAMBER CATASTROPHE OF 1976

The disrepute of hyperbaric oxygen therapy in Germany derived from a situation of manslaughter by culpable negligence when 5 patients were killed and several others severely damaged during and after a so-called "chamber therapy" without any oxygen breathing.

The chamber facility in Hannover went into service in January 1976 as another settlement of a nonmedical practicioner. It consisted of two chambers for 10 patients each, without entrance locks and, with regard to their compressed air supply, connected in series between each other, on-line with the only compressor, powered electrically, without any air banks. There was hyperbaric oxygen available, but not used for therapy. The chamber interior was totally covered by textile material, the seats were designed as comfortable lounge chairs.

When the facility started to treat patients there was an elderly physician available, without any training in diving medicine, no other trained personnel, but three doctor's receptionists without any experience at a chamber. There was no official inspection and certification of the entire system either.

Generally the hyperbaric exposures reached 30 meters depth for 90 minutes, with compressed air breathing exclusively. Only some exposures took place before in this facility, without any problems. On February 9, 1976, 20 patients, 10 in each chamber, 12 male aged between 47 and 79 years, 8 female aged between 51 and 78 years, entered the facility. They suffered from chronic obstructive bronchitis, lung emphysema, peripheral arterial perfusion deficits, heart insufficiency, and chronic headache. The same chronic health problems had been the indications of the physician on scene for their chamber treatment.

The chamber runs took place with 20 occupants but no inside attendant. The philosophy was that the most experienced patient became a senior patient with some responsibilities for the other occupants. After an uneventful compression and isopression one patient blacked out at the 9 meter decompression stop. After some confusion outside and a attempt to get advice what to do by phone the decision was made by the physician to recompress the chamber to 50 meters. Due to the fact that they were connected in series all 20 occupants had to perform a repetitive dive. The unconscious patient got basic life support by a female patient, who was exhausted extremely by doing this. The outside physician went into panic. During the next 3 hours he performed several yoyo-shaped dive profiles before he decided to surface the chambers. He tried to disconnect the two chambers, however, this resulted in a compressed air leakage from a valve he could not close any longer.

Eighteen patients, who had no immediate problems after surfacing, had been sent home by various means of transportation, some of them by bike, without any further advice. Three patients died of decompression sickness, several others got symptoms. Because they were distributed to different hospitals in Hannover, did or could not report on the previous exposition, no correct diagnose was possible for the following 12 hours.

At the chamber the physician tried to recompress the unconscious patient but had to surface again due to ear equalization problems of one of the receptionists who was advised to serve as an inside attendant. The role of the remaining two receptionists was to operate the chamber.

The female patient who had been engaged in BLS inside the chamber suffered severe decompression sickness problems before she left the facility. She, together with the almost dead patient, the nonmedical practicioner, and the physician were finally recompressed to 50 meters. Due to the still existing permanent compressed air leakage the electrical compressor went hot which resulted in a blow of the main fuse at about 4.30 p.m. The chambers could not be ventilated any more, the inside pressure went down steadily until a electrician was successful in re-establishing the compressor function. However, when the compressor was finally at work both patients inside the chamber were already dead. The victim who had the initial problems died of cerebral arterial air embolism due to the exposition; the female patient, who assisted him during the ongoing exposition, suffered fatal neurological decompression sickness.

During the trial expert witnesses showed several serious mistakes in the concept of the chambers:

- Patients with contraindications against hyperbaric exposure had been exposed because of those health problems for medically unaccepted "therapeutical" reasons.
- No thorough medical check for those exposed inside the chambers took place before.
- The chamber personnel was absolutely not qualified for their job.
- No official authority checked the chambers and gave the permission for safe operation.
- Personnel at the chambers was unexperienced. They did not know anything about chamber operating and the technical background of HBO therapy.
- There was no entrance lock available, transferring of occupants was impossible.
- The chambers could not be operated separately.
- No back-up compressed air bank was available. The entire technical concept was weak and without any back-ups.
- Lack of experience of the operating personnel resulted in panic, confused decisions and uncoordinated actions.

What lessons can be learned out of this catastrophe which happens to influence HBO therapy among the medical community persistently?

First of all, training of personnel dedicated for HBO therapy has to be vigorous. Safe operating of a hyperbaric chamber and its peripheral equipment requires a thorough understanding of operational procedures and engineering design as well. The various aspects of chamber safety include operating and emergency operating procedures, gas handling, pressure integrity, electrical safety, fire prevention, and control. Furthermore, physicians in charge and those who perform treatment in front or inside chambers have to be familiar not only with the entire chamber system, but also with accepted indications for HBO. Even patients in chronic stable conditions may require emergency medical assistance due to acute medical problems during HBO therapy or because of HBO therapy. Patients in a critical state require at least the same assistance as if they were on the intensive care ward (2).

OPERATIONAL SAFETY

Clearly defined supervision is essential to safe chamber operation.

This applies to HBO treatment universally whether the method is used for stable patients or patients in critical state. Hyperbaric facilities should be staffed with full-time experienced personnel, in hospitals ideally included in the anaethesiologic or intensive care department. Staff members must fully understand all aspects of the medical background and chamber operation.

Continuous patient care inside the chamber may require additional specialized staff as attendants. Emergency medicine physicians, surgeons, anaesthesiologists, nurse intensivists may be required in order to keep on with the intensive care but under pressure. Those who may be required on a case-by-case basis need extensive on-the-job training.

Emergency procedures must be internalized. All occupants, inside tenders as well as patients, must be briefed properly.

Continual failure identification, failure analysis, and emergency plans are essential to prevent panic reaction due to malfunction of systems. Safety systems are necessary which represent at least single back-up functions (3).

Operational Safety Requirements for Therapeutic Hyperbaric Chambers:

- clearly defined supervision
- experienced full-time personnel
- specialized inside attendants
- failure identification and analysis
- internalized emergency procedures
- back-up functions

HBO TREATMENT OF PATIENTS IN CRITICAL STATE

Patients in critical state who need acute hyperbaric therapy will usually suffer from health impairments which may more or less represent a threat for the vital functions.

Besides very special requirements on HBO therapy all principles of intensive care have to be followed. Crew proficiency is the crucial point for an uneventful treatment of a patient in critical state.

Adequate care of a critical patient under hyperbaric conditions needs to follow some peculiarities.

Limited space within the chamber may result in reduced freedom of movement so that therapeutic intervention and patient management is likely to be conducted from unfavourable positions.

When the chamber is under pressure, drugs and material may be available after some delay only because they need to be transferred through locks. Meticulous planning, adequate diagnostic and therapeutic equipment as well as an extended emergency kit not only stocked for cardiopulmonary resuscitation but for intensive care purposes also is mandatory to allow as much self sufficiency as possible inside the chamber.

Manual and mental performance may be impaired by heat or cold climate following pressure changes, high noise level and, especially in deep treatments, by inert gas narcosis (4).

HBO Treatment of Patients in Critical State—Peculiarities:

- vital functions impaired
- limited space, unfavourable conditions for management
- meticulous planning and extended emergency kit necessary
- manual and mental performance may be impaired

HBO TREATMENT OF PATIENTS IN A STABLE CHRONIC CONDITION

HBO therapy is known to have a supportive value for several usually chronic conditions. This is going to be a topic of workshop n°3.

Patients who apply for treatment may be of high age, have different underlying health disorders and accompanying symptoms. Elderly patients are likely to show concomitant pulmonary, cardiac, or endocrinal disorders. They need at least intensive visual monitoring ideally by an inside attendance, who can also react for oxygen induced problems, claustrophobia, or sudden general indisposition (3).

Breathing of hyperbaric oxygen following an accepted schedule with appropriate air breaks at a relatively low oxygen partial pressure compared to diving accident treatments does normally not cause any problems from oxygen toxicity, taken for granted that the monitoring personnel is trained to react early and sufficient for any warning signs. However, it will be impossible to reduce the risk of oxygen induced problems to zero, especially in elderly patients in chronic medical condition. For instance the so-called problem wound protocol which used to be introduced by the U.S. Air Force and became our standard protocol for non-emergency HBO therapy since more than 10 years, especially for long lasting HBO series, is known to have an oxygen induced problem rate of about 1 to 20.000 exposures.

In summary, although extremely seldom, oxygen problems such as cerebral convulsions may and will occur without too many preliminary symptoms. I cannot quote statistical data on this but I personally know from different sources about convulsions during ambulant HBO therapy in chambers without professional inside attendance, two of them with a fatal outcome. I'm not saying that the fatalities had been caused by unattended exposure, but I think the situation was possibly worse and legal questions may arise easily.

HBO treatment of patients in stable chronic conditions requires a minimum of monitoring depending on the individual status of the patient. It is strongly recommended not to leave the patients unattended. If the patient is at risk due to age or several accompanying health problems, monitoring requirements may also reach a maximum, likewise the treatment of patients in critical state.

HBO Treatment of Patients in a Stable Chronic Condition—Problems:

- elderly patients, multiple health problems
- concomitant pulmonary, cardiac, endocrinal disorders
- inside chamber attendance required
- oxygen-induced problems rare, but possible
- minimal up to maximal monitoring requirements

BASIC TECHNICAL REQUIREMENTS FOR HYPERBARIC FACILITIES

Hyperbaric chambers

Monoplace chambers for HBO therapy allow the entire body of the patient to be exposed to a specific gas environment with therapeutic gas breathing under increased atmospheric pressure. It is rated for single occupancy. Modern chambers are acrylic made and may be restricted to relatively low overpressurization for safe HBO purposes. If the patients situation allows to leave him unattended, most disorders which may require hyperbaric oxygen can be treated. Because a monoplace chamber has a pure oxygen environment, electrical equipment which is going to be introduced for use inside has to be intrinsically safe. Current versions offer a microprocessor control system, excellent communication, and the possibility to monitor EEG, ECG, blood pressure, breathing parameters, body temperature, transcutaneous blood gases via electrical pass-throughs. Monoplace chambers can be equipped with various respirators, drainage equipment from suction type, intravenous medications may be continued using a roller pump system.

Monoplace chambers have some advantages. They do not require as much space and peripheral installations as multiplace chambers. If the facility has only small staff available a monoplace may represent a real advantage.

It needs only a short period of time to train personnel to operate monoplace chambers. However, due to the 100 percent oxygen atmosphere, safety precautions against fire hazards are much more a problem compared to multiplace chambers. The fire safety can only be assured by the meticulous exclusion of any kind of ignition source, volatile material, oil, and grease. Textiles used have to be free of static charging. All materials have to be nonsparking and, if possible, noncombustible. Monoplace chambers need an emergency vent to allow quick depressurization within 20 to 30 seconds in order to reach the patient for emergency measures.

Dependent on national laws, monoplace chambers must meet the standards of medical technical regulations as well as construction standards set up by various classification agencies (5).

Hyperbaric Chambers—Monoplace Chambers:

- entire body exposed in oxygen atmosphere
- single occupancy
- electrical equipment used must be intrinsically safe
- complete monitoring and mechanical respiration possible
- need less peripheral installations
- need less personnel
- have to meet standards of medical technical regulations
- have to meet construction standards

The situation for multiplace chambers is comparable from the technical safety point of view.

International and national classification agencies used to look after the protection of outside personnel rather than inside chamber occupants. At the beginning a chamber used to be nothing more than a pressure hull for them, very much like a gas carrier or something like this.

Currently their safety codes do also reflect on the safety of the occupants. However, the interface between construction codes and medical regulations are not always clearly defined. For instance in Germany civilian hyperbaric facilities have to pass the substantial body of standards for the construction of diving systems and their components, the technical part of the authorization process. Because hyperbaric chambers represent a piece of treatment equipment which is energetically operated they belong to the highest class in the federal regulations for medical equipment. To obtain permission operating a chamber for hyperbaric treatment is based on condition to check on technical safety, to perform regular function tests, to designate a person responsible for safety and training (6).

Hyperbaric Chambers—Multiplace Chambers:

- have to meet standards of medical technical regulations
- have to meet construction standards
- belong to the highest class of medical equipment regulations

However, in case of hyperbaric chambers there are still important fields left open without regulation, for instance

- requirements of medical monitoring
- requirements for patient treatment inside hyperbaric chambers
- training and qualification of medical and paramedical personnel
- training and qualification of chamber operators

Gas storage and delivery equipment

Hyperbaric chambers may be compressed either directly from large low pressure, high volume compressors usually with small air banks, or, more likely, from high pressure compressors with high pressure storage tanks; both kinds of compressors may be oil-lubricated, not oil-lubricated, or non-lubricated.

In any case a pressurization system has to provide clean breathing air in sufficient quality and quantity. The definition of sufficient quantity may create a problem, as a general guideline compressed air back-up for at least one complete extended U.S. Navy Table 6A is accepted to be sufficient.

Air purity standards have to be met at any given time. The standards established by various agencies are in general agreement with each other. Since it is no problem to monitor oxygen and carbon dioxide in hyperbaric air constantly, this should be the standard.

Periodically checks on contaminants, mainly oil and carbon monoxide, are recommended every 4 or 8 weeks.

The breathing gases oxygen and oxygen mixtures as the therapeutic gases in HBO therapy are ideally administered using a built-in-breathing (BIBS) with overboard dump system for exhaled gas.

It is obligatory for therapeutic chambers to monitor BIBS gases continuously.

Hyperbaric Chambers—Gas Storage and Delivery Equipment:

- clean breathing air
- sufficient back-up for at least 1 complete extended USN 6A
- constantly monitoring of O_2 and CO_2
- periodically checks on contaminants

Safety devices

One of the most frightening emergency situation in hyperbaric chambers is fire.

Fire will be multifactorially caused by an elevation of oxygen concentration, flammable materials, insufficient extinguishing capacity and, especially significant, an ignition source. Almost all fires in hyperbaric chambers reported in the literature could have been avoidable by proper fire prevention. Precise elimination of possible ignition sources plays a major role in fire prevention.

A water deluge fire extinguishing system should be installed inside and outside each chamber compartment. A hand-held water or nitrogen hose which is always pressurized should be available in each compartment.

Chamber lights must operate even in case of fire fighting. Occupants should immediately breathe air through masks of the built-in-breathing system.

Plans for escaping have to be prepared including management thereafter, when decompression problems may arise because of the rush escape.

An accidental decompression due to excessive leakage may have fatal results for the chamber occupants. The pressure boundary of a chamber complex must be carefully examined and tested for gas tight integrity. Therapeutic chambers must have sufficient gas back-up to compensate for substantial air leakage. For emergency procedures the inside tender should be able to decompress the chamber to the surface, however, the chamber operator must be able to override this function from topside (3).

Hyperbaric Chambers—Safety Devices:

- fire hazard: Elevation of oxygen concentration, flammable materials, insufficient extinguishing capacity, ignition source
- elimination of ignition sources
- water deluge fire extinguishing system
- plans for escaping
- gas back-up to compensate for leakages

Monitoring devices

The chamber atmosphere concentration of oxygen and carbon dioxide should be continuously monitored. The same applies for breathing gases if it is not pure medical oxygen from oxygen banks. For instance production of a given oxygen/nitrogen mixture on-line needs a constant monitoring of the breathing gas. Continuous oxygen and carbon dioxide monitoring is also required when head tents are used in a closed or semi-closed circuit.

Visual and voice communication with inside tenders has to be maintained and recorded by cameras, monitors and videos, loudspeaker, emergency phone, and, as a back-up, emergency buttons.

Adiabatic temperature changes inside the chamber may be a problem for unstable intensive care patients. Continuous temperature monitoring is necessary in order to counter-regulate and maintain adequate inside ambient temperature quality.

Hyperbaric Chambers—Monitoring Devices:

- breathing gases and ambient atmosphere
- visual and voice communication
- temperature regulation

Ergonomics for medical used chambers

The European standard multiplace hyperbaric chamber is a double-lock, compressed air chamber with 4 to 10 occupants. Older chambers and those which are used primarily for diving support have usually 80 centimeter diameter entrance locks. Current chambers which are dedicated to HBO therapy and limited to HBO related maximum pressures have standard door-shaped entrance locks. Even disabled occupants may enter those facilities without major obstacles. For intensive care a standing cylinder with some 3 meter diameter can take a central operating theater table and offers sufficient space for medical equipment at the wall or ceiling.

Modern chamber design holds the interior free from unnecessary technical equipment. This results in additional space impression and enlarges the limited room for patients and tenders.

MEDICAL DEVICES IN HYPERBARIC CHAMBERS

Safety

For safety reasons electrically powered equipment beside low voltage cannot be allowed inside hyperbaric chambers. Equipment has to be adapted on hyperbaric conditions. In most cases this can be easily accomplished. For instance adaptation of respirators to the hyperbaric environment is mainly based upon the interest of the manufacturing company. It was only recently that we had been successful in adapting a brain mapping system to hyperbaric conditions. The crucial point is the separation of high voltage electricity and functional parts. Occasionally electrical components like blood gas analizers used inside chambers must be provided with a continuous nitrogen purge to avoid the fire risk in the event of arcing.

In modern therapeutic chambers nearly all medical equipment can be adapted. Modern medical devices may ask for special expert solutions, however, they are normally possible.

Safety of Medical Devices in Hyperbaric Chambers:

- no electrically powered equipment
- adaptation on hyperbaric environment
- most medical equipment can be adapted

Monitoring devices

An electrocardiogram monitor with connecting wires entering the chamber through penetrating contacts should be placed outside. The same electrodes may give on-line information about heart rate and respiration. Information about intravascular pressure and non-invasive arterial pressure may also be achieved using chamber ports. Respiratory signals may be obtained by the monitor but especially by the ventilator display which has to be located outside the chamber also. If the distance is moderate a standard EEG can be conducted off the chamber without signal loss (6).

Tissue oxygen measurements provide direct, continuous, and quantitative assessment of oxygen availibility to tissue. Transcutaneous polarographic oxygen electrodes provide a safe estimation of oxygen effectiveness especially in non-healing soft tissue wounds. The method is widely used without any problems. Intra-tissular oxygen measurement or different other methods under investigation are invasive or still too complex to calibrate or to handle for routine use (7).

Medical Monitoring Devices in Hyperbaric Chambers:

- ECG, HR, respiration
- intravascular and non invasive arterial pressure
- EEG
- tissue oxygen measurements

Therapeutic devices

The diagnostic and therapeutic material available to the intensive care ward is normally applicable to modern hyperbaric chambers, because they have sufficient penetration plates through the chamber hull for supply of gases or connector cables. Defibrillation however is not recommended inside a chamber. Transducers may be mounted inside the chamber without any problems, monitors and displays have to be mounted outside, but visible for the inside tenders.

For pressure monitoring devices (arterial, central venous, pulmonary artery, intracranial) and infusion systems the number of connections have to be minimized. Any gas entering the systems is likely to produce significant problems.

Plastic bags are preferred for infusion because they seldom require venting, but glass bottles do. During pressure changes extreme attention must be paid to infusions because of the risk of air entering the system. Pressure bags require thorough attention. Battery-powered perfusion pumps work properly under pressure, however, plastic covered keyboards sometimes need small pressure equalization holes because of malfunctioning under elevated pressure.

Suction is available easily by using the pressure difference between inside and outside through a pressure reducing regulator connected with a bottle trap. A venturi system powered by compressed air can also be used.

The cuffs on endotracheal or tracheostomy tubes must be blocked by fluids because of the gas volume changes during pressure alterations. Another possibility is using a cuff manometer, but this has to be monitored during pressure changing phases.

For ventilation inside, a chamber adapted self-inflating resuscitation bag is necessary as a back-up in case of mechanical ventilation failure.

Several ventilators have been tested for hyperbaric use, however, there is a tendency towards less complex and more reliable methods. Some facilities did their own adaptation together with the manufacturer. The ideal ventilator for hyperbaric use should be nonelectrical powered (or electrically/mechanically separated), volume cycled and unaffected be pressure changes. In Germany the Siemens 900 B or C ventilator is highly accepted for hyperbaric use. Evaluation of minute ventilation is accomplished by an expiratory volume spirometer corrected for high gas densities (3,4,6).

Therapeutic Devices in Hyperbaric Chambers:

- normally no adaptation problems
- monitors and displays outside
- tight pressure monitoring devices and infusion systems
- plastic bags better than glass infusion bottles
- cuffs on endotracheal tubes blocked by water
- self-inflating resuscitation bag
- (non)electrically powered, volume cycled respirator

CONCLUSION

I would like to read the four initial questions again and conclude my report with comments on them.

1. What requirements must be met for hyperbaric chambers to allow HBO treatment of patients in stable chronic conditions?

Patients in stable chronic condition may be treated in chamber systems which meet the basic standards of modern HBO systems. Personnel should have an intensive training and certification of an accepted national or international organization. Occupants should be monitored and chamber runs should be recorded. Never may occupants remain unattended inside multiplace hyperbaric chambers.

2. What requirements must be met for hyperbaric chambers to allow HBO treatment of patients in critical state?

Patients in critical state who have an absolute or relative indication for HBO therapy do literally need a pressurized intensive care unit rather than an upgraded pressure chamber. Since most medical material is equally applicable to HBO chambers, systems used inside the chamber should be compatible with those utilized in critical care units. Personnel must have expert medical and technical knowledge to ensure optimal safety. On-the-job training on a day-by-day basis is essential.

3. What safety requirements are needed in medical hyperbaric chambers?

Hyperbaric chambers are effective medical tools but may also be dangerous for the occupants. Safe operating procedures, fire prevention and control, electrical safety, integrity of pressure, purity of breathing gases, safe gas handling, and a high level of experience are indispensable prerequisites.

4. What safety and user requirements are needed for medical device to allow its use in hyperbaric chambers?

Any system used inside hyperbaric chambers has to be tested for malfunctions and certified for safe use by an appropriate national or international agency. The requirements my be high, but most systems normally used in operation theaters or intensive care units currently meet those standards. Beside technical safety, users must meticulously follow hand books and specific instructions set up for hyperbaric use of medical equipment. In hyperbaric medicine high professionality is required for optimal safety. Most of the problems will not be the result of technical failures but will be induced by the human factor.

REFERENCES

1. Drägerwerk, Lübeck, personal communication.
2. van Laak,U., Gesellschaft für Tauch- und Überdruckmedizin e.V.(GTÜM), Mitteilungsblatt CAISSON 7 Nr.4, 148 - 155, 1992.
3. Hamilton, R.W., P.J. Sheffield, Hyperbaric Chamber Safety. In: Davis, J.C., T.K. Hunt, Hyperbaric Oxygen Therapy, 47 - 60, 1988, UHMS, Bethesda, MD, USA.
4. Muth, C.M., Gesellschaft für Tauch- und Überdruckmedizin e.V.(GTÜM), Mitteilungsblatt CAISSON 7 Nr.4, 156 - 168, 1992.
5. Hart, G.B., E.P. Kindwall, Hyperbaric Chamber Clinical Support: Monoplace. In: Davis, J.C., T.K. Hunt, Hyperbaric Oxygen Therapy, 41 - 46, 1988, UHMS, Bethesda, MD, USA.
6. Sheffield, P.J., J.C. Davis, G.C. Bell, T.J. Gallegher, Hyperbaric Chamber Clinical Support: Multiplace. In: Davis, J.C., T.K. Hunt, Hyperbaric Oxygen Therapy, 25 - 39, 1988, UHMS, Bethesda, MD, USA.
7. Sheffield, P.J., Tissue Oxygen Measurements. In: Davis, J.C., T.K. Hunt, Problem Wounds - The Role of Oxygen, 17 - 53, Elsevier, New York, 1988.

MATERIAL AND SAFETY
—Final Report

P. Pelaia, University of Trieste, Italy

WHICH DESIGN AND SAFETY REQUIREMENTS FOR MEDICAL HYPERBARIC CHAMBERS?

Hyperbaric chambers are pressure vessels in which it is possible to breathe gas mixtures at pressures higher than the ambient atmospheric pressure.

Hyperbaric chambers are first of all pressure containers. As such, they have to be manufactured according to specific rules.

For medical use it is necessary to have comfortable and spacious vessels. The vessel should be well air conditioned, soundproof, with easy access and very efficient to operate. Such hyperbaric chambers are very expensive when one considers the global costs: manufacture, installation, specific room architecture, and overall running costs.

It is mandatory to define the best possible compromise in dimension, shape, running pressure in order to achieve the best and cheapest service as well as the best possible compromise in gas production and storage.

The volume of the hyperbaric chamber and the quantity of gas needed (production and storage) have to be defined according to the frequency of use and annual number of sessions.

In overall planning, it is also important to differentiate the so-called "chronic" patients from the "acute" ones. "Chronic" patients are part of a long term procedure and require only little monitoring. "Acute" patients require comprehensive support allowing resuscitation to be carried out without interruption before, during, and after hyperbaric treatment.

Thanks to better computer software, it is now possible to design hyperbaric chambers with large doors (oval and/or rectangular shape). This type of door allows better access for medical personnel. If it is large enough, it is even possible to enter a wheel-chair or a hospital bed directly into the chamber.

Above 2 ATA, physical effects of pressure are such that the only reasonable way to build a chamber is to make a cylinder with more or less rounded ends. Experience has shown that for "chronic" patients it is better to build chambers with horizontal axes. For emergency hyperbaric chambers, it is more convenient to have a cylinder with vertical axes. The diameter of the cylinder should be at least 3 meters.

In a horizontal cylinder with a diameter of 2 meters, it is possible to install a floor in such a way that there is a remaining height of 1.8 meter. This should be considered as the minimal acceptable height to allow easy circulation in the chamber. The introduction of a hospital bed into a hyperbaric chamber requires a 1 meter wide and 1,6 meter high door.

Intensive care specialists would like to use the hyperbaric chamber as an annex of the intensive care unit. The ideal situation would be to have a hyperbaric chamber for "acute" indications and one for "chronic" ones. For economical and space reasons, it is sufficient to have one common decompression lock to both chambers. The general layout of the chambers and of the lock depends on the space available.

Everything has to be done to give maximum comfort to the patients and maximum ease of work to the medical staff.

The partial pressure of CO_2 and O_2 in the chamber atmosphere must be constantly controlled in order to give maximum security to the occupants of the hyperbaric chamber.

Analysis of CO_2 remains a luxury in hospital based hyperbaric chambers. Analysis of O_2 however should be obligatory for a hyperbaric chamber in which pure oxygen is administered to 10 patients simultaneously.

Fire is the main hazard in a hyperbaric chamber. It is essential that any risk be avoided.

- The hyperbaric chamber must be built with fireproof materials. Paint and seats must be flame resistant;
- all types of combustible oil or grease must be avoided;
- oxygen must be expelled continuously from the chamber so that the concentration of oxygen does not increase in the chamber atmosphere.

If two chambers are connected by a common lock, it seems that 4 ATA for the "chronic" hyperbaric chamber and 6 ATA for the "emergency" and the lock are generally admitted.

For obvious security reasons, it will be necessary to have a reserve of air in case of unavailability of the compressors. This reserve must be large enough to make an emergency compression and to conduct an entire session.

Air can be compressed either with high (200 bars) or low (10 bars) compressors. The choice of the compressors depends on the quantity of air needed and on the available space for the air tanks.

Interventions at pressures different from the ambient pressure are potentially dangerous. The main task of prevention is to diminish the probability of accidents. This implies that the risk analysis has also to allow for modalities of assistance in cases where human or technical failure or even simple statistical rules could provoke an accident.

It is necessary to find individual solutions for each hyperbaric chamber because there are no universal security measures.

Risks of hyperbaric environments are very varied. They exist for the patients, for the personnel, or for both and are graded and treated accordingly. They come either from pressurization itself, from pressurization equipment or from the medical equipment used under pressure.

The comfort of the patient and of the personnel must also be taken in consideration.

The risk of human failure will never be entirely be eliminated. It is present in the medical action of the personnel, in the use of the medical equipment inside the hyperbaric chamber, or in the use of the hyperbaric chamber itself.

The only efficient prevention measures for human failures are:

- ergonomically designed medical equipment;
- teaching policies for the personnel involved inside and outside the hyperbaric chamber;
- use of systematic and written procedures.

Training must not only be obligatory for hyperbaric physicians but also for all those who have a responsibility in the organization and management of hyperbaric treatments.

WHICH SECURITY RULES SHOULD BE ADOPTED FOR MEDICAL EQUIPMENT IN A HYPERBARIC ENVIRONMENT? WHAT ARE THE MINIMAL REQUISITES FOR THE CONCEPTION OF HYPERBARIC CHAMBERS IN THE TREATMENT OF INTENSIVE CARE PATIENTS?

The emergency situations in which hyperbaric oxygen (HBO) have proved to be effective are numerous as are the potential applications in reanimation.

Loss of consciousness, respiratory failure, circulatory instability must not be an obstacle to the use of HBO. The patient must not suffer an interruption or a diminution in the quality of intensive care because he has to be pressurized. But on the other hand, he must not be refused the benefits of HBO with the argument that his situation requires continuous intensive care.

The normal access to an IV line, patient monitoring, HBO monitoring, hemodynamic support, patient ventilation, must be possible at all times during resuscitation in the hyperbaric environment.

This could only be achieved through the transfer of sophisticated equipment into the hyperbaric chamber. Unfortunately, equipment could implode during pressurization and explode during decompression. Further dangers for the equipment are flooding through condensed water, burning because of the use of materials and lubricants which are not adapted to an atmosphere of enriched oxygen. Fire could also be provoked by materials behaving as electrostatic accumulators or containing components susceptible to overheat.

These problems can be solved either by:

- the use of medical equipment specially designed for hyperbaric chambers;
- the adaptation of the standard equipment used in resuscitation to the hyperbaric environment;
- the transfer of all equipment outside the hyperbaric chamber, leaving only connections for electrodes or captors inside. The connection to the outside equipment is made with special plugs going through the walls of the hyperbaric chamber.

Assisted ventilation requires an adaptation to hyperbaric environments. The ideal respirator should be:

- very small using minimal space;
- easy to handle;
- supplied with a source of compressed air;
- without any electrical parts;
- without internal inflammable lubricants;
- without airtight compartment;
- able to be installed in the chamber only with minor modifications;
- have an output for expired gases connectable to the overboard-dumping system of the hyperbaric chamber;

- with a ventilation range of 0–20 l/min;
- with a frequency range of 1–40 cycles/min;
- with a volume of insuflation remaining stable during the changes in ambient pressure;
- with the possibility to change the FiO_2 (21–100%);
- with the possibility to realize a positive tele-expiratory pressure;
- the possibility to ventilate in CPPV as well as in IMV and/or SIMV and/or assisted/controlled mode.

Many respirators have been investigated under hyperbaric conditions. Some of those respirators fit many requisites of the ideal respirator except one: it is not possible to keep the respirator's parameters constant during the variations of pressure in the hyperbaric chamber.

The hyperbaric respirator should be built according to two technical principles:

- It should be a volumetric respirator (volume-cycled) fulfilling all the security standards required for hyperbaric environments. An electrical motor supplied with low-voltage should be realized. This motor should be very powerful.
- It should be a respirator following pneumatic principles, which allows it to function under hyperbaric conditions. The concept of the pneumatic system must allow the maintenance of the frequency delivered, the volume insuflat ed, and all the other parameters of ventilation up to a pressure of 6 ATA.

With these principles some hyperbaric ventilators have been developed. These ventilators work well under hyperbaric conditions, but they cannot yet provide the same quality of treatment as respirators working in the reanimation room, so that the ideal respirator has not yet been realized.

If the control systems for respirators are under development, respiratory monitoring is still experimental. Arterial gasometry is not routinely done because the measures are accurate only if they are made inside the hyperbaric chamber. The measuring instruments should be adapted to the hyperbaric environment and fulfill security standards. A scientific communication recently presented at the UHMS meeting in Denver-Colorado described a very small and simple device able to measure arterial gasometry in the hyperbaric chamber.

The measurement of transcutaneous oxygen during HBO objectivates the peripheral delivery of oxygen. It is a predictive test for the evolution of acute post-traumatic leg injury. It can help define the indications for hyperbaric oxygen and estimate precisely the therapeutic answer.

Transcutaneous oxygen measurement under HBO gives no information on central oxygenation but informs on the peripheral delivery of oxygen to hypoxic tissues.

Transcutaneous oxygen measurement under hyperbaric conditions can be made with the help of a miniaturized Clark electrode and a special calibration system.

Transcutaneous oxygen measurement can be modified by several factors like hemodynamic variations of the vascular system (micro- and macrocirculation), inadequate skin cleaning of the electrode site, horneous skin layers, tissue edema.

The use of a defibrillator in the hyperbaric chamber is connected with a risk of fire because of the voltaic arc on the electrodes.

To reduce the risks of fire, the defibrillator must be located outside of the hyperbaric chamber. It is connected to the electrodes through the wall of the chamber with a transmission cable. The electrical discharge is initiated outside the chamber and electricity is conducted to the electrodes through the transmission cables.

WHAT ARE THE MINIMAL REQUIREMENTS OF A HYPERBARIC CHAMBER IN THE TREATMENT OF CHRONIC PATIENTS?

Chronic patients are often elderly persons with many alterations of organs and extremities. For such patients, it is important to foresee possible complications of the hyperbaric treatment. Minimal monitoring, depending of the situation of each patient is necessary. The most essential monitoring is the non-invasive assessment of hemodynamic parameters.

Monitoring of transcutaneous oxygen and Doppler laser represent actually the best available assessment tools for the evaluation of the effects of hyperbaric therapy.

IS THERE ROOM FOR THE USE OF OXYGEN-PRESSURIZED HYPERBARIC CHAMBER?

It seems that hospital-based monoplace oxygen-pressurized hyperbaric chamber must be restricted to the treatment of "chronic" patients unless the patients need direct medical help.

Security constraints are very important and very high with the use of such oxygen-pressurized chambers.

WHICH SAFETY GUIDELINES COULD BE APPLIED WITHIN THE EUROPEAN COMMUNITY?

Hyperbaric chambers correspond to the definition of medical equipment. As such, they are regulated by the regulation 93/42/EC, dated 14 June 1993 for medical equipment's (J.O.C.E, 12 July 1993).

According to this regulation, equipment is certified as medical equipment if it is used for the purpose of diagnosis prevention or treatment of a disease, injury or handicap alone, or in combination with other equipment.

The fundamental principle of this regulation is that medical equipment can only be marketed if it does not jeopardize the security or the health of the patients or of any other person (medical staff).

Hyperbaric chambers are not quoted in the European regulations as such so that it is not easy to classify them in any of the existing categories.

They could be classified either under category IIa as non invasive equipment or under category IIb as active medical equipment.

In fact, European Health Authorities could also decide to create a distinct class for hyperbaric chambers and require a special certification label. Such a certification label should take the different use of hyperbaric chambers in account.

The standards should describe:

- the number and minimal volume of the chambers and of the locks;
- the size of the accesses;
- the number, the volume and the disposition of the material locks;
- the type of gas supply: volume of the reserve, pressure in the gas pipes and diameter of the gas pipes;
- the type of inhaled gas equipment and of overboard dumping systems;
- the parameters to use for the control of the chamber atmosphere, the control equipment necessary to regulate them as well as the minimal conditions of comfort for patients and staff;
- the anti-explosion and anti-fire equipment;
- the electrical connection to the equipment like maximal allowed voltage, connection type for standard and low voltage, connection type for transmission of biological signals.

A consensus exists for the classification of hyperbaric chambers into category IIb. Hyperbaric chambers located on tunnels and other building sites could be classified under category IIa regardless of the pressure used. This type of hyperbaric chamber should fulfill only the EC conformity regulations.

Medical equipment for use inside the hyperbaric chambers is submitted to the same regulations. It must consequently fulfill all the essential requisites for use in hyperbaric environments.

PERSONAL, PROFESSIONAL AND EDUCATIONAL REQUIREMENTS FOR THE STAFF OF A HYPERBARIC CENTRE
—Introductory Report

J. Desola, MD, Medicina Hiperbarica - Hospital Cruz Roya

INTRODUCTION

A hyperbaric centre must guarantee the best use of its equipment and services.

Depending on the kind of facility and of the final aim of its services, the hyperbaric centre can function on a continuous (24 hours a day) basis or intermittently, during periods of time scheduled in advance.

Depending on its technical availabilities, the location and the available medical services, the hyperbaric centre can be a hospital facility or an open self standing centre.

A hospital hyperbaric centre must guarantee its assistance 24 hours a day and must be able to offer adequate treatment for all kinds of diseases, including those requiring critical care inside the chamber.

A self-standing hyperbaric centre might have a certain work schedule and must limit its services to those patients not in emergency situation. It must be in functional relation or contact with a general hospital.

In cases that a transportable hyperbaric chamber is used, the schedules, profiles, staff, and regulations will be the same as a self-standing centre.

Staff requirements affecting these types of facilities should agree with the aforementioned conditions of availability and system of work.

This work aims to review the kind of staff needed by the hyperbaric centre, to define their behaviour and giving some general rules to be applied in each situation, depending on the conditions of each centre.

In order to develop its functions correctly, a hyperbaric centre needs different professional qualifications. These could be summarized as follows: doctors, the medical director, nurses, attendants, chamber operators, technicians, others.

Characteristics, functions, and background which should be followed by the whole staff will be reviewed. In each category the following items will be detailed: definition of functions, background, specific educational profile, academic requirements and degrees, continuous education, dedication.

DOCTORS - THE MEDICAL DIRECTOR

Functions

The medical director is responsible for all functions developed in the hyperbaric centre. This includes the following aspects:

1. Supervision of the correct operation of the hyperbaric facilities.
2. Medical care to the patients inside the chamber, if a multiplace facility is used

and whenever it might be necessary, due to reasons of critical care depending on the severity of the case, or special controls during therapeutical procedures.
3. Quality assurance.
4. Follow-up of patients.
5. Definition of protocol procedures for treatment.
6. Organization and participation in multi-centric over-all protocols and treatments.

The functions of the main medical director are complemented by a variable number of collaborators of the same or similar background and education, in which the medical director can delegate some responsibilities, but always under his control.

One or two people will not be enough to guarantee a 24 hours a day service, as the long stays inside the chamber (when a multiplace facility is used) that they must often endure renders them incapable of further decompressions in the following hours. A whole hyperbaric medical staff working in shifts would therefore be necessary.

Background

The medical director is a medical doctor with a wide multi-disciplinary education. Internal medicine, critical care and/or intensive medicine, reanimation, and anaesthesiology can provide the best background.

Other specializations might also be adequate if the candidate has documented experience and he has received the necessary education and training in hyperbaric medicine.

Sport or commercial diving can give to the medical director a great deal of additional knowledge. This also provides awareness of the whole problem concerning this specialization and it can add some complementary knowledge on diving and hyperbaric technology and practice. However this actual diving experience will not be required for the recognition of the medical director.

Educational profile

The medical director should have followed a full medical educational multi-disciplinary programme, in different fields of medicine, that must include at least the following matters:

1. Full medical education
2. Respiratory physiology and gas exchange theory
3. Critical care
4. Angiology
5. Traumatology
6. Neurology
7. ENT
8. Ophthalmology
9. Epidemiology
10. Diving medicine
11. Hyperbaric medicine
12. Diving technology
13. Hyperbaric technology
14. General principles of pneumatics

15. Safety and preventive measures in hyperbaric environment
16. Other aspects of both diving and hyperbaric medicine

Good knowledge in these matters is essential, although specific degrees will not be mandatory for recognition as medical director. In the near future the EUROPEAN COMMITTEE FOR HYPERBARIC MEDICINE (ECHM) will define more exactly the medical education exigible to the medical director.

Academic requirements and degrees

Even if medical directors have received a good self-trained education, they need a specific titulation degree, in order to avoid legal problems concerning the possible responsibilities deriving from the practice.

A medical doctorate in medicine is the basis. The medical education must be completed with postgraduate courses in both diving and hyperbaric medicine, preferably followed in University Departments of these specializations.

Other courses of similar level delivered by some well-known entities in hyperbaric and/or underwater medicine could also be accepted.

The medical director will be required to have specific educational and academic standards which will be defined by the Educational Committee of the ECHM in the near future.

The medical director, like all the medical staff in a hyperbaric centre, will be subjected to all regulations of work under pressure established by the European Community.

Continuous medical education

The medical director should undertake a periodic continuous education programme, about the main aspects of underwater and hyperbaric medicine. Participation in courses, workshops and conferences organized by International Societies well-known in this field, such as the European Undersea Biomedical Society (EUBS), the Foundation for the International Congress on Hyperbaric Medicine, the Undersea and Hyperbaric Medical Society (UHMS), or other courses approved or reviewed by the ECHM, could also be adequate.

Professional ethics and medical deontology oblige all medical directors to communicate their observations and improvements in the different fields of diving and hyperbaric medicine to their colleagues of the international scientific community. In addition, the medical director must take advantage of the experiences of his international colleagues and must take part in the wide-spread studies that might be performed.

The highest qualified hyperbaric centres should organize courses, workshops and periodical activities aiming to improve the education of specialized staff at all levels.

Dedication

All hyperbaric centres should have a permanent medical director, with partial or full-time dedication depending on the characteristics of each centre, complemented by a variable number of collaborators of the same or similar background and education. Hospital centre treating patients in situation of emergency will probably need more than three medical doctors.

NURSES

Functions
As in all fields of medicine, nurses complete medical treatment and they are responsible for the practical implementation of patient treatment.

The hyperbaric nurses perform the usual functions of their profession with some variations due to the characteristics of the hyperbaric activity:

1. Nursing measures belonging to the common pathologies of the hyperbaric therapeutics to be applied to the patients in a self standing chamber.
2. Nursing assistance of patients inside the hyperbaric chamber, taking special care of the specific conditions of the hyperbaric environment.
3. Adaptation of conventional medical techniques and specific treatments of each illness to the hyperbaric environment, so the other treatments that the patient is habitually receiving have not to be interrupted while in the chamber.
4. In some cases, operating the external controls of a monoplace hyperbaric chamber according to the compression and decompression schedules established.

Background
The hyperbaric nurse must have the corresponding degree of her profession. Specific education in critical care nursing will be very useful. Knowledge of other specializations like angiology, traumatology, and wound care will also be appropriate.

Special courses on diving and hyperbaric medicine are essential. The nurse may receive the necessary training in the same institution from the medical director.

Specific educational profile
Hyperbaric nurses should also receive a complementary education, according to their professional level, in the following matters:

1. General principles of decompression theory, diving technique, and pneumatics
2. Hyperbaric technique
3. Safety and preventive measures
4. Operation of monoplace hyperbaric chambers
5. Intensive critical care of patients
6. Other aspects inherent in both diving and hyperbaric medicine, concerning her profession

Academic requirements and degrees
A basic education and a nursing degree will be required. Special courses for hyperbaric nurses are highly recommended but they will not be strictly required.

The hyperbaric nurse will be subjected to the regulations on work under pressure established by the European Community.

Continuous education
As in all fields of health and medicine, hyperbaric nurses must complete and continue their education by reading specialized texts and attending courses and congresses. Their affiliation to specialized professional societies, such as the nurses

baromedical association or to other entities that might be created, would be of the greatest interest.

Dedication

All hospital based hyperbaric centres should have a permanent team of nurses with partial or full-time dedication depending on the needs of each centre. One or two people will not be enough to guarantee a 24 hours a day service, as the long stays inside the chamber that they must often endure (when a multiplace facility is used) renders them incapable of decompressions in the following hours. A whole team of hyperbaric nurses working in shifts would therefore be necessary.

ATTENDANTS

Functions

Patients inside a multiplace chamber need always to be under the control and supervision of trained personnel. Critical patients will always be joined by a doctor, a nurse or both.

Other patients however do not need such kind of direct and special medical and nursing assistance and in those cases the participation of a type of staff, specially trained, although not necessarily highly qualified may be adequate.

These are some of the activities attributed to attendants:

1. Patient care in non-invasive, non-specialized medical activities inside and outside the chamber.
2. Accompanying patients who are receiving treatment inside the multiplace chamber, but who do not need special assistance by doctors and nurses, but only by way of support, control and to give them confidence.
3. Other activities to develop inside or outside the chamber, indicated by the medical director or the nurse.

If monoplace chambers are used, the majority of these activities may be adopted by doctors and/or hyperbaric specialists and nurses.

Background

Attendants can come from different professions regarding underwater and hyperbaric medicine, such as:

1. Sport or commercial divers
2. Health auxiliaries, medical students, paramedics or assistants
3. Other professions preferably although not necessarily health/related

Items 1 and 2 are the most adequate conditions or origins for working as an attendant. However, these degrees should not be necessarily requested. Their education and training may be accomplished in the same hyperbaric institution.

Specific educational profile

At a level according to their capacity, previous experience and kind of work, attendants should be instructed in the following aspects:

1. General principles of medicine and therapeutics
2. Medical first aid
3. General principles of diving and hyperbaric medicine

Their basic education may be received in the same institution from a hyperbaric specialist and/or doctors and nurses.

As a result of this non-specific education programme, the attendants should meet the following requisites:

a. To feel comfortable in the hyperbaric environment
b. Excellent practice with hyperbaric techniques and necessary manoeuvres for adapting patients to the pressure
c. Sufficient knowledge of the main non-invasive medical instruments generally used under pressure
d. Capacity to interpret, but not to operate, the meaning of the control instruments placed inside the hyperbaric chamber. They must also be familiar with the pressure and control devices
e. To give first aid care in the case of an emergency

Academic requirements and degrees

There is no specific degree providing the requirements of an attendant. Some entities organize educational courses adapted to this activity. However only a course on medical first aid should be strictly required.

The attendants will be subjected to the regulations of work under pressure established by the European Community.

Continuous education

The attendants will be informed in the same institution, about any news on underwater and hyperbaric medicine and technique which could affect their activity. Their attendance at activities in the field of diving and hyperbaric medicine should be encouraged.

Dedication

All hospital and self-standing hyperbaric centres using multiplace hyperbaric chambers should have a permanent team of attendants, with partial or full-time dedication depending on the needs of each centre. One or two people will not be enough to guarantee a 24 hours/day service, as the long stays inside the chamber that they must often endure (if a multiplace facility is used) renders them incapable of further decompressions in the following hours.

If monoplace chambers are used, the attendants may not be necessary since all their functions are done externally by nurses and doctors and/or hyperbaric specialists.

CHAMBER OPERATORS

Functions

A hyperbaric facility may achieve a high level of sophistication that will require specialized attention and care.

The hyperbaric chamber itself, the air-compressors, other pressurized gas sources, or the gas reserves have some special devices whose manipulation might be very complex.

Monoplace chambers are handled sometimes by nurses and doctors and/or hyperbaric specialists.

When multiplace chambers are used, the hyperbaric centre must have qualified personnel to manage the hyperbaric facilities. These functions must be preferably carried out by specialized chamber operators.

The functions of the chamber operator of a multiplace facility will be:

1. Operation of the internal and external devices of the chamber.
2. Control and operation of the mechanisms for compression and decompression and for delivering gas mixtures and oxygen.
3. Control and application of the safety regulations concerning prevention of fire and oxygen toxicity.
4. Calculation, application, and control of compression and decompression schedules for patients, specialists and/or doctors, nurses, and attendants, applying decompression stops, when necessary.
5. Sometimes, interventions inside the chamber under pressure, in order to control or check the correct operation of determined parts of the pneumatic circuits or devices.
6. Adaptation and checking of the medical instruments carried by the patients before being introduced into the chamber, in order to assure their correct operation and to avoid dangerous or undesirable effects.
7. Control and checking of the operation of auxiliary facilities of the chamber air compressors, sources of compressed air or medical gases, air reserves, pneumatic circuits, control systems.
8. Maintenance of the facility. Small repair jobs or technical interventions due to problems which occasionally might occur, and which do not require the intervention of highly specialized technical staff.

Background

Hyperbaric operators usually come from a commercial diving environment, where often received specialized training. This is not indispensable and operators can come from other areas.

Despite the fact that they come from a non-health-related profession, they will need to learn elemental principles of health since they will be in contact with patients.

Some paramedical professions and health-related activities common in hospitals, may provide a good basis from which the candidate may be trained by the same institution to become a chamber operator.

Specific educational profile
Whatever their previous experience might be the hyperbaric operator needs good knowledge in the following subjects:

1. General pneumatics
2. General mechanics and electromechanics
3. Decompression theory, decompression schedules
4. Diving and hyperbaric technology
5. Medical first aid
6. General principles of medicine and medical therapeutics

Courses on diving and hyperbaric medicine for auxiliary staff will provide good training in all these matters.

Academic requirements and degrees
Some diving centres, off-shore facilities, and other specialized entities, result in some countries in specific degrees adapted to the activity of a chamber operator. However, this condition should not be regarded as indispensable until the European Community establishes a specific degree for chamber operators.

A degree in professional diving with a specialization in hyperbaric systems and facilities will be adequate.

A technical specialty degree in pneumatic systems or similar titulation would be of great benefit although it is not absolutely indispensable.

The chamber operators will be subjected to the regulations of work under pressure established by the European Community.

Continuous education
Hyperbaric operators will need to receive continuous education according to the advances in the field of hyperbaric technology and also in decompression theory. They must be regularly updated on the main aspects of the diseases that will be treated in the chamber.

For this reason, his periodical contact with other specialized centres is highly recommended.

Dedication
Since chamber operators are in charge of the operation of the multiplace hyperbaric chamber, their presence is absolutely essential in all hospital or self-standing multiplace hyperbaric centres.

A permanent chamber operator with partial or full-time dedication depending on the needs of each centre will therefore be needed.

In monoplace facilities, their services are also appreciated but their functions can be also attributed to other types of trained personnel.

TECHNICIANS

Functions
The hyperbaric centre needs to employ specialized technical staff, whose functions will be the checking and control of the chamber, pneumatic circuits, gas or compressed air reserves, air-compressors, and the rest of the technical parts of the facility.

Background

The hyperbaric technician must have a high level of knowledge in high, middle and low pressure pneumatics. They should also possess a deep knowledge of diving and hyperbaric technology. Some experience in the field of medical technology would be very suitable.

Some chamber operators can also be technicians.

Specific educational profile

In some areas, real specialists in diving systems or hyperbaric facilities will probably be very difficult to find. In many cases, a high pressure technician and some of the technical staff of a hospital will quite easily be able to adapt his knowledge receiving some additional instruction on pneumatics and high pressure.

Academic requirements and degrees

The hyperbaric technician must have either an official degree with specialty in pneumatic systems, or an official specific degree in hyperbaric technology, in the countries where these degrees exist. This activity should not be entrusted to persons or firms which, although experienced, might not be in a legal condition to give warranties and cover responsibilities in case of a possible disfunction, emergency, or even catastrophe.

Continuous education

The hyperbaric technician, being a high level specialist, must be aware of the latest technological advances and new changes which might occur in his sector, in order to use the most adequate systems.

Dedication

Depending on the amount of work and of the technical characteristics of each hyperbaric centre, maintenance of the facilities might be performed by full-time hyperbaric technicians or by subcontracted specialized firms or enterprises. Both conditions are equally acceptable.

OTHER STAFF

Many other professionals with different qualifications may and should be engaged with a hyperbaric medical centre, depending on the special characteristics of each and the hospital or institution where it is situated. Some of them are listed below.

1. Administrative
2. Statisticians
3. Rehabilitator
4. Fire specialists
5. Engineers
6. Others

Since the activities of these professionals do not adopt special characteristics or modifications by being carried out in a hyperbaric centre, and as their duties will be similar to their usual jobs, their functions, background, requirements, and dedication will not be detailed in this document. All these conditions will be developed as in other places or jobs.

ACCREDITATIONS AND CREDENTIALS

The European Committee for Hyperbaric Medicine (ECHM) will create a subcommittee for specialist assessment or accreditation, that will establish a credential document as explained in the aforementioned criteria in section 1 of this document. The selection and guarantee process will be established by the Subcommittee in a separate document in which the following items will be specified:

1. Educational criteria
2. Procedure for obtaining the credential
3. Usefulness and validity of the credential

In the meantime, lacking specific degrees in underwater and hyperbaric medicine, the aforementioned credential will be the guarantee for a hyperbaric specialist.

PERSONNEL EDUCATION AND TRAINING POLICIES
—Final Report

D. Elliott

The workshop was focused on the training needs for all staff associated with the pressure-related aspects of hyperbaric oxygen treatment.

It was acknowledged that while the majority of, if not all, such units are hospital based, there are many chambers which are not medical but which are used operationally for diving purposes and usually with no doctor present.

It was agreed that many of the basic training objectives for hyperbaric medicine and for diving medicine are the same, but not all.

It was also agreed that many hyperbaric doctors never see a diver except for those who attend for the treatment of a decompression accident and these are usually recreational divers. Similarly, most diving doctors with responsibilities for the health and safety of divers at work have no responsibilities for the treatment of patients in a hospital hyperbaric unit.

It was therefore recommended that there should be close liaison on training standards between the European Committee of Hyperbaric Medicine (ECHM) and the Medical Subcommittee of the European Diving Technology Committee (EDTC).

It was also concluded that the Report for the ECHM "EUROPEAN STANDARDS FOR HYPERBARIC MEDICINE, Section—Personnel, Professional, and Educational Requirements," which had been edited by Dr. Desola, was accepted in principle but with two conditions:

1. Removal of the subsection 8 on 'Minimal requirements' because this not an educational matter but one of operational safety, and
2. Incorporation of the conclusions of this meeting in Lille, with additional discussions and recommendations as necessary.

It was agreed that there should be a modular approach to training. There should be priority in this for the SAFETY module and that this should be the first to be given to all categories of personnel. Of the subsequent modules, some would be specified as compulsory for particular categories of staff and some could be optional.

It was agreed that the Medical Director of a Hyperbaric Unit should already have proved to be a competent hyperbaric specialist but that he or she should also have had appropriate management training.

It was agreed that for the Hyperbaric Specialist:

- a first degree in medicine is essential
- he or she can be from any medical specialty (by precedent, for example: intensive care, anaesthetics, occupational medicine, surgery, internal medicine, family practice, etc.
- the course of about one year should include some 200 hours of formal training

- a short research thesis ('memoire') is essential
- a final examination is essential and it should be validated by an University
- this diploma would be mandatory for hyperbaric doctors
- however there is also a need for trainee doctors (registrars/residents) to gain experience in a hyperbaric unit before beginning their formal training
- periodical 'update' training ("Continuing Medical Education") is also essential

It was agreed that nurses require some 120 to 160 hours of modular training and that there should be special emphasis on critical care.

It was agreed that Attendants are an optional category of staff not found in all units and, as they are not health professionals, should be trained for only non-invasive procedures.

It was accepted that the technical staff (the Technical Director, chamber operators, technicians) would require some qualifications not needed by the health professionals. Their specific training courses should be supplemented by appropriate modules on health-related issues.

It was noted that many non-routine technical tasks, such as maintenance, could be delegated to competent contractors.

It was recognised that there is a need for an International Institute of Baromedicine to bring together academically all categories of staff from the geographically separated units within Europe, particularly for the enhancement of the teaching of this diverse subject with the sparse resources available. The relationships will need to be developed between such an Institute and the other teaching centres using the various European languages.

It was agreed that there should be an authority, which would be separate from any teaching establishment, to harmonise and audit training standards within Europe. Such a body could be formed following discussion between the ECHM and the Medical Subcommittee of the EDTC.

RESEARCH IN HYPERBARIC OXYGEN:
A MEDLINE SURVEY OF TEN YEARS
—Introductory Report

Jörg Schmutz MD, Foundation for Hyperbaric Medicine, 177 Kleinhuningerstrasse. CH 4057 Basel

Daniel Mathieu MD, Service d'Urgence Respiratoire de Reanimation medicale et de medecine Hyperbare, Hopital Calmette, CHRU de Lille, F 59037 Lille Cedex

INTRODUCTION

The purpose of this document, is to give to the participants of the workshop an overview over the practice of research and publication done in Hyperbaric Oxygen Therapy (HBO) in the last 10 years. We will not make specific recommendations on research topics or scientifically unsolved problems. We consider that this must be discussed from case to case and within specific research projects between the highly specialised scientific involved.

METHODS

The following data have been obtained through searches in the MEDLINEO computer library (U.S. Department of Health and Human Services, National Library of Medicine) using the Silver Platter 3.11 Software. Key-words were found in the medical literature. Searches were done either with single or multiple key-words. Key-words were either selected by typing the desired key-word under the "find" prompt or by combining different key-words from the "index" prompt with the link "or," or with the link "and." A few examples are explained, the rest is listed below.

- gas gangrene—selects all the publications dealing with gas gangrene.
- multicenter or multicentre or multicentric study—selects a
  large group of publications dealing with multicentric research.
- gas gangrene and controlled—among the publications dealing with gas
  gangrene, select only those which are controlled.

For the key-word "hyperbaric oxygen," we have exploited all the subsets of the "Thesaurus" prompt. This means that all the publications dealing with HBO or in which HBO is even only quoted have been selected.

For the key-word "radiation injury," we took the following combination of key-words: radiation-injuries or radiation-injuries-drug-therapy or radiation-injuries-surgery or radiation-injuries-therapy or osteoradionecrosis.

The other key-words used were: Gas gangrene, carbon monoxide poisoning, decompression sickness, surgical flaps, air embolism, osteomyelitis, intensive care, surgery, therapy, drug therapy, surgery & therapy, controlled, prospective, retrospective, randomized, double-blind, experimental clinical, case reports, review, letter, oxygen toxicity, oxygen radical species, superoxide dismutase, free oxygen radicals, chemiluminescence, lipid peroxydation, reactive oxygen species, reperfusion injury, electron spin resonance, oxygen.

RESULTS

The number of scientific publications done in the last 10 years in HBO is of 160,9 per year with extremes ranging from 85 publications per year in 1992 to 203 in 1991. If we examine these publications with different key-words, we see that most HBO publications are dealing with the treatment of diseases (key-word: therapy). We have split our data in two 5-year periods (1983–1987 and 1989–1993) in order to show the evolution of research in HBO. Data are shown below in Table l.

Table 1 shows that the global number of HBO publications has slightly diminished and that the number of experimental publications has been reduced by more than 50%. On the contrary, the number of reviews, case reports, letters to the editor, and clinical articles is growing.

Table 1: Trends in HBO publications in two five year period: 1983-1987 and 1989-1993					
Key-words	1983-87	1983-87 in %	1989-93	1989-93 in %	increase in%
All FEBO	164,8	100,0%	157,0	100,0%	-4,7%
Experimental	26,3	16,0%	12,4	7,9%	-52,9%
Clinical	21,6	13,1%	25,6	16,3%	+18,5%
Case Reports	0,2	0,2%	0,6	0,4%	+140,0%
Review	13,0	7,9%	22,8	14,5%	+75,4%
Letter	10,6	6,4%	11,2	7,1 %	+5,7%
Therapy	118,4	71,8%	113,2	72,1%	-4,4%
Ox. Toxicity	7,2	4,4%	5,9	3,3%	-27,8%
Slulticentric	0,9	0,1%	0,2	0,5%	0%
Prospective	2	1,2%	2,8	1,8%	+40
Retrospective	1	0,6%	3,2	2,0%	+920%
Controlled	4,6	2,8%	5	3,2%	+10%
Randomized	2,2	1,3%	2,8	1,8%	+300%

Figure 2 examines the subset "therapy" of Table 1 with key-words representing the so-called "UHMS-accepted diseases" (decompression sickness, carbon monoxide poisoning, air embolism, gas gangrene, surgical flaps, osteomyelitis, radiation injury).

Within the HBO community, decompression sickness, carbon monoxide poisoning, gas gangrene, and air embolism are surely considered as the most proven indications for HBO. If we group the annual volume of HBO publications for all forms of treatment for these 4 diseases, we obtain a figure of 35,8 HBO publications per year out of a total of 85 publications per year (42%). This reflects the importance of HB0 in the treatment of these diseases. For chronic osteomyelitis, radiation injury and surgical flaps, also considered as "accepted indications" the situation is quite different. If we group again the data, we obtain a figure of 15,2 HBO publications per year out of a total of 349,2 publications per year (4,4%). This shows clearly that the interest and use of HBO in the treatment of chronic osteomyelitis, radiation injury and surgical flaps are small.

We will now use some of the key-words used in Table 1 to analyse the medical literature published in the last 5 years in intensive care, surgery, and HBO (Fig. 2). We see

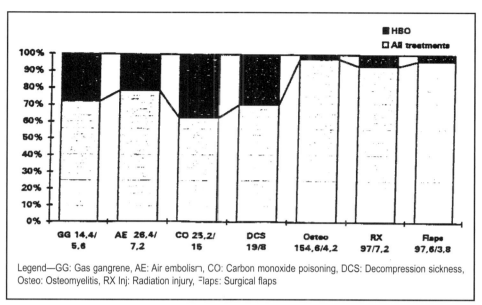

Legend—GG: Gas gangrene, AE: Air embolism, CO: Carbon monoxide poisoning, DCS: Decompression sickness, Osteo: Osteomyelitis, RX Inj: Radiation injury, Flaps: Surgical flaps

Figure 1. HBO in the treatment of "UHMS accepted diseases" (annual average 1989-1993).

in Figure 2 that the therapeutical aspect seems more important in the HBO literature than in intensive care and in surgery. This is not surprising since HBO is first of all a treatment modality (oxygen as a drug). Experimental research seems also very present in HBO: 7,9% of all publications compared with 1,7% for intensive care and 3,7% for surgery. The other types of publication are more or less the same than in surgery and in intensive care. Multicentric researches are at the contrary only scarcely used in HBO (0,5% of all publications) compared with 1,3% in intensive care and 0,9% in surgery.

For this purpose, we have combined key-words to obtain only the publications dealing with the therapeutical aspects of surgery, drug therapy, therapy in general, and the overall number of publications of each discipline.

Figure 3 compares the growth rate (indicated in percentage) of different type of medical studies, namely prospective, retrospective, controlled, randomized, and multicentric between two five-year periods (1983–7 and 1989–93) as well as the total number of publications done in each discipline. Each five-year period is presented as annual average of the period. We have looked at the research methodology done in four different forms of treatment: HBO therapy, surgical therapy, drug therapy and therapy in general.

Results show that the number of studies done in the 1989–93 period is growing compared to the 1983–87 period in surgical therapy, drug therapy, and therapy in general. HBO therapy in contrast shows a decrease in the overall number of publications, a less important growth in the other research methodologies except in retrospective studies where it has the largest growth of all treatment forms.

Table 2 shows the growth rates in surgical therapy, drug therapy, therapy in general, and HBO therapy in percentage of annual publications. We have applied these percentages to the baseline value of HBO (average of 83–79) in order to give an impression of the expected number of publications if HBO had the same growth rate. Table 2 shows that research is actually declining in HBO in comparison with surgical therapy, drug therapy, and therapy in general. This is in contrast to the often heard statement that HBO is expanding.

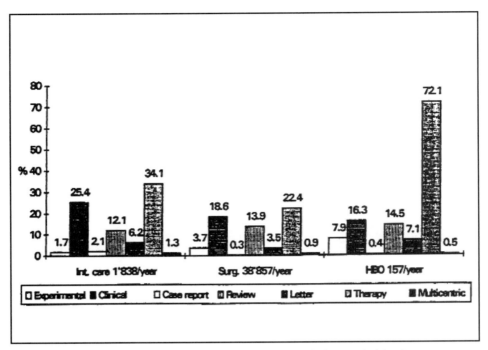

Figure 2. Type of publications done between 1989 and 1993 using the key-words: intensive care, surgery, and HBO.

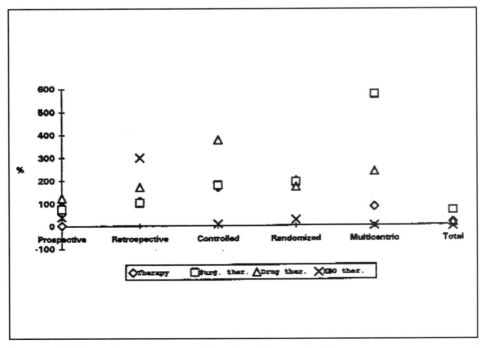

Figure 3. Evolution of the research methodology between two 5-year periods; 1983-1987 and 1989-1993 (increase in % of 83-87 value).

Table 2: Research methodology in HBO and & therapy. Some projection with other therapeutical disciplines.

	HBO 83-7 = baseline	HBO 89-93		Expected if therapy		Expected if surgery		Expected if drug	
		Abs.	in % ↗	Abs.	in % ↗	Abs.	in % ↗	Abs.	in % ↗
Total	118.4	113.2	-4.4	130	14.4	187.5	65.7	129.2	12.9
Prospective	2.0	2.8	0.5	5.2	4.0	24.8	13.2	2.2	1.7
Retrospective	1.0	3.2	1.3	4.7	3.6	14.8	7.9	3.2	2.5
Controlled	4.6	5.0	0.2	9.7	7.5	64.7	34.4	5.0	3.9
Randomized	2.2	2.8	0.4	8.0	6.2	56.4	30.1	5.0	170
Multicentric	0.2	0.2	0	3.1	2.4	3.9	2.1	4.1	3.2
Double-blind	0.01	0.06	?	0.7	0.5	0.2	0.1	1.2	0.9

Legend. Expected if = figures that would be expected if HBO would behave as the discipline mentioned. Abs = absolute figures in % = increase in percentage of the discipline named in the column.

Figure 3 already showed us that multicentric studies are not very frequently used by the HBO community. Figure 4 investigates now the type of multicentric research done in general in medicine. The annual average of each five-year period is indicated on the left X axis, the increase in annual number of publications for the 1989-93 period is indicated in percentage on the right X axis. We looked at the total number of multicentric studies registered in the MEDLINE(r) bank and how many of them were done as controlled, prospective, retrospective randomized, or double-blind studies.

Figure 4 shows an increase of about 600% in multicentric research between 1983–7 and 1989–93. Most multicentric studies are controlled, less randomized. The growing rate of retrospective and prospective studies is slightly greater as the one of multicentric studies. The increase in double-blind studies is slightly smaller. The increase in controlled studies seems to be three times greater and the increase in randomisation two times greater.

Multicentric research being the best way to reach the largest amount of data and the double-blind method (if possible) the most objective to evaluate the validity of a treatment method, we have decided to look at the actual use of multicentric research in H130 and in other therapeutic modalities. For this purpose, we have used the key-word multicentric alone or in combination with the key-word double-blind.

Figure 5 shows on the left X-axis the annual percentage of multicentric and multicentric & double-blind studies done in each field (1989–93). The right X-axis shows the percentage of increase between the 1983–87 and the 1989–93 period for multicentric and multicentric & double-blind studies. We have also indicated the increase rate in multicentric and multicentric & double-blind studies (line) in order to compare it with the growing rates in therapy in general, surgical therapy, drug therapy, and HBO therapy.

The data presented in Figure 5 show that the percentage of multicenter studies done in therapeutic modalities like HBO therapy, drug therapy, surgical therapy, or therapy in general, is growing except for HBO therapy. Surgical therapy is the only discipline where there is a real move towards more multicentric studies. The increase is twice as important as the general increase of all medical sciences. Therapy and drug therapy are keeping their relative number of multicentric study's stable. HBO is losing ground with the other disciplines. Regarding multicentric & double-blind studies, surgical therapy shows again the strongest growth even if it has actually a small number of multicentric & double-blind studies. Therapy and drug therapy are again stable and HBO is losing ground.

Since many scientists of the HBO community are considering HBO a drug that can be prescribed in a variable dosage, according to pressure, we investigated also how research was done on the level of oxygen itself. We have chosen to investigate some physiopathological mechanisms that we believe to be of interest for the field of HBO as well as the toxicity of oxygen.

Figure 6 shows the actual volume of research done in the 1989–1993 period (annual average) using key-words related to more basic research as free oxygen radicals and related topics.

Figure 6 shows that oxygen seems of concern to many scientists. Except for oxygen reactive species, the annual volume of publication is largely superior to the annual volume of publication in the whole field of HBO (see Table 2). All the other topics are much more researched than HBO. Since the HBO physicians are daily concerned with molecular oxygen, our next interest was to investigate how often the key-words HBO and oxygen were quoted in publications done in the same topics as above.

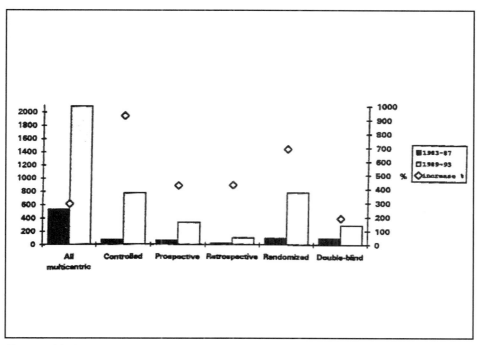

Figure 4. Multicentric research methodology: figures for 1983-1987 and 1989-1993, increase in % of the 1983-1987 figures.

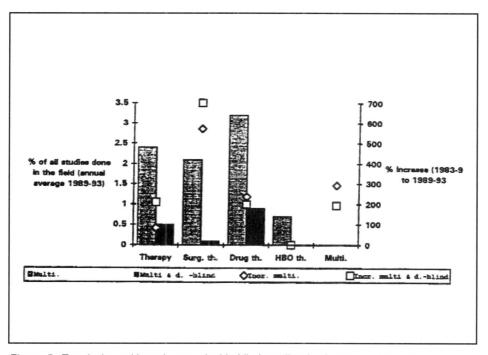

Figure 5. Trends in multicentric anc double-blind studies in therapy, surgical therapy, drug therapy, and HBO.

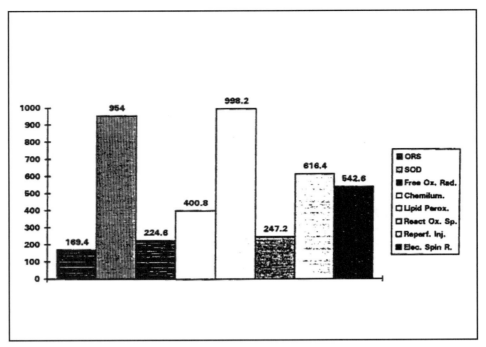

Figure 6. Free oxygen radicals and related research: annual average from 1989-1993.

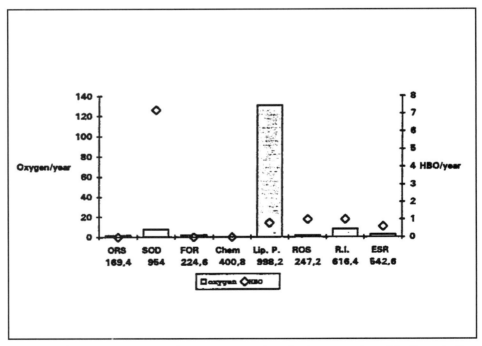

Figure 7. Comparative search of oxygen versus hyperbaric oxygen in publications dealing with molecular oxygen (annual average 1989-1993). Legend ORS: oxygen reactive species. SOD: superoxide dismutase. FOR: Free oxygen radicals. Chem: Chemiluminescence. Lip. P.: Lipid peroxydation. ROS: Reactive oxygen species. RI: Reperfusion injury. ESR: Electron spin resonance.

Table 3: Comparative search of oxygen versus hyperbaric oxygen in publications dealing with reactive oxygen species reperfusion injury.

	1983	1984	1985	1986	1987	1988	1989	1990	1991	1992	1993
ROS & Reperfusion Injury & HBO	0	0	0	0	0	0	0	0	0	0	0
ROS & Reperfusion injury & oxygen	0	1	1	1	0	4	6	11	16	11	64
ROS & Oxygen toxicity & HBO	0	0	0	0	0	0	0	0	1	1	1
ROS & Oxygen toxicity & oxygen	1	2	1	4	3	1	8	3	10	10	49

Figure 7 shows on the left X-axis the annual number of publications containing the key-word oxygen in relation to free oxygen and related topics. The right X-axis shows the same data but for the key-word HBO. The annual number of publications for each topic investigated (annual average of the 1989-93 period) is indicated for each topic on the Y-axis.

Figure 7 shows that most research done on molecular oxygen and its related topics is rarely related to oxygen; if it is, then it is mostly related to normobaric oxygen and only little to HBO.

As last search, we decided to investigate on the publications dealing with the role of reactive oxygen species in reperfusion injury and in oxygen toxicity with special reference to oxygen and to hyperbaric oxygen. The results are presented in Table 3.

Table 3 shows that there is a growing interest in the last years for oxygen toxicity and for reperfusion injury. Unfortunately, it seems that this interest is not reflected in the hyperbaric literature.

DISCUSSION

It is generally accepted in the medical community that controlled, prospective, randomized studies and large multicentric series provide the best way to prove the efficiency of a treatment. Our data show that there is a sustained trend in the last 1 0 years toward such studies in the medical literature. This type of generally well accepted study design is unfortunately not used enough in hyperbaric medicine. This evidence has led to the situation that even for disease entities like gas gangrene, air embolism, or CO poisoning the use of HBO is strongly contested, allowing some colleagues to speak of a "therapy in search of disease." Protestations of members of the HBO community in form of letters, advocating flaws or errors in studies showing that HBO is of little use, will not change the opinion of many scientists who pretend that there is no scientific proof for the efficacy of HBO in any other disease than decompression sickness.

The growing criticism about the quality of research in the scientific community, the data presented above clearly show that clinical research in HBO has to change towards more accepted forms of study designs. It will maybe be necessary to expand the volume of clinical research by creating international collaborative groups for clinical research with the support of governmental agencies and the volume of basic science by seeking more collaboration with scientist involved in oxygen physiology and biology.

FUTURE PROSPECTS IN RESEARCH FOR HYPERBARIC OXYGEN
—Final Report

D. Mathieu, Service d'Urgence Respiratoire, de Réanimation et Médecine Hyperbare, Hôpital A. Calmette, Centre Hospitalier Régional Universitaire, Bld du Professeur Leclercq, 59037 Lille Cedex, France

INTRODUCTION

Hyperbaric oxygen (HBO) therapy has gained a place now well recognized in the treatment of many diseases where it may be used either as the main therapy or as an adjunctive measure. However, controversy still persists about its use. Some of our colleagues keep on denying any interest in HBO despite numerous published studies. In many cases HBO indications and protocols remain largely empirical; even physiological bases and rationale for use of HBO are still unknown or unclearly understood. This leads to consideration of HBO in terms of certainty of clinical usefulness, safety for the patient and economic efficiency for the Society.

DIRECTIONS FOR FUTURE RESEARCH

Future research has to be directed towards four main objectives:
1. Determining the precise physiopathological basis of HBO
    a) Types of research
        i. Basic research:
            - In vitro
            - Animal study
        ii. Clinical research:
            - In patient
    b) Main subjects
        i. Tissular and cellular oxygen pressures and fluxes
        ii. Microcirculation
        iii. Oxygen free radicals
        iv. Cellular metabolic effects of hyperoxia
        v. Effect of hyperoxia on epithelium, bone or connective healing

2. Validating methods allowing assessment of HBO effects in patients
    a) Type of research
        i. Basic research: elaboration and validation of measurement methods
        ii. Clinical research: validation in patients of theses methods
    b) Main subjects
        i. Estimation of local oxygen status
            - Tissular or cellular oxygen pressures

- Regional or microvascular blood flows
- Derived parameters

ii. Estimation of hyperoxia-induced effects
- Metabolic effects
- Imaging consequences

All these techniques may be invasive or non-invasive, continuous or intermittent. The objectives are patient selection, prognosis, and oxygen delivery monitoring.

3. Evaluate clinical efficacy
   a) Type of research
      i. Clinical research: studies must follow actual rules for clinical evaluation: prospective, randomized, and/or not double blinded, and/or not in cross over, and/or not multicentric.
   b) Main subjects
      i. Clinical indications of HBO
   c) Problems to be solved
      i. Patient selection: homogeneity of patients between groups
      ii. Methodological problems: Double blind: false compression, hypoxic breathed mixture
         - Cross over
         - Multicentric studies
      iii. Evaluation criteria: Frequently, criteria for evaluation are non-existent or non-worldwide-recognized, e.g., Kurzke scale for multiple sclerosis, Wagner classification for diabetic foot lesions.

4. Evaluation of quality and pertinence of care
   a) Type of research
      i. Clinical, epidemiological, nursing, and economic research
   b) Main subjects
      i. Elaboration of standards (consensus conference)
      ii. Quality control of care:
         - Continuous (vigilance)
         - Intermittent (audit)
      iii. Cost/benefit analysis

METHODS FOR FUTURE RESEARCH

Basic Research

   a) Organization : university and research organization
   b) Problems to be solved
      i. Extensive methodological knowledge
      ii. Laboratory allowing in vitro and animal studies
      iii. Expensive and complex equipment
      iv. Difficulties to obtain proper fundings

   c) Action
      i. Need of a coordinated action to convince scientific committees of these organizations to obtain proper fundings
      ii. Association with basic research teams who already have the knowledge and experience
     iii. Development of research network between clinicians and research laboratories

Clinical Research

   a) Organization: university or team associated with university
   b) Problems to be solved
      i. Training in clinical research methodology
      ii. Close adherence to methodological rules in research protocol and follow-up in accordance with good clinical practices
   c) Actions
      i. Selection of topics where a sufficient knowledge exists to allow group homogeneity and proper patient evaluation
      ii. Association of hyperbaric specialists in multidisciplinary research team
     iii. Development of clinical research network on a national or international level

CONCLUSION

There is an urgent need for a great quality research to ensure credibility of HBO. This may be best achieved by an extensive training in basic and clinical research methodology for hyperbaric specialists, by promoting association of hyperbaric specialists with multidisciplinary research team and development of information and personal exchanges between hyperbaric centres. These are the preliminary steps allowing the development of a multicentric research study network. In that regard, the institution of a body for information exchange and coordination for HBO research will be very useful.

NOTES

EVOLUTION OF HYPERBARIC OXYGEN THERAPY IN EUROPE AND THE UNITED STATES (1994)

Enrico M. Camporesi, MD, SUNY HSC at Syracuse, NY, USA

Hyperbaric Oxygen therapy is relatively new, since it has evolved during the last 30 years from an experimental curiosity to a frequently employed therapeutic tool. It is, however, still only accepted by a small segment of medical practitioners throughout the world. In the early 60s, the application of oxygen breathing at increased barometric pressure promised to open new vistas in therapy, to the point that Dr. Jacobson of Mount Sinai Hospital described the new modality with the following words:

"... administration of oxygen at increased barometric pressure promises to be an advance comparable in importance to the therapeutic introduction of blood transfusion and antibiotics"(1).

Today, in the fall of 1994, hyperbaric oxygen therapy still remains as the passion of a few specialists, often unable to generate public and political support sufficient to promote widespread acceptance.

A historical review of the field demonstrates the European roots and the intermittent growth in the United States, with a noticeable exchange of leading characters across the Atlantic. An early ideation priority must date back to Henshaw in London, who expressed theoretical considerations in 1662 to the possible benefits of increasing breathing gas pressure. Junod in 1834 was first to utilize compressed air in France for therapeutic purposes. Paul Bert in 1873, and Haldane 1895, described in detail the principles and physiological bases for compressed air and oxygen treatments in France and in England. Finally, Boerema in Amsterdam established a systematic therapeutic approach and was able to bring hyperbaric oxygen into the surgical arena, with the idea to induce cardiac standstill in the hyperoxygenated heart, thus allowing for surgical repairs of significant shunts. At this time also (1961), Brummelkamp introduced hyperbaric oxygen in the therapeutic scheme for gas gangrene, which was at that time in full resurgence in Holland. The clinical growth continued with the exemplary text of Davis and Hunt published in 1977 under the auspices of the Undersea Medical Society (2). Today the Undersea and Hyperbaric Medical Society has changed its name to represent the wide interest for hyperbaric therapy, and has fostered critical applications of oxygen therapy, and the usual methods of publication and stringent review for papers in the field. The Committee Report on Hyperbaric Oxygen Therapy lists indications for treatment and is published periodically by the Undersea and Hyperbaric Medical Society. A reasoned review of several hundred well documented publications, summarizing the "science" behind HBO, was also recently edited and published by the society (3).

The field reached another significant stage when, in 1989, a meeting was held under the auspices of NIH to summarize in a Workshop (4) the views of the National Heart, Lung, and Blood Institute of NIH on the biological significance of this area and to focus the present status of Hyperbaric Oxygen Therapy on the biological studies centered in this field. The NIH Workshop published also on some peculiar aspects of the field; the diffusion of this therapy is still very limited, with a small number of patients (10,000 to 15,000 patients per year in the US treated during 1989) receiving 11 to 20 treatments each, at an average cost of $150 per treatment, for a total cost approaching $30 million per year. Clinical utilization figures published in the summary show that the rapid growth phase in the United States for Hyperbaric Oxygen Therapy started around 1978. At that time the number of patients treated per year approximated 1500, while today's rate approaches 18000. Another peculiarity of the field is that it requires a significant investment in equipment and in instructions to personnel in order to establish itself locally, however, it most often fails to maintain visibility due to lack of interest, time, or the lack of a dedicated specialist to maintain administrative excellency. Similar numbers are harder to obtain from the European colleagues: it appears, however, that multiplace clinical facilities are prevalent in Europe.

Hyperbaric oxygenation has a simple but brilliant rationale: a large group of diseases have a major component in intracellular oxygen insufficiency. Recovery from such a condition would reasonably be expected if oxygen availability can be improved. HBO represents a technically well-developed approach, able to enhance oxygenation.

The limitations to this straightforward application are many: if HBO increases tissue PO_2, at the same time it also increases generation of reactive O_2 species with potential toxicity. Moreover, tissue delivery of oxygen, which is enhanced by increased arterial O_2 and capillary PO_2, is altered by hyperoxic induced vasoconstriction which will reduce blood flow and reduce delivery of the response components, such as inflammatory response cells, nutrients, and clearance of metabolic by-products. The growth of several bacteria is inhibited by high oxygen concentration, but other bacteria may be enhanced. Furthermore, despite the increased safety record in delivering oxygen at 2–3 atmosphere absolute, the potential for mechanical accident, O_2 toxicity, and barotraumatic morbidity still exist.

Total cost of oxygen therapy in today's society is acceptably low, compared to the enormous cost of many medical applications. This additional cost has been expected to result in overall cost savings in many syndromes where a shorter recovery time and a total lower hospitalization cost is produced. Finally the limitation in number of published controlled clinical trials in HBO has been causing significant criticism by practitioners who are not utilizing HBO, as the larger medical community in this case lacks the capacity to readily test the reputed claims independently, since the use of HBO requires technical capabilities generally not available to the practitioner.

This year, in June of 1994, the Undersea and Hyperbaric Medical Society Meeting in Denver, Colorado, brought together approximately 100 clinical abstracts summarizing experiences on several hundred patients. The field is in active motion and significant critical debates are occurring within practitioners themselves. We have become very sensitive to the accusations of lack of scientific evidence and are striving to fill the gaps, although we are realizing there are only a few dozen practitioners in the world who have the support and capability to summarize in objective manner their experience in the field.

Another obstacle has been in our way: an indecisive attitude toward the best forum where to publish our results. Several years ago I was asked to assume the editorship of a new journal, "The Journal of Hyperbaric Medicine," which had survived some administrative problems after a few issues. After the fifth year of publication, I initiated procedures to have the journal indexed by the National Library of Medicine in order to achieve stature and visibility. However the journal was deemed by the National Library of Medicine to represent too narrow an interest to be indexed at that time. I support the subsequent decision by the Executive Committee of the Undersea and Hyperbaric Medical Society's to rename the other publication of the society, "Undersea Biomedical Research," (a Library of Medicine indexed publication), to a new comprehensive title reflecting significant participation by clinical practitioners to the hyperbaric field and to fuse the contents of the two journals. I am continuing to participate to its editorship. At this time, no other European or international publication exists which is electronically indexed by the Index Medicus. The new "Undersea and Hyperbaric Medicine" allows for rapid electronic retrieval of hyperbaric publications in our rapidly changing environment. In this new publication, hyperbaric clinical papers have been reviewed with the same emphasis as diving papers by an extended review board.

The growth and expansion of hyperbaric therapy activities in Europe, and in some way throughout the world, has been marked by similar observations which are valid for the North American continent, namely, clinical activities usually grow and become established in large tertiary referral hospitals, very often outside of the realm of University, very often due to the care and personal sacrifice of individual practitioners who are not at the center of academic productivity. The largest discrepancies between Europe and the US are represented by the success in Europe of treatments for sensory organ deficits, like sudden deafness, an area not popular for treatments in the US.

I have the good fortune to know most of you through several meetings in the past few years, both in Europe and the United States. I hope that this gathering be repeated in the future, creating a forum for publication of significant advances in the area. I am very grateful to the organizing committee and to Dr Wattel for our meeting today.

REFERENCES

1. J. Jacobson: Presidential Address - 8th International Congress on Hyperbaric Medicine, Long Beach CA, August 22-24, 1984.
2. Davis JC, Hunt TK: Hyperbaric Oxygen Therapy. Bethesda: Undersea Medical Society, 1977.
3. Hyperbaric Oxygen Therapy-A Critical Review, Camporesi EM, Barker AC, eds., UHMS, 1991.
4. NHLBI Workshop Summary, Hyperbaric Oxygenation Therapy. Am Re. Respir Dis, 144:1414 1421, 1991.

RECOMMENDATIONS OF THE JURY

The scope of this first European Consensus Conference was to establish an agreement on the situation of Hyperbaric Medicine in Europe in 1994 with regard to the different aspects that characterize a medical discipline: field of application, operational rules and procedures, training of dedicated personnel, effectiveness evaluation, research. Starting from these points the Jury, with the support of the Conference experts and rapporteurs, was called to formulate recommendations that could answer to the following six questions, after each one of them had been discussed and debated during monothematic workshops:

1. Which Treatment for Decompression Illness?
2. Which Acute Indications for Hyperbaric Oxygen Therapy?
3. Which Chronic Indications need Hyperbaric Therapy as an adjunctive treatment?
4. Which Safety Regulations for the design and use of medical hyperbaric chambers and of medical equipment for hyperbaric use?
5. Which initial Training and which Continuing Education for personnel employed in Clinical Hyperbaric Medicine?
6. Which Research to expect and plan for the next five year period?

E.M. Camporesi, New York (USA), A. Gasparetto, Rome (Italy), M. Goulon, Paris (France), L.J. Greenbaum, Bethesda (USA), E.P. Kindwall, Milwaukee (USA), M. Lamy, Liege (Belgium), D. Linnarsson, Stockholm (Sweden), J.M. Mantz, Strasbourg (France), C. Perret, Lausanne (Switzerland), P. Pietropaoli, Ancona (Italy), H. Takahashi, Nagoya (Japan), C. Voisin, Lille (France).

INTRODUCTION

The use of hyperbaric chambers in intensive care started in Europe more than 30 years ago; the present experience is sufficient to identify those clinical conditions where hyperbaric oxygen (HBO) has a therapeutical interest. Therefore the first scope of the Conference is to confront the obtained clinical results in order to reach a consensus in the definition of recognized indications for HBO, according to three levels of priority:

a) Situations where the transport to a hyperbaric facility is strongly recommended because it is recognized that HBO positively affects the prognosis for survival. This implies that the patient is transferred to the nearest hyperbaric facility as soon as possible (type 1 recommendation).

b) Situations where the transport to a hyperbaric facility is recommended because it is recognized that HBO constitutes an important part of the treatment of that given condition, which, even if it may not influence the prognosis for patient's survival, it is nevertheless important for the prevention of serious disorders. This implies that the transfer to a hyperbaric facility is made, unless this represents a danger to the patient's life (type 2 recommendation).

c) Situations where the transfer to a hyperbaric facility is optional, because HBO is regarded as a additional treatment modality which can improve clinical results (type 3 recommendation).

Establishing a similar list is not an easy task, as in almost the totality of cases, the choice of an indication for treatment is based on clinical experience and not on controlled studies. Is it necessary, in similar conditions, that the validity of a given indication is again put under discussion and that the results of controlled prospective studies are awaited before defining lists of indications for Hyperbaric Oxygen therapy? This Jury does not think that this is appropriate. Clinical experience has an unquestionable value when it is the result of multiple agreeing observations, collected during many years and independently confirmed by different groups. In other words, it seems justified that indications for which there is unanimous consensus of the leading experts are accepted without further evidence.

A criticism to a similar attitude, which can lead to accept a treatment without any formal evidence of its efficacy, is that it can expose the patient to unknown potential damage. But we can answer that the choice of any treatment modality, be it medical or surgical, is always based on a careful evaluation of its risk / benefit ratio as compared to the patient's specific conditions. There are circumstances where clinical experience shows that the benefits of treatment are of such magnitude that the potential side-effects can be considered negligible. Serious carbon monoxide intoxication, for instance, is a condition where it would seem unreasonable to withdraw HBO because of the potential pulmonary oxygen toxicity effects. In situations such as the latter, the choice is simple, but it may be more complicated when the expected advantage is not as evident. In these situations the issue is the objective evaluation of the real interest and usefulness of the treatment modality.

The Jury has attempted to identify those clinical situations for which the efficacy of Hyperbaric Oxygen Therapy is unanimously recognized and where the evidence of beneficial effects of the treatment is such that the treatment should not be ethically denied. In other situations, where sufficient evidence in favour of HBO is not available, it is necessary to start evaluation procedures based on multicentric studies and on clearly defined protocols, as approved by a suitable ethical committee. Only after the completion of such studies will it be possible to accept a new indication.

Professor Claude Perret
President of the Conference Jury

WHICH TREATMENT FOR DIVING DECOMPRESSION ACCIDENTS?

- The primary cause of DCI is the separation of gas in the body tissues (bubbles).
- The best prophylaxis is achieved by adequate ascent/decompression procedures.
- DCI is best classified descriptively.
- On-site 100% oxygen first aid treatment is strongly recommended (Type 1 recommendation).
- On-site fluid administration for the first aid of decompression accidents is recommended (Type 2 recommendation).

- Therapeutical recompression must be initiated as soon as possible (Type 1 recommendation).
- Aside from immediate recompression treatment tables which may be used on the site of the accident, the "low pressure oxygen treatment tables" are recommended as the treatment tables of first choice (Type 1 recommendation). High pressure oxygen/inert gas tables can be used in selected and/or recalcitrant cases (Type 3 recommendation). Deep, not sur-face-oriented, mixed gas or saturation diving accidents require special treatment protocols.
- Adjunctive pharmacological treatment is controversial but:
  - I.V. fluid therapy is recommended (Type 2 recommendation)
  - The use of steroids and anticoagulants, although widely adopted with out any apparent adverse effect, is considered optional (Type 3 recommendation).
- The continuation of a combined Hyperbaric Oxygen Therapy and rehabilitation treatment is recommended until clinical stabilization or no further amelioration is achieved (Type 2 recommendation).

COMMENTS

The minimal consensus obtained reflects the heterogeneous nature of the different conditions grouped under the definition "Decompression Illness," even if they share the same pathophysiological basis.

It must be remembered that the majority of the scientific papers on the subject refers to military or commercial diving. Considering the treatment results of these accidents, the role of pressure and the importance of the time factor in limiting the delay to recompression are unquestionable and consequently justify the need for hyperbaric chambers on the very site where commercial or military diving is performed.

The recent significant development of recreational diving, notwithstanding the stringent safety rules and procedures, is similarly accompanied by the occurrence of decompression accidents, based on the same pathophysiological mechanisms, but the situation is entirely different with regard to the start of therapeutical recompression pro-cedures, as the interval to recompression is consistently longer, with the consequence that the efficacy of recompression may be compromised and impaired.

As a further consequence the therapeutical procedures are applied at different stages of the same illness, characterized by a multi-factorial evolution.

Thus, a reliable comparative analysis of the therapeutical results becomes delicate and risky, as it deals with different procedures applied to heterogeneous conditions. Answering these pending questions will only be possible after further studies conducted with adequately modified approaches.

WHICH ACUTE INDICATIONS FOR HYPERBARIC OXYGEN THERAPY?

I - General

- Hyperbaric Facilities accepting emergency indications in potentially Intensive Care requiring patients should be hospital based and located in or immediately near-by the hospital Intensive or Emergency Care Department.

- Technical competence and personal skills at the hyperbaric facility must be adequate and such that any potential accident—derangement—problem will not be likely to interfere with the decision to accept an indication for Hyperbaric Oxygen Therapy.
- Hyperbaric Oxygen Therapy must be seen as part of a therapeutical continuum, without any interruption of the chain of treatment. It cannot be considered as an isolated treatment modality.
- Hyperbaric Oxygen Therapy implies the administration of oxygen under pressures not lower than 2 ATA and for times not shorter than 60 minutes.

II - Carbon Monoxide (CO) Intoxication

- Carbon monoxide intoxications must be treated with normobaric oxygen as a first aid treatment (Type 1 recommendation).
- Carbon monoxide intoxications presenting with consciousness alterations, clinical neurological, cardiac, respiratory, or psychological signs must be treated with Hyperbaric Oxygen Therapy, whatever the carboxyhemoglobin value may be (Type 1 recommendation).
- Pregnant women must be treated with Hyperbaric Oxygen Therapy, whatever the clinical situation and the carboxyhemoglobin value may be (Type 1 recommendation).
- In minor carbon monoxide intoxication cases there is a choice between normobaric oxygen therapy for at least 12 hours and HBO. Until the results of randomized studies are available HBO remains optional (Type 3 recommendation).

III - Gas Embolism

- Whatever is the symptomology of air embolism, Hyperbaric Oxygen Therapy is strongly recommended; the minimal treatment pressure must not be lower than 3 ATA (Type 1 recommendation).

IV - Anaerobic or Mixed Bacterial Necrotizing Soft Tissue Infections

- Hyperbaric Oxygen Therapy is strongly recommended in the treatment of anaerobic or mixed bacterial necrotising soft tissue infections (myonecrosis, necrotizing fasciitis, necrotizing cellulitis, etc.). HBO therapy should be integrated in a treatment protocol comprising adequate surgical and antibiotic therapy (Type 1 recommendation). The sequential order for HBO, antibiotics, and surgery is a function of the conditions of the patient, of the surgical possibilities, and of hyperbaric oxygen availability.

V - Acute Soft Tissue Ischemia

- HBO is recommended in limb crush trauma and reperfusion post-traumatic syndromes (Type 2 recommendation).
- HBO is optional in post-vascular surgery reperfusion syndromes (Type 3 recommendation).

- HBO is recommended in compromised skin grafts and myo-cutaneous flaps (Type 2 recommendation).
- HBO is optional in the re-implantation of traumatically amputated limbs (Type 3 recommendation).
- In every case the measurement of transcutaneous oxygen pressure is recommended as an index for the definition of the indication and of the evolution of treatment (Type 2 recommendation).

VI - Post-anoxic Encephalopathy

- HBO is optional for the treatment of cerebral anoxia (Type 3 recommendation).

VII - Burns

- HBO is strongly recommended when the burn is associated to carbon monoxide intoxication (Type 1 recommendation).
- In the absence of a carbon monoxide intoxication, HBO is optional when burns exceed 20% of body surface and are of 2nd degree or more (Type 3 recommendation).
- If Burned areas are less than 20% of body surface, HBO therapy is not advised.

VIII - Sudden Deafness

- HBO, together with other treatment measures, such as hemodilution, is recommended in sudden deafness (Type 2 recommendation). However, the respective efficacy of the two treatment modalities is not known at the moment.

IX - Ophthalmological Disorders

- HBO is optional in acute ophthalmological ichemia (Type 3 recommendation).

WHICH CHRONIC INDICATIONS NEED HYPERBARIC OXYGEN THERAPY AS AN ADJUNCTIVE TREATMENT?

I - Ischemic lesions (ulcers or gangene) without surgically treatable arterial lesions or after vascular surgery

- In the diabetic patient, the use of HBO is recommended in the presence of a chronic critical ischemia as defined by the European Consensus Conference on Critical Ischemia, if transcutaneous oxygen pressure readings under hyperbaric conditions (2.5 ATA, 100% Oxygen) are higher than 100 mmHg (Type 2 recommendation).

- In the arteriosclerotic patient the use of HBO is recommended in case of a chronic critical ischemia, if transcutaneous oxygen pressure readings under hyperbaric conditions (2.5 ATA, 100% Oxygen) are higher than 50 mmHg (Type 2 recommendation).
- Chronic Critical Ischemia: periodical pain, persistent at rest, needing regular analgesic treatment for more than two weeks, or ulceration or gangrene of foot or toes with ankle systolic pressure <50 mmHg in the non-diabetic or toes systolic pressure <30 mmHg in the diabetic (Second European Consensus on Critical Ischemia: Circulation 1991, 84, IV, 1-26).

II - Radionecrotic lesions

- HBO is strongly recommended in osteoradionecrosis (Type 1 recommendation). The most frequently adopted treatment protocol implies 20 HBO sessions pre-surgery and 10 sessions post-surgery.
- HBO is strongly recommended as a preventive treatment for dental extraction in irradiated or osteonecrotic bone (Type 1 recommendation). The most frequently adopted treatment protocol implies 20 HBO sessions pre-extraction and 10 sessions post-extraction.
- HBO is strongly recommended in soft tissue radionecrosis (Type 1 recommendation), except in radionecrotic lesions of the intestine where HBO has to be considered only as optional (Type 3 recommendation).
- HBO is optional in spinal cord radionecrosis (Type 3 recommendation).

III - Osteomyelitis

- HBO is recommended in chronic refractory osteomyelitis defined as osteomyelitic lesions persisting more than six weeks after adequate antibiotic treatment and at least one surgery (Type 2 recommendation).
- In cranial (except the mandible) and sternal osteomyelitis, HBO should be started simultaneously with antibiotics and surgical treatment (Type 2 recommendation).

IV - Other Indications

- Multiple sclerosis and pigmentous retinitis are not recognized indications for Hyperbaric Therapy at the moment, but various research protocols are currently underway.

COMMENTS

Only the indications generally accepted by the leading representatives of the discipline have been discussed.

Other Consensus Conferences, dedicated to the evaluation of certain particular aspects of the treatment of a disease for which HBO is already used or to new indications, seem already necessary. In fact the present recommendations should not prejudice the possible extension of the indications for Hyperbaric Oxygen Therapy. For example, chronic ophtalmological disorders, foeto-placentar insufficiencies, certain mycotic and parasital infections, peripheral arteriopathies, certain dermatological disorders, spinal and cerebral contusions are part of the HBO indications for which the evaluation is being currently conducted.

WHICH SAFETY REGULATIONS FOR THE DESIGN AND USE OF MEDICAL HYPERBARIC CHAMBERS AND OF MEDICAL EQUIPMENT FOR HYPERBARIC USE?

I - Minimal prerequisites for the design of medical hyperbaric chambers and for medical equipment aimed at the emergency or intensive treatment of a patient under hyperbaric conditions

- Conscience troubles, respiratory insufficiency, hemodynamic instability should not constitute an obstacle to the administration of Hyperbaric Oxygen Therapy (Type 1 recommendation).
- Accepting a patient for hyperbaric treatment, in a situation requiring emergency or intensive care treatment, requires that the following is assured, even under hyperbaric conditions: administration of parenteral perfusion treatment, hemodynamic monitoring and treatment, respiratory monitoring, possibility to assure adequate ventilation to respiratory compromised patients, hyperbaric oxygen effect monitoring, with special regard to transcutaneous oxygen pressure monitoring (Type 1 recommendation).
- In order to minimize the risk of fire, no medical equipment and instrumentation should be used in a hyperbaric chamber unless:
  - it has specifically been designed for this use and its safety has been adequately controlled
  - it has been specifically modified for use under hyperbaric conditions and its safety has been adequately controlled
  - the equipment and instrumentation not specifically adapted for hyperbaric use is kept outside the hyperbaric chamber and only parts of the equipment, such as electrodes and probes, are used inside, with appropriate and safety-controlled trans-hull penetrations to assure electrical connection (Type 1 recommendation)
- Mechanical ventilation under hyperbaric conditions requires special adaptations. No specific ventilator which can assure all the possibly required ventilatory modes and can be considered ideal for hyperbaric use presently exists.

II - Minimal prerequisites for the design of medical hyperbaric chambers and for medical equipment for the treatment of chronic patients under hyperbaric conditions

- A minimal monitoring capability, adequate for the conditions of any given patient, is necessary for the administration of Hyperbaric Oxygen Therapy to chronic patients. In particular it is strongly recommended that the principal hemodynamic parameters are non-invasively monitored (Type 1 recommendation).

- Transcutaneous oxygen pressure monitoring, intratissular oxygen pressure monitoring, Laser Doppler flow monitoring are presently considered as the most valid monitoring instruments to evaluate the efficacy of hyperbaric oxygen therapy (Type 2 recommendation).

III - Use of oxygen-pressurized hyperbaric chambers

- Their use is possible, but only if very stringent safety measures are adopted (Type 1 recommendation).

IV - Safety recommendations to be foreseen at European Union level

- Hyperbaric Chambers are considered as type II b instruments and are subject to directive 93.42CE of 14 June 1993 regarding medical instrumentation (Type 1 recommendation).

V - Safety regulations must be respected upon designing and using hyperbaric chambers and all medical instrumentation used in hyperbaric chambers

- Fire is the principal danger in hyperbaric conditions. Every preventive measure must be taken to avoid the risk:
  - the chamber must be built with non-burning materials
  - any greasy or oily materials must be avoided inside the chamber
  - the concentration of oxygen in the chamber must be kept at normal levels (outboard dumping systems, forced ventilation, etc.)
    (Type 1 recommendation)
- Maximized fire prevention must be adapted to any given case and hyperbaric installation, as no universally valid system exists at the moment.

WHICH INITIAL TRAINING AND WHICH CONTINUING EDUCATION FOR PERSONNEL EMPLOYED IN CLINICAL HYPERBARIC MEDICINE?

- The identity of the physical and physiological phenomena involved in both diving and hyperbaric medicine allows us to strongly recommend that a common training curriculum is designed for medical personnel involved in diving as well as in hyperbaric medicine. In this regard the European Committee for Hyperbaric Medicine and the Medical Sub-Committee of the European Diving Technology Committee are invited to cooperate (Type 1 recommendation).
- The respect of the European Standards concerning the initial training and the continuing education of personnel, contained in the attached document, is strongly recommended (Type 1 recommendation).
- The initial training should be planned in a modular fashion. Initial training of medical doctors should last not less than 200 hours. Certain teaching modules should be the same for diving medicine and hyperbaric medicine students. The first common module concerns safety. Other optional modules

should be added as a function of the specific orientation of the course towards diving or hyperbaric medicine. Hyperbaric Medicine candidates may come from different medical specialities, but should undergo a testing stage in hyperbaric medicine before starting the official training. The preparation and discussion of a thesis or paper in hyperbaric medicine is a necessary pre-requisite for the completion of the training. The final diploma must be released by an University (Type 1 recommendation).

- The Medical Director of a Hyperbaric Medicine Facility, being responsible for all the activities performed in the Center, should have adequate training in both hyperbaric medicine and enterprise management (Type 2 recommendation).
- It is strongly recommended that the European Committee for Hyperbaric Medicine and the Medical Sub-Committee of the European Diving Technology Committee closely cooperate with the goal to constitute a European Authority to control and validate training in diving and hyperbaric medicine (Type 1 recommendation).
- There should be at least one Training Center for each European linguistic area (Type 1 recommendation).
- The possibility to create a European Baromedical Institute should be considered.

WHICH RESEARCH TO EXPECT AND PLAN FOR THE NEXT FIVE YEAR PERIOD?

- It is strongly recommended that quality research protocols are put in place to assure and reinforce the credibility of hyperbaric oxygen therapy (Type 1 recommendation).
- It is strongly recommended that doctors operating in hyperbaric centers are trained to basic and clinical research methods (Type 1 recommendation).
- It is strongly recommended that hyperbaric facilities and specialists associate into multidisciplinary teams (Type 1 recommendation).
- It is strongly recommended that information and personnel exchange policies between hyperbaric facilities are implemented (Type 1 recommendation).
- It is strongly recommended that a network of multicentric clinical research is implemented (Type 1 recommendation).
- It is strongly recommended that a structure for coordination and information is created (Type 1 recommendation).
- It is strongly recommended that Reference Centers as well as a European Ethical and Research Commission are constituted, within the European Committee for Hyperbaric Medicine (Type 1 recommendation).

COMMENTS

The implementation of these recommendations suggest the need to create a European Ethical and Research Commission as well as of a Coordination and Information Structure with the following primary goals:

1. establishment of a directory of centers and teams involved in Hyperbaric Medicine Research
2. establishment of a network of consultants (epidemiologists, methodologists, engineers, etc.)
3. organization of seminars and workshops dedicated to clinical research training
4. coordination of Reference Centers, after approval of the same by the European Ethical and Research Commission (EERC)
5. monitoring and assuring the achievement of the planned goals, as defined by the EERC

SECTION I – PART 2

The 2nd European Consensus
Conference on Hyperbaric Medicine

The 2nd European Consensus Conference on

Treatment of Decompression Accidents in Recreational Diving

Section I – Part 2
May 9–11, 1996—Marseille, France

ORGANISED BY THE EUROPEAN COMMITTEE FOR HYPERBARIC MEDICINE
F. Wattel, President—Lille, France

CONTENTS

SCIENTIFIC COMMITTEE

B. Gardette, Marseille (France)   JM. Sainty, Marseille (France)
A. Marroni, Ancona (Italy)   J. Seyer, Rouen (France)
D. Mathieu, Lille (France)   F. Wattel, Lille (France)

JURY CONSENSUS

P. Pelaia, Trieste (Italy), President
D. Bakker, Amsterdam (Netherlands)   JM. Meliet, Toulon (France)
P. Carli, Paris (France)   G. Oriani, Milano (Italy)
D. Elliot, London (United Kingdom)   M. Sarrias, Barcelona (Spain)
B. Grandjean, Ajaccio (France)   PH. Unger, Genève (Switzerland)
M. Lamy, Liège (Belgium)   U. Van Laak, Kiel (Germany)

EXPERTS

A. Barthelemy, Marseille (France)   J. Ross, Aberdeen (United Kingdom)
E. Bergmann, Toulon (France)   W. Sterk, Zindwolde (Netherlands)
A. Brubakk, Trondheim (Norway)   J. Wendling, Vienne (Switzerland)
J. Desola, Barcelona (Spain)   J. Wolkiwiez, Nice (France)
R. Moon, Durham (USA)   D. Zannini, Genova (Italy)

UNDER THE AEGIS

- Université de la Méditerranée
- Assistance Publique de Marseille
- Faculté de Médecine de Marseille
- Institut de Médecine Navale du Service de Santé des Armées
- DAN Europe
- Fédération Française d'Etudes et de Sports Sous-Marins

SPONSORED BY

- Société de Physiologie et de Médecine Subaquatique et Hyperbare
- European Underwater and Baromedical Society
- Undersea and Hyperbaric Medical Society
- Societa Italiana di Medicina Subaquea e Iperbarica
- Societa Italiana di Anestesia Anagesia Rianimazione e Terapia Intensiva
- Comite coordinator de Centros de medicina Hiperbarica
- British Hyperbaric Association
- Nederlandse Vereniging voor Duikgeneeskunde
- Gesellschaft für Tauch und Uberdruckmedizin
- Société Suisse de Médecine Subaquatique et Hyperbare

WITH THE PARTICIPATION OF

- Centre Océanographique de Marseille
- COMEX
- UCPA Niolon

TREATMENT OF RECREATIONAL DIVING DECOMPRESSION ACCIDENTS
Methodology of the Conferences

The scope of the Second European Consensus Conference on Hyperbaric Medicine was to establish an agreement on the treatment of decompression accidents in recreational diving. More than 200 specialists from 17 different countries participated at this conference. An international jury, assisted by a panel of 10 experts was called to formulate recommendations that could answer to the questions selected by the Scientific committee of the Conference (D.J. Bakker, A. Marroni, D. Mathieu, G. Oriani), after each of those has been discussed and debated during general session.

To reach a consensus between European Hyperbarists on these questions and to facilitate the work of the jury, the Scientific Committee elaborated instructions for jury members and experts.

It was proposed that jury members note and grade relevant arguments and recommendations made by each expert. It was suggested that the same scale than in consensus conference in other medical disciplines would be used to assess the weight of their recommendations:

A : Recommendation based on at least 2 concordant, large, double-blind, controlled randomized studies with no or only weak methodological bias.

B : Recommendation based on double-blind controlled, randomized studies but with methodological bias, or concerning only small sample, or only a single study.

C : Recommendation based only on uncontrolled studies: (historic control group, cohort study).

As large scale double-blind controlled, randomized studies are often lacking in HBO Medicine, it was suggested that facts, arguments, and recommendations presented at the conference would be divided in three groups and graded as follows:

- Basic studies (tissular, cellular or subcellular level)
  4. strong evidence of beneficial action
  3. evidence of beneficial action
  2. weak evidence of beneficial action
  1. no evidence of beneficial action or methodological or interpretation bias preclude any conclusion

- Animal studies with control group
  4. strong evidence of beneficial action
  3. evidence of beneficial action
  2. weak evidence of beneficial action
  1. no evidence of beneficial action or methodological or interpretation bias preclude any conclusion

- Human studies
  4. strong evidence of beneficial action (equivalent to A in the previously exposed classification)
  3. evidence of beneficial action (equivalent to B in the previously exposed classification)
  2. weak evidence of beneficial action (equivalent to C in the previously exposed classification)
  1. no evidence of beneficial action (Case report only) or methodological or interpretation bias preclude any conclusion

Considering these grading scales, the jury elaborated his recommendations according to 3 levels of priority:

- Type 1 recommendation
  The jury considers that the implementation of this type of recommendation will be of critical importance for the future knowledge about decompression accident or, in case of clinical recommendation, for the final outcome of the patient.

- Type 2 recommendation
  The jury considers that the implementation of this type of recommendation will positively affect the future knowledge about decompression accident or, in case of clinical recommendation, will avoid serious consequences for the patient.

- Type 3 recommendation
  The jury considers that the implementation of the type of recommendation is optional.

SUMMARY OF THE RECOMMENDATIONS OF THE JURY

After listening to the presentations by the Experts and the following floor discussion, the Jury met to answer the six questions posed by the Conference Scientific Committee. The recommendations of the jury were based on the analysis of the clinical and experimental studies, according to the current scientific standards, although considering the limited data provided by the—otherwise scientifically correct—clinical studies presented. The jury evaluated the data on the basis of their general concordance and of the fact that the studies refer to several years of observations by many independent international groups. The jury also considered that its recommendations are intended as aimed at recreational diving performed in European waters and that, regarding logistical conditions of other diving sites that may not allow for the full respect of the Jury's recommendations, rather than downgrading the Jury's conclusions, its recommendations should be taken as a stimulus towards optimal diving safety worldwide.

IS THERE A DIFFERENCE BETWEEN RECREATIONAL AND COMMERCIAL DIVING DECOMPRESSION ACCIDENTS ?

Whatever the reasons and the methods for diving, they all share similar risk (the same decompression profile after the same dive will bring about the same decompression risk), similar physicpathology (a decompression accident will generate similar disorders in both circumstances) and similar results (if the delay to treatment is similar).

The observed differences between decompression accidents in the two types of diving essentially regard the degree of risk (fitness to dive, training, work load, depth, environment, safety standards) and the delay before treatment (symptom recognition, hyperbaric chamber availability).

The recommendations of the jury (Type 1 recommendation) are the following:
- implementing fitness to dive standards, both for recreational and commercial diving
- implementing an adequate classification of Decompression Accidents
- implementing a coordinated network for the collection and the retrospective analysis of data concerning decompression accidents
- improving the recreational diving safety standards to approach the current standards applied in commercial diving, with special regard to:
  - availability of oxygen on every dive site
  - availability of a recompression chamber within a delay of 4 hours
  - preparation of an emergency plan before any dive
- recreational divers should be trained, like commercial divers are, to recognize signs and symptoms of decompression accidents

HOW TO CLASSIFY DECOMPRESSION ACCIDENTS ?

Depending on the intended utilization objective, there are three possible ways to classify decompression accidents:
- immediate clinical use, need for rapid and efficient communication between divers and Emergency Services, on site first aid and medical evacuation of injured divers, data selection and availability for clinical studies
- epidemiological use for the retrospective analysis of data and of treatment results
- description of lesions based on Anatomo-Pathological observations

The recommendations of the Jury (Type 1 recommendation) are the following:
- immediate use classification should be simple and objective. The jury recommends that it is based on that adopted by the UHMS (Smith and Francis)
- epidemiological use classification for retrospective analysis should allow for the institution of a data bank collecting the observations from a great numbers of countries. To this purpose, harmonization between national classifications should be established in order to allow transcodification. This classification should:
  - be multithematic in its conception
  - include the type of diving, chronological data, clinical manifestations and a two-year follow-up

WHICH EXPERIMENTAL MODEL FOR DECOMPRESSION STUDIES ?

Considering the complexity of the question and the difficulty in conducting rigorous clinical studies with sufficient numbers of experimental subjects, the Jury agreed that animal studies are still needed.

The recommendations of the jury (Type 1 recommendation) are the following:
- experimental studies are necessary for more information on decompression accidents
- the variables to study are many and include:
  - the bubble phenomenon
  - central neurological manifestations
  - bone and skin manifestations
  - pulmonary disorders
  - cardio-vascular disorders
- as a general principle in vitro studies should precede in vivo studies, and ex vivo studies should be done before in vivo ones
- among the animal models so far used, small animals (rodents) do not seem to adequately reproduce the human observations. Among the larger animals, the dog is less and less used, sheep and ewes are mainly used for pulmonary studies, while the pig seems to be the animal that better reflects human reactions to decompression

Concerning methodology, the Jury recommends that studies:
- consider clinically significant parameters,
- consider experimental conditions, particularly when anesthesia modalities may interfere with the observations, and
- include a detailed description of the animal model in each published paper.

WHICH INITIAL RECOMPRESSION MODALITY ?

Decompression accidents are true medical emergencies that must benefit from treatment in specialized centers as soon as possible. A specialized center is considered as a hospital based facility, having not only a hyperbaric chamber but also a permanent and adequately trained medical and paramedical staff.

The victims of a decompression accident should be immediately directed from the site of the diving accident to the closest specialized center (Type 1 recommendation).

Minor decompression accidents (pain only) should be treated with oxygen recompression tables at 18 meters depth maximum (Type 1 recommendation).

Regarding more serious decompression accidents (neurological and vestibular accidents), the jury observed that there are presently two acceptable protocols, as neither one has been proved better by any scientifically valid study to date:
- oxygen recompression tables at 2.8 ATA (with possible extensions)
- hyperoxygenated breathing mixtures at 4.0 ATA

The choice between the two may depend on personal experience and on local logistics. However, under no circumstance the un-availability of one of the two accepted modalities should delay the treatment (Type 1 recommendation).

The jury also considered the following optional treatment modalities (type 3 recommendation):

- compression to 6 ATA in case of cerebral arterial gas embolism, with the condition that this compression is performed using hyperoxygenated mixtures and not compressed air and that the delay to treatment is not more than a few hours
- saturation treatment tables in case of persistent symptoms

Finally the jury recommends that:

- in water recompression should never be undertaken as the initial recompression modality for a decompression accident (Type 1 recommendation)
- all decompression accidents should be the object of a standardized recording method aimed at the creation of database for epidemiological studies (Type 1 recommendation)

WHICH FLUID REPLACEMENT PROTOCOL AND WHICH ROLE FOR DRUGS IN THE TREATMENT OF DECOMPRESSION ACCIDENTS?

Fluid Treatment

Victims of decompression accidents generally suffer from a certain degree of dehydration, depending on decreased fluid input, increased urinary output, capillary fluid leakage, and disorder-related relative hypovolemia.

The degree of dehydration should be evaluated:

- on site: history, dive conditions, thirst, clinical evaluation of neurological conditions, hemodynamics, temperature, vasoconstriction, dryness of mucosae, urinary output
- at hospital: urinary output, hemodynamics to include CVP, hematocrit, plasma proteins, and electrolytes

Recommended hydration protocols:

a) On site:

- oral hydration is recommended only if the patient is conscious (Type 1 recommendation)

Contra-indications to oral re-hydration are stringent and include:

- any consciousness abnormality
- nausea and vomiting
- suspected lesions of the gastro-intestinal tract

Oral re-hydration should be done with plain water, possibly with the addition of electrolytes but with no gas. The administered fluid should be cold if the patient is hyperthermic. Sugar is not recommended. The amount of fluids administered should be adapted to the patient's thirst and acceptance.

- venous re-hydration should be preferred if a physician is present. Recommended procedures are as follows:
    - use a peripheral venous catheter (18 gauge) and preferably Ringer Lactate as the infusion fluid. Glucose containing solutions are not recommended.
    - the addition of colloids can be considered if large quantities of fluids are needed. Recommended colloids, in order of preference, are starch-containing solutions, gelatines, haptene added dextranes (Type 3 recommendation).

b) At the hospital:
    - intravenous rehydration is recommended while controlling the routinary physiological parameters: urinary output, hemodynamics, CVP, standard laboratory tests.

Drug Treatment

a) Strongly recommended (Type 1 recommendation):
    - normobaric oxygen

The administration of normobaric oxygen allows for the treatment of hypoxemia and favours the elimination of inert gas bubbles. Oxygen should be administered with an oro-nasal mask with reservoir bag, at a minimal flow rate of 15 l/min, or with CPAP mask circuit, using either a free flow regulator or a demand valve, in such a way to obtain a FiO_2 close to 1.

In case of respiratory distress, shock or coma, the patient should be intubated and ventilated with a $FiO_2 = 1$ and setting the ventilator to avoid pressure and volume trauma. Normobaric oxygen should be continued until hyperbaric recompression is started (with a maximum of 6 hours when the FiO_2 is 1).

b) Recommended (Type 2 recommendation):
    - any necessary drug for the support treatment of an intensive care patient (adequate first aid kit)

c) Optional (Type 3 recommendation):
    - on site
        - any way to prevent hyperthermia
        - aspirin: 500 mg orally in the adult patient (contra-indications similar to oral re-hydration)
    - at the hospital: use drugs having no significant collateral effects, such as:
        - aspirin: 500 mg if not already administered or contraindicated
        - lidocaine
        - low dose heparin (avoid complete decoagulation)
        - steroids, calcium channel blockers, antioxydants

WHICH TREATMENT PROTOCOL FOR PERSISTENT SYMPTOMS AFTER THE INITIAL RECOMPRESSION?

The Jury concluded that there are no scientifically valid data to allow for a recommended approach to this issue.

More studies are necessary as well as the adoption of standardized evaluation methods. Concerning spinal cord injuries, a specific scoring system (such as the ASIA scale) is recommended for pre- and post treatment evaluation and during the two-year follow up.

Randomized prospective studies are needed to better evaluate the efficacy of hyperbaric oxygen therapy and of rehabilitation before any protocol can be proposed or recommended. However, in analogy with any other neurological injury, rehabilitation should be started as soon as possible (Type 1 recommendation).

Hyperbaric oxygen treatment is recommended to a maximum of 10 treatment sessions after the initial recompression, in combination and during rehabilitation therapy. The continuation of HBO therapy can be accepted if objective improvement is observed under pressure during the hyperbaric treatment sessions (Type 3 recommendation).

NOTES

EPIDEMIOLOGY, SYMPTOMATOLOGY, AND TREATMENT RESULTS OF DECOMPRESSION INCIDENTS IN PROFESSIONAL DIVING AND CAISSON WORK

W. Sterk, I. Nashimoto, R. Takashima, T. Mochizuki

In The Netherlands we have about 20 to 30 cases of decompression illness per year. In a population of about 15 million people this makes a very low incidence. Although all these people can be considered as exposed to pressure changes, these changes due to weather variations or commercial flying are not sufficient to cause decompression illness (DCI). About 40,000 persons in our population are involved in diving or caisson work, which creates sufficient pressure changes to induce the risk of DCI. Counting only these people, still the incidence is not even one per mil. However, many of these people are only diving occasionally, for instance during a holiday in tropical surroundings. There are about 3,000 professional divers in Holland, but also these are not always diving regularly or to significant depths. We do not know the magnitude of the hard core of recreational divers, diving every weekend, even in winter time, but let us assume that the total number of regular divers is about 3,000; then the incidence of DCI would be 1%. This is by many considered as a too high risk (Vann and Thalmann 1993). We do not know if the frequent divers produce the most cases of DCI. If we look only at the probabilistic nature of DCI, which by the way is the reason that we prefer to speak of decompression "incident" rather than "accident," this is likely to be true. However, most of the cases of DCI treated at the Diving Medical Centre of our Navy are recreational divers. It seems reasonable to assume that even the sports diving die-hearts dive less frequently than many professional divers. On the other hand, the risk of DCI is not only a matter of bottom pressure and time, but also of the decompression procedures as well as many environmental and individual factors.

The above mentioned trivialities indicate that many more data are necessary than a collection of cases of DCI when considering epidemiology. Apart from the numerator we should also know the denominator, which means data of dive and decompression profiles, divers, and environmental circumstances. In 1990 we had a workshop on the collection and analysis of such data (Sterk and Hamilton, 1991), where we made many plans how to achieve this in the future. However, nothing much happened after that in this respect.

Still, the collection of cases of DCI is also important. It can tell us about symptomatology and treatment results. From such data bases we know now that the division of DCI in Type I or minor, and Type II or serious manifestations, is an oversimplification. Therefore, Sykes et al. (1994) have proposed a more descriptive approach to the decompression illnesses. This is valuable for treatment considerations and looking at treatment results, but makes epidemiological investigation more difficult. Therefore, in this presentation we will still use the terms Type II or I for indicating more or less serious cases of DCI.

EPIDEMIOLOGY IN PROFESSIONAL DIVING

Published dive and decompression data for the North Sea area are still relatively scarce. The survey of Shields and Lee (1986) on commercial dives in the UK sector during 1982 and 1983 revealed 79 cases of DCI in nearly 26,000 dives, an incidence of 3 per mil. Decompression tables used are almost exclusively U.S. Navy standard air tables. Shields and Lee observed that the frequency of DCI increased with the severity of hyperbaric stress, in terms of the depth and time of the dive, and they considered this the most powerful factor involved. Their data, obtained from dive logs, show a six to four distribution of Type I against Type II at all depths, and a reversal of this proportion for all dives with bottom times longer than 90 minutes, irrespective of depth. This finding became the reason for the Department of Energy to limit bottom times. The results of the 1982/83 report were confirmed in the report of Shields et al. (1990), dealing with commercial dives in the UK sector from 1982 to 1988. In total the data from 126,980 dive logs were entered into the survey, including 333 episodes of DCI, so an overall incidence of 2.6 per mil and a Type I Type II ratio of 6 to 4. Limiting the bottom times did indeed bring down the incidence of DCI. In 1988, only 17 cases of DCI were found in over 17,000 dives, but 6 were classified as Type I and 11 as Type II, i.e., a four to six ratio.

Results from the Netherlands Diving Centre (NDC) database, consisting of data from Dutch diving companies, showed a different picture. The decompression tables used were all based on the computational model that generated the Dutch NDC tables. Here, the choice was made to make decompression more conservative instead of limiting bottom times. The series published in 1991 (Sterk and Hamilton) consisted of 25,902 dives, many of them much longer than in the UK 1982/83 report, with 11 cases of DCI. Of these cases, 8 were of Type I and 3 Type II, or a 7 to 3 ratio. There was no relationship between the incidence of DCI and the decompression stress in terms of dive depth and time. The differences with the findings of Shields and Lee in a comparable sample size are remarkable. The reason could be that NDC decompression tables are more conservative than the U.S. Navy air tables used in the UK. Logically, decompression stress is not only defined by dive depth and time, but also by the decompression procedure.

The trend of the NDC database was confirmed in the years thereafter. In the years from 1990 until now 10 more cases of DCI were reported, with 27,259 dives added to the database and some 10,000 data waiting to be included. Due to a lack of funding, this has to be done in spare time and may therefore take a while. Still we can say that in well over 60,000 dives we had in total 21 cases of DCI as shown in Figure 1, 17 of them of Type I and 4 of Type II, a 8 to 2 ratio. It should be noted that DCI, even of Type II, did also occur well within the no-stop diving range.

In 1994 NDC decided to drop the obligation for the users of the tables to report all dive data and to allow them to do this on a voluntary basis. This decision was made since they thought over 50,000 data sufficient to demonstrate the reliability of the tables. This of course is a wrong conclusion. In the first place an overall incidence of DCI does not tell the whole story. In fact it is the incidence per single decompression schedule, in terms of depth and time, that counts. Therefore, conclusions about the reliability of

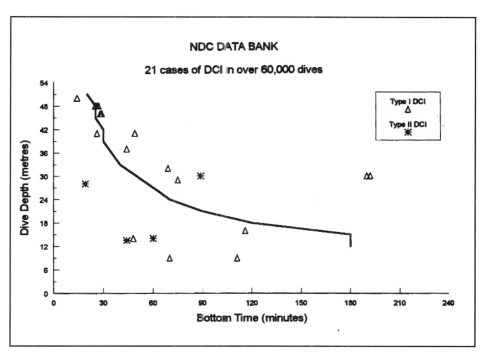

Figure 1. Cases of DCI plotted in terms of depth and time of the dives. The continuous line represents the Department of Energy (DOE) bottom time limits according to DSM 7/86 and 5/88.

decompression tables require many more data. Furthermore, changes in diving circumstances or diving populations may cause tables to fail that were reliable in the past. Among the many factors that may facilitate the occurrence of DCI, also the dive history as well as mistakes in following the procedures may play a role.

In 1992 we had a small cluster of 4 cases of DCI at a particular job using surface decompression, which caused concern. Figure 2 shows all cases of DCI after surface decompression at that time, including this cluster. It displays the number of dives in the database at the schedules at stake, as well as the sequence number of the event of DCI; the statistical evaluation regarding table reliability was tested using an open sequential method described by Homer and Weathersby (1985). From this test it can be concluded that statistically there was no reason to assume that our demand of a DCI incidence of less than 0.5% was violated. However, this cluster of DCI made us also look into the dive history and it appeared that in 3 of the 4 cases the procedures were not followed properly in preceding dives and or the dive that caused DCI. This demonstrates that a continuous feedback of all dive and decompression data, as well as all cases of DCI, promotes diving safety by enabling to analyze factors that may be a cause of DCI. Although the collection of data from dive logs may give valuable information, it is a clumsy way to do it. With modern computer technology it should be possible that every diver has his personal black box, which records all pressure—time events as well as gas switches. Apart from diving, also flying or mountaineering could be detected from such recorders, and related to possible pressure diseases. This would be much better than the online dive profile recorders that at present tend to turn up in North Sea diving.

date	table time minutes	table depth metres	symptoms DCI Type I	DCI Type II	treat-ment	residual symptoms	number of dives on schedule	temporary sequence number
25/09/1989	30	51	pain shoulder	-	table 5	no	264	119
27/09/1989	30	51	pain l. Arm	-	table 5	no	264	138
12/09/1991	40	42	pain r. Elbow	-	table 5	no	36	15 **
10/05/1992	50(70)*	42(33)*	skin abdomen	-	table 5 + 6	red spots	55 (191)*	54 (167)*
13/05/1992	50	39	pain both knees	-	table 5 + 6a	no	20	18
10/07/1992	70	33	pain elbow	-	table 5	no	191	>191 **
11/07/1992	80	30	skin breast	-	table 5	no	179	>179 **

Figure 2. All cases of DCI, using surface decompressing according to the NDC tables, reported until August 1992. * symptoms started already at previous dive, with table time and depth within ( ) ** dives not reported to database up till now.

Although these online recorders can accurately log the events at the diving site, it does not follow the diving history of free-lancers that move from site to site, nor does it record flying after diving. It is hoped that the introduction of a personal black box for professional divers will be enforced by future diving regulations.

EPIDEMIOLOGY IN CAISSON WORK

At the UHMS workshop "What is Bends?" in 1990, Nashimoto (1991) gave an extensive overview of the occurrence of DCI in compressed air work in Japan at 8 construction sites. Maximum working pressure was around 4 bar, but at one site even up to 5 bar. In total 6,447 decompressions were involved, using Japanese air tables, firmly prescribed by law, and based on the RN standard air tables 11. This ended up in a total of 253 cases of DCI, ranging from 0 to 130 per working site. The overall incidence rate was therefore 3.9%, with a clear prevalence of Type I, being 216 cases. Nashimoto suggested that long exposure to moderate pressure would exert an influence upon this prevalence of Type I DCI. However, this is not supported by the results from the NDC database. It is very likely, that also the dive profile, the decompression table used, and the delay before treatment may be of importance in this respect.

Last year, there was a caisson work at Nagoya, Japan, with a maximum working pressure of 5.5 bar. The work was performed by remotely controlled robots, but still workers and engineers had to go down for maintenance, repairs and finally disassembly of the machinery. To avoid nitrogen narcosis in the compressed air filled caisson, the workers breathed trimix, consisting of 50%N2-25%He-25%O2, by full face mask at working pressures greater than 4 bar. Working times ranged from 42 to 120 min. Decompressions were carried out according to Sterk's tables. During decompression the workers switched to ambient air breathing and began oxygen breathing in 20 min cycles interrupted by 5 min air breaks from 2.2 bar up to the surface. In 470 cases out of the total of 1,055 man exposures on trimix, precordial bubble detection was performed during the first 2 hours after decompression using an ultrasound pulse Doppler detector. Details of this research will be presented elsewhere, but we found a clear correlation between work rate and bubble grade. In total 9 cases of DCI were reported, only 1 being Type II (Figure 3). At least in 3 cases there were gross violations of the proper procedures, particularly in the case ending up with neurological DCI. Here, the worker was decompressed directly to the surface, passing all prescribed stops, because of a mistake of an inexperienced chamber operator. When this was discovered after several minutes, the worker was recompressed to the pressure of the first stop and thereafter recompressed according to the normal table. But even in the other cases, some minor deviations from the supposed decompression profile were recorded. In contrast to most diving jobs, pressure-time recording is a routine in caisson work, which allows more accurate analysis. However, deviations in gas switches may still go unnoticed, despite video control and elaborate notes in the supervisor's log. Furthermore, recording DCI depends largely on the cooperation of the workers.

At this job, these reports reached us only because there was a doctor at the site, performing the measurements for our research, who gained the trust of the workers and

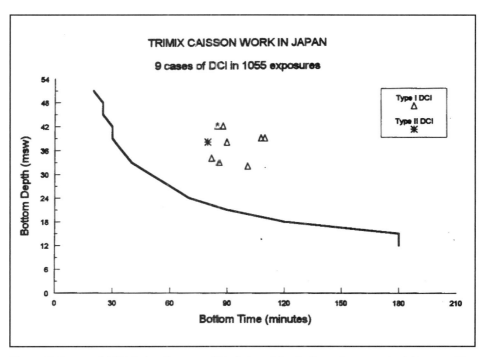

Figure 3. Cases of DCI during the use of trimix breathing in the caisson work at Nagoya. The continuous line represents the DOE bottom time limits.

had no formal ties with the construction company. It appeared that the caisson workers, employed by a subcontractor at the bottom of the complex organization ladder of companies that deal with such large projects in Japan, were very reluctant to admit to their boss that they suffered from DCI. They said it could mean they would lose their job. Therefore, they all refused recompression treatment as proposed by our colleague at the job site. Some way or another they came away with it, at least on the short run, even the case with clear neurological DCI. In the hours or days after the occurrence of symptoms, they all became symptom free without treatment, but while still continuing their work in the caisson. Maybe the conservative decompressions have helped to cure these symptoms.

We fear that under-reporting of DCI is not only happening at compressed air work in Japan, but also elsewhere and possibly also in professional diving. For commercial diving in the North Sea, we have been stressing the importance of prevention and proper treatment of DCI, particularly in the last decades. Divers received proper training, acquired knowledge of diving physiology, and were bound to governmental rules. A golden rule imposed by diving doctors was "in case of doubt if there is DCI, treat it as such." However, we doctors were also concerned about the possible danger of returning to dive after suffering from DCI. Depending on the policy of the doctor that treats DCI, and of course the seriousness of the case, it may take days to as much as 6 weeks before such a diver is declared fit for diving again.

Particularly for free-lance divers this might be a reason not to report minor symptoms. But also other reasons can be thought of, such as a waiting helicopter at the end of an offshore term.

SYMPTOMATOLOGY AND TREATMENT RESULTS

In caisson work there seems to be a clear prevalence for minor symptoms of DCI like limb pain and skin manifestations. But also in professional diving, provided more conservative decompression tables are used, this seems to be the case as demonstrated by the NDC database results. Still, the shore based institutes that treat DCI see much more Type II than Type I cases, particularly in recreational divers. Amongst other reasons, this could be due to the delay between onset of symptoms and treatment, where pain-only could turn into neurological manifestations as well. By now it is clear that the division in minor (Type I) and serious (Type II) DCI is highly artificial.

During the workshop "What is bends" (Nashimoto and Lanphier, 1991) it was concluded that talking about limb bends might have been confused by addressing different types of pain. Therefore, Sterk (1993) constructed a pain questionnaire to investigate the modality and intensity of pain in DCI. Although these pain questionnaires were made available in various languages, only two British diving medical centres responded so far. From the small number of completed questionnaires it became clear that "pain-only" limb bends is hardly seen in those institutes. The majority showed clear neurological involvement. This raises the question if the limb bends diagnosed and treated in the field could not be, at least in part, manifestations of pain from neurological origin. In the attempt to achieve a more descriptive approach to DCI, the term "limb pain" (Sykes et al., 1994) is not sufficient to describe the pain involved. The phenomenon of pain in DCI has to be investigated in more detail, for which the mentioned pain questionnaire seems to be a useful tool.

Finally some words about treatment results. In professional diving, there is always a compression chamber at site. Therefore, most cases of DCI are treated promptly and nowadays usually with USN Table 6, sometimes with extensions. The use of USN Table 5 for the treatment of DCI has been abandoned and serves only as a backup in cases of decompression irregularities. All cases of DCI in the NDC database were symptom free after treatment. For the cases treated in diving medical centres, there is usually a delay and results may be different.

Nevertheless, the cases sampled with the pain questionnaires were also treated with USN Table 6 and were symptom free except for one. Here, repeated treatment was necessary, but still residual neurological symptoms remained.

In caisson work, at least in Japan, DCI is under-reported and goes sometimes untreated, as during the trimix caisson work at Nagoya. Still, the workers got away with it. This raises once more the question: if skin bends and "niggles" do need recompression treatment. Also it questions whether we should prohibit divers, successfully treated for DCI, to return to work without much delay. Our safety rules, although with the best intentions, might make them reluctant to report minor symptoms.

REFERENCES

1. Homer LD, Weathersby PK, 1985. Statistical aspects of the design and testing of decompression tables. Undersea Biomed Res 12(3); 239-249.
2. Nashimoto I, 1991. Epidemiology of bends: The actual situation in japan. In: Nashimoto I, Lanphier EH, eds., 1991. What is bends? UHMS Publ. 80(Bends) 06/01/91. Bethesda, Md: Undersea Hyperbaric Medical Soc; 25-33.
3. Nashimoto I, Lanphier EH, eds., 1991. What is bends? UHMS Publ. 80(Bends) 06/01/91. Bethesda, Md: Undersea Hyperbaric Medical Soc.
4. Shields TG, Lee WB, 1986. The incidence of decompression sickness arising from commercial offshore air-diving operations in the UK sector of the North Sea during 1982/83. Hyperbaric Medicine Unit. Robert Gordon's Institute of Technology.
5. Shields TG, Duff PM, Wilcock SE, 1990. Decompression sickness from commercial offshore air-diving operations on the UK continental shelf during 1982 to 1988. Department of Energy (Giles R). Robert Gordon's Institute of Technology.
6. Sterk W, Hamilton RW, eds., 1991. Operational dive and decompression data: Collection and analysis. EUBS Report (DATA)17-8-90. Amsterdam: Foundation Hyperbaric Med.
7. Sterk W, 1993. What is pain in bends pain? In: Reinertsen RE, Brubakk AO, Bolstad G, eds. Proceedings XIXth Annual Meeting of European Undersea Biomedical Society. Sintef Unimed, Trondheim, Norway: 274-277.
8. Sykes JJW, Smith DJ, Francis TJR, 1994. A descriptive approach to the decompression illnesses. In: Jardine FM, McCallum RI, eds. Engineering and health in compressed air work. CIRIA book 16. London, E&FN Spon; 381-384.
9. Vann RD, Thalmann ED, 1993. Decompression physiology and practice. In: Bennett PB, Elliott, DH, eds. The Physiology and Medicine of Diving. 4th ed. London: W B Saunders Co; 376-432.

EPIDEMIOLOGY, CLINICAL MANIFESTATION AND TREATMENT RESULTS OF RECREATIONAL DIVING ACCIDENTS

Jürg Wendling, Bienne, Switzerland

The best treatment procedures for dive accidents are still to be defined. The professional and recreational diving community has to a certain extent developed its own approach to face the problems of diving incidents. A comparative review of data concerning this topic can help to define the common denominators and to get to a consensus on how to manage dive accidents in general.

EPIDEMIOLOGY

To investigate the incidence and prevalence of diving accidents related to the diver's population or total population of a geographical area we first need to define the elements. The term "diving accident" includes many other pathologies which are not related to decompression, and as the most dangerous and most specific diving accident is the decompression illness (DCI), we try to select those cases from the evaluable statistics. The problematic of the DCI definition will be discussed later in detail. The main difficulty to start on is the definition of the diving population in relation to an accident statistics. As there is no official regulation for the collection of diving accident data nor do recreational divers have to be certified and registered, the exact relationship of accidents to divers is always a rough estimate.

In Switzerland we have for instance about 15'000 sports divers, about 700 active diving instructors, 20 scientific divers, 100 police divers and about 20 occupational divers (inshore air diving). The total number of diving accidents collected by DAN EUROPE Suisse are about 30 per year. I would estimate the total number to be about 50 cases. However we have to consider that more than 50% of our cases happened abroad, so they could be registered as well in the country of the dive holiday. As occupational divers dive several hours almost every day and more than 50% of the licensed recreational divers have probably less than 20 dives a year, the calculation of accidents per diver is of no value in this small population.

DAN EUROPE has the most accurate epidemiologically valid statistics actually available, which was presented by Marroni at the EUBS Congress in Istanbul 1994 (Fig. 1) (1). As DAN members have to indicate every year the number of dives they performed during the last 12 months, the total number of dives of the population of members per year is known. DAN members very probably use the DAN Hotline and rescue service in case of a diving accident so we can use the DAN accident statistics to get the incidence rate of dive accidents. For the period of 1989–93, during which 442'500 man dives were performed by DAN members (average 25 dives per year), 67 DCI cases (out of the 202 total cases) were collected. Figure 1 shows the incidence per dive which is 1 to 6'604 dives considering any dive profile, 1 to 40'228 dives for no decompression dives to depth of less than 30 meters. The average risk per diver and year corresponds quite well with the case number we have in Switzerland and that of many other reporters.

CLINICAL MANIFESTATION

What Pathology are we Looking For?

Diving accidents are not a well defined entity. For insurance companies they are just harmful events during the activity of diving, thus including minor and major trauma while going in or out of the water. Included are also incidents at the water surface including complications of sea sickness, near drowning, and so on. If we want to compare diving accident data of divers performing different activities as for instance sports divers and professional divers, we have to get data which are independent of those additional incidents. We need data about decompression related accidents excluding small ear barotraumas and other true diving related minor pathologies. For many years it was usual to distinguish DCS I, DCS II, and AGE as pathogenetically different entities, which were believed to need different treatment procedures. Today we know that even mild neurological symptoms need a full HBO Therapy as is used for the more serious symptoms. On the other hand many minor and localized symptoms change in character and intensity to become more serious ones. Thus the scientifically most valuable way to analyse decompression related accidents will be to use the descriptive method as proposed by Francis (2). Doing that, DAN USA notes the first symptoms and their onset time after surfacing against the total occurrence of the particular symptoms during the entire observation period of all the decompression illnesses in the Diving Accident Report (3). In this study the authors realized that not only the old classification does not reflect the severeness of an accident but that the emergency doctors treating the cases even misdiagnosed many cases. Final evaluation of the case studies showed that about 50% of the DCS I cases (which is 1/8 of all DCI cases) were found to have suffered from neurological complains during their observation period. Nine percent of the divers misdiagnosed as DCS I had even severe neurological symptoms. The group formation into mild and severe neurological and the others (including pain, skin, non-specific) is proposed as a better way to find outcome predicting factors (Fig. 2).

N = 17700 divers, 442500 dives	risk per diver	risk per dive
all dives (any depth or time)	0,38%	0,015%
< 30 meters and No-Deco dives	0,06%	0,0025%

Figure 1 : DCI risk in recreational divers. A statistical analysis of the DCI cases involving DAN EUROPE members in the 1989-1993 period (from Marroni [1]).

DCI Group N = 566	Symptoms	First Symptoms	Total Occurence
pain, skin, non specific S.	difficult breathing, pain, extreme fatigue, headache, itching, rash, restlessness, muscletwitch, hemoptysis	313 55.3 %	106 18.7 %
mild neurological S	numbness, dizziness, decreased skin sensation, personality change, weakness	205 36.2 %	307 54.2 %
severe neurological S	paralysis, visual disturbance, difficulty walking, semiconsciousness, bowel problem, speech disturbance, bladder problem, convulsions	25 4.4 %	153 27 %
ambiguous and others (excluded)	hearing loss, ringing in ears, stiffness, hot/cold flashes, cramps, swelling, pressure sensation, amnesia, fullness, muscle ache/soreness, euphoria, discoloration of skin, unequal pupils, coughing up mucus	12 2.4 %	34 6.2 %

Figure 2: Most frequent symptoms of DCI in 1994 (from DAN's report on diving accidents and fatalities, 1996 [3])

An other important question is: when a particular symptom or sign is it called a "DCI case." Everybody working with divers knows that the grey zone of non-reported cases is very high. This concerns particularly the mild symptoms which really are difficult to interpret conclusively in the first instance and which often show a spontaneous resolution even if no treatment is given. Circulating bubbles during or immediately after the decompression phase of a dive are known to be a very common finding. Mostly these bubbles remain silent bubbles, some produce symptoms, some may set subclinical organ damage that result in a long term effect or later-arising pathology as for instance bone necrosis. Many symptoms, even typical neurological ones can arise from impingement situations that have nothing to do with the decompression of the diver but eventually with the mechanical stress induced by the diving suit or the posture. These faulty positive symptoms should be treated as a DCI when differential diagnosis is not possible and omission of immediate treatment could have invalidating consequences. However they may erroneously contribute to the total number of DCI cases in the statistics. One should discuss as well whether the expression of "diving accident" is still to be accepted, as first of all in several countries the typical diving accidents are not recognized as accident by the national legislation and furthermore the uprising of symptoms is rather a consequence of a probabilistic situation in relation to decompression stress, so we should rather speak of "diving incidents" instead.

The mortality of diving accidents is not known exactly for the reasons described above. DAN is collecting fatality reports from 1989 on and, while now cooperating with NUADC, the data collected are quite representative for the USA. Over 25 years, 2'682 scuba deaths were collected (US residents only). The death rate is quite constant over the years (about 100 cases a year). The 97 scuba deaths of 1994 don't show a particular prevalence as to a diving activity or level of experience. If we assume that DAN USA gets about the same percentage of DCI cases reported as they got fatality reports from all USA, the mortality of diving would be about 10% of the DCI risk.

Prevalence of Diving Habits

DAN USA has a comprehensive data bank of pure recreational dive incidents (3). Over 100'000 divers in need have been assisted in the last 15 years. In 1994, they received 1'951 emergency calls of which 858 were DCI cases. The following data come from the 566 cases which had completed data sheets. Closer look at the certification level or the years of experience of divers did not show a prevalence for any particular subgroup. Only 3/4 of the injured divers were found to be completely fit and free from other illness; only about 1/2 of the victims had a history without past health problems. However a prevalence of DCI related to a particular risk factor is not evident.

Analyses as to dive habits or technical risk situations showed, that only about 11% were diving outside the decompression limits of the table or dive computer (Fig. 3). Other factors generally assumed to be particularly risky like multiday diving and others are shown to be non-significant. Three-fourths of the DCI were found after no-decompression dives; 1/2 were single dives. Rapid ascent is found in 1/2 of the AGE cases and in 1/4 of the DCS cases. Two-thirds of the DCI happened after dives deeper than 24 meters.

Modern Trends?

As we know, diving habits are changing, primarily due to the use of dive computers which allow irregular dive profiles and due to introduction of new diving gear. Striking is the increase of the percentage of injured divers who dived within the limits (56 to 87%) and that did no-stop dives (78 to 83%). Depth, multiday, and other factors show no particular trend. This trend is probably due to the wide acceptance of the computer as a dive planner in the rather shallow American dive sites.

AGE cases show a trend to happen in situations of extreme physical effort (exertion climbed from 19 to 65%, current from 33 to 63% during the last five years).

Most interesting is the distribution of DCI cases in relation to the use of computers or tables. The number of computer users increased by a factor of 10 (41 to 313) while the number of table users remained stable during the last 7 years. In 1994, the percentage of computer users was 55% of all DCI cases. The only obvious trend is a reduction of AGE to about 1/2 the incidence of table users (Fig. 4). This probably shows that the use of the computer is an important contribution in extraordinary situations when ascent is urgent but a rapid ascent (blow up) is to be avoided.

Is There a Difference between USA and Europe?

The DAN EUROPE study (1), including data of accidents between 1989–93 (202 cases), shows that the most important risk factors are deep diving (81% of DCI cases dived deeper than 30 meters) and decompression dives (79%) which is in contrast to the US study. Other factors did not show to be significant. The majority of DCS cases was found to occur after dives "within the limits" (51% DCI cases DAN EUROPE 1989-93) in contrast to the 87% of DCS cases in DAN USA (1994). The difference suggests that the diving habits in the different continents are not the same. In the Mediterranean Sea

Traits	1994	1993	1990-92	1988-89
outside of limits	10.8 %	18.2 %	22.6 %	23.4 %
> 24 meters	55.5 %	53 %	60.8 %	52.1 %
repeat dives	61.3 %	62.1 %	61.6 %	55.2 %
square dives	56.9 %	63.3 %	50.9 %	55.2 %
rapid ascent	31.4 %	32.3 %	35.6 %	42.2 %

Figure 3: New diver profile traits (from DAN's report on diving accidents and fatalities, 1996 [3])

	COMPUTERS USERS							
	1994	1993	1992	1991	1990	1989	1988	1987
	Percent	Percent	Percent	Percent	Percent	Percent	Percent	Percent
DCS I	27.8	27.1	22.3	20.1	28.1	31.0	31.0	26.8
DCS II	66.1	66.9	71.4	73.4	64.0	62.7	60.7	61.0
AGE	6.1	6.0	6.3	6.5	7.9	6.3	8.3	12.2
TOTAL	100.0	100.0	100.0	100.0	100.0	100.0	100.0	100.0
	n = 313	n = 266	n = 224	n = 199	n = 203	n = 126	n = 84	n = 41

	TABLE USERS							
	1994	1993	1992	1991	1990	1989	1988	1987
	Percent	Percent	Percent	Percent	percent	percent	Percent	Percent
DCS I	22.9	18.6	12.9	16.0	17.2	18.5	18.5	15.8
DCS II	62.8	67.8	75.1	66.8	61.3	64.9	60.3	63.6
AGE	14.2	13.6	12.0	17.2	21.5	16.6	21.2	20.6
TOTAL	100.0	100.0	100.0	100.0	100.0	100.0	100.0	100.0
	n = 218	n = 242	n = 241	n = 238	n = 256	n = 256	n = 184	n = 228

Figure 4. DCI Symptoms in computer users and table users (from DAN's report on Diving accidents & fatalies, 1996 [3])

divers tend to go deeper as most of the biologically interesting places are deeper than 20 meters, while in the USA the most visited places are coral reefs which are most beautiful in the uppermost 10 to 15 meters. In consequence, the risk factor depth and decompression diving are more pronounced in the European statistics. Divers never diving deeper than 30 meters and never going into decompression, have a 6x lower risk for decompression illness than the general average of all divers (1 DCI per 40'228 dives against 1:6'604 total average; see Fig. 1).

Long Term Effects

In discussing the incidence of diving accidents, I would like to add a remark on further decompression induced pathologies, that is the long term effects of diving. Apparently divers with a very high degree of diving activity over many years show a very low incidence of pathologies that are related to the decompression stress. While slight effects on lung vital capacity, small airway changes, neuropsychological findings are rather debated, the existence of aseptic bone necroses is generally accepted. The highest incidence rate is found in tunnel workers, which accumulate the greatest decompression stress over long working periods, even without being inside the water. However divers, professional as well as sport divers, occasionally have bone necroses. McCallum (4) reported in a survey of 5015 divers 210 definitive bone lesions (=4,2%) and 102 suspected lesions (2%). Sixty-four percent of patients with decompression induced bone necroses had been treated once in their active diving period for bends. However only a extremely low percentage developes major joint pathology that is incapacitating or which needs surgery. We do not know how many DCI cases end in a long term invalidity or produce an occupational problem. Brubakk (11) found a significant prevalence of cerebral symptoms in divers which is analysed in the discussion (Fig. 10).

Treatment Results

The DAN USA statistic shows a total release of symptoms in 56% of the 566 cases in 1994. Twenty-eight percent still had some neurological symptoms, 17% residual pain. The DAN EUROPE statistics showed 85% cases with complete relief of symptoms (N = 202 DCI cases 1989–93). The statistics are not analyzed for the different treatment tables, most divers however were treated with US Navy Table 6 or similar procedures. The quite important difference in outcome does not reflect a different quality standard of hyperbaric treatment but shows how poor the information is that we can extract from such general data. Even more different than the diving habits of the regional diving populations is the behavioural pattern during diving accidents. The two main factors influencing the final outcome are the immediate treatment with normobaric oxygen and giving liquids. On the other side the delay to the recompression therapy is of eminent importance. About 70% of the patients with milder neurological symptoms or pain as pre-recompression symptoms still were symptomatic after the treatment when the delay was more than 12 hours, while the percentage of residual symptoms is only 20% for a delay between 4 and 12 hours and about 10% for a delay of less than 4 hours (Fig. 5). Surprisingly, the severe neurological symptoms do not show the same characteristics, but the interpretation is not easy, as the exact incidence of severe symptoms for the delay groups is not given. The American case study shows that the median delay before HBO-treatment start in AGE cases was about 7 hours, while a more important delay of 26 hours for DCS I and 20 hours for DCS II cases is found (median delay = 50% of cases had a shorter, 50% a longer delay). DAN EUROPE does not give the equivalent figures, but shows that the delay to call for assistance after onset of the first symptoms has a median time of about 3 hours (21% below 1 hour, 40% 1 to 4 hours, 24% 4 to 12 hours, 12% more than 12 hours), while the DAN USA study notes 22 hours for DCS I, 9 hours for DCS II and 3 hours for AGE respectively. As the number of AGE cases is quite low, the delay to call and accordingly the delay to treatment is quite longer in the US than in Europe by a factor of about 3. This could be a factor for the better overall outcome of treated cases.

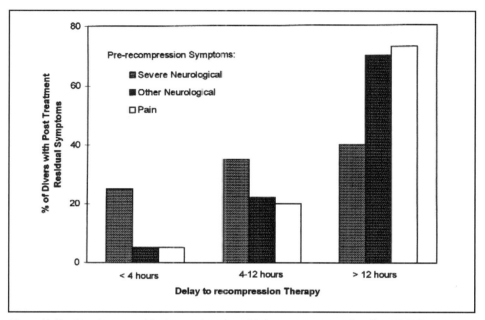

Figure 5. Post-treatment residuals as a function of delay to recompression (from DAN's report on diving accidents and fatalities, 1996 [3])

In Australia the mean delay was even longer with 28h in Gorman's analysis who found also much more residual symptoms. Gorman (12) described a 100% total relief of symptoms after the first HBO-recompression in divers with a pretreatment delay of less than 24 hours. Two-thirds however relapsed and required repeat HBO treatments and 1/2 of these patients remained with sequelae after the last treatment. If the delay was more than 24 hours 2/3 of the patients remained with sequelae, of which 1/4 were neurological deficits.

The importance and effectiveness of normobaric oxygen treatment is documented in several accident statistics. DAN USA shows that 33% of DCI cases used oxygen as first therapy during the transport (which is an increase of about 1/4 since 1993, when only 26% of DCI got oxygen). Only 6% of all DCI cases got oxygen and fluids. Oxygen pre-clinical treatment increased the symptom release rate before recompression (that is symptomatic patients that arrived at the chamber without symptoms) by a factor of 2 to 8, as shown in Figure 6. Less impressing, but still very clear is the effect on the general outcome after recompression treatment (see Fig. 6). The data of the DAN EUROPE statistics are even more striking: while 99% of the no oxygen group remained symptomatic, 55% of the oxygen group showed net improvement and 12% complete release of symptoms at arrival of hyperbaric facility. The release rate after HBO treatment is 70% for the no oxygen, 96% for oxygen group. Very similar results were found by Wolkiewiez 1983 (5). These figures show that the oxygen first aid therapy is not just a additive to the overall treatment, but an important contribution with a significant effect on the final outcome. If we consider that the majority of cases that got oxygen did not really get 100% ($FiO_2 = 1.0$) due to inappropriate oxygen breathing devices and that many of them did not get oxygen during all the transport time, the difference in outcome could even be much more important. Neither of the statistics gives any indication about the effect of a fluid therapy.

DIAGNOSIS	RELIEF BEFORE RECOMPRESSION		RELIEF AFTER RECOMPRESSION	
	No Oxygen	Oxygen	No Oxygen	Oxygen
AGE	7.2	13.8	55.4	58.0
DCS-II Severe	3.7	16.4	56.2	66.7
DCS-II Mild	2.1	10.6	49.0	73.2
DCS-I	1.5	12.1	54.8	70.1
All DCI	2.9	12.4	52.4	69.3

Figure 6. Relief of Symptoms in divers with / without preclinical normobaric O_2 - treatment (from DAN's report on Diving accidents & fatalities, 1996 [3])

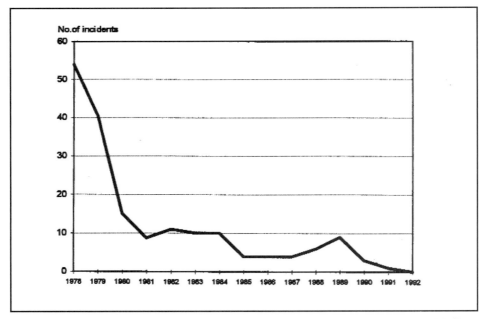

Figure 7. Evolution of DCI incidence in the Norwegian shelf offshore divers 1978–92 (from Brathens [7])

Sainty, et al. 1984 (6) report total relief of symptoms after the first HBO treatment in 60% of treated cases, increasing to 71% after the final treatment of the HBO series. However half (14%) of the 29% with residual symptoms still had major invalidating neurological symptoms. This shows the value of continuing the treatment until the clinical findings are stable. Nevertheless the 14% with severe residual symptoms are a heavy socio-economical burden for the population and a nightmare for the diver's population.

DISCUSSION

Difference Between Recreational and Professional Divers?
Epidemiology
It is difficult to find data bases that include all professional divers and all diving accidents of a particular region. Many professional working sites are offshore and so the official supervision by a governmental office is not assured. Many platforms are owned by companies of different nations, sometimes introducing their data to the data banks of their own nation. The few statistics indicating number of working hours and the specific working conditions of professional divers, for instance in UK and Norway, do not include all the very many "low grade" professionals like police divers, scientific divers, fish farming divers. The status of diving instructors who are also "man working under pressure," so in a certain sense professionals, is still debated. Diving accident reports generally do not distinguish between professional and recreational diver's accidents. Brathen from Stavanger reviewed the situation of the Norwegian Continental Shelf in the 1993 Consensus Conference on long term health effects (7), where he reported 2'252 surface oriented professional dives per year with an average diving time of 1,8 hours (generally hose bounce diving with air or mixed gas). Saturation diving, which is difficult to quantify, was represented with 14'004 bell runs of an average stay of 5,9 hours, average saturation period of 12,3 days and a total of 177'211 man hours under saturation per year. In terms of decompression, this means about 2'850 man decompressions. Decompression sickness in that diver's population decreased from 54 incidents in 1978 to 0 in 1992. These figures are representative for offshore oil companies, where the occupied divers have to dive a maximum of what is allowed by security regulations. The divers population is rather young and represents a selection of physically well trained persons. They stop their diving activity in general after a couple of years, about the age of 32-35. This study, that looks only at offshore divers, shows that we must be careful comparing incidence rates of professional divers with others. The trend in DCS incidence (Figure 7) shows that in the beginning of industrial diving activity the DCS risk was exceedingly high, and that by a learning effect and by more and more restrictive regulations, the security level gets to the modern standard, which is comparable to other occupational risks and also to the recreational diving incidence rate. So if we want to compare, we have to compare recreational divers with the very actual figures of professional diving incidents.

In another study of Oceaneering International Service LTD of Scotland (8) and a comparison with the UK Diving Industry Review of the North Sea, we find a DCS incidence going from 0,383% (which means 1 case DCI per 261 dives) in 1984 to a DCI incidence of 0,023% (1 DCI case per 4'174 dives) in 1995. This shows again the learning curve mentioned in the Norwegian study (Fig. 8).

	1990	1995	1990-1995
Air dives	25222	16696	133250
Depth aver (m)	19.5	22	20.2
Bottom time (min)	56.2	67.6	62.3
No deco dives	15705	8959	74922
Stand air decompr.	4187	3690	28511
DCS < 30 m	7	2	30
DCS > 30 m	3	2	29
% incidence of DCS	0.039 %	0.024 %	0.044 %
Dives per DCS	2556	4174	2258

Surface mixed gas dives	893	363	3993
Depth aver (m)	65.4	61.2	63.3
Bottom time (min)	31	34	36
DCS incidents	1	0	4
% incidence of DCS	0.112 %	none	0.100 %
Dives per DCS	893	-	898

Bell mixed gas dives	8	0	110
Bottom time (min)	38.3	0	42
DCS incidents	0	0	0

Man saturations	442	59	1040
Man hours under pressure	159904	15553	312800
DCS incidents	5	0	7

Tot. dives and lockouts	30625	17384	144933
DCS incidents	16	4	70
% incidence of DCS	0.052 %	0.023 %	0.048 %
Dives per DCS	1914	4346	2070

Figure 8. Dive incidents using different diving techniques; an oceaneering survey 1990–1995 (from Holland [7])

More interesting is the splitting of the professional divers into groups as air bounce dives, which are generally performed with hose from a diving platform, into surface supplied mixed gas dives with the same technique but using mixed gas (Nitrox or Trimix), into bell bounce dives, which are like surface mixed gas dives but technically a different entity, and finally into a group of saturation dives with the divers staying in a habitat on a working pressure and performing work by transfer under pressure to a diving bell, leaving the bell for their work and decompressing inside the bell up to pressure of the habitat. Of course, this group gives us the biggest number of hours under pressure, but as this technique is very different from what we look at in recreational divers the data gotten from this diving type are not reliable for other types of diving. Figure 8 shows the DCI incidence rate for the mentioned subgroups over the last 6 years. If we compare only the air diving and surface mixed gas diving group, we find that in respect to the small numbers there is no significant difference in DCI probability (even if it looks like being more dangerous to go on mixed gas using only the calculated percentage). The statistics do not distinguish between decompressions performed in water, by transfer under pressure (TUP), or by surface transfer to a decompression chamber (SURD). Standard in-water decompression and surface decompression in the air diving group are performed with about the same frequency; mixed gas diving is probably done with surface decompression (not indicated). This would be an interesting point to analyse, in order to know whether the delicate phase of complete decompression to ambient pressure before going into the surface decompression chamber does not induce any pathologies. Surface decompression is normally done on oxygen tables. Knowing that after excessive diving with a certain decompression stress and specially after surfacing without decompression many silent circulating bubbles could be found, the decompression under oxygen in the chamber could as well be considered as being a prophylactic HBO treatment.

	Air TUP	Air SURD	Nitrox
No of dives	7835	24831	8045
DCS I incidence	11	25	6
DCS II incidence	7	19	1
Dives per DCS (all)	435	564	1149
Dives per DCS II	1119	1306	8045

Figure 9. DCI risk in different diving techniques (a Department of energy analysis 1987 - 90, from Holland [8])

A differential evaluation of the Dept. of Energy 1987–90 shows that the nitrox diving group has a considerably lower DCI risk, particularly for type II DCS than the divers performing surface decompression or TUP. The incidence rate on the cumulated 8'045 nitrox dives was 6 DCS type I and 1 DCS type II which corresponds to a risk of 1 DCS I per 1'149 dives, respectively one DCS II per 8'045 dives. The other 2 divers groups had a markedly higher risk with 1 DCS I per about 500 dives, respectively 1 DCS II per 1'200 dives (Fig. 9). This leads to the conclusion that nitrox diving is a big advantage for the professional divers security while diving in the shallower depth range. The cumulated statistics of Oceaneering Ltd from 1989–96 shows even better results on 9'076 nitrox dives: 2 DCS cases in the dives of more than 30 meters depth during all these years, which gives an incidence of 0,022% (1 DCS per 4'538 dives). For working divers, nitrox is also of evident economical advantage compared to air, because it allows much longer stays.

Very little is known about the risks of all the different inshore professional divers, that is, police divers, Navy divers, harbour divers, and fish farming divers as well as scientific divers. Most of them have less than 50 dives per year so they have a completely different pattern of decompression stress, on the other hand they have much less training and routine than the full time professionals. Many of those inshore professionals are self-employed and thus have another notion as to the risk they like to take to assure their financial income. In many countries, including Switzerland, there is no medical control of those self-employed divers. I found the small statistics, presented by Minsaas 1985 (9), who showed that in the Norwegian onshore chambers, they treated each year about 30 inshore divers, mainly sports divers, but 12% were military divers, 25% were occupational divers. No further data about clinical signs and other circumstances are given, so that a further analyse is impossible.

Clinical manifestations

As the majority of working hours under pressure are performed in saturation and using mixed gas and pressures up to 30 bars and more, the clinical signs and frequency distribution is supposed to be completely different from what we see in recreational divers. This is obvious, if we consider the phenomenon of HPNS, temperature management problems, exposure to unusual humidity, and other technically induced environmental factors over many days living under pressure. If we don't want to compare apples with pears, we have to look at the subgroup of surface supplied divers using air or nitrox. The statistics of Oceaneering International Ltd. gives only the relation of DCS I and II cases for nitrox, surface decompression and TUP dives (see Figure 9), which shows about 2 to 3 relation between DCS II and DCS I for air divers, 6 to 1 for nitrox dives, which is however not representative looking at the very small numbers of DCI cases.

LONG TERM EFFECTS IN HEATHLY DIVERS (vs controls)

	Office worker	Fire-men	Sports-divers	Profes hose D	Profes bell D
History N =	342	92	740	365	112
Total accidents in diving	-	-	7	15	22
Deco problems treated	-	-	3	13	28
Deco problems untreated	-	-	19	50	63

Actual findings :

	Office worker	Fire-men	Sports-divers	Profes hose D	Profes bell D
Lung function changes %	-	-	3	3	6
Auditory Imparement %	-	34	30	37	51
CNS Symptoms %	10	15	14	19	28

CORRELATION OF CNS SYMPTOMS WITH SPECIFIC RISK FACTORS

	Office worker	Fire-men	Sports-divers	Profes hose D	Profes bell D
Risk factors : N =	342	92	740	365	112
Cranial trauma	n.s.	n.s.	n.s.	++	n.s.
Deco problems treated	-	-	n.s.	n.s.	n.s.
Deco problems untreated	-	-	++++	+++	+

+ p < 0.1, ++ p < 0.05, +++ p < 0.001, ++++ p < 0.001

Figure 10. Long term effects in healthy divers (from a study of Brubakk et al., Sintef UNIMED, Trondheim 1994 [11])

A great majority of mild symptoms is certainly hidden to all statistics, because the professional divers are very anxious to lose their job by admitting they have symptoms and would need a diving accident treatment. So they help each other and treat themselves, e.g., by prophylactic recompressions which are not going to the medical statistics. Many mild symptoms are just neglected or treated by other methods. Thus the frequency of hyperbaric treatment might be too high for unnecessary prophylactic treatments if the use of recompression chambers is accurately logged, on the other hand, the incidence rate will be too low if looking at the medical reports only. However, looking at the long term effects, examining divers that stopped diving activity or divers still continuing after many years does not show significant pathologies besides the well known and already mentioned aseptic bone necrosis. However the Todnem study (10), performed on divers of the 80s when the DCI incidence rate was still very high, shows a higher incidence of neurological symptoms and signs, including abnormal EEG which correlate with exposure to saturation diving, as compared to the non-diving control group.

Brubakk (11) found in a epidemiological study on experienced divers in Norway, that although 98% declared to feel themselves as perfectly healthy, 20 to 30% of the professional, 15% of sport divers had signs of cerebral dysfunction (frequent problems of concentration, irritation, depression, memory). Four-tenths of one percent of sports divers and 3.5–22% of professional compressed air divers had a history of DCI treatment (average diving experience 7 years), and 2.5% of sports divers respectively 15 - 55% of professionals had decompression problems that were never treated! Most strikingly the CNS symptoms correlated significantly with untreated decompression problems in the past (Fig. 10). Diving depth and antecedents of DCI however were not significant factors. Future studies will have to elucidate the importance of these light symptoms for the individual diver.

Treatment results

The treatment results of DCI in professional diving are not comparable directly to analogous results on recreational divers, as the diving techniques require quite different treatment procedures, specially when helium is involved. As our knowledge about the gas lesion disease, called decompression illness, as well as its treatment mechanism is still very limited and the actual theoretical basis were developed only in the last decades, treatment results are improving as a general trend during the last years while more and more the low pressure oxygen tables are used, at least for air and nitrox divers.

Professional divers including surface supplied compressed air divers usually are treated immediately when symptoms arise, so the treated pathology is not the same as in recreational divers who come to the chamber only after 7–20 hours, with important secondary metabolic reactions around the bubbles and the ischaemic zone. For that reason the best hyperbaric treatment procedures might eventually be different for the two diver's populations.

CONCLUSION

Similar Features in Recreational and Professional Dive Accidents

1. *The Risk of Inadequate Recording of Diving Incidents*
    Recreational divers often ignore the problematics of DCI and its symptoms and thus do not feel necessary to alert the buddy or supervising person. Others are too convinced of their correct behaviour that they believe it was impossible they could have symptoms of DCI, as they followed the tables or the computer indications correctly. A third group is just too fascinated with what they see every day in diving, that they don't want to stop the diving group con tinuing its dive trip, or they are ashamed to accept, that they are victim of a DCI. These inappropriate reactions are responsible for the unregistered cases, on the other hand they contribute to the much too long delay in call or trans port to the hyperbaric facilities. Professional divers, specially employed off shore divers, have another reason to hide their symptoms, as mentioned. The recorded incidence rate for professionals might even be virtually too low because concealed prophylactic treatments were performed without informing the medical adviser. Even in recorded cases, the diagnosis is made on the base of the symptoms reported from the diving platform crew, as generally no doc tor can be brought into the zone of the dive accidents where the therapy chamber is placed. So pre-treatment diagnosis is very coarse and cannot be completed later.

    Divers are generally not aware of the fact that the diving accident is a prob abilistic event and that the more they go to the limits, more they risk to be hit. How important that point is as to the recording of accident conditions, and so for the epidemiologic analysis, can be shown from the DAN EUROPE data (1): the 11 DCI cases found in the low risk group which dived less than 30 meters and within no-stop time were all cases that would be outside the limit if we take modern dive tables as the DCIEM recreational diving tables of Canada. The attribute "within the limits" means the victim was diving not exceeding the limits of his particular tables or computer. Still too many divers look for the "best" tables leaving them the highest degree of freedom.

2. *Similar Risks for Same Dive Techniques*
    As mentioned the population of professional and recreational divers have to be subdivided into groups using the same dive technique. If this is done, we will be able to show that the DCI risk is in the same range for both groups.

The Differences
Motivation
As we know specially from recreational diving accidents, motivation is one of the most important reasons for producing or avoiding incidents. The recreational divers are diving mostly for fun, sometimes also to demonstrate their social state or courage. They are free to decide whether they want to go to a certain depth or not, however, the temptation to stay a little longer or go a little deeper is obvious and it is only in the end of the dive that some get punished. The typical employed professional diver is generally more conscious of the importance of the various security regulations.

They don't dive for fun, their work is hard and mostly not very pleasant, but well paid. The main problem is not to lose the job. In that view the sports diver tends to dive with more ease to take a higher risk than a professional.

Planning

Recreational divers tend to dive in an uncontrolled way, what means exploring the ground and rather than performing an online planning with the dive computer, sometimes they just rely on the technical equipment, for instance the reserve valve of the diving tanks. Professional divers have very strict regulations and more conservative dive tables. They are obliged to plan the dive and they have a supervising person on the platform while the dives and the conversations are logged continuously.

First aid procedures and pre-clinical therapy

Recreational divers are advised to give oxygen at 100%, to give liquids and put the victim in flat position in case of DCI symptoms, CPR being applied in first priority if necessary. Next they have to phone a medical hotline to get further advice and to organize emergency evacuation if indicated. As shown by the statistics, only about 1/3 uses oxygen and not all of oxygen users apply 100%. The percentage for the other treatment elements is even worse. In reality too many divers do not care about the next telephone or the facility to get to a hyperbaric chamber, nor do they know the symptoms of DCI or take an oxygen delivery system with them. Fortunately the percentage of oxygen users is increasing each year in the DAN statistics, which is probably a result of the intensive promotion and information campaign accompanying the oxygen courses. The professional diver is not himself cared about treatment procedures, but he knows that the appropriate equipment would be close by and that well trained and experienced first aid personal and recompression specialists will be ready in case of need. Indeed most of the professional diving accidents offshore are treated with a very short time delay and thus with the best conditions of a complete relief of symptoms. This comparison shows that again recreational divers take much more risk than professional divers. Scientific divers, police divers, and many other sporadic professional divers such as the diving instructors are rather in the higher risk group of the recreational divers. The situation will probably be better in a few years, when the consensus decisions of the EDTC of the Luxembourg meeting 1994 will be applied. The consensus decision was that for each professional diving site, the next hyperbaric treatment facility should be at least within a range of two hours transport time and that every professional diver must have appropriate oxygen delivery systems at the diving site.

The use of prophylactic HBO treatment

As mentioned earlier recreational divers as well as professional divers hesitate to go to the hyperbaric chamber if the question is to treat officially a decompression illness. However the effectiveness of recompression and HBO is quite well known to all professional divers and they are stimulated and practise recompression also in case of doubt or suspicious symptoms. So many recompressions might be done as prophylactic recompressions which even in spite of the costs weighs much less than a case more of DCI that could have been avoided. Recreational divers still hesitate even to use the normobaric oxygen in a situation of doubtful symptoms, for example in the case of omitted decompression, but still with absence of symptoms. It seems to be a shame to admit that one could have symptoms of DCI. Many believe that every case of DCI can be explained by an incorrect diving technique. Recreational divers also dive generally in quite remote places, which are the most interesting ones for exploring coral reefs or wrecks, so that often the next treatment facility is at a distance of many hundreds of kilometers. This partly explains the long delay between the first symptoms to the start of recompression, which is a primary condition for a good outcome. Overall, again, recreational divers show a situation that gives according to the known statistics a higher risk for unreleased symptoms or residual incapacity.

Due to the different risk situations that in many cases cannot be changed in the future, the recreational diver has probably a higher risk of DCI and for incomplete symptom relief after treatment than the modern professional diver in the offshore platform. The high risk period of the professionals is over. Police divers, scientific divers, and other rather sporadic professionals such as many diving instructors will probably be within the risk zone of recreational divers.

REFERENCES

1. Marroni A., Recreational diving to-day: Risk evaluation and problem management, In: Proceedings of the EUBS Congress Istanbul, 1994.
2. Francis TJR, Smith DJ, Describing Decompression Illness, 42th UHMS Workshop, Bethesta, 1991.
3. DAN, Report on diving Accidents and Fatalities. The annual review of recreational scuba diving injuries and deaths based on 1994 data, Edition 1996.
4. McCallum R.I., The current status of hyperbaric bone necrosis in the UK, In: Hope A., Lund T., Elliott D.H., Halsey M.J., Wiig H., Long term health effects of diving - International Consensus Conference, Godøysund, Norway, June 1993, Bergen, Norway, 1994.
5. Wolkiewiez J, 1983, cited in 1.
6. Sainty J.M. et al., Tables suroxygénées et accidents neurologiques de decompression, In : F. Wattel, D. Mathieu, Proceedings of the 1st European Consensus Conference on hyperbaric medicine, Lille, September 1994.
7. Bråthen R., Diving operations on the Norwegian continental shelf, In: Hope A., Lund T., Elliott D.H., Halsey M.J., Wiig H., Long term health effects of diving - International Consensus Conference, Godøsyund, Norway, June 1993, Bergen, Norway, 1994.
8. Holland R.H., Oceaneering International Services Limited, Aberdeen, Scotland, (Personal communications).
9. Minsaas B., Requirements for medical services to support diving operations, In: Safety of diving operations- Part I: Proceedings of the International Symposium on safety and health in diving operations, Luxembourg, May 1985., Graham and Trotman Ltd., London, 1986.
10. Kvåle G., Nyland H., Duration of employment for saturation in divers in Norway, In: Hope A., Lund T., Elliott D.H., Halsey M.J., Wiig H., Long term health effects of diving-International Consensus Conference, Godøysund, Norway, June 1993, Bergen, Norway, 1994.
11. Brubakk A.O., Bolstad G. and Jacobsen G., Health effects in compressed air diving amateurs and professionals, Sintef UNIMED study, Trondheim, Norway 1994.
12. Gorman D.F., Pearce A. and Webb R.K., Disbaric illness treated at the royal adelaide hospital 1987 - a factorial analysis, SPUMS journal 18: 95-101 (1988).

NOTES

DESCRIPTIVE CLASSIFICATION OF DIVING ACCIDENTS

J. Desola, MD, PhD
Coordinating Committee of Hyperbaric Medical Centres
(CCCMH) Spain

All diving disciplines are exposed to a high potential of serious accidents, which can be considered inherent to this underwater activity. Some modalities or specialties imply a higher level of hazard, like deep mixed gas-diving in off-shore industry, or cave/speleological diving usually done by divers with a recreational or sport diving license.

Another important risk factor is imposed by the underwater environment, which by itself may convert into a tragedy an incident that would have been irrelevant in the land. This is the case of the people being able to have a normal activity but with a silent or hidden disease that can produce a loss of consciousness underwater.

Different etiopathogenic factors are responsible for a quite wide variety of disorders. Some depend on the underwater environment and the physiological mechanisms of adaptation required of the human body. Others are linked to the variation of pressure implicit to any diving activity.

Almost all parts of the body can suffer from the consequences of a Diving Disorder (DD), so signs and symptoms can be extremely varied (Table 1). There is usually a coincidence of these different symptoms and pathophysiological mechanisms in a diving disorder, and similar signs and symptoms may be due to different origins (Table 2).

As a result of this combination of factors, a wide range of diving disorders exists, and diving medical specialists frequently have difficulties in adequately classifying apparently similar diseases which are, however, produced by different mechanisms.

An additional factor to this classifying difficulty may come from the fact that diving injuries have been excessively associated with diving activity in itself, and therapeutical procedures were designed to be applied by divers, or by diving supervisors, usually in diving facilities, sometimes in non-medically controlled hyperbaric chambers, generally forgetting basic medical disciplines, and avoiding routine procedures usually followed in medical centres.

A person suffering from a Decompression Disorder is not a diver that has omitted a decompression step, or an individual that has suffered an interruption of his underwater job, and he[1] does not need to be placed in a hyperbaric chamber just to complete his decompression schedule. An injured diver is a patient suffering from a multifactorial systemic disease, with a complex pathological mechanism of multifocal gas microembolism, frequently with haemodynamic and rheological alterations, affecting different structures of his body, and producing a wide range of symptoms, some of them paradoxical. He does not need "to be recompressed" but he must be sent

---

1.- In order to simplify the text and its reading, we will avoid the use of expressions like he/she, he and she, and we are using the masculine personal pronoun he in its impersonal neutral meaning. The reader will understand that we are always referring to men and women divers.

TABLE 1
MOST COMMON SYMPTOMS
OF DYSBARIC DISORDERS

SYMPTOM	%
Limb bends	31.20
Vertigo	20.90
Paraparesis	19.30
Consciousness alteration	14.50
Bladder paralysis	13.80
Skin rash	12.50
Monoparesis	10.00
Lumbar pain	8.00
Bronchoaspiration	5.10
Paraplegia	5.10
Subcutaneous emphysema	4.50
Tympanic barotrauma	4.80
Pneumomediastinum	4.50
Hemiparesis	4.80
Haemoptysis	2.90
Rhinolalia	2.60
Shock	2.30
Hemiplegia	1.30
Tetraparesis	1.30
Tetraplegia	1.00
Pneumothorax	1.00
Other symptoms	1.60

(Source : CRIS - Unitat de Terapèutica Hiperbàrica - Barcelona)

TABLE 2 - COMMON CLINICAL MANIFESTATIONS OF DIVING DISORDERS
Otalgia during immersion
Frontal headache after diving
Skin pruriginous rash initiated some minutes after surfacing
Pain in one arm some minutes after diving
Limb bends + skin rash
Subjective neurological symptoms
Subjective neurological symptoms + limb pain
Paraparesis + bladder paralysis
Paraplegia + haemodynamic/rheological alterations
Chest pain + cervical emphysema after a rapid ascent
Hemiparesis after a free ascent
Hemiplegia + pneumomediastinum + haemodynamic/rheological alterations
Tetraplegia + thoracic and/or abdominal impairment + dysbaric shock
Vertigo initiated during ascent
Vertigo initiated after surfacing

to a Hyperbaric Medical Centre where he will be examined, studied, and analyzed, and as a result of all that, he will receive the most adequate treatment for his complex disease, which usually will include, among other therapeutical procedures, the application of Hyperbaric Oxygenation (HBO) within a Hyperbaric Chamber. Obviously some high level diving medical centres have always existed in some countries, but this not generally the case.

Historically, Diving Disorders were classified in two wide categories (type I and type II) corresponding to minor and major cases. In Type I those cases with only skin or limb pain symptoms were included. Type II corresponded to the rest of the symptoms, where a large variety of conditions were mixed.

This classification not only made it impossible to separate different etiopathogenic mechanisms coinciding in one single patient, but in fact both types of disorders (type I and type II) very frequently coincide in the same diver. When we were listening to an expression like "a diver suffering from a type II decompression sickness" we could not know what kind of process the patient was suffering.

Many persons had mentioned their disagreement with this inexpressive classification, which was a common topic of discussion at any meeting of diving medicine. Some expert diving medical centres had developed their own classification based on their knowledge and experience. Meetings of EUBS and UHMS frequently showed those different attitudes.

An important contribution was given by FRANCIS & SMITH who a few years ago proposed a new approach to the description of diving disorders, more based on medical practice, introducing the term Decompression Illness, widely used after that. Experience demonstrated, however, that some problems remained unsolved and we did not manage to adopt an unified classification criteria at that point.

European countries have a long tradition of diving medicine, and some centres have their own well-established protocols. The different European languages have difficulties in accurately translating some anglo-saxon words; few European languages, for instance, can translate in different words illness, sickness and disease.

Adopting an unique common scientific language is certainly very difficult, but this is one of the main reasons why the European Committee for Hyperbaric Medicine (ECHM) wished to propose a mainly Descriptive Classification of Diving Disorders that can be used in different European areas, using different languages, in which basic concepts, more than technical words, will be introduced.

It is not an easy job, really, but here is an attempt to establish a common and unified approach to diving disorders, following approximately the same system usually adopted to describe the great majority of diseases that appear in books of medical pathology. This is a preliminary report that will be discussed in this II European Consensus Congress. Results of general discussion will be later incorporated and the resulting classification will be newly discussed if necessary.

METHOD

These are the general rules followed for this classification.

Diving disorders can be classified according to different criteria. Some of these criteria are compatible and can be consequently incorporated. We have chosen five different groups that will not be excluding ones to others but, on the contrary, may be accumulated.

We have given special attention to concepts, more than to words, in order to establish similar classifying groups, in spite of the fact that a word or a technical concept may need to be expressed with different words when it is translated into another language.

TABLE 3 - DIVING DISORDERS Classification Criteria
• Morphologic • Clinical • Etiopathogenic • Chronologic • Evolutional
• SIMPLIFIED

We have used English words but international concepts, trying overall to produce a classification that can be used, with minor changes, in all European languages. We have chosen basic English words, selecting those more grammatically close to other languages. In some cases you possibly will find a description or a sentence that is not exactly the most commonly used in English medical literature, but the reason is that among other synonyms or equivalent words, we have selected those with the same initial or similar pronunciation in other European languages.

As an attempt to establish an standard, we have finally suggested an alpha-numeric code that would represent any of the most important groups of phenomena, and that would be used as a reference to be included in reports and communications, like is done, for instance, with the international classification of pneumoconiosis. These codes may have some special utility when an exact criterion is needed, for instance in order to establish therapeutical protocols, to join groups of patients, or to define reimbursement policies from insurance companies. This is not a classification to be used for short clinical reports in operational diving centres, or to be included in the brief information given in the emergency room to the patients. For that purpose we have included at the end a simplified classification, very easy to follow, that will permit a non-specialized diving doctor (at least we hope so) to descriptively summarize the main pathogenic and clinical aspects of the most common diving disorders.

PRELIMINARY REMARKS

Terminology

Diving disorders have been nominated of different forms. Recently the term DECOMPRESSION ILLNESS has become common. There are some reasons for which we consider this term inadequate. This opinion is mainly based in three facts:

1. Not all diving disorders are pressure related; some are underwater related independently of the pressure.
2. Not all pressure relate disorders are decompressive; some happen during the compression phase.
3. The translation of Illness and Sickness to the majority of European languages corresponds to a single word. In consequence, this difference between sickness and illness can not be established. We believe more appropriate to reserve the word Decompression for the so called Decompression Sickness, so we will not make any difference between illness and sickness.

Pathophysiology of Diving Disorders

Many references to etiopathogenic fundamentals are done in the pages that follow, but obviously not all basic concepts are mentioned but only directly related to terminology and/or classification. The reader must understand all unmentioned principles of diving pathophysiology.

Key-codes and Abbreviations

In order to make easier the use of these codes, we will follow a mnemonic guide using when possible the initial of the word, or the letter more closely related to the concept that the word is representing. For instance, A and V are the keys corresponding to the words Arterial and Venous, but X and M have been selected as keys for the

TABLE 4 MORPHOLOGICAL CLASSIFICATION OF DIVING DISORDERS	Code	Description
Cutaneous	*(cut)*	
Petechial	*pet*	C.pet
Infiltrative	*inf*	C.inf
Maculous	*mac*	C.mac
Emphysematous	*emp*	C.emp
Muscular	*mus*	
Osteo-articular	*ost*	
Neurologic	*(N)*	
Cerebral	*cer*	N.cer
Cerebellar	*crb*	N.crb
Medullar	*med*	N.med
Peripheral	*per*	N.per
Neuropsychic	*psy*	N.psy
Systemic	*(S)*	
Haemodynamic	*hem*	S.hem
Rheologic	*rhe*	S.rhe
Coagulopathic	*cgl*	S.cgl
Dysbaric shock	*shk*	S.shk
Somato-Splanchnic		
Otologic	*oto*	
Tympanic		*tym*
Vestibular		*ves*
Sinusal		*sin*
Dental		*den*
Thoraco-respiratory	*res*	
Pulmonary		*pul*
Pleural (pneumothorax)		*pnt*
Mediastinal (pneumomediastinum)		*pnm*
Abdomino-gastrointestinal		*abd*

concepts eXplosion and iMplosion, instead of their initials. When two main words have the same initial, we have given preference to the most important one, in terms of frequency of use, more than in relevancy of the disease. For small locations, or few frequent concepts, we have used their three first letters, or the three more representative ones, shown in lower cases and separate by a point (ex.: mus.abd.neu). In two special situations we have considered it more useful to indicate a zero (Ø) after a letter in order to better remark its negative or antagonistic effect. The code for DYSBARIC is the letter D and for NON-DYSBARIC is DØ (D-zero). The code for BUBBLE-RELATED is B and for NON-BUBBLE-RELATED is BØ (B-zero). This number zero should not be confused with the letter O. In order to avoid this kind of confusion, and taking more specially into account the common practice in some areas of saying O when they are reading a zero, we are using the sign Ø referred to the zero key code, and the conventional 0 for numbers, like 2000.

CLASSIFICATION OF DIVING DISORDERS

Five different criteria have been adopted for classifying diving disorders (Table 3).

1. MORPHOLOGICAL. Attending to the affected part of the body.
2. CLINICAL. Based on the main syndromic groups of symptoms.
3. ETIOPATHOGENIC. According to the cause and to the mechanism of the disorder.
4. CHRONOLOGICAL. Depending on the phase of the diving activity in which the disorder occurs.
5. EVOLUTIONAL. Relative to the outcome of the patient.

Any diving disorder can, and must, be classified according to the five criteria. No group excludes another one. On the contrary, any case can, and should, be entered in each one, and the final expression will include the five linked conditions. A SIMPLIFIED CLASSIFICATION for general use is also included at the end.

TABLE 5 CLINICAL CLASSIFICATION OF DIVING DISORDERS	Abbreviation (DD)
Decompression Sickness	DCS
Dysbaric Osteonecrosis	DON

Intrathoracic Hyperpressive syndrome
    Thoraco-pulmonary syndrome
    Abdomino-gastrointestinal barotraumatism
    Arterial Gas Embolism
    Systemic syndrome
	IHS
	TPS
	AB
	AGE
	SS

Inert gas narcosis	IGN
High Pressure Neurologic syndrome	HPNS
ENT Barotraumatism	ENTBT or ORLBT
Breath-hold anoxic syncope of emersion	BASE
Extreme depth apnoeic pulmonary oedema	EDAPO or EDAPE

Morphological Classification

Depending on which part of the body is affected, the diving disorder will be cutaneous, muscular, osteo-articular, neurologic, systemic, or resident in other somato-splanchnic locations (Table 4). Cutaneous lesions may be petechial, infiltrative, maculous, or emphysematous. Neurologic forms may be cerebral, cerebellar, medullar, peripheral, or neuropsychic. Systemic forms can be haemodynamic, rheologic, coagulopathic, or all at the same time producing a new kind of shock that will be later discussed. Somatosplanchnic forms may be otologic, sinusal, dental, thoraco-respiratory and abdomino-gastrointestinal. In the otological area either the general code oto can be used, relative to a general location, or a most concrete one relative to a single organ, like tympanic, or vestibular. Similarly the code res can be generally used for all thoraco-respiratory locations, but more specific codes can be used for pulmonary (pul), pleural (pnt) or mediastinal (pnm) locations; the particles ple or med have been avoided in order to prevent confusion with other terms, specially taking also into account that pneumothorax or pneumomediastinum are the principal, or may be the only, disorders associated to this area in diving medicine.

Clinical Classification

The well known major syndromes are included in this area, generally respecting the expression by means of which are widely known (Table 5). However some few ones need an explanation.

Decompression Sickness (DCS). We have already discussed the reason why we reserve the words decompression and sickness just for this disease.

Intrathoracic Hyperpressive Syndrome (IHS). A lot of different names are used among different areas in relation to the barotraumatism of the chest. The terms arterial gas embolism, brain embolism, traumatic air embolism, pulmonary overexpansion, burst lung, only refer to some elements of the syndrome. Gas embolism not always occurs in every kind of barotraumatic lesions of the lung; lung rupture due to over-expansion is not always seen in cases of gas embolism; the brain is not the only target organ for gas embolism although it is the more serious and frequent; some patients have pneumothorax and/or pneumomediastinum with no other neurological or respiratory signs or symptoms. All these factors however are conditioned by the relative increase of the intrathoracic pressure that the chest experiences when the external pressure is reduced and respiratory air is not adequately drained, which converts the thoracic cage into a pressure container. Gas embolism, pleural or mediastinal ruptures, subcutaneous emphysema are caused by a mechanism of intrathoracic increase of tension.

However the word hypertension should be avoided in order to prevent confusion with the vascular pulmonary hypertension.

There are at least four different pathophysiological mechanisms that usually coincide in these patients although they may happen separately: the thoraco-pulmonary syndrome (TPS), the abdomino-gastrointestinal syndrome (AB), the arterial gas embolism (AGE), and a systemic syndrome (SS). Consequently, this is not a disease but a syndrome and we have considered that Intrathoracic Hyperpressive Syndrome (IHS) is the expression that more closely explains all mechanisms of this most serious diving disorder.

- *E.N.T. (or O.R.L.) Barotraumatisms.* They can be described using the generic syndromic terms common in medical practice, and the well known Edmonds classification. The use of English (Ear-Nose-Throat) or Greek-Latin derived initials (Oto-Rhino-Laryngology) will vary according different areas; both should be accepted.
- *Breath-hold Anoxic Syncope of Emersion (BASE).* This has been given in the past different names to the lost of consciousness that some breath-hold divers can suffer during the ascent. The more widely diffused is the French "Rendez-vous sincopel des 7 mètres." This term may be confusing since the loss of consciousness, during the ascent in a breath-hold dive, does not appear exactly at 7 m. but may occur at any moment, if the necessary

conditions are done. The term BASE seems more closely descriptive for this frequent, serious, and often undiagnosed entity.

- *Extreme Depth Apnoeic Pulmoary Oedema (EDAPO or EDAPE)*. Although it is not a widely practised diving activity, some individuals are diving at extreme depths, and making possible the development of pulmonary alterations as a result of the paradoxal mechanism of adaptation to this out of limit activity.

Etiopathogenic Classification of Diving Disorders

Diving Disorders are here classified according to their origin and pathophysiological mechanism. Two main preliminary groups exist. Those mainly related to changes in the environmental pressure (DYSBARIC), and those other ones that would be irrelevant if they occurred in the land but they become serious while diving due to the implication of the underwater environment.

NON-DYSBARIC DIVING DISORDERS (Abbrev.: NDDD - Code: DØ). They are not specific of diving, but they can be classified in three wide groups. Some may occur after suffering an aquatic traumatism (boats, rocks, propellers) or an aggression from aquatic animals (Table 6), or after catastrophic damage caused by the diving apparatus (explosion of air cylinders, rupture of high pressure pipes, or hyperbaric chamber defects).

A second group of NDDD result as a failure of the individual mechanisms of adaptation to the underwater environment, like hypothermia, thermo-differential shock, or kinetosis.

The disorders included in the final group are caused by the appearance of non-diving related disorders or diseases that will be a real hazard if they are coincidental with diving. They can be pre-existent silent diseases, which must be considered as a cause of unfitness to dive (seizures, diabetes, asthma, cardiac disorders). Other groups of disorders remain hidden or unknown, but when they coincide with diving, the drowning of the diver can result, like is the case of any situation that can produce a loss of consciousness.

The most important group of Diving Disorders are directly related to changes in environmental pressure, either hyper or hypobaric (Table 7). Some deal with bubble formation in the body and in other ones this phenomenon does not occur, in spite of the fact that all are pressure related, so they properly constitute the group of DYSBARIC DISORDERS (Abbrev.: DD - Code: D).

The first group correspond to NON-BUBBLE-RELATED (or NON-BUBBLE-FORMING) disorders in which no bubble is formed so there is no embolic or infiltrative pathogenic factor (Code: BØ). These changes will cause modifications in both the solution and the morphology of all organic gases. Some gas soLution dependent disorders (Code L) are Breath-hold anoxic syncope of emersion (BASE), Extreme depth apnoeic pulmonary oedema (EDAPE), Inert gas narcosis (IGN) and High pressure neurologic syndrome (HPNS). All disorders produced by the toxical effects of breathing gases will also be included in this group, like the Acute Cerebral Oxygen Toxicity (ACOT), or Carbon monoxide or Carbon dioxide poisonings (CMI or CDI), in the relation to which the word Intoxication should be preferred over Poisoning because its initial coincides with its translation into the majority of European languages.

In the gas volume dependent subgroup, the reduction of gas volume during the compression phase, is the cause of iMplosive traumatisms; the contrary effect during

TABLE 6 - Etiopathogenic Classification of Diving Disorders - I		
NON-DYSBARIC Diving Disorders	Code	Description
Traumatic Aquatic animals injury Static jolt or impact Diving systems caused damage	R	DØR
Adaptive Hypothermia Thermo-differential shock Kinetosis	P	DØP

Coincidental
Pre-existent silent diseases
   Seizures
   Hypoglycaemia
   Asthma attack
   Cardiac attack
 	
Unknown or hidden
   Loss of consciousness
   Any disorder causing drowning
	C	DØC

TABLE 7 - Etiopathogenic Classification of Diving Disorders - II		
NON-DYSBARIC Diving Disorders	Code	Description
Non-bubble-related	BØ	DBØ
Gas **Solution** Dependent *Breath-hold anoxic syncope of emersion (BASE)* *Extreme depth apnoeic pulmonary oedema (EDAPE)* *Inert gas narcosis (IGN)* *High pressure neurologic syndrome (HPNS)* *Acute cerebral oxygen toxicity (ACOT)* *Carbon monoxide intoxication (CMI)* *Carbon dioxide intoxication (CDI)*	L	DBØL
Gas **Volume** Dependent (Barotraumatisms) Implosive Explosive	M X	DBØM DBØX
Bubble-related - (Combined, solution and volume dependent)	B	DB
Infiltrative/ischaemic (extravascular or intratisular bubbles)	I	DBI

Embolic (gas embolism)
   Arterial (due to pulmonary gas explosion)
   Venous (mainly) + arterial (due to tissue gas saturation)
	
	A
	V
		
		DBA
		DBV

Systemic (due to gas-liquid interphase interaction)	S	DBS

decompression produces eXplosive barotraumatisms. When this phenomenon occurs within the chest, the first part of the Intrathoracic Hyperpressive Syndrome (IHS) appears, although not always the intrathoracic hyperpressurized air enters into the blood stream, so it is a non-bubble-related disorder yet.

Other group of Dysbaric disorders are BUBBLE-RELATED (Code: B). Decompressive bubbles remain intratisular, interstitial or extravascular causing by Infiltration compressive or ischaemic effects that will produce varied clinical forms of DCS, some of which were included in the old type I group.

In some southern European areas, divers and also some physicians usually give the name "embolia" to all kind of decompression symptoms, even limb bends; on the contrary, in some anglo-saxon areas the term "neurological, cerebral or vestibular bends" are sometimes employed. If, perhaps, we are obliged, by history and by tradition, to continue using this inadequate and medically inexpressive word, the term bends should be only applied to the bubble-related infiltrative non-embolic limb pain, and embolism should not be applied to the infiltrative/ischaemic bubble-related decompressive minor incidents.

Bubbles will enter into the blood stream producing gas embolism of arterial or venous vessels; this implies not only an etiopathogenic but an important clinical difference. The air bubbles released from a hyperpressurized chest will enter into the arterial system and this will define the predominant encephalic extension of the disease, although other areas can also be embolized.

Bubbles formed in tissues are drained through the venous system and for years this was considered the only mechanism of decompression sickness. It has been proved that arterial embolization is almost always present in DCS, although it can be difficult to detect. This group of embolizing disorders is actually mixed, which means mainly venous plus arterial, and target organs are the spinal cord, the inner ear, and the brain.

Other group of dysbaric bubble-related disorders do not depend, or do not only depend, on their infiltration in tissues or on their embolizing action, but on the haemodynamic and rheological alterations developed over the plasm/bubble interphase causing a real systemic disease. Depending on the importance of these mechanisms, the patient can be in a very specific and peculiar kind of shock. It is not a cardiogenic shock, in spite of the fact that some of its required factors have been developed; it is not a pure neurogenic shock although the clinical presentation may be really similar; it is strictly not a hypovolemic shock since no blood lack has occurred, although haemoconcentration due to hypovolemia sometimes reaches in DCS the highest value that can be seen in human pathology. It is a new type of shock, different, specific, characteristic, that we can properly qualify as DYSBARIC SHOCK.

Chronological Classification

According to the phase of the immersion in which the accident has happened, five different situations may be differentiated (Table 8). The non-dysbaric diving disorders can happen in the surface or at any moment while in the water. Implosive barotraumatisms, for instance, are compressive/descent disorders. Non-bubble-related gas-solution-dependent disorders are developed during the underwater stay at depth.

Bubble-related infiltrative/ischaemic, and embolizing accidents are initiated during the ascent and they continue during the first hours after surfacing. Systemic signs or symptoms are mainly prominent after surfacing. Dysbaric osteonecrosis and other long term effects of diving are post-dive or after-surfacing diving disorders.

TABLE 8 - CHRONOLOGICAL CLASSIFICATION OF DIVING DISORDERS

In the surface (and/or at any moment while in the water)
Aquatic animals injury
Static jolt or impact
Diving systems damage
Hypothermia
Thermo-differential shock
Kinetosis
Seizures
Hypoglycaemia
Asthma attack
Cardiac attack
Loss of consciousness
Any disorder causing drowning

During descent/compression
Implosive barotraumatism
Squeeze
Dental
Tympanic and sinusal
Oval and round window
Pulmonary

During stay at depth
Inert gas narcosis (IGN)
High Pressure Neurologic Syndrome (HPNS)
Extreme depth apnoeic pulmonary oedema (EDAPE)

During ascent/decompression
Explosive barotraumatism
Dental
Sinusal and tympanic
Alternobaric vertigo
Gastro-intestinal
Intrathoracic Hyperpressive Syndrome (IHS)
Decompression Sickness (DCS)
Breath-hold anoxic syncope of emersion (BASE)

After surfacing
Decompression sickness (DCS)
Dysbaric Osteonecrosis (OND)
Neurological sequels of DCS or IHS
Long term effects of diving

Evolutional Classification

Diving Disorders can be finally classified according to their outcome and clinical evolution (Table 9). The majority of dysbaric disorders are acute in the strict sense of this word. Some divers may follow a relapsing outcome. Some rare forms experience a recurrent evolution. Some few disorders, like Dysbaric osteonecrosis (DON), can be considered as chronic.

TABLE 9

EVOLUTIONAL CLASSFICATION OF DIVING DISORDERS

- Acute
- Relapsing
- Recurrent
- Chronic or Long Term

Simplified classification

If all these different groups are placed in one single table that includes all diving disorders, the result can be discouraging (Table 10). Obviously this extended classification, although being very flexible, is not immediately easy to use and require some reflection, a good analysis of the actual condition of the patient, and a good knowledge of dysbaric/diving physiology. For general practice, and for the majority of situations common in medical centres, such deep description is not necessary. For those routine cases we have developed a last synthesizing classification (Table 11). It will bring together, in one single group, the few major factors, syndromes, and pathogenic mechanisms, that must be noted when dealing with a diver who has suffered a diving disorder, because they condition not only some parts of the treatment, but even the final prognosis of the disease. Abbreviations are the same as already explained.

Final remarks

As the final part of this preliminary report we have applied this classification to those situations defined in Table 2 as commonly seen in injured divers, in order to verify its utility and practice. These cases are explained in the pages that follow. On the right of the last line of any case the corresponding alpha-numeric code is annotated. We suggest that readers use these examples trying to establish the utility, or not, of this approach to descriptively classify Diving Disorders.

Obviously we are not only fully open to accept all kind of comments and constructive criticisms, but we actually will appreciate receiving your suggestions in order to improve this classification. You will decide if it can be useful for our common purpose.

TABLE 10		
CLASSIFICATION OF DIVING DISORDERS	Code	Description
NON DYSBARIC	DØ	DØ
Traumatic *Aquatic animals injury* *Static jolt or impact* *Diving systems caused damage*	R	DØR
Adaptive *Hypothermia* *Thermo-differential shock* *Kinetosis*	P	DØP

Coincidental
Pre-existent silent diseases
   Seizures
   Hypoglycaemia
   Asthma attack
   Heart attack
Unknown or hidden
   Loss of consciousness
   Any disorder causing drowning
	C	DØC

DYSBARIC	D	D
Non-bubble-related or Non-bubble-forming	BØ	DBØ

Gas **Solution** Dependent
   Breath-hold anoxic syncope of emersion
   Extreme depth apnoeic pulmonary oedema
   Inert gas narcosis
   High pressure neurologic syndrome
Acute oxygen cerebral toxicity
Carbon monoxide intoxication
Carbon dioxide intoxication
	L
	BASE
	EDAPE
	IGN
	HPNS
	ACOT
	CMI
	CDI
		DBØL

Gas **Volume** Dependent (Barotraumatism)
   Implosive
      Squeeze
      Dental
      Sinusal
      Tympanic
      Oval and round window
   Explosive
      Dental
      Sinusal
      Tympanic
      Alternobaric vertigo
      Gastro-intestinal
      Respiratory or Thoraco-pulmonary
         Cutaneous
         Pleural
         Mediastinal
         Pulmonary
	M
	squ
	den
	sin
	tym
	win
	X
	den
	sin
	tym
	alt
	int
	res
	cut
	pnt
	pnm
	pul
		DBØM
		DBØM.squ
		DBØM.den
		DBØM.sin
		DBØM.tym
		DBØM.win
		DBØX
		DBØX.den
		DBØX.sin
		DBØX.tym
		DBØX.alt
		DBØX.int
		DBØX.res
		DBØX.cut
		DBØX.pnt
		DBØX.pnm
		DBØX.pul

TABLE 10 (continued)		
CLASSIFICATION OF DIVING DISORDERS	**Code**	**Description**
Bubble-related or **Bubble-forming** (Combined, solution and volume dependent)	B	DB
Infiltrative/ischaemic (extravascular or intratisular bubbles)	I	DBI
Cutaneous	cut	DBI.cut
Muscular	mus	DBI.mus
Osteo-articular	ost	DBI.ost
Neural	neu	DBI.neu
Embolic (gas embolism)		
Arterial (due to pulmonary gas explosion)	A	DBA
Encephalic		
Cerebral	*cer*	DBA.cer
Cerebellar	*crb*	DBA.crb
Coronaric	*cor*	DBA.cor
Venous (mainly) + arterial (due to tissue gas saturation)	V	DBV
Medullar	*med*	DBV.med
Vestibular	*ves*	DBV.ves
Cerebral	*cer*	DBV.cer
Cerebellar	*crb*	DBV.crb
Systemic (due to gas-liquid interphase interaction)	S	DBS
Haemodynamic	hem	DBS.hem
Hypovolemia		
Haemoconcentration		
Dysbaric shock	*shk*	DBS.shk
Rheologic	*rhe*	DBS.rhe
Consumptive coagulopathy	*cgl*	DBS.cgl
Disseminate Intravascular Coagulation	*dic*	DBS.dic

TABLE 11 SIMPLIFIED CLASSIFICATION of Diving Disorders	Abbreviation
NON-DYSBARIC DIVING DISORDERS	NDDD
DYSBARIC DISORDERS	DD
Non-embolizing or non-bubble-related	
Gas Solution Dependent:	
Breath-hold anoxic syncope of emersion	BASE
Inert gas narcosis	IGN
Acute Cerebral Oxygen Toxicity	ACOT
Carbon monoxide intoxication	CMI
Carbon dioxide intoxication	CDI
Gas Volume Dependent - Barotrauma	
Implosive (of the descent):	
Sinusal	
Medium ear	
Inner ear	
Explosive (of the ascent):	
Sinusal	
Tympanic (few frequent)	
Alternobaric vertigo	
Thoraco-pulmonary	Intrathoracic Hyperpressive Syndrome IHS
Bubble-related	
Arterial Gas Embolism	
Mixed venous (mainly) + arterial embolizing bubbles:	Decompression
medullar, cerebral, vestibular	Sickness
Infiltrative/ischaemic (extravascular bubbles):	DCS
cutaneous, muscular, neural	
Systemic (due to the bubble gas/liquid interphase interaction):	
dysbaric shock	

NEW DESCRIPTIVE CLASSIFICATION OF DIVING DISORDERS

EXAMPLES

Otalgia during immersion.
Dysbaric, non-bubble-related, implosive, otologic.
Tympanic barotrauma
Descent - Acute

DBØM.oto

Frontal headache after diving.
Dysbaric, non-bubble-related, explosive, sinusal.
Sinusal barotrauma
Ascent - Acute

DBØX.sin

Skin pruriginous rash initiated 45 minutes after surfacing.
Dysbaric, bubble-related, infiltrative, cutaneous (petechial
infiltrative, maculous, or emphysematous).
Cutaneous Decompression Sickness (old type)
Ascent - Acute

DBcut (pet,inf,mac, or emp)

Pain in one arm 15 minutes after diving.
Dysbaric, bubble-related, infiltrative, muscular.
Muscular Decompression Sickness
Ascent - Acute

DBI.mus

Limb pain + with small non-confluent haemorrhagic skin lesions.
Dysbaric, bubble-related, infiltrative, muscular and cutaneous.
Cutaneous and muscular Decompression Sickness
Ascent - Acute

DBI.mus.cut.pet

Subjective neurological symptoms in one arm.
Dysbaric, bubble-related, infiltrative-ischaemic, neurologic, peripheral.
Neural (or peripheral neurologic) Decompression Sickness
Ascent - Acute

DBI.neu

Subjective neurological symptoms + limb pain.
Dysbaric, bubble-related, infiltrative-ischaemic, neurologic, peripheral, and muscular.
Muscular and neural (or peripheral neurologic) Decompression Sickness
Ascent - Acute

DBI.neu.mus

Paraparesis + bladder paralysis.
Dysbaric, bubble-related, venous embolizing, neurologic, medullar.
Medullar neurologic Decompression Sickness
Ascent - Acute

                                                                                    DBV.med

---

Paraplegia + dysbaric shock.
Dysbaric, bubble-related, venous embolizing, neurologic, medullar, systemic.
Medullar neurologic and systemic Decompression Sickness
Ascent - Acute

                                                                                    DBV.med.S

Chest pain + cervical emphysema after a rapid ascent.
Dysbaric, non-bubble-related, explosive, thoracic and cutaneous.
Pulmonary barotrauma due to Intrathoracic Hyperpressive Syndrome
Ascent - Acute

                                                                                    DBØX.pul.cut.emp

---

Hemiparesis after a free ascent.
Dysbaric, bubble-related, arterial embolizing, neurologic, cerebral.
Arterial cerebral gas embolism due to Intrathoracic Hyperpressive Syndrome
Ascent - Acute

                                                                                    DBA.cer

---

Hemiplegia + pneumomediastinum + dysbaric shock.
Dysbaric, bubble-related, arterial embolizing, neurologic, cerebral, systemic,
and explosive, thoracic.
Arterial cerebral gas embolism and pleuro-pulmonary barotrauma due to Intrathoracic
Hyperpressive Syndrome
Ascent - Acute

                                                                                    DBA.cer.SXT

**Tetraplegia + dysbaric shock + gastric distension + pneumothorax + pneumoperitoneum, after a free ascent
from deep and long dive.**
Dysbaric, bubble-related, arterial and venous embolizing, neurologic, cerebral and medullar,
systemic, explosive, pulmonary, and abdominal.
Arterial and venous cerebral and medullar gas embolism, pleuro-pulmonary and gastrointestinal barotrauma due to
both Decompression Sickness and Intrathoracic Hyperpressive Syndrome
Ascent - Acute

                                                                                    DBAV.cer.med.SX.pul.abd

---

Vertigo with facial pain initiated during ascent from a short and swallow dive.
Dysbaric, non-bubble-related, explosive, otological.
Alternobaric vertigo
Ascent - Acute

                                                                                    DBØX.oto

---

**Vertigo initiated five minutes after surfacing from a long and deep immersion with normal ascent and correct
ears equalization, and no other neurological impairment.**
Dysbaric, bubble-related, venous-combined embolizing, vestibular.
Vestibular Decompression Sickness
Ascent - Acute

                                                                                    DBV.ves

WHICH ANIMAL MODELS ARE TO BE USED TO STUDY DECOMPRESSION ACCIDENTS?

Alf O. Brubakk

Department of Physiology and Biomedical Engineering, Medical Faculty, Norwegian University of Science and Technology, Trondheim, Norway.

"Contribution of animal experimentation to the formulation of rational compression schedules must necessarily take the form of identification of potentially relevant phenomena and mechanisms, rather than the determination of numerical values of tolerance limits or development of specific pressure/time profiles directly applicable to man"

—Brauer (1)

"In the decompression literature on humans there appears to be an irresistible urge to pretend knowledge based on a few DCS cases or a few uneventful exposures"

—Weathersby (2)

Decompression accidents can be defined as unwanted effects of decompression. These are quite varied, from bubble formation in the vascular system without any acute clinical symptoms (silent bubbles) to paraplegia and death. The main aim of using animal models to study this problem is to describe the mechanisms involved, not to develop specific procedures for use in a clinical situation. Thus, the animal model chosen should allow us to draw conclusions about mechanisms representative for these effects in man. As far back as 1626, Francis Bacon suggested in his book "New Atlantis" that "trials may be conducted on animals for the purpose of learning what may be wrought upon the body of man" (3).

The animal studies of Robert Boyle (4) and Paul Bert (5) are mentioned in every textbook on decompression as evidence that the basis for decompression sickness is gas separation. Since then, a large number of animal studies have been performed to study decompression. However, even if the perhaps most influential study in decompression research, namely that of Boycott et al. (6), relied heavily on animal studies, animal studies have had relatively little impact on both the development of procedures and methods for treatment of accidents. The reason for this is not quite clear. Perhaps one of the reasons is that diving research has mainly been aimed towards practical goals, "what works, works," with little need for a better understanding of basic details. It can also have something to do with the fact that a large majority of procedures have been developed by the world's navies. They do not operate under the same restraints regarding human studies as for instance universities and they are willing to accept higher risks.

As an example, testing of the US Navy excursion tables were performed on humans (7) in spite of the observation that similar excursions produced gas bubbles in the carotid artery in the majority of exposures (8).

In some cases, animal studies can alert us to potential serious problems. Lehner et al. (9) pointed out that fatal respiratory decompression sickness (chokes) can be provoked if an altitude exposure is performed shortly after a shallow air saturation (to 13 msw). The animal studies of the same group also alerted us to the fact that deep short dives tend to produce central nervous symptoms, while chokes were common with both long and short exposures (10).

Two main questions have to considered when evaluating the use of animals to study decompression accidents. One concerns the most suitable animal species to use, the other the experimental setup. The answer to both these questions will have to depend upon the nature of the problem under study. If, for instance, the basic mechanisms for bubble formation are to be studied, then in vitro models like gels may be quite suitable (11). If bubble formation in the organism is to be evaluated, then animal models that have a similar uptake and elimination of gas as man have to be used. Clinical syndromes, like for instance extreme fatigue, can probably only be studied in man. It is always important to bear in mind that any study will involve a bias, in the sense that experimental conditions will influence the results. When evaluating the result from any study this has to be borne in mind. For example, Vik et al. (12) found in their study in pigs that breakthrough of bubbles in the lungs occurred after 12–20 minutes in four out of six animals during infusion of air at a rate of 0.1 ml min-1kg-1. However, if the animals had received a small infusion of air prior to the experiment, the time to breakthrough was increased to 29 minutes and only occurred in 1 out of 7 animals.

ADVANTAGES OF AN ANIMAL MODEL

Ethical Problems Related to Human Experiments Can Be Avoided

Most of the testing performed to evaluate decompression procedures have been performed using clinical symptoms as an end point. One of the basic principles of using healthy individuals for testing procedures is that no harm shall come to the individual (13). Thus, testing in man must be based on the assumption that no harm will come to the diver if he is treated immediately after clinical symptoms have been observed. However, this has never been properly documented. On the contrary, it is probably true that there is a certain risk of permanent injury even if rapid treatment is initiated. A recent consensus conference on decompression injury stated that changes could be found in divers that had not been involved in decompression accidents (14). The theoretical study of Beckman and Kunkle points out the time to resolution of a bubble with treatment is longer than the survival time of neurons (15).

Conditions of the Experiment Can Be Controlled

When performing testing in humans, it is often difficult to control all environmental conditions. Thus, mechanisms are difficult to elucidate properly.

Animal Testing Allows the Use of Objective End-Points

In order to study mechanisms of injury, objective end points are needed. For instance, the understanding that autochonous bubbles may be responsible for the damage of the spinal cord in serious decompression sickness is based on studies in dogs (16), as is the relative importance of oxygen and pressure in treatment schedules (17). Only animal experiments could have yielded this kind of information.

Cost

Developing new and improved decompression procedures is an increasingly expensive business. The reason for this is that modern decompression procedures have a low incidence of treated decompression sickness, probably in the range of 0.1 to 0.5%. This makes these procedures very difficult to test as a very large number of dives will have to be performed in order to have meaningful statistics about the risk. In fact, if a particular depth / time combination is tested with no case of DCS in 10 dives, this only means that it is unlikely that the next 100 dives will have more than a 31% incidence of DCS (18). The recent revision of the French air tables required 65.000 dives to establish a DCS incidence of 0.3% (19). To determine if a new table would improve this incidence to 0.1% would require the evaluation of about 500.000 dives (20), a nearly impossible task. Preliminary testing in a suitable animal model with objective end points can greatly reduce the need for human testing, by identifying the "best" table, for instance the table that produces the least amount of separated gas.

Extensive Measurements Can Be Performed

To understand the mechanisms between decompression and injury, it is of value to know about the physiological responses involved. For instance, if one wishes to judge the risk for arterial gas embolisation in individuals with an open foramen ovale, one has to know about the relationship between bubble formation and increases in right atrial pressure. This can be studied in an animal model (21). Furthermore, a variety of morphological and biochemical methods can be used to study the mechanisms of injury.

PROBLEMS IN USING ANIMAL MODELS

If clinical endpoints, like for instance pain, are used, it is important to appreciate that animals will respond to training. For instance, it is told that some of the goats in the Royal Navy studies, after a number of bend-inducing dives, lifted their leg in response to the noise of gas escaping the chamber, probably because they knew that this would induce the desired behavior in the researcher, namely ordering recompression.

Species Differences

It is difficult to compare the results from different experimental animals, using different experimental preparations in different laboratories. However, species differences clearly exist. For instance, the alveolar and capillary surface area relative to weight is smaller in the sedentary pig than in the athletic dog (22–24). Air infusion rates of 0.30-0.35 ml kg-1 min-1 have been tolerated in dog experiments (25,26), whereas infusion rates of only 0.10 and 0.20 ml kg-1 min-1 induced cardiovascular collapse in pigs (27). Direct extrapolation of the results from dog experiments to humans may be questioned, as humans are grouped together with the "sedentary" animals. Wolffe and Robertson concluded that the amount of air necessary to produce death in rabbits and dogs when injected intravenously, seemed to be directly proportional to the size of the pulmonary artery and its branches (28).

The autonomic inervation of pulmonary vasculature varies to a certain degree in different species (29), which may explain differences in response. In addition, pigs and other animals such as sheep, goats, cows, and cats have intrapulmonary macrophages in the pulmonary circulation. These cells may release thromboxane A2, a potent vasoconstrictor, when exposed to particles of different kinds in the pulmonary circulation (30). This fact could also contribute to the difference in response between dogs and pigs, since only few intrapulmonary macrophages have been found in dogs. Such cells have been observed in humans, although it appears that their number is relatively small in the normal lung (31).

Many different species have been exposed to pressure and decompressed to study bubble formation. Small-sized animals such as guinea pigs, cats, rats, mice, hamsters, frogs, and crabs have been used in experimental studies (32-38). Boycott et al. (6) argued that larger animals, e.g., goats, were preferable as models for humans, since both the uptake and elimination of gas, and therefore bubble formation, would be dependent on the relationship between cardiac output to weight.

Several species of larger animals have been used to study the effects of venous gas embolism (VGE). The dog has been used most frequently, both in experiments using gas infusion or gas injection and after decompression (39-46). VGE studies have also been performed using sheep (47–50), pigs (27,51,52) and goats (53).

Size

The problem of size is related to the relationship between blood flow and tissue volume. In small animals, there is a considerable higher blood flow relative to tissue volume than in bigger animals, by about a factor of 2. Small animals also have a relatively higher metabolism than bigger animals (54). If cardiac output is related to metabolism, larger animals have a relatively higher flow.

This is demonstrated in Table 1.

Table 1. Cardiac output in relation to size. Adapted from (55)					
Animal	Weight kg	C.O. l./min.	C.O./Wt. l./kg/min.	C.O./Wt.$^{3/4}$	C.O./Wt.$^{2/3}$
Rat	0.18	0.047	0.26	0.17	0.15
Rabbit	2.6	0.139	0.11	0.14	0.15
Cat	3.1	0.33	0.11	0.14	0.15
Dog	19.3	2.3	0.12	0.24	0.31
Goat	23.7	3.1	0.13	0.29	0.37
Sheep	40	4	0.10	0.25	0.34
Man	70	6	0.09	0.25	0.35
Pig+	32	4.5	0.15	0.33	0.44
Horse+	342	24	0.07	0.3	0.49
Pig*	23.6	5.4	0.23	0.50	0.66

Wt.$^{3/4}$ is proportional to metabolism (54)
Wt.$^{2/3}$ is proportional to body surface area (55)
+ Data from (56)
* Data from (21). Anesthetized and after insertion of catheters.

The relationship between weight and cardiac output can be described by the formula :

$$C.O. = 0.1017W^{0.9988}$$

where W is weight in kg and C.O. is cardiac output in liters/min (56). As can be seen this will give slightly different values for cardiac output than the values given above. Furthermore, it must be considered that quite different values can be obtained depending upon the experimental conditions. For instance, values of C.O./Weight varies from 0.14 to 0.41 in the data given for various strains of rats in Biological Handbooks (56). Our own data from the pig also shows this (see above).

Berghage (56) collected some data on the saturation time for various species and their susceptibility for decompression sickness. Some of these are shown in Table 2.

Table 2.			
Animal	Weight, kg	Time to Sat., min	ED_{50} Sat.pressure. ATA +
Mouse	0.022	40	13.8
Hamster	0.091	90	7.6
Rat	0.25	130	6.8
Guinea pig	0.52	163	6.0
Dog	12	250	3.3
Goat	33	300	2.7
Man	78	720	2.2
Pig*	24	600?	?

+ ED_{50} sat. pressure is the saturation pressure from which 50% of the individuals will suffer decompression sickness if they are decompressed rapidly to 1 ATA
* Preliminary data from (58). n=8, anesthetized. Extrapolation from nitrogen content in the pulmonary artery measured for 5 hours.

There is probably considerable variation in saturation and desaturation time within the same species, depending on many variables. For instance, Dick et al. (59) showed that regular exercise will considerably increase the rate of gas elimination. This mechanism may be the basis for the reduction in the incidence of neurological decompression sickness in exercised pigs (60). Our own study, based on measurement of the nitrogen content in the pulmonary artery in the pig, shows a considerably longer saturation time than would be expected from the weight of the animal, but there are considerable uncertainties due to a large variation between individuals (59).

The ED_{50} pressure difference is related to weight and the absolute value of the saturation pressure by the formula:

$$\Delta ED_{50} = (19W^{-0.215}) + (1.64W^{-0.221}) * (P - 19W^{-0.215})$$

where W is weight in grams and P is the saturation pressure (57). These values are established for nitrogen as the inert gas.

As can be seen from the formula, this means that a small animal like a rat will have a large increase in ΔED_{50} with an increase in saturation pressure, while the saturation pressure has less effect on this value in man (57). For instance, over the whole range of practical diving (1–31 ATA), the ΔED_{50} increases from 2.2 to 5.1 ATA (131%) in man, while it increases from 6.8 to 19.1 (181%) ATA in the rat. A similar relationship exists for helium (57).

Lin et al. (61,62) showed that bubble formation in the venous system was independent of animal size. Eckenhoff et al. (63) demonstrated that bubbles could be detected in the pulmonary artery in man after saturation to 3.7 meters on air. Hope et al. showed bubbles in 2 out of 4 rats after saturation at 3 msw on heliox (64), and bubbles were detected in 2 out of 8 divers saturated at 5 msw on heliox (Risberg et al. 1995, unpublished). In pigs, we found bubbles in the pulmonary artery in six out of seven animals after 3 hours at 5 meters on air (Brubakk et al. 1996, unpublished). All these data together indicate that at least for the vascular bubbles in the pulmonary artery, animal size does not seem to matter. This is not too unexpected, because blood in the pulmonary artery is a mixture of blood from all parts of the body. Relative differences in flow will therefore only influence the total saturation/desaturation time of the whole body which will be quicker in a smaller than a larger animal.

These results are in contrast to the data shown in Table 2 and to the study of Kindwall (65), who demonstrated that cats, rabbits, guinea pigs, and rats all were very resistant to decompression sickness after saturation exposure. This can be explained by differences in flow to the different tissues. A relatively lower flow to a particular tissue will reduce the ability of that tissue to remove gas, thus giving the bubbles more time to grow.

If one relates cardiac output to metabolism, then this will be relatively higher in a big rather than a small animal. The reason for this is probably related to temperature regulation, as a bigger animal has a bigger surface area.

Anesthesia

Most experimental studies of gas uptake have been performed in anesthetized animals. Thus, the effect of anesthesia may be of importance. It is often stated that barbiturates reduce cardiac output and decreases cardiac function. However, in light barbiturate anesthesia no effect on cardiac output has been noted (55). In dogs, no circulatory effects of morphine, ether, barbital, urethane, chloralosone, or pentobarbital could be detected (66). In another study in the same species, no effect of (-chlorates and pentobarbital on cardiac output could be detected (67). Ketamine generally leads to a slight increase in cardiac output (68), but may also lead to a redistribution of flow between the organs (69).

Even data from awake animals or even man may be seriously affected by differences in temperature, activity, stress, physical fitness, all factors that influence circulation (55). For instance, a 1° C increase in body temperature will increase cardiac output by 25% (70) while changing from the supine to the standing position may decrease cardiac output by 20% (71). Immersion in thermoneutral water will increase cardiac output by approximately 40%; if the water temperature is decreased to 20° C, cardiac output will decrease by 30% (72).

The studies that use spontaneously-breathing animals may give different results from the studies using mechanically ventilated animals (73), since the first group may increase their ventilation and thereby are able to prevent an increase of carbon dioxide in the arterial blood.

Activity Level

Exercise may increase cardiac output five to six times in a well trained athlete. However, even much more limited exercise will influence bubble formation and the incidence of decompression sickness.

Harvey et al. (33) studied the limits for bubble formation in cats, both at rest and after electrical stimulation and tissue injury. The conclusion from these studies was that at marginal exposures, stimulation or injury was needed for bubble formation. At higher supersaturations, bubbles will occur at rest; the time of occurrence will be determined by the fat content. Essentially the same results have been obtained in frogs and rats (34). These results are of particular importance for modern diving procedures.

Based on these studies, the authors concluded that gas bubbles are chiefly intra-vascular and that they are responsible for nearly all important phases of the syndrome of decompression sickness. Only in very severe cases did extravascular bubbles play a role and then only in lipid rich structures.

CHOICE OF ANIMAL MODEL

As mentioned previously, a large number of species have been used for decompression studies. In choosing an animal, there seems to be little appreciation about possible species differences, most choices seem to have been made by convenience. Boycott et al. point out that " ...*for regular use goats were selected chiefly because they were the largest animals that could be conveniently dealt with and which could be obtained in considerable numbers*" (6). The important question is then if this is adequate or if a more thorough study is warranted into species differences.

Another question that has to be considered is the availability of data from one particular animal species, like the response to anesthesia, circulatory and ventilatory data, hematology a.s.o. If immunological methods are to be used, suitable antibodies have to be available.

As far as we know today, decompression accidents will lead to changes and/or symptoms in mainly the following organ systems (14): lungs, central nervous system, blood vessels, bone, tendons, and muscle. At least for the mammalian species, differences exist, but they are generally of a quantitative not a qualitative nature.

Bubble Formation in Tissue and Blood

For evaluating this an animal model with similar gas dynamics features as man is needed. As was pointed out above, size is of importance if bubble formation in tissue is to be studied, but not if bubbles in the pulmonary artery is used as an end point. Study of changes in the skin or the effect of changes in temperature require an animal without fur.

Central Nervous System Injury

The central nervous system shows large similarities in all mammals. Some differences in vascular supply exist, but this will only influence the distribution of gas bubbles.

Bone

Lanphier and Lehner have pointed out (74) that sheep are well suited for studies of bone necrosis. Although probably other mammals can be well suited for such studies, these authors have demonstrated that bone necrosis can be produced even after one single saturation exposure.

Blood Vessels and Lungs

Damage to the endothelial layer of the blood vessel probably represents the initial insult in all decompression accidents, as vascular bubbles is a regular feature. In the study by Smith et al. (75), endothelial damage could be demonstrated in pigs exposed to severe decompressions. Endothelial damage has also been observed in several other studies (76,77). The endothelial system and its response to bubbles has been inadequately described, but there is probably few species differences between mammals. Resident macrophages adhering to the endothelium (Pulmonary Intravascular Macrophages, PIM) have been identified in the lungs of several mammalian species (78). Such macrophages have been identified both in the baboon (79) and in man (31), although they seem to be much less numerous than in other species like pig or sheep. In sheep they occupy approximately 15% of the capillary blood volume, while they are found in only 2% of that volume in the baboon (79). However, PIMs may be induced by breathing high doses of oxygen (79), as well as other stimuli. The most important secretory product of these macrophages is thromboxane (30).

Flick et al. (80) examined the role of leukocytes in capillary damage in sheep. The authors accept that the role of leukocytes may be species dependent but believed that leukocytes play a role in humans and that the clotting cascade and platelets serve an augmenting role by trapping leukocytes in the pulmonary vasculature.

CONCLUSIONS

Most, if not all, practical decompressions will lead to some degree of gas bubble formation in the organism. The exact threshold for this bubble formation is not known, but it is probably in the range of 50–70 kPa in the tissue (81) and even lower in the vascular system as mentioned above. There are data indicating that there may be a large difference in susceptibility to decompression sickness not directly related to the amount of vascular gas bubbles observed (82).

The basis for all decompression injury is considered to be gas separation. Furthermore, one considers gas nuclei to be the basis for the growth of bubbles, as "pure" solutions have a very high resistance to bubble formation (83). Thus an animal model should be chosen that has a similar circulatory and ventilatory system to that of man and preferably a similar amount of gas nuclei. To my knowledge, no information about possible species differences in the number of nuclei exist, but the fact that all animals, regardless of size, seem to bubble at the same level of supersaturation (see above) makes large differences unlikely. There are few instances where similar decompression profiles have been compared between man and experimental animals. Comparisons between man and the pig have shown that the incidence of bubble formation in blood is similar (84) and that these animals develop decompression sickness after the same exposures as man (85).

Generally it can be stated that in mammals, differences in physiological and biochemical responses are of a quantitative and not a qualitative nature. However, as has been documented in many studies, these differences can be of importance and must be considered if any conclusions about the applicability of the data to man is to be reached.

REFERENCES

1. Brauer RW. The contribution of animal experimentation toward the development of rational compression schedules for very deep diving. In Lin Y-C, Shida KK (eds). Man in the sea, Vol I. San Pedro; Best Publishing Company 1990:pp 1-22.
2. Weathersby PK. Effect of different gases on decompression sickness. In: Vann RD (ed). The physiological basis of decompression. Bethesda,MD; Undersea & Hyperbaric Medical Society 1989:pp 107-116.
3. Bacon F. New Atlantis. London 1626.
4. Boyle R. New pneumatical experiments about respiration. Philos Trans 1670;5:2011-058.
5. Bert P. La pression barometrique. Paris. G. Masson 1878.
6. Boycott AE, Damant GCC, Haldane JS. The prevention of compressed-air illness. J Hygiene, London 1908; 8:342-443.
7. Thalman ED. Testing of revised unlimited-duration upward excursions during helium-oxygen saturation dives. Undersea Biomed Res 1989;16:195-218.
8. Brubakk AO, Peterson R, Grip A, Holand B, Onarheim J, Segadal K, Kunkle TD, Tønjum S. Gas bubbles in the circulation of divers after ascending excursions from 300 to 250 msw. J Appl Physiol 1986; 60:45-51.
9. Lehner CE, Will JA, Lightfoot EN, Lanphier EH. Decompression sickness in sheep: fatal chokes after 24-hour dives with altitude provocation. In: Bachrach AJ, Matzen MM (eds). Underwater Physiology VIII. Bethesda, MD; Undersea Medical Society 1984:pp191-200.
10. Lehner CE, Lanphier EH. Influence of pressure profile on DCS symptoms. In: Vann RD (ed). The physiological basis of decompression. Bethesda, MD. Undersea & Hyperbaric Medical Society 1989:pp 299-322.
11. Yount DE. Growth of bubbles from nuclei. In Brubakk AO et al (Eds.). Supersaturation and bubble formation in fluid and organisms. Tapir Publishers; Trondheim 1989:pp 131-164.
12. Vik A, Brubakk AO, Hennessy TR, Jenssen BM, Ekker M, Slørdahl SA. Venous air embolism in swine: transport of gas bubbles through the pulmonary circulation. J Appl Physiol 1990; 69:237-244.
13. Lanphier EH. Ethical aspects of validation. In: Schreiner HR, Hamilton RW (eds). Validation of decompression tables. Bethesda, MD;Undersea & Hyperbaric Medical Society 1989:pp 119-123.
14. Hope A, Lund T, Elliott DH, Halsey MJ, Wiig H (eds). Long term health effects of diving. Bergen; NUTEC 1994.
15. Kunkle T, Beckman EL. Bubble resolution physics and the treatment of decompression sickness. Med Physics 1983;10:184-190.
16. Francis TJR, Pezeshkpour GH, Dutka AJ, Hallenbeck JM, Flynn ET. Is there a role for the autochothonous bubble in the pathogenesis of spinal cord decompression sickness. J Neuropath Exp Neur 1988; 47:475-487.
17. Sykes JJW, Hallenbeck JM, Leitch DR. Spinal decompression sickness: A comparison of recompression therapies in an animal model. Aviat Space Environ Med 1986;57:561-568.
18. Weathersby PK, Homer LD, Flynn ET. On the likelihood of decompression sickness. J Appl Physiol Respirat Environ Exercise Physiol 1984; 57:815-825.
19. Imbert J, Bontoux M. A method for introducing new decompression procedures. In: Schreiner HR, Hamilton RW (eds). Validation of decompression tables. Bethesda, MD;Undersea & Hyperbaric Medical Society 1989: pp 97-105.
20. Imbert J. Decompression safety. In: Subtech 93. London; Kluwer Academic Publishers;pp 239-249.
21. Vik A, Jenssen BM, Brubakk AO. Arterial gas bubbles after decompression in pigs with patent foramen ovale. Undersea & Hyperbaric Med 1993; 20:121-132.
22. Burri PH and Weibel ER. Ultrastructure and morphometry of the developing lung. In: Hodson WA (ed) Development of the lung. (Lung Biol Health Dis Ser). New York; Dekker 1977:pp 215-268.
23. Weibel ER. Oxygen demand and the size of respiratory structures in mammals. In: Wood SC, Lenfant C (eds) Evolution of respiratory processes: A Comparative Approach. (Lung Biol Health Dis Ser). New York; Dekker 1979:pp 289-334.
24. Weibel ER. The Pathway for Oxygen. Cambridge, MA: Harvard Univ Press, 1984.
25. Butler BD, Leiman BC, Katz J. Arterial air embolism of venous origin in dogs: effect of nitrous oxide in combination with halothane and pentobarbitone. Can J Anaesth 1987; 34:570-575.
26. Butler BD, Hills BA. Transpulmonary passage of venous air emboli. J Appl Physiol 1985; 59:543-547.
27. Vik A, Brubakk AO, Hennessy TR, Jenssen BM, Ekker M, Slørdahl SA. Venous air embolism in swine: transport of gas bubbles through the pulmonary circulation. J Appl Physiol 1990; 69:237-244.
28. Wolffe JB, Robertson HF. Experimental air embolism. Ann Intern Med 1935; 9:162-165.
29. Harris P, Heath D. The Human Pulmonary Circulation. 2nd edition. Edinburgh: Churchill Livingstone 1977.
30. Warner AE, Brain JD. The cell biology and pathogenic role of pulmonary intravascular macrophages. Am J Physiol 1990; 258 (Lung Cell Mol Physiol 2) L1-12.
31. Dehring DJ, Wismar BL. Intravascular macrophages in pulmonary capillaries of humans. Am Rev Respir Dis 1989; 139:1027-1029.
32. McDonough PM, Hemmingsen EA. Bubble formation in crabs induced by limb motions after decompression. J Appl Physiol 1984; 57:117-122.
33. Harvey EN. Animal experiments on bubble formation. Part I. Bubble formation in cats. In: Fulton JF (ed) Decompression sickness. Philadelphia, PA; Saunders, 1951:pp 115-144.
34. Blinks LR, Twitty VC, Whitaker DM. Animal experiments on bubble formation. Part II. Bubble formation in frogs and rats. In: Fulton JF (ed) Decompression sickness. Philadelphia, PA; Saunders, 1951:pp 145-164.
35. Lynch PR, Brigham M, Tuma R, Wieceman MP. Origin and time course of gas bubbles following rapid decompression in the hamster. Undersea Biomed Res 1985; 12:105-114.
36. Wolffe JB, Robertson HF. Experimental air embolism. Ann Intern Med 1935; 9:162-165.

37. Lever MJ, Miller KW, Paton WDM, Smith EB. Experiments on the genesis of bubbles as a result of rapid decompression. J Physiol 1966; 184:964-969.

38. Powell MR. Gas phase separation following decompression in asymptomatic rats: visual and ultrasound monitoring. Aerospace Med 1972; 43:1240-1244.

39. Bove AA, Hallenbeck JM, Elliott DH. Circulatory responses to venous air embolism and decompression sickness in dogs. Undersea Biomed Res 1974; 1:207-220.

40. Butler BD, Katz J. Vascular pressures and passage of gas emboli through the pulmonary circulation. Undersea Biomed Res 1988; 15:203-209.

41. Catron PW, Thomas LB, Flynn ET, McDermott JJ, Holt MA. Effects of He-O2 breathing during experimental decompression sickness following air dives. Undersea Biomed Res 1987; 14:101-111.

42. Catron PW, Thomas LB, McDermott JJ, Smallridge RC, Lake CR, Kinzer C, Chernow B, Flynn ET. Hormonal changes during decompression sickness. Undersea Biomed Res 1987; 14:331-341.

43. Gottdiener JS, Papademetriou V, Notargiacomo A, Park WY, Cutler DJ. Incidence and cardiac effects of systemic venous air embolism. Echocardiographic evidence of arterial embolization via noncardiac shunt. Arch Intern Med 1988; 148:795-800.

44. Katz J, Leiman BC, Butler BD. Effects of inhalation anesthetics on filtration of venous gas emboli by the pulmonary vasculature. Br J Anaesth 1988; 61:200-205.

45. Verstappen FTJ, Bernards JA, Kreuzer F. Effects of pulmonary gas embolism on circulation and respiration in the dog. l. Effects on circulation. Pflügers Arch 1977; 368:89-96.

46. Yahagi N, Furuya H. The effects of halothane and pentobarbital on the threshold of transpulmonary passage of venous air emboli in dogs. Anesthesiology 1987; 67:905-909.

47. Atkins CE, Lehner CE, Beck KA, Dubielzig RR, Nordheim EV, Lanphier EH. Experimental respiratory decompression sickness in sheep. J Appl Physiol 1988; 65:1163-1171.

48. Deal CW, Fielden BP, Monk I. Hemodynamic effects of pulmonary air embolism. J Surg Res 1971; 11:533-538.

49. Neuman TS, Spragg RG, Wagner PD, Moser KM. Cardiopulmonary consequences of decompression stress. Resp Physiol 1980; 41:143-153.

50. Spencer MP, Oyama Y. Pulmonary capacity for dissipation of venous gas emboli. Aerospace Med 1971; 42:822-827.

51. Black S, Cucchiara RF, Nishimura RA, Michenfelder JD. Parameters affecting occurrence of paradoxical air embolism. Anesthesiology 1989; 71:235-241.

52. Vik A, Jenssen BM, Brubakk AO. Effect of aminophylline on transpulmonary passage of venous air emboli in pigs. J Appl Physiol 1991; 71:1780-1786.

53. D'Aoust BG, Swanson HT, White R, Dunford R, Mahoney J. Central venous bubbles and mixed venous nitrogen in goats following decompression. J Appl Physiol 1981; 51:1238-1244.

54. Klieber M. Body size and metabolic rate. Physiol Rev 1947;27:511-541.

55. Guyton AC, Jones CE, Coleman TG. Circulatory physiology: Cardiac output and its regulation. London; WB Saunders Company 1973.

56. Altman P, Dittmer DS (eds). Biological Handbooks: Respiration and Circulation. Bethesda, MD; Fed Am Soc Exp Biol 1971.

57. Berghage TE, David TD, Dyson CV. Species differences in decompression. Undersea Biomedical Research 1979; 6:1-13.

58. Flook V, Brubakk AO, Holmen IM, Koteng S, Ustad A-L. Effect of decompression bubbles on nitrogen concentration. SINTEF Report STF78A96102. Trondheim; SINTEF 1996.

59. Dick AP, Vann RD, Mebane GY, Feezor MD. Decompression induced nitrogen elimination. Undersea Biomed Res 1984;11:369-380.

60. Broome JR, Dutkc AJ, McNamee GA. Exercise conditioning reduces the risk of neurologic decompression illness in swine. Undersea Hyperbaric Med 1995;22:73-85.

61. Lin YC. Species independent maximum no-bubble pressure reduction from saturation dive. In: Bacharach AJ, Matzen MM (eds). Underwater Physiology VII. Bethesda, MD; Undersea Medical Society 1981:pp 699-706.

62. Lin YC, Mack GW, Watanabe DK, Shida KK. Experimental attempts to influence the bubble threshold from saturation dives in animals. In: Bacharach AJ, Matzen MM (eds). Underwater Physiology VIII. Bethesda, MD; Undersea Medical Society 1984:pp 259-268.

63. Eckenhoff RG, Olstad CS, Garrod G. Human dose-response relationship for decompression and endogenous bubble formation. J Appl Physiol 1990;69: 914-918.

64. Hope A, Segadal K, Sundland H. Gas bubbles in awake, free roaming rats after rapid decompression from shallow heliox saturation (in Norwegian). NUTEC Report 26-95. Bergen; Norwegian Underwater Technology Centre 1996.

65. Kindwall EP. Metabolic rate and animal size correlated with decompression sickness. Am J Physiol 1962; 203:385-388.

66. Wiggers HC. Cardiac output and total peripheral resistance measurements in experimental dogs. Amer J Physiol 1944;140:519-522.

67. Van Citters RL, Franklin DL, Rushmer RF. Left ventricular dynamics in dogs during anesthesia with alpha-chloralose and sodium pentobarbital. Am J Cardiol 1964;13:349-354.

68. Lanning CF, Harmel MH. Ketamine anesthesia. Ann Rev Med 1975;26:137-141.

69. Traber DL, Wilson RD, Priano LL. The effect of alpha-adrenergic blockade on the cardiopulmonary response to ketamine. Anesth Analg 1971;50:737-742.

70. Brendel W, Albers C, Usinger W. Der Kreislauf in Hypothermie. Pluegers Arch ges Physiol 1958;266:341-345.

71. Bevegard S, Holmgren A, Jonsson B. The effect of body position on the circulation at rest and during exercise, with special reference to the influence on the stroke volume. Acta Physiol Scand 1960;49:279-282.

72. Pendergast DR, Olszowka AJ. Effect of exercise, thermal state, blood flow on inert gas exchange. In: Vann RD (ed). The physiological basis of decompression. Bethesda,MD. Undersea & Hyperbaric Medical Society 1989: pp 37-51.

73. Verstappen FTJ, Bernards JA, Kreuzer F. Effects of pulmonary gas embolism on circulation and respiration in the dog. II. Effects on respiration. Pflügers Arch 1977; 368:97-104.

74. Lanphier EH, Lehner CE. Animal models in decompression In: Lin YC, Shida KK (eds) Man in the Sea, Vol I. SanPedro; BestPubl Co 1990:pp 274-216.

75. Smith KH, Stegall PJ, Harker LA, Slichter SJ, Richmond VL, Hall MH, Huang TJ. Investigation of Hematologic and Pathologic Response to Decompression. Virginia Mason Research Center, Seattle. Final report Project #N00014-71-C-0273,1978.

76. Catron PW, Flynn ET, Yaffe L, Bradley ME, Thomas LB, Hinman D, Survanshi S, Johnson JT, Harrington J. Morphological and physiological responses of the lungs of dogs to acute decompression. J Appl Physiol 1984; 57:467-474.

77. Levin, LL, Stewart GJ, Lynch PR, Bove AA. Blood and blood vessel wall changes induced by decompression sickness in dogs. J Appl Physiol 1981; 50:944-949.

78. Staub NC. Pulmonary intravascular macrophages. Ann Rev Physiol 1994; 56:47-67.

79. Fracica PJ, Bertram T, Knapp M, Crapo JD. Pulmonary intravascular macrophages in normal and oxygen injured baboon lung tissue. Clin Res 1988; 36:A591.

80. Flick MR, Perel A, Staub NC. Leucocytes are required for increased lung microvascular permeability after microembolization in sheep. Circ Res 1981; 48:344-351.

81. Daniels S. Ultrasonic monitoring of decompression procedures, Phil Trans R Soc Lond 1984; B304:153-175.

82. Ward CA. Identification of individuals susceptible to decompression sickness In: Bove AA et al (eds). Underwater Physiology IX, UHMS, Maryland, USA 1987: pp 239-247.

83. Hemmingsen EA. Nucleation of bubbles in vitro and in vivo. In: Brubakk AO, Kanwisher J, Sundnes G (eds) Diving in animals and man. Trondheim; Tapir Publishers, 1986:pp 43-59.

84. Brubakk AO. A laboratory for the study of decompression. In: Reinertsen RE, Brubakk AO, Bolstad G (eds). Prodeedings EUBS 1996. Trondheim 1996;pp 302-307.

85. Fife WP, Mezzino MJ, Naylor R. Development and operational validation of accelerated decompression tables. In: Shilling CW, Beckett MW (eds). Underwater Physiology VI. Bethesda MD; FASEB 1978: pp359-366.

NOTES

WHICH INITIAL RECOMPRESSION TREATMENT?

Richard E. Moon, MD

Duke University Medical Center - Durham, NC, USA

The central role of tissue bubble formation in decompression illness (DCI) is indisputable. Initially it was assumed that all of the signs and symptoms of decompression illness are due either to direct tissue damage by bubbles or a reduction in blood flow due intravascular gas.

In recent years, however, it has been recognized that while bubbles are the initiating factor in decompression illness, they also produce secondary changes, which may amplify their direct effects. Platelet depletion and complement activation have both been observed. Also described was a late reduction in cerebral flood flow after arterial gas embolism even after the bubbles had moved distally. This has been attributed to leukocyte accumulation on damaged endothelium and the release of their toxic products into surrounding tissue. In other forms of neural injury secondary damage due to reperfusion of ischemic tissue, mediated by oxygen free radicals and neurotoxic neurotransmitters, has been described. The choice of a recompression treatment must therefore take into account possible beneficial or detrimental effects of recompression on these other mechanisms.

The important descriptors of a recompression table are pressure, time, and breathing gas.

PRESSURE AND TIME

That the ambient pressure should result in a reduction in bubble volume, and resolution of symptoms has been confirmed by observation. Over 100 years ago compressed air workers noticed that bends symptoms, which initially occurred after decompression from the high pressure environment, would often disappear when they re-entered the environment on the next shift. The efficacy of recompression treatment was systematically examined by Keays (1909) and since then this has been supported by clinical experience.

This led people to believe that bubble volume reduction and, ultimately, elimination of the constituent gases of bubbles, constituted the major therapeutic role of recompression therapy. Based upon such a hypothesis one would predict the most efficacious treatment would be one which would result in the largest bubble volume reduction and the most rapid elimination of bubble inert gas. If one assumes that tissue bubbles must be made as small as possible, as rapidly as possible, then it follows that the ideal recompression table should use the highest practical pressure.

Several recompression schedules (commonly referred to as "treatment tables") have been empirically developed. The most widely used of these are USN Treatment Table 5 and USN Treatment Table 6, or similar equivalents. The two-step algorithm, with periods of oxygen breathing at 18 meters of sea water equivalent depth (msw) and 9 msw. USN Table 6 can be "extended" to provide additional breathing cycles at both depths, the extreme example of which is the "Catalina" Table (Pilmanis, 1987), in which up to 8 cycles of oxygen can be administered at 18 msw, and 18 cycles at 9 msw.

Several reports have examined the issue of the best treatment depth. Using anesthetized dogs Leitch et al. (1984b) examined the efficacy of a range of treatment depths from 18 to 90 msw for gas embolism and found that none were superior to 100% oxygen breathing at 18 msw. Leitch & Hallenbeck (1985) performed a similar study in dogs with spinal cord decompression sickness, using 20, 40, and 60 msw treatment depths with an inspired PO_2 of 202 kPa, or 18 msw breathing 100% oxygen (inspired PO_2 282 kPa). Using somatosensory evoked potential amplitude as the measure of outcome, there were no significant differences in any of the groups. Leitch & Green (1985) retrospectively examined a series of divers and concluded that pressurization deeper than 18 msw was rarely required.

US Navy guidelines for the use of Table 5 include the requirement that it be used only for pain only or skin bends, and that symptoms must resolve within ten minutes of reaching 18 msw depth. When applied according to these criteria Green et al. found that a single treatment using USN Table 5 was effective in 95.7% of cases (Green et al., 1989).

For all other situations, a different table is generally used, such as USN Table 6. The vast majority of decompression illness in dives originating at the surface (e.g., non-saturation dives) can be managed using Table 5, Table 6, or Table 6 with additional oxygen breathing periods. Workman (1968) reported that of 110 military divers treated with these oxygen tables, 106 (96%) had complete relief of symptoms and 4 had substantial relief.

Divers with major neurological abnormalities who continue to improve during treatment, but for whom the maximum time limit at 2.8 ATA has been reached, or in whom major deterioration occurs during decompression, can be considered for saturation treatment. In this form of treatment the chamber pressure is maintained until clinical stability has been reached, typically for 12 hours or more. Once saturation treatment has been initiated, decompression must occur at a considerably reduced rate, and oxygen cycles have to be administered using a different schedule in order to reduce pulmonary oxygen toxicity. Saturation treatment at a chamber depth of 2.8 ATA allows the chamber atmosphere to consist of air. The US Navy implementation of saturation at 2.8 ATA is referred to as Table 7 (Navy Department, 1993).

Other saturation depths have been proposed (Miller et al., 1978), and may be imperative for individuals decompressing from either deep bounce dives or saturation dives. In such situations the treatment gas must be specially mixed such that the partial pressure of oxygen does not exceed 3 atmospheres.

Shorter tables, such as those designed for use in monoplace chambers, also appear to be effective (Hart et al., 1986; Kindwall, 1996). The monoplace table designed by Hart specifies 100% oxygen administration at 3 ATA for 30 minutes followed by 2.5 ATA for 60 minutes (Hart, 1974; Hart et al., 1986). These shorter, shallower tables appear to be effective in most cases (Kindwall, 1996), although they have not been prospectively compared with the more commonly used schedules such as USN Table 6, and their equivalence to the longer oxygen tables in severe decompression illness has not been confirmed.

The initial US Navy experience with oxygen recompression at an equivalent depth of 18 meters (60 feet, 2.8 ATA) was so successful that it has become the mainstay of modern recompression therapy (Workman, 1968), both for recreational and military diving accidents. At a pressure of 2.8 ATA 100% oxygen can be breathed with a low probability of oxygen toxicity, and both the diver being treated and the tender accompanying him inside the chamber can be decompressed relatively quickly. Most cases of DCI in diving which commenced at the surface can be satisfactorily managed by compression to 18 meters equivalent depth while breathing 100% oxygen. US Navy Table 5 can be used if the diver's symptoms are pain only, and all symptoms resolve completely within 10 minutes of reaching pressure. Most other cases can be managed using Table 6, often with additional oxygen cycles. When only a monoplace chamber is available, if it is equipped with a BIBS which can deliver air to the diver, standard USN tables can be administered. If there is no mechanism to deliver air breaks, a monoplace table (e.g. Hart, Kindwall tables: see above) is an option.

If the chamber complex and staff are capable of supporting saturation therapy, then it can be considered for divers with severe neurological DCI and either continued improvement at 18 msw even after a maximum number of oxygen cycles has been administered, or significant deterioration during decompression (Davis et al., 1996).

Deeper recompression (e.g., to 50 msw) can be considered for severe cases with incomplete response at 18 msw. While animal studies (Leitch et al., 1984a; Leitch et al., 1984b) and a published case review (Leitch & Green, 1985) provide little evidence in favor of treatment at pressures greater than 2.8 ATA, the clinical experience of experienced commercial diving physicians is that a trial of additional recompression often produces additional improvement. This is most likely to occur shortly after the onset of symptoms, at which stage symptom relief is most related to a reduction in bubble volume. After bubbles have initiated secondary pathophysiological processes, reduction in bubble size is only one component of multifactorial therapy, which may include rehydration, hyperoxygenation, and administration of adjunctive pharmacotherapy. In addition to reducing the volume of existing bubbles, increasing the pressure to equal or exceed the tissue inert gas partial pressure may prevent the evolution of new ones.

Lee et al. (1991) have published retrospective data reporting treatment using four 15 minute cycles consisting of 40% oxygen-60% nitrogen breathing (10 minutes) then air breathing (5 minutes) at 6 ATA (50 meters, 165 feet), followed by staged decompression over 40 minutes to 2.8 ATA (18 meters, 60 feet) and then USN Table 6. Using this table to treat divers with neurological or cardiorespiratory bends cure was obtained in 70 of 99 divers (70.7%) despite delays in treatment of up to 96 hours. The authors report that this table is superior to USN Table 6A, although the study was retrospective and not randomized, and insufficient details are provided to determine comparability of the patients in each group. Immediate recompression has the greatest success, with delays resulting in a worse prognosis in both professional divers (Ball, 1993) and recreational divers.

BREATHING GAS

The original treatment tables used air as the breathing gas. Recompression would reduce bubble volume and resolve symptoms, which would then be followed by a slow decompression, allowing excess inert gas to be eliminated.

It was acknowledged that recompression with a breathing mixture containing nitrogen would result in additional uptake of inert gas, which theoretically could augment bubble growth and result in new symptoms during the subsequent decompression.

This led to the development of oxygen tables. Since oxygen is metabolized by tissues, it therefore does not accumulate as does an inert gas. This results in a reduction of total gas pressure in the tissues surrounding the bubble, enhancing the rate of diffusion of inert gas from the bubble into the surrounding tissue. This is referred to as the "oxygen window."

Hyperbaric oxygen administration has other potentially beneficial effects, such as oxygenation of ischemic tissue, reduction of CNS edema, and possibly inhibition of endothelial leukocyte accumulation (Zamboni et al., 1993).

Oxygen can be administered safely in a dry hyperbaric chamber at ambient pressures up to around 3 atmospheres absolute (ATA), above which there is a significant risk of central nervous system oxygen toxicity. Oxygen treatment tables (e.g., USN Tables 5 and 6) were designed to allow 100% oxygen breathing at the highest practical ambient pressure while avoiding oxygen toxicity.

Under some circumstances, when recompression is required to depths at which 100% oxygen can safely be administered, it may be preferable to use helium as the inert gas diluent, rather than nitrogen. There is some evidence that in divers who have breathed helium-oxygen (heliox) and decompressed all the way to the surface using this gas, nitrogen breathing can exacerbate the symptoms of decompression illness (Barnard & Elliott, 1966). It therefore seems logical that if a diver develops symptoms after surfacing from such a dive, then he should be recompressed using either oxygen or heliox.

Some diving physicians have suggested that heliox may be superior to oxygen as a breathing gas. Indeed, the work of Hyldegaard and co-workers provides evidence that at I ATA heliox breathing might result in faster bubble resolution than air or oxygen breathing (Hyldegaard & Madsen, 1994; Hyldegaard et al., 1994; Hyldegaard & Madsen, 1989; Bennett, 1965). This suggests the hypothesis that for first aid or transportation of the injured diver, heliox may be superior to oxygen. However, in animal studies, when the effects of different gases were examined during recompression, there was no clear advantage of heliox over oxygen (Hyldegaard & Madsen, 1996).

A comparison of air and heliox recompression of guinea pigs with DCI after air dives was reported by Lillo et al. (1988). Heliox breathing was associated with a slower recovery from tachypnea. Catron et al. (1987) reported that heliox breathing caused an increase in pulmonary artery pressure when administered to dogs with experimental DCI.

There are few published cases in which heliox was used to treat DCI in air divers. Douglas & Robinson (1988) and Kol et al. (1993) reported the use of heliox in small series of cases of spinal cord DCI. Neither report included a control group.

It is theoretically possible that inert gases may affect the outcome of decompression illness by virtue of different pharmacological effects. Indeed, Bennett (1965) observed in anesthetized cats exposed to an ambient pressure of 11 ATA (100 msw) that cortical oxygen tension was greater when breathing $He-O_2$ than when breathing N_2-O_2 (see Table 1).

While the relevance of such observations to the treatment of DCI is speculative, they suggest that investigations of different inert gases in DCI should look beyond their effects on bubble volume.

In conclusion, the preponderance of experience and experimental evidence supports the traditional use of 18 msw as an initial treatment depth for recreational divers. While shallower initial treatment may also be efficacious, unless the treatment pressure is constrained by the available equipment, there is little reason to change the traditional recommendation. The ability to deliver 100% is widely available, and use of USN Tables 5 and 6 according to their guidelines are highly successful when treatment is not delayed. When serious symptoms fail to resolve with USN Table 6, deeper or longer treatment (e.g., Catalina Table, saturation) are options which can be used at the discretion of the diving physician. While it is interesting to speculate whether heliox should be used routinely during recompression for DCI experienced during air dives, there is insufficient evidence available as yet to recommend it routinely. The answer to the question can be provided by a randomized trial, which is currently in progress (Drewry & Gorman, 1994).

REFERENCES

1. Ball R. Effect of severity, time to recompression with oxygen, and retreatment on outcome in forty-nine cases of spinal cord decompression sickness. Undersea Hyperb Med. 20:133-145, 1993.
2. Barnard EEP, Elliott DH. Decompression sickness: paradoxical response to recompression therapy. Br Med J. 2:809-810, 1966.
3. Bennett PB. Cortical CO2 and O2 at high pressures of argon, nitrogen, helium and oxygen. J Appl Physiol 20:1249-1252, 1965.
4. Catron PW, Thomas LB, Flynn ET Jr, McDermott JJ, Holt MA. Effects of He-O2 breathing during experimental decompression sickness following air dives. Undersea Biomed Res 14: 101-111, 1987.
5. Davis P, Piantadosi CA, Moon RE. Saturation treatment of decompression illness in a hospital based hyperbaric facility. In: Treatment of Decompression Illness, RE Moon, PJ Sheffield, Eds. Kensington, MD: Undersea and Hyperbaric Medical Society, 1996 (in press).
6. Douglas JD, Robinson C. Heliox treatment for spinal decompression sickness following air dives. Undersea Biomed Res 15:315-319, 1988.
7. Drewry A, Gorman DF. A progress report on the prospective, randomized, double-blind controlled study of oxygen and oxygen-helium in the treatment of air-diving decompression illness (DCI). Undersea Hyperb Med. 21 (Suppl):98, 1994.
8. Green JW. Tichenor. J. Curley MD. Treatment of type I decompression sickness using the U.S. Navy treatment algorithm. Undersea Biomed Res 16:465-470, 1989.
9. Hart GB. Treatment of decompression illness and air embolism with hyperbaric oxygen. Aerosp Med. 45: 1190-1193, 1974.
10. Hart GB, Strauss MB, Lennon PA. The treatment of decompression sickness and air embolism in a monoplace chamber. J Hyperbaric Med. 1: 1-7, 1986.
11. Hyldegaard O, Madsen J. Influence of heliox, oxygen, and N2O-O2 breathing on N2 bubbles in adipose tissue. Undersea Biomed Res. 16:185-193, 1989.
12. Hyldegaard O, Madsen J. Effect of air, heliox, and oxygen breathing on air bubbles in aqueous tissues in the rat. Undersea Hyperb Med. 21:413-424, 1994.
13. Hyldegaard O, Madsen J. Effect of different breathing gases on bubble resolution in lipid and aqueous tissues. Animal experiments. In: Treatment of Decompression Illness, RE Moon, PJ Sheffield, Eds. Kensington, MD: Undersea and Hyperbaric Medical Society, 1996 (in press).
14. Hyldegaard O, Moller M, Madsen J. Protective effect of oxygen and heliox breathing during development of spinal decompression sickness. Undersea Hyperb Med. 21:115- 28, 1994.
15. Keays FL. Compressed air illness, with a report of 3,692 cases. Dept Med Publ Cornell Univ Med Coll. 2:1-55, 1909.
16. Kindwall EP. Use of short versus long tables in the treatment of decompression sickness and air embolism. In: Treatment of Decompression Illness, RE Moon, PJ Sheffield, Eds. Kensington, MD:Undersea and Hyperbaric Medical Society, 1996 (in press).
17. Kol S, Adir Y, Gordon CR, Melamed Y. Oxy-helium treatment of severe spinal decompression sickness after air diving. Undersea Hyperb Med 20:147-154, 1993
18. Lee HC, Niu KC, Chen SH, Chang LP, Huang KL, Tsai JD, Chen LS. Therapeutic effects of different tables on type 11 decompression sickness. J Hyperbaric Med. 6:11-17, 1991.
19. Leitch DR, Green RD. Additional pressurization for treating nonresponding cases of serious air decompression sickness. Aviat Space Environ Med. 56:1139-1143, 1985.
20. Leitch DR, Hallenbeck JM. Pressure in the treatment of spinal cord decompression sickness. Undersea Biomed Res 12:291-305, 1985.
21. Leitch DR, Greenbaum LJ, Jr., Hallenbeck JM. Cerebral arterial air embolism: I. Is there benefit in beginning HBO treatment at 6 bar? Undersea Biomed Res. 11:221-235, 1984a.
22. Leitch DR, Greenbaum LJ, Jr., Hallenbeck JM. Cerebral arterial air embolism: 11. Effect of pressure and time on cortical evoked potential recovery. Undersea Biomed Res. 11:237-248, 1984b.
23. Lillo RS, MacCallum ME, Pitkin RB. Air vs. He-O2 recompression treatment of decompression sickness in guinea pigs. Undersea Biomed Res 15:283-300, 1984.
24. Miller JN, Fagraeus L, Bennett PB, Elliott DH, Shields TG, Grimstad J. Nitrogen-oxygen saturation therapy in serious cases of compressed air decompression sickness. Lancet. 2:169-171, 1978.
25. Navy Department. US Navy Diving Manual. Vol 1: Air Diving. NAVSEA 0994-LP-001-91 10. Flagstaff, AZ: Best, 1993.
26. Pilmanis A. Treatment for air embolism and decompression sickness. SPUMS J. 17:27-32, 1987.
27. Workman RD. Treatment of bends with oxygen at high pressure. Aerosp Med. 39:1076-1083, 1968.
28. Zamboni WA, Roth AC, Russell RC, Graham B, Suchy H, Kucan JO. Morphological analysis of the microcirculation during reperfusion of ischemic skeletal muscle and the effect of hyperbaric oxygen. Plast Reconstr Surg. 91:1110-1123, 1993.
29. Reproduced in part from Moon, RE. Treatment of Decompression Illness. In: AA Bove (Ed) Diving Medicine, Philadelphia: WB Saunders, 1996 (in press).

FLUID INFUSIONS IN THE ADJUNCTIVE TREATMENT OF DECOMPRESSION ACCIDENTS IN RECREATIONAL DIVING: WHICH PROTOCOLS?

J. Ross
Department of Environmental and Occupational Medicine
University of Aberdeen, Scotland. United Kingdom

Fluid intake is an essential part of the body's homeostasis and the treatment of any medical condition must take it into consideration to some extent however fleetingly. The problems of fluid balance become more of a focus in therapy when the normal mechanism of fluid intake is disrupted or in conditions where there are abnormal losses or where capillary permeability breakdown causes tissue oedema. All three of these factors may be relevant in an injured diver. However, the commonest reason for a diver presenting for treatment after an accident is the onset of decompression sickness or the diagnosis of cerebral gas embolus and both these conditions warrant immediate recompression therapy. Many recompression chambers, however, are not hospital based and do not have the facilities for the complex management of fluid balance which may in any case be difficult even in a hospital based recompression chamber for environmental reasons. In this context a discussion of the management of fluid balance is of interest both in terms of what may constitute ideal management and what is practical and politic at the time of recompression therapy.

FACTORS AFFECTING FLUID BALANCE IN DIVING

Normal diving practice is quite likely to cause dehydration in the normal course of events and such dehydration may be a causative factor in decompression illness.

Cold Diuresis
Many divers are exposed to cold conditions while on an outing either during the dive itself or while in the boat before and after diving. The major response to cold is peripheral vasoconstriction and the resulting increase in central blood volume induces a diuresis which is due to a failure of tubular resorption of sodium and water. There is contraction of the extracellular fluid volume which remains isotonic (Lloyd 1986).

Immersion Diuresis
Both head out and total immersion induce a diuresis which is potentiated by cold and this is associated with sodium and potassium loss. Furthermore, the fluid loss occasioned by this effects does not seem remediable by a prophylactic fluid load before immersion (Arnall and Goforth, 1993).

Fluid Loss During Exercise and to the Breathing Gas

Moisture is also lost through respiration and the volume lost is increased by exercise and further increased by breathing cold dry air. Exercise, even in the cold, induces sweating and further fluid loss is occasioned by this route.

All these factors may be further amplified by the impracticability of fluid replacement while diving.

IMPORTANCE OF THE INITIAL DIAGNOSIS

The outcome of a diving accident is of importance in the subsequent fluid balance management. Of course the commonest outcome encountered at a medical recompression facility is decompression illness or cerebral gas embolism, but others are possible and should be considered. Intercurrent illness such as myocardial ischaemia, diabetes, or asthma can be the cause of an accident or can be exacerbated by an accident. In the author's experience, however, near drowning and carbon monoxide poisoning with their potential to present with unconsciousness and convulsions on surfacing should be considered prior to initiating a fluid therapy programme. Similarly, the unconscious patient should be examined for traumatic injury prior to recompression since fractures and haematoma formation are important causes of hypovolaemia.

FACTORS AFFECTING FLUID BALANCE IN VICTIMS OF DECOMPRESSION ILLNESS

Serious decompression sickness leads to the symptoms and signs of hypovolaemia in man (Barnard et al., 1966; Kindwall and Margolis; 1975, Norman et al., 1979) and in animals (Jacey et al., 1974; Leitch and Hallenbeck, 1984). The human incidents described required the correction of hypovolaemia by intravenous fluids and in one study on spinal decompression illness in dogs (Leitch and Hallenbeck, 1984) it was found that, after precipitous decompression, animals could be prevented from going into shock by giving intravenous fluids.

The cause of acute hypovolaemia is certainly a breakdown in endothelial cell permeability and this has been repeatedly demonstrated in animal models of decompression illness and gas embolism and which has been reviewed (Francis and Gorman, 1993).

THE HAEMATOCRIT

A raised haematocrit has been observed in animal models of decompression illness and it has been demonstrated to be due the hypovolaemia caused by capillary leakage (Jacey et al., 1974; Bove et al., 1974).

A raised haematocrit has also been regularly observed with hypovolaemia in decompression illness in man and this has been reviewed (Philp, 1974). In milder cases of decompression illness, however, the change in haematocrit has been slight (Philp et al., 1972) or absent (Neuman et al., 1976) and no change in haematocrit has been observed after repetitive air dives which produced venous gas emboli with occasional pruritis and fatigue in the experimental group. Indeed, in this study, a reduction in red cell mass was described over the 12 days of the study. A more recent study also found no overall difference in haematocrit in a group of divers who had sustained neurological decompression sickness in comparison to a control group of divers (Blanc et al., 1995). On the other hand, these workers did find that haematocrit in divers who went on to show neurological sequelae after treatment was significantly raised. They went on to conclude that a haematocrit of more than 48% was significantly correlated with seque- lae after treatment. When haematocrit was more than 48% the incidence of sequelae was 53% and compared to an incidence of 13% when haematocrit was lower.

A high haematocrit seems to be typical of more serious decompression illness and probably indicates some degree of hypovolaemia. It is possible to have decompression illness with a haematocrit in the normal range and without a rise in haematocrit. Significant hypovolaemia, therefore, need not be an inevitable concomitant of decom- pression illness.

WHEN TO GIVE FLUIDS

The infusion of fluids is the fundamental treatment of acute hypovolaemia and is probably the most important advance in the treatment of trauma this century. It is logical if not mandatory, therefore, to correct hypovolaemia if this is identified in the course of treating decompression illness and the beneficial effects of this have been anecdotally demonstrated in man (Barnard et al., 1966; Kindwall and Margolis, 1975; Cockett et al., 1979; Norman et al , 1979) and animals (Leitch and Hallenbeck, 1984). Correction of hypovolaemia has been regarded as part of the routine adjuvant therapy of decompression illness for some years (Bove, 1982; Catron and Flynn, 1982).

Degrees of dehydration that stop short of producing hypovolaemia are probable in the victims of any decompression accident simply due to the physiological process at work which have been described briefly above. It might seem logical therefore to give fluids to every case. There is no evidence, however, that this practice is beneficial. On the other hand if dehydration is identifiable on clinical examination it seems logical to reverse it in the same manner as is hypovolaemia.

If the ability of the patient to take oral fluids is impaired either due to impaired consciousness, trauma, intestinal barotrauma or intercurrent illness the fluid balance must be maintained by the administration of intravenous fluids using an appropriate maintenance regime.

THE ROUTE OF ADMINISTRATION

There are two realistic routes for fluid therapy in the context of decompression accidents: oral and intravenous. Whereas there is a considerable degree of evidence supporting the benefits of intravenous fluids, administration of oral fluids are of unproven benefit. The oral route is the only realistic way of giving fluids in the first aid treatment of decompression illness however, and is worth some consideration especially since a degree of dehydration is likely after most significant dives.

ORAL REHYDRATION

The area of oral rehydration has been the subject of much attention in recent years. Initially as a treatment for infantile diarrhoea but more recently in the context of rehydration after exercise (Walker-Smith, 1992; Maughan, 1991). The physiological fluid loss accompanying diving is associated with loss of electrolytes and the serum remains isotonic. Capillary leakage allows electrolytes and components of plasma to leak out of the extravascular space and, at least in the short term the plasma in this condition also remains isotonic. Under such conditions of electrolyte loss, if the extravascular fluid loss is replaced with water intake without sodium there is a danger of hyponatraemia (Nose et al., 1988). Rehydration with water alone, with or without the addition of glucose, is also less effective than if electrolyte solutions are ingested. If fluid loss due to exercise is replaced with water very much more of the intake is lost as urine than if electrolyte is given when using output is lower as more fluid is retained. If urine output during rehydration is being monitored then the increase in urine output observed in water alone rehydration may lead to a false sense of achievement as the body excretes the rehydration fluid in an attempt to restore isosmality.

In post exercise rehydration in man better rehydration is obtained from electrolyte solutions than from water and there is no added benefit to be gained from adding potassium as well as sodium, nor is there a difference between isotonic and hypotonic solutions when the difference in tonicity is due to glucose in the drink (Maughan et al., 1994). In a trial studying the impact of varying concentrations of sodium in oral rehydration fluid, the amount of fluid retained related directly to sodium content (Maughan and Leiper, 1995). Interestingly, in this study 100 sodium was required to maintain serum osmolalty at the pre-exercise control level. The beverages used in this study also contained 90 m mol l-1 glucose with the addition of sugar free lemon squash as flavouring.

If oral fluids are to be used a decompression accidents then they should contain sodium to promote fluid retention. The amount of sodium for rehydration after exercise is known but it may differ from that required after the onset of decompression illness. The component of dehydration caused by diving would be appropriately tackled, however, and the danger of hyponatraemia avoided. In addition, a water induced diuresis would not mislead the attending clinician with regard to the patient's true fluid balance. Oral fluids might prove a useful first aid measure in the treatment of decompression illness and if this were so oxygen administration equipment could be modified to aid their ingestion.

INTRAVENOUS FLUIDS

The clinician has some choice in what intravenous fluid to use but the choice falls broadly into one between colloid only, crystalloid only or a combination of both. Solutions containing free water are not advised in the treatment of acute hypovolaemia since hyponatraemia may result and this will aggravate cerebral oedema (hypo-osmotic oedema) in patients with cerebral injury. It is the author's practice to avoid glucose containing or hypotonic fluids in this context.

Crystalloids
Glucose solutions
Glucose solutions essentially provide free water. Since body water constitutes 60% of body weight and plasma volume only 5%, less than 10% of an intravenous injection of glucose solution remains in the plasma. They are ineffective and potentially dangerous if used in an attempt to expand plasma volume.

Saline solutions

Saline solutions are distributed throughout the extracellular space which constitutes one third of body water. Therefore 25% of an intravenous dose of normal saline remains in the plasma. If massive infusions are required, Ringer lactate solution containing sodium lactate which is metabolised to bicarbonate, may be preferred since large quantities of normal saline can induce a hypernatraemic, hyperchloraemic acidosis.

Isotonic saline solutions are conventionally used as plasma expanders and hypotonic solutions are ineffective intravenously.

Hypertonic saline solutions : Recent years has seen an increasing interest in hypertonic saline solutions for the treatment of hypovolaemia (Vincent, 1991). Their use, however, has important side effects and careful management is required. This technique remains experimental and is not yet appropriate in the management of a decompression accident.

Colloids

These solutions are aqueous solutions of high molecular weight compounds. Initially natural colloids only were available, but now there are a range of synthetic preparations available; enough to cause a degree of bewilderment when it comes to choice.

Blood

This will not be discussed here as blood loss is highly unusual following a diving accident. In addition, the treatment of acute blood loss is replacement of the circulating volume lost rather than of haemoglobin. If the haemoglobin is more than 100 g l-1 transfusion is rarely indicated.

Albumin

5% albumin solution is prepared from pooled human plasma by fractionation, then sterilized by heat treatment and adjusted to a pH of 6.9. Albumin is also available as a hyperoncotic preparation of 25% in normal saline. The 5% solution is an effective short term plasma expander and since 40% of the body's albumin is held in the circulating blood with rest be distributed throughout the extravascular compartment it offers a long term expansion of about 50% of the volume administered.

Dextran

Dextrans are prepared from glucose polymers. Dextran 40 has a weighted average molecular weight of 40,000 Daltons while for Dextran 70 this is 70,000 Daltons. Dextran 40 is hyperoncotic and produces a short lasting plasma expansion of more than the volume infused as extracellular fluid is pulled into the circulating blood volume. However, the smaller molecules rapidly escape from the plasma and the volume effect decreases. Dextran 40 has a plasma half-life of 2.5 hours. Dextran 70 has a plasma half life of 6 hours. Their general pharmacology has been reviewed (Dollery, 1991).

Dextrans, particularly dextran 40, have been advocated as specifically indicated for the treatment of decompression illness (Norman et al., 1979; Cockett et al., 1970). Animal experiments (Wells et al., 1971) have shown reduction of capillary blood flow in decompression illness with red blood cell aggregation and an increase in capillary blood viscosity. Low molecular weight dextrans are reported to reduce blood viscosity due to inhibition of red cell aggregation (Dollery, 1991) although some clinical studies have failed to demonstrate this (Dormandy, 1971).

Dextran in doses of more than 20 ml kg-1 may increase the bleeding time. High urinary concentrations of dextran accompany the excretion phase of dextran 40 and high doses have been associated with renal failure in patients with sepsis or other complications.

Hetastarch

Hydroxyethyl starch (HES) is a polydisperse colloid with a weighted average molecular weight of 450 Daltons. HES is a natural starch of highly branched glucose polymers derived from amylopectin. It has a plasma half life of about 17 days. The volume replacement effect of the commercially available 6% solution in normal saline is about the same as for 5% albumin. Administration of large volume of HES can disrupt coagulation and there is in addition a specific lowering of factor VII. This subject has been reviewed (Imm and Carlson, 1993).

Gelatin plasma substitutes

A number of variants are available. Succinylated gelatin solution is prepared by heating and hydrolysis and the resulting polymers are linked using succinic hydrochloride as a coupling agent to produce polymers with an average molecular weight of 35,000 Daltons. Urea linked gelatins are similarly produced by heating but cross linking is brought about with hexamethylene di-isocyanate, which forms urea bridges and polypetides of 35,000 Daltons mean molecular weight. The general pharmacology of these compounds has been reviewed (Dollery, 1991). The plasma half life of gelatins is 2–3 hours which is the shortest of the synthetic agents discussed but the initial plasma expansion effect is similar to that of albumin. Large volumes can be given without affecting haemostasis.

Anaphylactoid reactions to plasma expanders

Anaphylactic reactions to all fluids used as plasma expanders have been reported including isolated reactions occurring after crystalloid solutions. The incidence of reactions, however is higher after colloids with there being no real distinction between them in this respect. The subject has been reviewed (Ring, 1985). The overall incidence is in the order of 0.1% to 1.0% of patients treated.

Reactions to dextrans are caused by antibodies to dextran and these can be blocked by the administration of a low molecular weight dextran which acts as a hapten (Ljungstrom, 1993) and markedly reduces the incidence of anaphylactoid problems.

Reactions to gelatin infusions are predominantly related to histamine release and pre-treatment with H1-receptor and H2-receptor antagonists has been reported to substantially reduce the incidence of problems (Ring, 1985).

Choice of Colloid

There is little to choose between the colloid solutions available if moderate quantities (up to 1.5 l) are to be used. Gelatin solutions have the advantage of being cheapest and are advocated in the author's unit for this reason. They have the further advantage of being relatively short acting and this may fit the time scale of recovery in the course of decompression illness under effective recompression therapy. One should be aware, however, that gelatin may not be the choice of those patients that are vegetarians and albumin may not be acceptable to certain religious groups.

Colloid versus crystalloid

A more controversial topic is whether to choose crystalloid solutions rather than colloid solutions for the resuscitation of shocked or hypovolaemic patients. A full review of this subject is beyond the scope of this paper and the subject has been reviewed elsewhere (Gould et al., 1993; Imm and Carlson, 1993; Vincent, 1991).

Colloids have the advantage in that lower volume can be given and three times the volume of normal saline or Ringer's solution needs to be given for an equivalent effect. On the other hand, it is easier to overload the circulation with colloids and there is the ever-present problem of an anaphylactoid reaction. The subject is unlikely to be resolved in the near future but there are two meta-analysis studies that are of interest. Bisonni (Bisonni et al., 1991) compared mortality rate in severe hypovolaemia with and without complications and found that outcome was independent of the solution used but that the cost of colloid resuscitation was thirty times more expensive. Velanovich (Velanovich 1989) found that there was a 5.5% difference in mortality in favour of crystalloid solutions if all type of resuscitation were considered. This rose to 12.3% if only trauma patients were considered.

Intravenous fluids in hypovolaemia associated with increased permeability

In patients with no compromise of endothelial integrity, colloid resuscitation is associated with less radiographic evidence of pulmonary oedema although there may be no difference in gas transfer (Rackow et al., 1985).

Moderate to severe decompression illness is associated with vascular endothelial leakage and this also occurs in a number of other conditions which include the adult respiratory distress syndrome and sepsis. In conditions of failure of capillary permeability, colloid solutions are as liable to cause oedema as crystalloid. In addition, colloidal solutions are at a theoretical disadvantage in these conditions, since the osmotically active component can leak out into the tissues pulling fluid out of the vascular space so causing oedema although this has not been demonstrated clinically.

Concern has been expressed that one type of fluid or the other may promote the onset of adult respiratory distress syndrome but again there is no conclusive evidence that this is so. There is also an increasing body of evidence to suggest that it is inadequate resuscitation with resulting hypoxia of lung tissue that is the most important factor in the genesis of this condition (Shoemaker et al., 1993). In other words, it does not matter what fluid is used as long as haemodynamic stability is maintained and oxygen delivery to the tissues is sufficient to meet oxygen consumption.

COMPLICATIONS OF FLUID RESUSCITATION

Complications secondary to fluid loading are common vary greatly in severity. The most commonly studied problems are an overloaded circulation and pulmonary oedema although cerebral oedema is also a problem that is of relevance to the treatment of decompression accidents.

Pulmonary Oedema

If the pulmonary capillary endothelial cell layer is not compromised, pulmonary oedema will not develop if fluid overload is avoided and moderate degrees of fluid overload may be well tolerated.

If the pulmonary capillary endothelial layer is compromised and there is increased fluid leakage, then interstitial pulmonary oedema develops and this will be greatly aggravated by fluid overload. Two conditions associated with diving accidents cause an increase in pulmonary capillary permeability and should be considered as risk factors for pulmonary oedema formation. These are partial drowning and pulmonary oxygen toxicity. Cerebral oedema Severe decompression illness can present as acute pulmonary oedema, the chokes, and this also should be considered.

Partial Drowning

Inhalation of either salt water or fresh water causes pulmonary oedema although the mechanism of oedema formation may differ in each case (Tabeling and Modell, 1983) and partial drowning while diving is no exception (Harris et al., 1995). The pulmonary oedema of drowning may clear rapidly with appropriate therapy but may recur as an inhalation pneumonitis develops at a later stage. Aggressive fluid therapy may exacerbate the situation and, if required due to hypovolaemia, is an indication for intensive therapy which may be required in any case if the pulmonary problem is severe.

Pulmonary Oxygen Toxicity

Administration of 100% oxygen at increased atmospheric pressure is the mainstay of treatment for decompression illness. The most commonly used recompression table is the United States Navy table 6 or a close equivalent. The permissible amount of oxygen given during treatment of severe decompression illness or cerebral gas embolism might cause a 10% reduction in pulmonary vital capacity. In the author's unit the incidence of symptoms and signs attributable to pulmonary oxygen toxicity is about 10% of patients treated. The underlying lesion in pulmonary oxygen toxicity is a breakdown in pulmonary endothelial cell permeability with the formation of interstitial pulmonary oedema (Weir et al., 1994). Aggressive fluid therapy may aggravate this condition.

Pulmonary Decompression Illness

Pulmonary decompression illness (chokes) is thought to be due to impaction of inert gas bubbles in the pulmonary microcirculation and may present as pulmonary oedema. Tracheobronchial inflammation is reported as being common in this condition and breakdown of endothelial permeability is likely. Any necessary correction of hypovolaemia should proceed with caution.

Cerebral Oedema

The effect of bubbles on the cerebral vasculature has been reviewed (Francis and Gorman, 1993). The passage of bubbles through the cerebral vasculature results in a breakdown in endothelial cell permeability and a number of mechanisms have been suggested. The effect is described as transient in experimental animals but this is no guarantee that the same applies in a decompression accident victim. Fluid overload may exacerbate any oedema formation and hyponatraemia should be avoided as should the administration of free water. Small decreases in serum osmolality can lead to increased cerebral oedema formation. If cerebral injury is diagnosed then hypovolaemia must be corrected. Diffuse brain injury after trauma is managed by correction of hypovolaemia and fluid restriction to maintain a slightly elevated plasma osmolality (Manara, 1994; Midgely and Dearden, 1994; Sutin et al., 1992). Although there has been no specific study of this aspect of recompression illness, it seems logical to adopt a similar regime.

In spite of these cautionary words it is generally accepted that cases of micro-vascular injury are made worse by inadequate fluid resuscitation. Complications should be anticipated and dealt with appropriately. Attempts to avoid these complications by inadequate fluid resuscitation should not be made.

A PROTOCOL FOR FLUID ADMINISTRATION

First Aid
Divers with decompression illness should be encouraged to take oral fluids as a first aid measure if there are no contra-indications to this. The oral rehydration solution should contain sodium and 100 mmol l-1 has been shown to be an effective rehydration fluid after exercise. Glucose solutions are likely to be much less effective and may complicate the assessment of fluid balance on admission to hospital. Fluid administration should not interfere with administration of 100% oxygen.

At the Recompression Facility
If recompression is possible within minutes of the diagnosis of decompression illness then the patient should be quickly compressed with fluid therapy used as an adjunct in the chamber if required.

Usually, however, the patient arrives at the chamber some time after diagnosis. Any microcirculatory disturbance has had time to establish itself and assessment of fluid balance is an important part of the pre-compression examination.

Global dehydration can be recognised relatively easily by clinical examination of the teguments and confirmed by estimation of plasma osmolality, urea or sodium.

The clinical signs of hypovolaemia are not reliable. Early changes may be a reduction in pulse pressure or postural changes in arterial pressure. An increased heart rate and reduced arterial pressure may be present but neither of these signs is reliable. Peripheral vasoconstriction with slow capillary filling in the skin of the feet and hands is a valuable sign and this can be monitored by skin temperature measurement. Urine output may be reduced and there may be an increase in urine osmolality. In decompression illness hypovolaemia is due to plasma loss and estimation of haemoconcentration by measuring haematocrit will be useful.

Intravenous access should be established prior to compression and if there is clinically overt hypovolaemia then correction should be started immediately by the infusion of Ringer lactate solution. The amount of fluid to be given can be estimated by the fluid challenge technique (Weil and Hanning, 1979). Having decided on Ringer l actate, the rate of infusion should be related to the severity of the patient's condition. Criteria for reducing the infusion to a maintenance rate should be established and satisfaction of any one of three criteria should stop the fluid challenge (Vincent, 1991).

A. Reduction in pulse rate to a stipulated level
   Return of blood pressure to an acceptable value
   Acceptable urine output
B. A maximal filling pressure, e.g. central venous pressure (CVP) reaches 13 mmHg.
C. Fluid challenge rules in response to regular assessment perhaps every 10 minutes. e.g. CVP < 3 mm Hg then continue infusion: CVP 3-5 mm Hg interrupt infusion for 10 minutes and re-assess: CVP > 5 mm Hg stop infusion.

Once initial resuscitation has been started with an electrolyte solution the use of colloids may be considered. This should be left to the preferences and experience of the clinician in charge. Gelatin solutions may be adequate and have the benefit of being cheapest. Dextrans have been advocated but there is no evidence that they have any specific benefit.

Monitoring Fluid Balance in Hypovolaemia

In clinically overt hypovolaemia an intravenous cannula which allows estimation of the CVP is required. A technique of insertion which ensures no risk of pneumothorax should be adopted. A long line inserted from the medial aspect of the antecubital fossa is acceptable and can be set up in the chamber. The line need only lie in the large veins close to the chest and need not be intrathoracic so avoiding the need for confirmatory radiology. A short cannula inserted into the internal jugular using an extrathoracic insertion site high in the neck is also acceptable but in this instance head-down tilt is required which may not be possible in the chamber.

Severely ill patients may require intensive care and if this is available for application in the chamber it should be instituted. The lack of intensive care facilities, however, should not prevent recompression.

A fluid balance chart should be started and the urine output measured. If aggressive fluid therapy is required, a urinary catheter should be inserted to allow hourly urine volume measurement. Again this can be inserted in the chamber.

Measurement of peripheral and core temperature gives a valuable indication of return of peripheral blood flow as hypovolaemia is corrected.

Measurement of blood pressure and pulse should be routine with a measurement interval dictated by the clinical situation.

Respiratory rate should be measured since a rising rate is an early indicator of pulmonary oedema formation. The lung bases should be regularly auscultated but one should be aware that interstitial pulmonary oedema may form without the presence of pulmonary crepitations.

Complicating Factors

The presence of factors likely to complicate fluid therapy should be identified early. In particular any requirement for artificial ventilation of the lungs should be foreseen as the logistics or arranging this may be complex if the chamber is not already equipped and appropriately staffed.

If fluid overload is identified then this may be treated with diuretics. Low dose dopamine also promotes a diuresis and is more controllable.

Correction of Dehydration

Mild dehydration can be dealt with by oral rehydration
Dehydration causing hypovolaemia can be dealt with as above.

REFERENCES

1. Arnall D.A., Goforth H.W. (1993) Failure to reduce body water loss in cold-water immersion by glycerol ingestion. Undersea and Biomedical Researches 20:309-320.
2. Barnard E.E.P. et al (1966) Post-decompress on shock due to extravasation of plasma. British Medical Journal 2:154-155.
3. Bisonni R.S., Holtgrave D.R., Lawler R , Marley D.S. (1991) Colloids versus crystalloids in fluid resuscitation. Journal of Family Practice 32:387-90.
4. Blanc Ph. et al (1994) Neurological decompression illness: the value of the hematocrit level assessment. In: Proceedings of the XXIst Annual Meeting of European Underwater and Baromedical Society. Helsink. The Finnish Society of Diving and Hyperbaric Medicine. pp241-245.
5. Bove A.A. (1982) The basis for drug therapy in decompression illness. Undersea Biomedical Researches. 9:91-111.
6. Bove A.A., Hallenbeck J., Elliott D.H. (1974) Changes in blood and plasma volumes in dogs during decompression sickness. Aerospace Medicine 45:49-55.
7. Catron P.W., Flynn E.T. (1982) Adjuvant therapy for decompression sickness: a review. Undersea Biomedical Researches. 9:161-174.
8. Cockett A.T.K., Saunders J.C., Depenbusch F.L., Pauley S.M. (1970) Combined treatment in decompression sickness. In: Proceedings of the Fourth International Congress on Hyperbaric Medicine. Eds Wada J., Takashi I. London. Balliere Tindall and Cassell. pp 89-99.
9. Dollery C., ed. (1991) Therapeutic Drugs. Edinburgh, Churchill Livingstone.
10. Dormandy J.A. Influence of blood viscosity on blood flow and the effect of low molecular weight dextran. British Medical Journal 4:716-719.
11. Eckenhoff R.G., Hughes J.S. (1984) Hematological and hemostatic changes with repetitive air diving. Aviation, Space and Environmental Medicine. 55:592-7.
12. Epstein M. (1992) Renal effects of head-out water immersion in humans: a 15-year update. Physiological Reviews 72:563-621.
13. Francis T.J.R., Gorman D.F. (1993) Pathogenesis of the decompression disorders. In: The Physiology and Medicine of Diving. Eds. Bennett P., Elliott D. London. W.B. Saunders Company Ltd. pp 454-480.
14. Gould S.A. et al (1993) Hypovolaemic shock. Critical Care Clinics 9:239-259.
15. Harris J.B., Stern E.J., Steinberg K.P. (1995) Scuba diving accident with near drowning and decompression sickness. American Journal of Roentgenology 164:592.
16. Imm A., Carlson R.W. (1993) Fluid resuscitation in circulatory shock. Critical Care Clinics. 9:313-333.
17. Jacey M.J., Tappan D.V., Ritzler K.R. (1974) Hematologic responses to severe decompression stress. Aerospace Medicine 45:417-421.
18. Kindwall E.P., Margolis I. (1975) Management of severe decompression sickness with treatment ancillary to recompression: a case report. Aviation, Space and Environmental Medicine 46:1065-8.
19. Leitch D.R., Hallenbeck J.M. (1984) A model of spinal cord dysbarism to study delayed treatment: I. producing dysbarism. Aviation, Space and Environmental Medicine 55:584-91.
20. Ljungstrom K.G. (1993) Safety of dextran in relation to other colloids - ten years experience with hapten inhibition. Infusiontherapie and Transfusionsmedizin 20:206-210.
21. Lloyd E.L. (1986) Hypothermia and cold stress. Beckenham. Croom Helm Ltd. Manara A. (1994) Postoperative care and aspects of intensive care. In: Anaesthesia and Intensive Care for the Neurosurgical Patient. Eds. Walters F.J.M., Ingram G.S., Jenkinson J.K. Blackwell Scientific Publications. Oxford. pp 404-434.
22. Maughan R.J. (1991) Fluid and electrolyte loss and replacement in exercise. Journal of Sports Sciences 9:117-142.
23. Maughan R.J., Leiper J.B. (1995) Sodium intake and post-exercise rehydration in man. European Journal of Applied Physiology. 71:311-319.
24. Maughan R.J., Owens J.H., Shirreffs S.M., Leiper J.B. (1994) Post-exercise rehydration in man: effects of electroyte addition to ingested fluids. European Journal of Applied Physiology. 69:209-215.
25. Midgely S., Dearden M. (1994) Head injuries. In: Anaesthesia and Intensive Care for the Neurosurgical Patient. Eds. Walters F.J.M., Ingram G.S., Jenkinson J K. Blackwell Scientific Publications. Oxford. pp 373-403.
26. Neuman T.S., Harris M.G., Linaweaver P.G. (1976) Blood viscosity in man following decompression: correlations with hematocrit and venous gas emboli.
27. Norman J., Childs C.M., Jones C., Smith J.A.R., Ross J., Riddel G., McIntosh A., McKie N.I.P., McAuley I., Fructus X. (1979). Management of a complex diving accident. Undersea Biomedical. Researches. 6: 209-216.
28. Nose H, Mack G.W., Shi X., Nadel E.R. (1988) Role of osmolality and plasma volume during rehydration in humans. J Appl Physiol 65: 325-331.
29. Philp R.B. (1974) A review of blood changes associated with compression-decompression: relationship to decompression sickness.
30. Philp R.B. et al (1972) Changes in the hemostatic system and in blood and urine chemistry of human subjects following decompression from a hyperbaric environment.
31. Rackow E.C., Falk J.L., Fein I.A., Seigel J.S., Packman M.I., Haupt M.T., Kaufman B.S., Putnam D.(1983) Fluid resuscitation in circulatory shock: a comparison of the cardiorespiratory effects of albumin, hetastarch and saline solutions in patients with hypovolaemic and septic shock. Critical Care Medicine 11:839-50.

32. Ring J. (1985) Anaphylactoid reactions to plasma substitutes. International Anesthesiology Clinics. 23:67-95.
33. Shoemaker W.C., Appel P.L., Bishop M.H. (1993) Temporal patterns of blood volume, haemodynamics and oxygen transport in pathogenesis and therapy of postoperative adult respiratory distress syndrome. New Horizons 1:522-37.
34. Ring J. (1985) Anaphylactic reactions to plasma substitutes. International Anesthesiology Clinics 23:67-95.
35. Sutin K.M., Ruskin K.J., Kaufman B.S. (1992) Intravenous fluid therapy in neurologic injury. Critical Care Clinics 8:367-408.
36. Tabeling B.B., Modell J.H. (1983) Drowning and near drowning. In Care of the Critically Ill Patient. Eds Tinker J., Rapin M. Springer Verlag. Berlin. pp697-706.
37. Velanovich V. (1989) Crystalloid versus colloid fluid resuscitation: a meta-analysis of mortality. Surgery 105:65-71.
38. Vincent J.-L. (1991) Fluids for resuscitation. British Journal of Anaesthesia 67:185-193.
39. Walker-Smith J.A. (1992) Recommendations for composition of oral rehydration solutions for the children of Europe: report of an ESPGAN Working Group. Journal of Paediatric Gastroenterology 14:113-115.
40. Weil M.H., Henning R.J.(1979) New concepts in the diagnosis and fluid treatment of circulatory shock. Anaesthesia and Analgesia 58:124-132.
41. Weir K.L., O'Gorman N.S., Ross J.A.S., Godden D.J, Woo J., McKinnon A.D., Johnson P.W. (1994). Lung capillary albumin leak in oxygen toxicity: a quantitative immunocytochemical study. American Journal of Respiratory and Critical Care Medicine. 150: 784-789.
42. Wells C.H., Bond T.P., Guest M.M., Barnhart C.C. (1971) Rheologic impairment of the microcirculation during decompression sickness. Microvascular Research 3:162-169.

DRUGS IN THE ADJUNCTIVE TREATMENT OF DECOMPRESSION ACCIDENTS IN RECREATIONAL DIVING: WHAT ROLE?

Richard E. Moon, MD

Duke University Medical Center - Durham, NC, USA

While recompression therapy remains the most definitive component of the treatment of DCI, adjunctive treatment modalities may contribute to successful outcome. It is from new developments in the neurosciences that advances in the treatment of DCI are likely to occur.

OXYGEN

The initial adjunctive treatment, which can be administered whenever symptoms develop, is oxygen. Supplemental oxygen administration is appropriate to treat hypoxemia caused by pulmonary abnormalities such as aspiration of water or vomitus, pneumothorax, ventilation/perfusion abnormalities due to venous gas embolism or hypoventilation. Even in the absence of lung pathology hyperoxygenation of the blood augments oxygen delivery to underperfused tissue. Finally, when breathing 100% oxygen, the absence of inert gas in the inspired mix enhances washout of inert gas from tissues, thus increasing the partial pressure gradient for diffusion of inert gas from bubble into tissue. Theoretical calculations predict that the PN2 gradient from bubble to surrounding tissue can be increased from 142 mmHg breathing air to 713 mmHg breathing 100% O_2 (Moon & Gorman, 1993). When 100% oxygen is administered to experimental animals, bubbles shrink more rapidly (Hyldegaard & Madsen, 1994; Hyldegaard et al., 1994). In recreational diving accidents reported to the Divers Alert Network, spontaneous resolution of symptoms occurs in 3% of divers breathing air, versus 12% of divers who breathe surface oxygen. Surface oxygen administration during transport to the chamber also results in a greater probability of complete resolution after recompression treatment (69% vs. 52% with no surface oxygen) (Moon et al., 1995).

While any increase in inspired oxygen concentration is probably helpful, it is likely to be most efficacious when administered at a concentration of 100%, using a tightly fitting mask, either from a demand valve regulator or closed circuit apparatus.

BLOOD GLUCOSE CONTROL

There is evidence that central nervous system injury in both brain (Pulsinelli et al., 1983) and spinal cord (Drummond & Moore, 1989) can be worsened by hyperglycemia, due to accelerated production of lactate and the resulting intracellular acidosis. Evidence from series of human head injury patients (Lam et al., 1991) and rats undergoing global ischemia (Li et al., 1994) suggests that the effect becomes significant above a threshold plasma glucose of around 200 mg/dI. There is also evidence that administration of even small amounts of glucose, for example one liter of intravenous 5% dextrose solution, may worsen neurological outcome, even in the absence of significant hyperglycemia (Lanier et al., 1987). Therefore, unless it is necessary to treat hypoglycemia, it is advisable to avoid the administration of intravenous solutions which contain glucose, and to measure plasma glucose if there is reason to suspect that it may be elevated (e.g., if high dose corticosteroids are prescribed).

FLUIDS

Fluid administration may be beneficial by replenishing intravascular volume and reversing hemoconcentration. Blood pressure may therefore be maintained and microcirculatory flow augmented. There is indirect evidence that aggressive hydration can result in more rapid elimination of anesthetic gases (Yogendran et al., 1995), suggesting that a similar approach in divers with decompression illness may accelerate the washout of excess inert gas. Indeed, interventions which increase central blood volume and cardiac preload such as supine position (Balldin et al., 1971), head down tilt (Vann & Gerth, 1990) and head out immersion (Balldin et al., 1971; Vann & Gerth, 1990) significantly increase the rate of inert gas washout. Therefore there may be an advantage of fluid administration even in divers who are not dehydrated.

Rapid intravenous administration of fluids which have an osmolality less than plasma can cause swelling of the central nervous system (Kaieda, 1989). Reduction in oncotic pressure with unchanged osmotic pressure has no effect, however, and there is no advantage of colloidal solutions over crystalloids (Zornow, 1988; Kaieda et al., 1989). Therefore isotonic fluids without glucose, such as normal saline, lactated Ringer's solution or Normosol-RTM (Abbott Laboratories, North Chicago, IL), are recommended.

CORTICOSTEROIDS

Pharmacological doses of glucocorticoids have often been administered in decompression illness. In a retrospective review of AGE Pearson & Goad (1982) reported that after initial improvement secondary deterioration occurred less often in divers who had received glucocorticoids. However, glucocorticoids have not been shown to be beneficial in the treatment of head injury (Gudeman et al., 1979; Cooper et al., 1979; Braakman et al., 1983), or in animal models of decompression illness (Dutka, 1990) In a series of AGE cases analyzed retrospectively for a possible relationship between glucocorticoid administration and outcome, no benefit was evident (Gorman, 1984). However, in traumatic spinal cord injury there is evidence that early administration (within 8 hours after injury) of very high doses of methylprednisolone (30 mg.kg-1 intravenously over one hour followed by 5.4 mg.kg-l.h-l for 23 hours) can improve outcome six months after injury (Bracken et al., 1990). Such high doses have not yet been specifically tested in DCI, either in animals or humans. Moreover, the only systematic animal studies have used only short term outcomes, with somatosensory evoked responses as the end point, a measurement which, in humans, correlates poorly with clinical neurological function. Therefore, while there is no definitive evidence that corticosteroids effect an improved outcome in decompression illness, the question remains open.

LIDOCAINE

Intravenous administration of lidocaine appears extremely promising as an adjunctive treatment for DCI. In models of AGE in both cats (Evans et al., 1989) and dogs (Dutka et al., 1992), lidocaine administration designed to achieve standard clinical plasma drug levels has improved short term neurological outcome. Randomized trials of lidocaine in humans have not yet been reported, although an anecdotal report supports its use in decompression illness (Drewry & Gorman, 1992). Intravenous lidocaine therefore holds some promise as an adjunctive agent.

ANTICOAGULANTS

Because of evidence that bubble-blood interaction may cause platelet deposition and vascular occlusion refractory to recompression, there is some reason to believe that agents which inhibit platelet function and soluble clotting factors might be beneficial in DCI. Administration of aspirin and other anti-platelet drugs reduces the mild drop in platelets observed after dives (Philp et al., 1974; Philp et al., 1979). A single case report of heparin administration to a patient with neurological bends indicated neither benefit nor harm (Kindwall & Margolis, 1975) However, animal studies in which single agents were administered have shown no benefit of anticoagulants, except for one study (Hallenbeck et al., 1982), in which only a triple combination of indomethacin, PGI2, and heparin resulted in a beneficial short term effect in a canine model of AGE.

Furthermore, histological evidence of hemorrhage has been described in arterial gas embolism (Waite et al., 1967), inner ear decompression sickness (Landolt et al., 1980) and spinal cord decompression sickness (Elliott & Moon, 1993; Palmer et al., 1978). Thus there is little evidence that antiplatelet agents or other anticoagulants alter the neurological outcome in decompression illness and reason to believe that some lesions actually may be made worse. However, in individuals with severe neurological bends and leg weakness, deep vein thrombosis (DVT) and pulmonary embolism have been described (Spadaro et al., 1992). Therefore in these patients some form of prophylaxis against DVT, which may include low dose heparin, is recommended.

Whatever their benefits (if any) on platelet function, the analgesic and anti-inflammatory properties of nonsteroidal anti-inflammatory drugs (NSAIDS) and aspirin are useful for the treatment of pain only bends. However, in order that their analgesic properties not obscure the effects of recompression, it may not be advisable to administer them until after recompression treatment.

BODY TEMPERATURE

Animal models of CNS injury have shown that outcome is significantly worsened by hyperthermia (Wass et al., 1995). Thus fever in a patient with DCI should be vigorously treated.

FUTURE DEVELOPMENTS

Mechanisms of cell death in CNS injury have been investigated vigorously in recent years. While prolonged anoxia can produce cell death within minutes due to depletion of intracellular energy sources, if cell death does not immediately occur, reperfusion of ischemic brain can result in rapid recovery of cellular respiration and ATP synthesis and return of electrical activity. However, increased production of oxygen free radicals can lead to lipid peroxidation and other mechanisms of free radical injury, and delayed neuronal death. Further understanding of the mechanisms of secondary tissue damage may lead to the development of pharmacological interventions to prevent these effects.

In ischemic or traumatic brain injury there is release of excitatory neurotransmitters such as glutamate. Increased extracellular glutamate facilitates the entry of calcium into cells, which can be neurotoxic (Choi, 1987). Calcium can enter the cell via voltage dependent calcium channels which open upon neuronal depolarization. Blockade of these channels using nimodipine and nicardipine has been shown to ameliorate somewhat the damage due to subarachnoid hemorrhage and ischemic stroke (Mohr, 1994).

Calcium entry can also occur with activation of specific glutamate receptors, such as N-methyl-D-aspartate (NMDA), a-amino-3-hydoxy-5-methyl-4-isoxazole propionate (AMPA) and 1-aminocyclopentyl-trans-1,3-dicarboxylic acid (t-ACPD). After an ischemic insult, blockade of these receptors might reduce entry of calcium into the cell and help to preserve neuronal function. These concepts have been reviewed by Warner (1996).

The next major advances in the treatment of neural injury due to decompression illness is likely to be the development of appropriate agents to reduce the effects of reperfusion injury and delayed cell death. Cross fertilization of diving medicine is likely to occur from other areas in the neurosciences. We must carefully follow studies which are investigating methods by which neuronal damage due to injuries other than DCI.

REFERENCES

1. Balldin Ul, Lundgren CEG, Lundvall J, Mellander S. Changes in the elimination of 133Xe from the anterior tibial muscle in man induced by immersion in water and by shifts in body position. Aerosp Med. 42:489-493, 1971.
2. Braakman R, Schouten HJA, Dishoeck MB-V Minderhoud JM. Megadose steroids in severe head injury. Results of a prospective double-blind clinical trial. J Neurosurg. 58:326-330, 1983.
3. Bracken MB, Shepard MJ, Collins WF, Holford TR, Young W, Baskin DS, Eisenberg HM, Flamm E, Leo-Summers L, Maroon J, et al. A randomized, controlled trial of methylprednisolone or naloxone in the treatment of acute spinal-cord injury. Results of the Second National Acute Spinal Cord Injury Study. New Engl J Med. 322:1405-1411, 1990.
4. Cooper PR, Moody S, Clark WK, Kirkpatrick J, Maravilla K, Gould AL, Drane W. Dexamethasone and severe head injury. A prospective double-blind study. J Neurosurg. 51:307-316, 1979.
5. Choi D. Ionic dependence of glutamate neurotoxicity. J Neurosci. 7:369-379, 1987.
6. Drewry A, Gorman DF. Lidocaine as an adjunct to hyperbaric therapy in decompression illness: a case report. Undersea Biomed Res. 19:187-190, 1992.
7. Drummond JC, Moore SS. The influence of dextrose administration on neurologic outcome after temporary spinal cord ischemia in the rabbit. Anesthesiology. 70:64-70, 1989
8. Dutka AJ. Therapy for dysbaric central nervous system ischemia: adjuncts to recompression. In: Diving Accident Management, PB Bennett, RE Moon, Eds. Bethesda, MD: Undersea and Hyperbaric Medical Society, pp. 222-234, 1990.
9. Dutka AJ, Mink R, McDermott J, Clark JB, Hallenbeck JM. Effect of lidocaine on somatosensory evoked response and cerebral blood flow after canine cerebral air embolism. Stroke. 23:15 15-1520, 1992.
10. Elliott DH, Moon RE. Manifestations of the decompression disorders. In: The Physiology and Medicine of Diving, PB Bennett, DH Elliott, Eds. Philadelphia, PA:WB Saunders, pp. 481-505, 1993.
11. Evans DE, Catron PW, McDermott JJ, Thomas LB, Kobrine Al, Flynn ET. Therapeutic effect of lidocaine in experimental cerebral ischemia induced by air embolism. J Neurosurg. 70:97-102, 1989.
12. Gorman DF. Arterial gas embolism as a consequence of pulmonary barotrauma. In: Diving and Hyperbaric Medicine, J Desola, Editor. Barcelona: European Undersea Biomedical Society, pp. 348-368, 1984.
13. Gudeman SK, Miller JD, Becker DP. Failure of high-dose steroid therapy to influence intracranial pressure in patients with severe head injury. J Neurosurg. 51:301-306, 1979.
14. Hallenbeck JM, Leitch DR, Dutka AJ, Greenbaum U, Jr., McKee AE. Prostaglandin 12, indomethacin and heparin and heparin promote postischemic neuronal recovery in dogs. Ann Neurol. 12:145-156, 1982.
15. Hyldegaard O, Madsen J. Effect of air, heliox and oxygen breathing on air bubbles in aqueous tissues in the rat. Undersea Hyperb Med. 21:413-424, 1994.
16. Hyldegaard O, Moller M, Madsen J. Protective effect of oxygen and heliox breathing during development of spinal decompression sickness. Undersea Hyperb Med. 21:115-28, 1994.
17. Kaieda R, Todd MM, Cook LN, Warner DS. Acute effects of changing plasma osmolality and colloid oncotic pressure on the formation of brain edema after cryogenic injury. Neurosurgery. 24:671-678, 1989.
18. Kaieda R, Todd MM, Warner DS. Prolonged reduction of colloid oncotic pressure does not increase brain edema following cryogenic injury in rabbits. Anesthesiology. 71:554-560, 1989.
19. Kindwall EP, Margolis I. Management of severe decompression sickness with treatment ancillary to recompression: case report. Aviat Space Environ Med. 46:1065-1068, 1975.
20. Lam AM, Winn HR. Cullen BF, Sundling N. Hyperglycemia and neurological outcome in patients with head injury. J Neurosurg. 75:545-551, 1991.
21. Landolt JP, Money KE, Topliff ED, Nicholas AD, Laufer J, Johnson WH. Pathophysiology of inner ear dysfunction in the squirrel monkey in decompression. J Appl Physiol. 49:1070-1082, 1980.
22. Lanier WL, Stangland KJ, Scheithauer BW, Milde JH, Mitchenfelder JD. The effect of dextrose solution and head position on neurologic outcome after complete cerebral ischeimia in primates: examination of a model. Anesthesiology. 66:39-48, 1987.
23. Li PA, Shamloo M, Smith ML, Katsura K, Siesjo BK. The influence of plasma glucose concentrations on ischemic brain damage is a threshold function. Neurosci Lett. 177:63-65, 1994.
24. Mohr J, Orgogozo JM, Harrison MJG, Hennerici M, Wahlgren NG, Gelmers JH, Martinez-Vila E, Dycka J, Tettenbom D. Meta-analysis of oral nimodipine trials in acute ischemic stroke. Cerebrovasc Dis. 4:197-203, 1994.
25. Moon RE, Gorman DF. Treatment of the decompression disorders. In: PB Bennett & DH Elliott, eds. The Physiology and Medicine of Diving. Philadelphia: WB Saunders, 1993, pp. 506-541.
26. Moon RE, Uguccioni D, Dovenbarger JA, Dear G de L, Mebane GY, Stolp BW, Bennett PB. Surface oxygen for decompression illness. Undersea Hyperb Med 22(Suppl):56, 1995.
27. Palmer AC, Blakemore WF, Payne JE, Sillerce A. Decompression sickness in the goat: nature of brain and spinal cord lesions at 48 hours. Undersea Biomed Res. 5:275-286, 1978.
28. Pearson RR, Goad RF. Delayed cerebral edema complicating cerebral arterial gas embolism: Case histories. Undersea Biomed Res. 9:283-296, 1982.
29. Philp RB, Bennett PB, Andersen JC, Fields GN, McIntyre BA, Francey 1, Briner W. Effects of aspirin and dipyridamole on platelet function, hematology, and blood chemistry of saturation divers. Undersea Biomed Res. 6:127-146, 1979.
30. Philp RB, Inwood MJ, Ackles KN, Radomski MW. Effects of decompression on platelets and hemostasis in men and the influence of antiplatelet drugs (RA233 and VK744). Aerosp Med. 45:231-240, 1974.

31.   Pulsinelli WA, Levy DE, Sigsbee B, Scherer P, Plum F. Increased damage after ischemic stroke in patients with hyperglycemia with or without established diabetes mellitus. Am J Med. 74:540-544, 1983.

32.   Spadaro MV, Moon RE, Fracica PJ, Fawcett TA, Saltzman HA, Macik BG, Massey EW. Life threatening pulmonary thromboembolism in neurological decompression illness. Undersea Biomed Res. 19 (Suppl):41-42, 1992.

33.   Vann RD, Gerth WA. Physiology of decompression sickness. In: Proceedings of the 1990 Hypobaric Decompression Sickness Workshop, AA Pilmanis, Editor. Brooks Air Force Base: Armstrong Laboratory, pp. 35-51, 1990.

34.   Waite CL, Mazzone WF, Greenwood ME, Larsen RT. Cerebral air embolism I. Basic studies. US Naval Submarine Medical Center Report No. 493. 1967, US Navy Submarine Research Laboratory: Panana City, FL.

35.   Warner DS. Principles of resuscitation in CNS injury and future directions. In: Treatment of Decompression Illness, RE Moon, PJ Sheffield, Eds. Kensington, MD: Undersea and Hyperbaric Medical Society, 1996 (in press).

36.   Wass CT, Lanier WL, Hofer RE, Scheithauer BW, Andrews AG. Temperature changes of $\geq 1\,^\circ C$ alter functional neurological outcome and histopathology in a canine model of complete cerebral ischemia. Anesthesiology. 83:325-335, 1995.

37.   Yogendran S, Asokumar B, Cheng DC, Chung F. A prospective randomized double-blinded study of the effect of intravenous fluid therapy on adverse outcomes in outpatient surgery. Anesth Analg. 80:682-686, 1995.

38.   Zomow MH, Scheller MS, Todd MM, Moore SS. Acute cerebral effects of isotonic crystalloid and colloid solutions following cryogenic brain injury in the rabbit. Anesthesiology. 69:180-184, 1988.

39.   Reproduced in part from Moon, RE. Treatment of Decompression Illness. In: AA Bove (Ed) Diving Medicine, Philadelphia: WB Saunders, 1996 (in press).

TREATMENT OF RECREATIONAL DIVING DECOMPRESSION ACCIDENTS
Recommendations of the jury

Jury Consensus
P. PELAIA, Trieste (Italy), President

D. BAKKER, Amsterdam (Netherlands)   JM. MELIET, Toulon (France)
P. CARLI, Paris (France)   G. ORIANI, Milano (Italy)
D. ELLIOT, London (United Kingdom)   M. SARRIAS, Barcelona (Spain)
B. GRANDJEAN, Ajaccio (France)   PH. UNGER, Genève (Switzerland)
M. LAMY, Liège (Belgium)   U. VAN LAAK, Kiel (Germany)

The 1st European Consensus Conference on Hyperbaric Medicine had the ambition to establish the state of the art of Hyperbaric Medicine in Europe in 1994 with regard to its possible applications, its implementation, the training of personnel and the possibilities for its evolution and for further research in the field.

Based on this, the Jury answers the questions proposed at the conference and formulate specific recommendations. These recommendations are the first base of consensus and also serve as the starting point for new advances and evaluation.

At the end of the Lille Conference, it was proposed to consider the theme of decompression accident treatment for the next European Consensus Conference.

Marseille and the Conseil General des Bouches du Rhone, whose interest in diving is well known, spontaneously offered their kind hospitality to the event.

Decompression is usually considered safe as long as it does not involve clinical manifestations requiring medical treatment.

There is probably no disagreement to consider abnormal decompression as a potential illness which is likely not to develop if appropriately and rapidly treated. The scope of our efforts should be to keep the abnormal decompression manifestations at the stage of a transient disorder. To reach this goal we need a much better knowledge about decompression and its biological effects.

Hyperbaric research is mainly based on experimental and clinical studies. During the last five years, unfortunately, the experimental and controlled studies decreased, while retrospective studies increased. Controlled, prospective, multicentric studies are not increasing in diving medicine at the same pace as in other medical disciplines. This lack of methodologically acceptable studies caused a increasing gap between the hyperbaric community and the rest of the scientific community.

In order to answer the posed questions, the Jury had to keep the above considerations in mind, although the undisputable value of clinical experience cannot be forgotten, especially when it generates from concordant observations by many independent groups and during many years.

The best reward will be to see our efforts generating recommendations which will help improving the results of our treatment of decompression injuries.

IS THERE A DIFFERENCE BETWEEN DECOMPRESSION ACCIDENTS IN RECREATIONAL AND PROFESSIONAL DIVING ?

The jury acknowledged the fact that there are differences between decompression accidents in recreational and professional diving, but there an also similarities.

SIMILARITIES

Decompression accidents both in recreational and in professional diving lead to the same illness. The incidence of decompression accidents is not so much dependent on recreational or professional diving than as on the diving profile.

Evolution of symptoms and the clinical course of the disease is the same in both types of diving.

Treatment is the same in both types of diving and depends on signs and symptoms.

DIFFERENCES : THERE ARE NUMEROUS OF CONCERN

a. Medical and physical fitness to dive. The jury likes to recognize the often existing difficulty for recreational divers to find a doctor for examination for fitness to dive. For professional divers, this is not a problem.

b. Age. In recreational diving there are divers under the age of 18 years which does not happen in professional diving. This can have consequences for medical, ethical and legal aspects in treatment of decompression accidents.

c. Environment. The environment in recreational diving is mostly less hazardous than in professional diving.

d. Training. Professional divers in general are better trained in underwater stay than recreational divers.

e. Work load. The professional diver dives to work in contrast with the recreational diver.

f. Depth. Depth in professional diving is often greater than in recreational diving.

g. Diving technique. There is a wide variety in diving techniques in professional diving from compressed air to saturation diving. This is far less so in recreational diving.

h. Incidence of accidents. The difference in incidence depends on the variation in diving techniques used in professional diving (see simil.a). However the incidence in decompression accidents seems to be lower in professional diving than in recreational diving.

i. Recognition of symptoms. The recognition of symptoms of decompression accidents is better in professional diving than in recreational diving, because of better training. The reasons to deny symptoms after diving can be very strong but completely different in recreational and professional diving. The consequences for a decompression accident for the professional diver can be far greater than for the recreational diver.

j. Symptomatology. The symptoms of decompression accidents are more serious in recreational diving than in professional diving.

k. Availability of treatment. In professional diving there is a better availability of immediate treatment facilities than in recreational diving. The major difference is that in professional diving there is a plan when something goes wrong. There is a decompression chamber on the spot or one in the immediate vicinity. Surface oxygen is almost always imediate available in professional diving.

l. Treatment delay. Because of the above, treatment delay in decompression accidents in recreational diving is always longer than in professional diving, usually over 2 1/2 hours with virtually no upper limit. Denying symptoms is another factor that causes delay in treatment but that happens both in professional and in recreational diving (see diff. j)

The jury recognizes the wide variety that exists in professional diving and mentions this only in general terms (for instance saturation diving on the Continental Shelf versus "low grade" professional police or fire department divers). There is a gliding scale between the "low grade" professional divers and the recreational divers, therefore the recommendations given for recreational diving can be applied as well to "low grade" professional diving.

The jury also recognizes the fact that the lack of an adequate classification makes it more difficult to see the existing differences and similarities between professional and recreational diving.

RECOMMENDATIONS (TYPE 1 RECOMMENDATIONS)

1. It is necessary to standardize the rules for fitness to dive both in professional and in recreational diving but more so in recreational diving.
2. Develop an adequate classification system for decompression accidents with international validity.
3. Both professional and recreational divers must be trained in the same way in recognition of symptoms of decompression accidents.
4. The safety measures in recreational diving should be the same as in professional diving.
    - Whenever diving takes place there must be a plan made in advance what to do when something goes wrong.
    - Oxygen must be available on the diving spot in sufficient quantities.
    - A qualified hyperbaric treatment center must be within 4 hours travelling distance from the diving spot.

5. There must be a central collection of all data on decompression accidents, available for retrospective analysis. The incidence of decompression accidents is too low for any treatment center alone to draw valid conclusions.

HOW TO CLASSIFY DECOMPRESSION ACCIDENTS DESCRIPTIVELY?

A descriptive classification of decompression accidents is in contrast to the conventional categorisation which is according to the pathology thought to be present. There is no need to change the traditional classification which includes decompression sickness ("dissolved gas disease"), pulmonary barotrauma and gas embolism, combinations of these two, plus the more recently described PFO (patent foramen ovale or intra-atrial septal defect) which appears to cause a different syndrome. This conventional classification is correct for use in pathology in which the cause is know but it is wrong to apply it to clinical cases in whom the underlying pathology cannot be confirmed. Such presumptions have led to many errors of diagnosis and management.

There is need to adopt a classification which is both practical and accurate. In fact there are two distinct reasons for requiring a dynamic classification which will not introduce the errors of classification by clinical guesswork of pathology:
- for immediate use in acute clinical cases
  - for communication between divers and doctors, and between doctors
  - for clinical management decisions, particularly if the manifestations are not static but changing
  - for the selection of suitable candidates for clinical trials
- retrospectively
  - for epidemiological study of decompression accidents
  - for the analysis of treatment outcomes

Recommendations
Type 1 recommendation

1. For immediate clinical use, adopt a classification based upon "Describing Decompression Illness" already accepted by UHMS (42nd Undersea & Hyperbaric Medical Society Workshop. T.J.R. Francis, D.J. Smith, eds. UHMS Publication Number 79(DECO)5/15/91. 1991).

2. For epidemiology and retrospective analyses, employ a wider multi-thematic classification which will include the descriptive classification but also, when known, the pathological findings. These need to be associated with the dive data and the clinical progression of the illness in relation to the treatments given. A two-year follow up of all cases of decompression illness should be required. This will allow to form a large database by collecting case reports from numerous countries provided that national classifications have been properly transcoded.

CHOICE AND VALIDITY OF EXPERIMENTAL MODELS FOR DECOMPRESSION ACCIDENTS

We recommend an intensification of animal research in the field of decompression accidents because of the rarity of observed cases and of the dangers of studying healthy volunteers.

It is therefore necessary to develop controlled and comparable models. It appears that the experimental models may be very useful for physiopathological studies, but that their result are less applicable to man when it comes to therapy.

Experimental studies regard a vast range of applications. Certain physical phenomena may be revealed by in vitro or ex vivo models. In vivo animal studies can also be performed.

Animal models have been used to study bubbles, central nervous system (particularly motor system), joints, bone and muscles, skin, lung, and the cardio-vascular system.

Among the proposed animals we should distinguish :
- the small animals : rats, mice, rabbit, which frequently behave differently than man
- larger mammals, like the dog, the sheep, the ewe and the pig, which are closer to human physiology

The dog is the older model. However this animal is very resistant to decompression accidents. It is still used by certain research teams, but current regulations tend to limit its use in many countries.

Sheep and ewes are also common models, particularly for pulmonary and bone effects.

The pig offer many advantages. Its availability and cost, its characteristics, quite similar to man's, and the fact this animal is also a very common model in cardiovascular research. On the contrary, the pig shows differences from man for what concerns the pulmonary function. However its advantages are more that the disadvantages and the pig is becoming the animal model of choice for decompression research.

Whichever animal is chosen, it should be kept in mind that the human compara-bility should be more qualitative than quantitative.

Recommendations
Type 1 recommendation

1. It is recommended that animal experimentation is based on simple parameters, as close as possible to those clinically accessible in humans.
2. Anesthesia is generally mandatory for animal experimentation. This influences ventilation, circulation and neurological conditions. The anesthesiology protocol should be selected in a way to minimally influence the studies parameters. Similarly, the use of anesthetic gases is not recommended.
3. It is recommended that the experimental models are described in detail in every scientific paper. This description should include at least the type of animal, its age and maturity, its weight, ventilation method and temperature.

Type 2 recommendation

In order to improve the adequacy of the experimental studies, the pig seems to be the model of current preferred choice, in view of its good advantage / disadvantage ratio.

WHICH MODALITY FOR INITIAL RECOMPRESSION?

Recommendations

Type 1 recommendation

1. The efficient management of Decompression Accident (DCA) in recreational diving should only be done at a specialized center defined as follows : hospital based hyperbaric chamber-trained medical and paramedical team.

2. Decompression Accident (DCA) is a true medical emergency which should be treated with recompression in the shortest possible time, therefore DCA patients should be immediately and directly addressed to the closest specialized treatment center.

3. In water recompression should never be performed as the initial recompression.

4. Minor DCA (pain only) should be treated with oxygen recompression tables at 2.8 ATA maximum. This type I recommendation is based on the experience and the good results observed in commercial diving.

5. For serious DCA (neurological : cerebral, spinal or vestibular) reliable data are lacking that allow to define which of the two more frequently adopted recompression protocols is better. At this stage two treatment protocols are acceptable:
   - Hyperoxygenated tables (FiO_2 = 1) at 2.8 ATA and possible extensions, as guided by clinical evolution during treatment.
   - Hyperoxygenated breathing mixtures tables at 4 ATA. The optimal PiO2 (maximum 2.8 ATA), and the kind of inert gas to be used cannot at this stage be recommended due to the lack of scientific evidence.

When the choice of either modality may depend on personal experience and preference, as well as on local availability, under no circumstance this choice should cause any delay in starting recompression with the more readily available modality.

The jury recommends that the current European comparative multicentric clinical study is continued (2.8 ATA O2 vs 4 ATA Hyperoxygenated tables), and proposes a study to better define the nature of the "selected recalcitrant cases," such as described during the 1st European Consensus Conference in Lille (September, 1994).

Type 2 recommendation

6. Initial recompression of cerebral arterial gas embolism accidents can be performed at 6 ATA with hyperoxygenated breathing mixtures, but not

compressed air, only if the delay to treatment is less than a few hours (type III recommendation). There are not, anyway, sufficient data to define :

- the nature and PiO2 of the hyperoxygenated mixture
- the maximum acceptable delay after which not to start this procedure

7. In case of persistent clinical signs, during the initial recompression, the continuation of treatment with a therapeutic saturation table may be useful.

WHICH PROTOCOL FOR REHYDRATION AND WHICH ROLE FOR DRUGS?

Rehydration Protocol

I. There are many causes leading to dehydration in victims of decompression accidents:
- reduced liquid input during diving,
- increased fluid loss during diving due to dry gas breathing, cold and immersion induced diuresis, sweating due to physical exercise,
- capillary plasma leakage caused by the decompression disorder itself,
- relative hypovolemia due to neurological disorders induced vasoplegia.

II. Diagnosing dehydration:
    A. On the site of the accident :
- History : last drink, dive conditions, thirst, etc.
- Clinical :
  - state of skin and mucosae, vasoconstriction
  - neurological : confusion, hyperthermia
  - hemodynamics : tachycardia, arterial hypotension, postural hypotension
  - urinary output and characteristics (volume, colour)

    B. At the hospital :
- history and clinical evaluation
- laboratory: hematocrit, serum proteins, plasma osmolality, urea, creatinin, pH
- physiology: diuresis, CVP monitoring and hemodynamic evaluation

III. If signs, even minimal, of dehydration are observed, rehydration is mandatory (Type I recommendation)
    A. Oral rehydration—this should be started on the site of the accident. The patient should be encouraged to drink, with the following exceptions :
- un-cooperative patient, confused or unconscious, whose oropharyngeal reflexes may be compromised (risk of pulmonary fluid inhalation)
- nausea or vomiting
- suspected lesion of the gastro intestinal tract

Type of fluid: plain water, preferably containing salt, 50 to 100 mmoles/liter (this is the type of rehydration suggested for athletes and diarrhoic children), not containing (too much) sugar (risk of increasing blood glucose, possibly dangerous when neurological problems are present).

The temperature of the administered water should be cold in case of hyperthermic patients.

> B.   Venous rehydration—this is mandatory when a physician is present (and the necessary materials are available). It should be performed with a peripheral 18 gauge (minimum) cathether.

Type of fluid: a cristalloid, preferably Ringer Lactate or hyperosmolar saline. Avoid glucose containing solutions (may be dangerous in case of neurological injury).

Colloids may also be administered, especially when large quantities of fluids are needed, to reduce the total volume of infused fluids and the degree of interstitial edema. In this case starch containing fluids should be preferred (low or no risk of anaphylaxis), followed by gelatines (more frequent anaphylaxis ?). Dextrans should always be administered with promiten and can be useful as anti-platelet aggregation agents.

Rehydration Monitoring:

- On site: according to clinical evolution, as a general rule not more than 2 liters in the adult.
- At hospital: clinical signs, diuresis (> 50 ml/hr in the adult), CVP and other hemodynamic indexes, laboratory biology. Titration according to the fluid challenge principles.

PHARMACOLOGICAL TREATMENT

> I.   Normobaric oxygen (Type I recommendation)
> A.   Rationale:
> 1)   Prevention and/or treatment of hypoxemia (due to respiratory or circulatory causes and with possible compromising of oxygen transport) and/or of tissue hypoxia due to the presence of inert gas bubbles
> 2)   More rapid elimination of inert gas from tissues, blood and the lungs

Administration modalities: $FiO_2 = 1$ during all the inspiratory phase, while spontaneously breathing: through a facial mask with reservoir bag with O_2 flow rate of 15 l/min minimum in the adult patient, through a high seal facial mask (with continuous flow and CPAP circuit or a with demand valve). In case of respiratory or circulatory distress, or coma, controlled ventilation is mandatory with $FiO_2 = 1$ and according to accepted Lung Protective Ventilation modalities (tidal volume 8 ml/kg bw, plateau airway pressure 30 cm H_2O).

In case of neurological distress $PaCO_2$ should be kept at levels 40 mmHg.

The administration of 100 % oxygen should be continued until therapeutic recompression is started. This should take place within the maximum interval of 6 hours, in order to reduce the possibility of oxygen toxicity manifestations.

II. Other Drugs
- For seriously ill patients, any drug or therapeutic procedure will be adopted in first priority according to current intensive care criteria.
- No drug can be strongly recommended due to the lack of acceptable scientific evidence.
- The prevention of hyperthermia (dangerous in case of neurological injury) is recommended (Type 2 recommendation) by ways of physical methods or with drugs (paracetamol, non-steroid anti-inflammatory drugs)
- Other drugs are optional (type 3 recommendation):
  - on the site of the accidents aspirin 500 mg orally in the adult
  - at the hospital: aspirin 500 mg orally or IV
- The following drugs, when used, should be administered early and in dosages not likely to cause negative collateral effects : lidocaine, steroids, antiplatelet drugs, anti-coagulants (low dose heparin, to avoid/reduce central nervous system bleeding), non-steroid anti-inflammatory drugs (humoral or cellular), antioxydant drugs, calcium channel blockers, other neuronal protectants, vasodilators, fluorocarbons, etc.

WHAT IS THE PROTOCOL FOR PERSISTENT SYMPTOMS AFTER AN INITIAL TREATMENT ?

The problem of the treatment in case of persistent symptoms following initial recompression is current and of primary importance.

It is not possible to deduce a unique therapeutic approach from the analysis of international literature, nor to extract objective data supporting a specific line.

Decompression accident, especially in its most severe expression, is always accompanied by disturbances of central (medullar) and peripheral nervous system with functional muscular and sphincter disturbances.

In any type of decompression accident, the need of a classification, both relative to the primary damage and its consequences, has to be stressed. Concerning the medullar syndromes, a simple evaluation scale, in stages by level of damage and recovery, is recommended. This evaluation scale, even if it may be completed by more sophisticated neurological examinations, must be able to easily code for the initial symptoms, remaining manifestations after the first recompression and possible further recovery. This evaluation scale has to be simple and quick to use and the jury recommends the ASIA scale used for medullar trauma.

The continuation of the treatment seems to be logical but prospective studies including long term follow up are needed to answer at this question. However, it is strongly recommended (type 1 recommendation) that the treatment is continued but it is not possible to indicate a unique therapeutic schema.

Starting from the pathophysiological knowledge and clinical studies carried out in similar situations of neurologic damage, as well as from the results obtained in the neurologic rehabilitation area, it may be recommended that kinesiatherapy and physiotherapy must be started as soon as possible after the initial recompression (type 1 recommendation) in order to prevent the subsequent stage of flaccidity or spasticity and with the scope of recruiting all the active or recoverable fibers.

Because recovery has been reported during this period of time, close follow-up must be done for, at least, 2 years after the accident. Continuation of hyperbaric treatment seems to be acceptable, even if further prospective randomized multicentric studies are still needed to establish the exact modalities of hyperbaric treatment, as well as of kinesiatherapy and of the association kinesiatherapy-hyperbaric treatment.

Recommendations
Type 1 recommendation

1. Prospective, randomized, multicentric studies are needed and must include long term follow-up (at least 2 years).
2. In case of persisting neurologic symptoms after the initial recompression, continuation of the treatment by hyperbaric oxygen sessions together with rehabilitation measures is recommended.
3. Hyperbaric oxygen treatment is only recommended up to 10 sessions and if done simultaneously with rehabilitation.
4. Continuation of hyperbaric oxygen treatment after 10 sessions is only permitted if an objective functional improvement has been observed during hyperbaric oxygen session.

SECTION I – PART 3

The 3rd European Consensus
Conference on Hyperbaric Medicine

The 3rd European Consensus Conference on
The Role of HBOT in Acute Musculo-Skeletal Trauma

Section I – Part 3
September 7, 1996—Milano, Italy

ORGANIZED BY THE EUROPEAN COMMITTEE FOR HYPERBARIC MEDICINE

CONTENTS

RECOMMENDATIONS OF THE JURY

JURY

- P.G. Marchetti, Bologna (Italy); President
- A. DUQUENNOY, LILLE (FRANCE)
- D. Linnarson, Stockholm (Sweden)
- F. Malerba, Milano (Italy)
- R. MARTI, AMSTERDAM (THE NETHERLANDS)
- C. MARTIN, MARSEILLE (FRANCE)
- J. NIINIKOSKI (FINLAND)
- R. VILADOT, BARCELONA (SPAIN)

RECOMMENDATIONS

- HBO therapy has to be considered as an adjunctive treatment modality.
- Optimal surgery and resuscitation have to be done before or simultaneously.

Question 1
Can HBOT prevent post-traumatic Bone hypoxia and post-traumatic Edema?

Until now there is not sufficient evidence to definitively state that HBO can prevent bone hypoxia, and edema. However there is experimental and clinical evidence supporting that HBO act to correct post-traumatic tissue edema and delayed bone healing (Type 2 statement).

Question 2
Which is the role of HBOT in prevention of reperfusion injury?

There is some experimental evidence showing a positive effect of HBO in preventing reperfusion injury, but there is not sufficient clinical evidence.

However, no study showed a detrimental effect of HBO in increasing the oxidative stress, in injured tissue (Type 3 statement).

It is strongly recommended that well conducted clinical studies have to be undertaken, because of the existing experimental evidence (Type 1 recommendation).

Question 3
Which is the role of HBOT in prevention of post-traumatic superimposed infections?

The procedure of choice is surgery (repeated if necessary), but HBO can be recommended as an adjunctive treatment to enhance antibiotic efficacy, to improve tissue oxygenation and prevent superinfections (Type 2 statement).

Questions 4 and 5

Which is the role of HBOT in improving tissue salvage after acute and subacute musculo-skeletal trauma?

In case of severe tissue damage, with dubious vitality, there is experimental and clinical evidence that HBO improves tissue salvage and clinical outcome (Type 2 statement).

Question 6

What is the role of HBOT in improving the final clinical outcome in acute and subacute musculo-skeletal trauma?

In cases of open fractures with extensive soft tissue and/or vascular damage (corresponding with type III B/C of Gustillo's classification) adjunctive HBOT is recommended (Type 2 recommendation).

In less severe cases HBOT adjunctive to surgery can be used in compromised hosts (Type 3 recommendation).

In every cases HBO is considered, measurement of transcutaneous oxygen pressure is recommended as an index for the definition of the indication and of the evolution of treatment (Type 2 recommendation).

The cost of the use of adjunctive HBO will be at least compensated by the decrease in morbidity in these patients (e.g. lower amputation rate) (Type 2 statement).

CAN HBOT PREVENT POST-TRAUMATIC BONE HYPOXIA AND POST-TRAUMATIC EDEMA?

G. Bouachour
Service de Réanimation Médicale, Unité de Médecine Hyperbare, Centre Hositalier Universitaire, 49033 ANGERS CEDEX 01, FRANCE

INTRODUCTION

Severe post-traumatic limb injuries may associated bone lesions (as open fractures), neurological lesions, vascular lesions (as arterial disruption or compression), and soft tissue (cutaneous and/or muscular) lesions (as edema, infection...). Acute ischemia of the limb resulting from crush injury leading to amputation, local infection of open fracture are for example the most common and severe complications of post-traumatic injuries. A high morbidity (as an amputation rate of 60%) can occur in spite of appropriate surgery (1, 2, 3). Hyperbaric oxygen therapy may be indispensable for the management of severe limb injuries. Numerous experimental and clinical studies had given arguments for the use of hyperbaric oxygen therapy (HBOT), because HBOT allows the immediate consequences of trauma to be fought against: cutaneous ischemic, soft tissue ischemic damage and bone hypoxia, compartment syndrome and infection (4, 5).

EFFECTS OF HYPERBARIC OXYGEN ON BONE HYPOXIA

Alteration in oxygen supply is a limiting factor in the healing of fractures, and recovery from osteomyelitis. Normal oxygenation is fundamental to cause a differentiation to osseous tissue from multipotent mesenchymal cells, whereas hypoxia result in cartilage formation (6). It is known that the alternance of hyperoxia and hypoxia such as is achieved by HBOT favors the synthesis of collagen (7) and proliferation of fibroblasts (8) enabling a support for neovascularization (9), thus allowing accelerated tissue repair and a shortening of the healing period (10).

Bone tissue culture in 30% oxygen has a maximum synthesis of hydroxyproline (11). In a physiological point of view, oxygen is essential in bone tissue for the synthesis of collagen hydroxyproline. Collagenous matrix formation and mineralisation (as enhanced accumulation of calcium, magnesium and phosphorus) in bone fracture of rats are accelerated in animals exposed to pure oxygen at 2.5 ATA compared with control rats treated at atmospheric pressure (12). Moreover intermittent HBOT results in a greater uptake of 45Ca and a higher breaking strength in fractured femur of rats (13). Exposure to 100% oxygen in healing rabbit tibias injured by an operation results in a gradually increase of the bone PO_2 from 75 to 230 mmHg (14). This level is obtained progressively between the sixth and the fifty-seventh day of exposure, with no further increase between the fifty-seventh and the ninetieth day. Moreover the oxygen tension in the tibia of the control group breathing air are markedly lower (14). These experiments suggest that the healing process is retarded partly by an extremely unfavorable oxygen environment. Supply of oxygen and consequently local circulation play a important role in bone growth. Compact bone tissue, which is diaphysial, has endosteal and periosteal vascularization. Endosteal vascularization which depends on the diaphysial nutritive artery can be compromised by a simple fracture. Periosteal vascularization is preserved in simple fractures but is destroyed in traumas of high energy forces, due to lesions in soft tissue, especially muscles. Blood vessels are crucial to achieve normal osteogenesis (15). The main process of callous formation is occurring within the marrow cavity possibly because of the good intramedullary blood supply. An experimental study (16) on the healing process of fractured femurs in rats showed that the group of rats treated with hyperbaric oxygen (100% oxygen at 3ATA for one hour twice a day) had fractures completely remodeled compared to the control group. Microradiography showed abundant medullary canal and subperiosteal new bone in HBO-treated animals at a time when there was incomplete bony union in the control animals. The development of vascularisation in regenerating tissue is achieved by hyperoxia and appears to be a direct consequence of HBOT leading to bone healing. HBOT increases periosteal thickness, trabecular bone outgrowth, and number of capillaries in the fractures region. Thus vascular bed and blood flow on the proximal and distal site of the fracture are earlier restored to normal values by HBOT (17).

In summary, HBOT, by inducing systemic hyperoxia, is responsible for a better oxygen supply to the bone stimulating the neovascularization. Consequently, local microcirculation and the nutritional supply to the bone are restored, leading to osteosynthesis with collagenous matrix formation and bony mineralisation.

INDICATIONS OF HYPERBARIC OXYGEN THERAPY IN POST-TRAUMATIC BONE HYPOXIA IN MAN

There are few published human studies concerning particularly the results of HBOT in the management of post-traumatic bone injuries without considering the effect of HBOT on soft tissue injuries. Yet, HBOT should acts again a lack of bone consolidation. Incidence of nonunion can be as high as 75% in displaced tibia fractures. In long bone fractures, primary healing occurs in 100% of the patients when HBOT is started within 10 days of the fractures (18). In case of pseudarthosis which requires surgery such as bone grafting, HBOT seems to be a useful adjunct to surgery both preoperatively an postoperatively (19 and personal data).

EFFECTS OF HYPERBARIC OXYGEN ON POST-TRAUMATIC EDEMA

In traumatized tissue autoregulatory mechanisms increase blood flow to compensate hypoxia. In a damaged microcirculation this autoregulation causes undesirable swelling. Edema occurs, increasing the diffusion distance of oxygen from the vessels to the injury area. All the conditions necessary to compromise wound repair are present : microcirculatory alteration, swelling and hypoxia leading to a compartment syndrome. Compartment syndrome is connected to the pressure increase of the intramuscular interstitial space exceeding capillary perfusion pressure. Thus, when intramuscular pressure exceeds 30 mmHg the microcirculatory perfusion flow collapses. Muscular edema linked to the crush injuries is the cause of this increased pressure and it gives rise to muscular necrosis, vascular and neurological compression.

In addition when HBOT is started, local hemodynamic effects also occur through hyperoxia-related vasoconstriction. This vasoconstriction is probably induced by the direct action of the increase in the partial pressure of oxygen in blood vessel walls (20, 21). This vasoconstricting effect affects only healthy vessels and brings about a 20 to 30% reduction in peripheral blood flow counterbalancing in this way the vasodilatation reflex in ischemic tissues. This vasoconstriction does not change local oxygen delivery which is maintained thanks to hyperoxygenation. Furthermore, vasoconstriction results in a diminution of the post-traumatic edema (22). Reduction of capillary transudation flow rate will bring about a diminution of the post-traumatic edema the immediate effect of which is an improvement in microcirculatory local blood flow rate. This effect is the factor offering an explanation to the efficacy of hyperbaric oxygen therapy in compartment syndrome. In an experimental model of canine compartment syndrome (23, 24), hyperbaric oxygen reduced the formation of the edema by roughly 20% in injured muscular tissue as well as muscular necrosis estimated on the uptake of technetium-99m pyrophoshate. The reduction of intramuscular water content during compartment syndrome is all the more effective when hyperbaric oxygen therapy is started early (22).

Moreover HBOT appears to protect the microcirculation by reducing venular leukocyte adherence and inhibiting progressive adjacent arteriolar vasoconstriction (25). As regards tissue metabolism, hyperbaric oxygen enables cell reserves of adenosine triphosphate (ATP) to be maintained, thus allowing cell membranes to keep control over osmolarity and therefore limiting cellular damage resulting from water movement induced by ischemia (26). In a rat hindlimb model, after four hours of ischemia, the changes in levels of the intracellular muscle compounds adenosine triphosphate, phosphocreatine and lactates were less in the hyperbaric oxygen-treated rats than in the untreated animals (27). In an other study, the same authors showed that HBOT also decreased edema formation in the postischemic muscle following three hours of ischemia and reperfusion when compared to untreated rats, moreover the loss of total glutathione was less in HBO treated animals (28).

In conclusion, all the results of these experimental data conclude to the beneficials effects of HBOT: it decreases muscle edema, stimulates intracellular aerobic oxidation, restores energy content and probably maintains the transport of ions and molecules across the cell membrane, explaining the diminished degree of skeletal muscle injury after severe trauma of the limbs.

CLINICAL RESULTS OF HYPERBARIC OXYGEN THERAPY IN CRUSH INJURIES

The main interest in using HBOT in emergency cases will be to prevent or restrict skin necrosis in order to prevent secondary exposure of joints, bone fractures, blood vessels and neural structures. Exposure of these various major structures radically modifies trauma prognosis. Nevertheless, in cases of occlusion of major vessels with no collateral circulation, HBOT is not expected to help anoxic tissue to survive. But in such cases HBOT is helpful to separate viable from non viable tissues and to limit the excision of ischemic tissue. Moreover another role of HBOT which is very useful in severe limb injuries, distant in time from the acute stage, is the healing effect of hyperoxygenation.

Published clinical studies, showing the interest in using HBOT in the surgical management of severe limb injuries are very limited. The first published data was undertaken in 1961 (29), where the beneficial effect of HBOT was reported in a patient with ischemic near avulsion of foot. HBOT is considered useful, with 60 to 85% of case results being judged positive (30-33). Indications considered for HBOT involved vascular injury, soft tissue injuries, and anaerobic infection combined with open fractures (31). Several authors underscore the interest of using HBOT in patients suffering from persistent limb ischemia, in spite of the reestablishment of effective arterial perfusion after surgery. HBOT has, in the majority of cases, enabled amputation to be avoided, and the limb to be saved thanks to distal oxygenation sustained by HBOT in tissues having suffered from prolonged ischemia (5, 32, 34).

However no study showed indisputably the place of HBOT in the management of severe limb traumas. We conducted a prospective random clinical study over a 2-year period, comparing hyperbaric oxygen therapy with placebo in the management of crush injuries (35). Thirty-six patients with crush injuries were assigned in a blinded randomized fashion, within 24h following surgery, to treatment with HBO (session of 100% O_2 at 2.5ATA for 90min, twice daily, during 6 days) or placebo (session of 21% O_2 at 1.1ATA for 90 min, twice daily, during 6 days). All the patients received the same standard therapies (anticoagulant, antibiotics, wound dressings). The two groups (HBO group: n=18; placebo group: n=18) were similar in terms of age, risk factors, vascular injuries, fractures and type, location or timing of surgical procedures. Complete healing was obtained in 17 patients in the HBO group versus 10 patients in the placebo group (p<0.01). New surgical procedures (such as skin flaps and grafts, vascular surgery or even amputation) were performed in one patient in the HBO group versus 6 patients in the placebo group (p<0.05). Systematic evaluation of the injured extremities before each session showed that edema was present, at the first session in 12 patients in the HBO group and 11 patients in the placebo group, whereas, at the end of treatment, three patients in the HBO group and six patients in the placebo group had persistent edema of the injured extremities. Cyanosis was present initially in four patients in the HBO group and five patients in the placebo group. During the following HBO sessions, only one patient had persistent skin cyanosis, whereas in the placebo group two additional patients developed skin cyanosis at the injury site (p<0.05). Analysis of groups of patients matched for age and severity of injury showed that in the subgroup of patients older than 40 with Grade III soft-tissue injury, wound healing was obtained in seven patients (87.5%) in the HBO group versus three patients (30%) in the placebo group (p<0.05). This study shows the effectiveness of HBOT in improving wound healing and reducing repetitive surgery when perioperative wound management fails. According to the results of this clinical trial, HBOT should be recommended in the management of severe trauma (Grade III soft-tissue injuries) in patients over 40 years old.

Furthermore HBOT accelerates healing and helps to prevent functional sequelae necessitating expensive equipment and the financial charge of patients suffering from heavy functional incapacities. An advantage in terms of the cost of hospitalization for complicated limb fractures is highly probable. In the USA, for example, early care with hyperbaric oxygen therapy of compartment syndrome associated with crush injuries, prior to surgical decompression indications being necessary, enables the estimated cost of treatment to be divided by four (36).

CONCLUSION

HBOT has an important role to play as an adjuvant to surgery in the management of severe limb injuries. It enables skin, skeletal muscles and bone to resist ischemic damage. It prevents the constitution of compartment syndrome by reducing post-traumatic edema, it prevents the risk of infection notably to anaerobic germs in the case of open fracture, and enables healing phenomena to be induced more rapidly. Certainly not every patient with trauma of the extremities requires HBOT. In our study the benefits of HBOT in improving healing and limb survival are in close relationship with age and severity of the injury. Traumatic injury treating centers should have easy access to the use of hyperbaric oxygen so as to start this treatment as early as possible for the greater benefit of patients with recognized risk factors, clinical compromise or a history of impaired wound healing.

REFERENCES

1. Drapanas T, Hewitt RL, Weichert RT, et al (1970). Civilian vascular injuries. A critical appraisal of three decades of management. Ann Surg 172: 351.
2. Keeley SB, Sydner WH, Weigelt JA (1983). Arterial injuries below the knee: Fifty one patients with eighty two injuries. J Trauma 23: 285.
3. Lange RH, Bach AW, Hansen ST, et al (1985). Open tibial fractures with associated vascular injuries: Prognosis for limb salvage. J Trauma 25: 203.
4. Strauss MB (1981). Role of hyperbaric oxygen therapy in acute ischemias and crush injuries- An orthopedic perspective. HBO Review 2: 87.
5. Shupak A, Gozal D, Ariel A, Melamed Y, Katz A (1987). Hyperbaric oxygenation in acute peripheral post-traumatic ischemia. J Hyperbaric Med 2: 7.
6. Basset CAL, Herrmann I. (1961). Influence of oxygen concentration and mechanical factors on differentiation of connective tissue in vitro. Nature 190: 460.
7. Hunt TK, Pai MP (1972). The effect of varying ambient oxygen tensions on wound metabolism and collagen synthesis. Surg Gynecol Obstet 135: 561.
8. Hunt TK, Niinikoski J, Zederfeldt BH, Silver IA (1977). Oxygen in wound healing enhancement : cellular effects of oxygen. In: Davis JC, Hunt TK (ed) Hyperbaric Oxygen therapy. Undersea Medical Society, Bethesda, pp 111-122.
9. Manson PN, Im MJ, Myers RAM (1980). Improved capillaries by hyperbaric oxygen in skin flaps. Surg Forum 31: 564.
10. Kivisaari J, Niiniskoski J (1975). Effects of hyperbaric oxygenation and prolonged hypoxia on the healing of open wounds. Acta Chir Scand 141: 14.
11. Stern B, Glimcher MJ, Goldhaber P (1969). The effect of various oxygen tensions on the synthesis and degradation of bone collagen in tissue culture. Proc Soc Exp Biol Med 121: 869.
12. Niinikoski J, Penttinen R, Kulonen E (1970). Effect of hyperbaric oxygenation on fracture healing in the rat. Calcif Tissue Res Suppl, 4:115.
13. Coulson DB, Fergusson AB, Diehl RC, (1964). Effect of hyperbaric oxygen on the healing femur of the rat. Surg Forum, 17: 449.
14. Niinikoski J, Hunt TK (1972). Oxygen tension in healing bone. Surg Gynecol Obstet, 134: 746.
15. Trueta J (1963). The role of the vessels in osteogenesis. J Bone Joint Surg, 45B: 402.
16. Yablon IG, Cruess RL (1968). The effect of hyperbaric oxygen on fracture healing in the rats. J Trauma, 8: 186.
17. Granstrom G, Nilsson LP, Rockert HOE, Magnusson BC (1989). Experimental mandibular fracture. Effect on bone healing after treatment with hyperbaric oxygen. Proceeding of the XV annual Meeting of the European Undersea Biomedical Society. Eilat, Israel, 1989 sept. 17-21: 290.
18. Strauss MB, Hart GB (1977). Clinical experiences with HBO in fracture healing. In: Smith G (ed). Proceedings of the 7th international congress on hyperbaric medicine. University of Aberdeen Press, Aberdeen, pp 329-332.
19. Oriani G, Barnini C et al. (1982). Hyperbaric oxygen treatment in various orthopedic disorders. Minerva Med 73: 2983.
20. Bird AD, Telfer ABM (1965). Effect of hyperbaric oxygen on limb circulation. Lancet 1: 355.
21. Sullivan SM, Johnson PC (1981). Effect of oxygen on blood flow autoregulation in cat sartorius muscle. Am J Physiol 241: H807.
22. Nylander G, Lewis D, Nordstrom H, Larson J (1985). Reduction of postischemic edema with hyperbaric oxygen. Plast Reconstr Surg 76: 595.

23. Skyhar MJ, Hargens AR, Srauss MB, Gershuni DH, Hart GB, Akeson WH (1986). Hyperbaric oxygen reduces edema and necrosis of skeletal muscle in compartment syndromes associated with hemoraghic hypotension. J Bone Jt Surg 68A: 1218.

24. Strauss MB, Hargens AR, Gershuni D, Greenberg DA, Crenshaw AG, Hart GB, Akeson WH (1983). Reduction of skeletal muscle necrosis using intermittent hyperbaric oxygen in a model of compartment syndrome. J Bone Jt Surg 65A: 656.

25. Zamboni WA, Roth AC, Russell RC, Graham B, Suchi H, Kucan JO (1993). Morphologic analysis of the microcirculation during reperfusion of ischemic skeletal muscle and the effect of hyperbaric oxygen. Plast Reconstr Surg 91: 1110.

26. Nylander G, Nordstrom H, Lewis D, Larsson J (1987). Metabolic effects of hyperbaric oxygen in postischemic muscle. Plast Reconstr Surg 79: 91.

27. Haapaniemi T, Nylander G, Sirsjo A, Larsson J (1996). Hyperbaric oxygen reduces ischemia-induced skeletal muscle injury. Plast Reconstr Surg 97: 602.

28. Haapaniemi T, Sirsjo A, Nylander G, Larsson J (1995). Hyperbaric oxygen treatment attenuates glutathione depletion and improves metabolic restitution in postischemic skeletal muscle. Free Radical Research 23: 91.

29. Smith G, Stevens J, Griffiths JC, et al (1961). Near avulsion of foot treated by replacement and subsequent prolonged exposure of patients to oxygen at two atmospheres pressure. Lancet 2: 1122.

30. Slack WK, Thomas DA, De Jode LRJ (1966). Treatment of trauma, ischemic disease of limbs and varicose ulceration. In: Brown IW Jr, Cox BG (ed) Proceedings of the third international congress on hyperbaric medicine. Washington, DC: National Academy of Sciences, National Research Council; pp 621-624.

31. Szekely O, Szanto G, Takats A (1973). Hyperbaric oxygen therapy in injured subjects. Injury 4: 294.

32. Monies-Chas I, Hashmonai M, Hoerer D, et al (1977). Hyperbaric oxygen treatment as an adjunct to reconstructive vascular surgery in trauma. Injury 8: 274.

33. Loder RE (1979). Hyperbaric oxygen therapy in acute trauma. Ann R Coll Surg Engl 61: 472.

34. Schramek A, Hashmonai M (1977). Vascular injuries in the extremities in battle casualties. Br J Surg 64: 644.

35. Bouachour G, Cronier P, Gouello JP, Toulemonde JL, Talha A, Alquier P (1996). Hyperbaric oxygen therapy in the management of crush injuries: A randomized, double-blind, placebo controlled clinical trial. J Trauma 41:(August; in press).

36. Strauss MB (1988). Cost-effective issues in HBO therapy: complicated fractures. J Hyperbaric Med 3: 199.

WHICH ROLE FOR HBO THERAPY IN THE PREVENTION OF REPERFUSION INJURY?

A.J. van der Kleij
Department of Surgery, Academic Medical Center, University of Amsterdam,
PO Box 22700, 1100 DE, Amsterdam, The Netherlands

INTRODUCTION

When a disease possesses a point in time between the moment that the usual clinical diagnosis is made and the early diagnosis is possible it can be shown that a new treatment modality e.g. hyperbaric oxygen therapy may play a role in the prevention of an injury or the improvement of the final outcome (Sacket, et al., 1991). These authors presuppose four stages within the "natural history" of a disease: the biologic onset, the stage at which point early diagnosis is possible, the stage at which point the usual diagnosis is made, and finally the outcome stage. In addition, several critical points between the stages of the natural history of a disease have to be identified. In order to determine the optimal point of timing for HBO therapy to prevent a reperfusion injury we have to define the characteristics of an early diagnosis.

Revascularization of ischemic tissue may cary the risk for serious complications. These complications can be systemically as well as localized in the revascularized tissue itself. Reperfusion of an ischaemic limb may result into pulmonary leuco-sequestration (Anner et al., 1987) and initiate pulmonary dysfunction caused by oxygen derived free-radicals (Nelson et al.,1992). Furthermore, an ischemic leg can also be the source of complement activation associated with a systemic inflammatory response (Bengtson et al., 1987; Hickley et al., 1992).

Revascularization of a previously ischemic area initiates a sequence of events that causes additional cell injury. It has been shown that 3 hours of enteric ischemia followed by 1 hour of reperfusion results in more tissue damage compared with 4 hours total ischemia (Parks et al., 1986). The local tissue damage is characterized by increased microvascular permeability to macromolecules, increased leukocyte adherence to post-capillary venular endothelium and areas of no flow and are referred to as the ischemic-reperfusion (R-I) injury.

The biologic onset of a localized reperfusion injury occurs within a few minutes after reperfusion of ischemic tissue. The magnitude and duration of the ischemic insult determine the initial injury. The final overall sustained injury is composed by an ischemic component and a reperfusion component. The reperfusion component, also with its own time course, is receptive for preventive therapy and will only be effective within the treatment window (Figure 1). The approach of "the treatment window" (Bulkley, 1987) provides insights in the dynamics of the ischemic-reperfusion injury. An attenuation of the total sustained injury curve can be achieved by a reduction of the reperfusion component

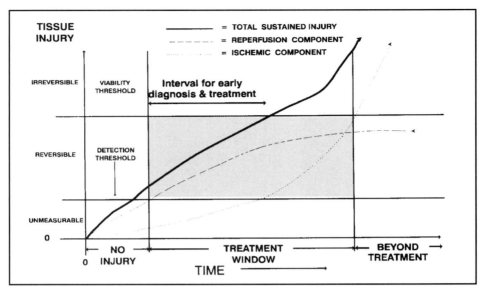

Figure 1. Treatment window adapted from Bulkley (Br J Cancer. 1987; 55:Suppl. VIII,66-73). Therapy directed to the reperfusion component will only be effective within the treatment window.

which means that any preventive measure can only be effective when it is   initiated at the left side within the treatment window below the tissue viability threshold. This small time interval is the stage at which point early diagnosis is required. The right side of the treatment window represents the time interval in which the usual clinical diagnosis is made but not more receptive for preventive measures.

Biological events and early symptoms of a reperfusion injury.

In order to cope with free radical biochemistry the organism is equipped with oxidants and antioxidants residing in specific cellular compartments (Bast et al., 1991). Oxygen derived free radicals are often associated with their potential damaging properties but they do also play an essential role in normal cellular functions (Figure 2). For this reason it is advocated to use HBO treatment to restore cellular defense mechanisms.

Intravital (fluorescence) microscopy is used to study the microcirculation and provides information about mechanisms of damage and can be used to test therapeutic modalities (Kleij van der A.J et al., 1994; Zamboni et al., 1993; Suval et al., 1987). As mentioned before the local complications are characterized by increased microvascular permeability to macromolecules, increased leukocyte adherence to postcapillary venular endothelium and areas of no flow. Carden and Korthuis (1989) studied the microcirculatory alterations after reperfusion of ischemic skeletal muscle tissue and identified two major events which play a role in the final post-ischemic reperfusion injury:

1) Xanthine oxidase and oxygen derived free radicals,
2) Activation of neutrophils.

At the onset of ischemia there is a rapid proteolytic conversion of xanthine dehydrogenase to xanthine oxidase. Lack of molecular oxygen causes excess accumulation of the substrate hypoxanthine and the activated enzyme xanthine oxidase. The biologic onset of

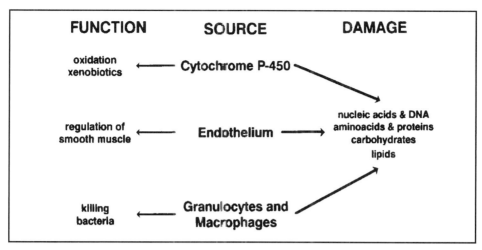

Figure 2. Source of oxygen derived free radicals with the beneficial physiological functions and potential damaging properties. Adapted from Bast et al., 1991.

the reperfusion injury, the sudden supply of molecular oxygen, results in a rapid production of the superoxide free radical. The iron-catalyzed reduction of $H2O_2$ and O_2 results in very toxic hydroxyl radicals inducing lipid peroxidation of cellular membranes.

The role of the neutrophils in the post-ischemic injury explains the low- and no-flow events in the microcirculation. During reperfusion platelet aggregating factors (PAF) and LTB4 (a chemoattractant for neutrophils promoting neutrophil adhesiveness), are two factors among many others, which are activated by the xanthine oxidase derived oxidants and augment the final post-ischemic injury. It is generally accepted that leukocyte adhesion molecules such as GMP-140, ELAM-1, and VCAM reside within the endothelial glycocalyx and interaction of neutrophils with ELAM-1, increase microvascular permeability. After binding to the endothelial adhesion molecules, leucocytes might influence permeability either by secreting stored cationic proteins or by producing free radicals such as superoxide anions (Defouw et al., 1994).

Limited reperfusion in experimental models has revealed a significantly reduction of the reperfusion injury (Walker et al., 1987; Anderson et al., 1990). The period of limited reperfusion was employed only for the first hour of reperfusion implicating that the critical events occurs within 1 hour of reperfusion. Malcolm and Fantini (1987) reported that the endogenous superoxide radical scavenger enzyme, superoxide dismutase, prevents in a rat hind limb model of ischemic-reperfusion injury the progressive deterioration of cell membrane electrical potentials. Carden et al. reported that reperfusion with anoxic blood results in a reduced microvascular permeability compared with normoxic blood indicating that the ischemic reperfusion injury is an oxygen-dependent process.

It is clear that the biochemical events and interactions between the activated intraluminal leucocytes and the endothelial cells are governed by complicated mechanisms which are not completely understood. However, molecular oxygen plays a substantial role in the ischemic reperfusion injury.

This brings us back to the question: how to diagnose early a reperfusion injury?

Increased microvascular permeability is one of the first symptoms and is clinically expressed by edema. For example the existence of an reperfusion injury after a revascularization procedure for the lower limb can clinically be detected by measurements of the calf circumference (van der Kleij, 1985, own observation). In the same study the investigators were unable to detect biochemical (e.g., ceruloplasmine) alterations in post-ischemic venous blood samples. Edema, however, may be also associated with other   diseases which means that the clinician cannot merely rely on this symptom to identify an early reperfusion injury. When organ dysfunction such as paralysis, myocardial stunning, failure of limb reimplantation becomes obvious the stage at which point the usual diagnosis is made has been reached and during this stage reperfusion is not more receptive for preventive measures.

It is evident that using the microcirculatory characteristics of an early reperfusion injury the clinician is unable to make an early diagnose of an ischemic-reperfusion injury, unless he is informed about the time point of the reperfusion event.

Is there any proof in the literature that hyperbaric oxygen attenuates ischemic-reperfusion injury?

Since hyperbaric oxygen therapy is associated with an increased production of oxygen derived free-radicals (Sinclair et al., 1990) and free radicals themselves are the mediators of the reperfusion injury it seems to be controversial to use HBO treatment to prevent a reperfusion injury. However, more evidence is accumulating that reperfused tissue may benefit by pretreatment with hyperbaric oxygen. The beneficial effects of hyperbaric oxygen on ischemic myocardium has been shown by Thomas et al.(1990). A single exposure to 90 minutes hyperbaric oxygen (2 ATA and 100% O_2) after 2 hours of coronary artery occlusion resulted in a 36% restoration of myocardial oxidative enzyme activity in ischemic myocardium despite persistent occlusion by a thrombus. Treatment with rt-PA resulted in restoration of 48% oxidative enzyme activity and the combined treatment, hyperbaric oxygen and rt-PA restored 97% of enzyme activity versus the control group (p<.001) and 94% restoration versus the thrombolysis alone group.

Mink and Dutka (1995) found in rabbits, which were subjected to a 10 minutes global cerebral ischemia, a significantly reduced brain vascular permeability in gray matter (16%) as well as in white matter (20%) in the HBO group. HBO was initiated after 30 minutes reperfusion. HBO attenuates the reperfusion injury of the small intestine in rats (Yamada et al., 1995). In these experiments HBO was immediately initiated after the reperfusion event.

Zamboni et al. (1993) evaluated the morphologic events in the microcirculation of the rat's gracilus muscle. During the last hour of 4 hours ischemia, the first hour during reperfusion, and the second hour during reperfusion a hyperbaric oxygen treatment was given. These authors observed no exacerbation of the reperfusion injury rather a protection as expressed by a reduced number of leukocytes adherence to postcapillary venular endothelium. Furthermore, it was noticed that the HBO treatment during the second hour of reperfusion was less effective compared with the group animals receiving HBO treatment during the first hour of reperfusion and the last hour of 4 hours ischemia.

These experimental data indicate that the beneficial effect of hyperbaric oxygen is effective immediately after a reperfusion and/or during the first 60 to 90 minutes of a reperfusion.

However, we must realize that during an experimental approach the investigator can make his own exact time schedule to study the effect of a treatment modality whereas in clinical situations timing is much more difficult.

SUMMARY

The efficacy of a prevention of an ischemic reperfusion injury is primarily influenced by the magnitude and duration of the ischemic insult. Within the limitations of the treatment window there is experimental evidence for a place to use HBO to reduce the reperfusion injury. Furthermore, it appears that only when it is initiated just briefly before the reoxygenation of the ischemic tissue or within the first hour after the reoxygenation one can expect positive results.

However, there are no clinical trials or series to support the experimental findings. It seems to me advisable to perform this therapy only in a multi-centric prospective trial to prevent disappointments. Moreover, recently (Tibbles and Edelsberg, N Engl J Med 1996:334:1642-48) it has been emphasized that the lack of randomized controlled trials is a limiting factor for the assessment of the efficacy of hyperbaric oxygen in most diseases.

During the consensus meeting the following subjects will be highlighted.

1. Define to which organs we restrict ourselves.
2. The characteristics of an early diagnosis of an reperfusion injury for the involved organ.
3. Experimental evidence of the beneficial effects of HBO (pre) treatment.
4. Define exactly the timing for HBO treatment in clinical settings.
5. Is restriction for this type of therapy to special centers needed?

REFERENCES

1. Anderson RJ, Cambria RA, Dikman G. Role of eicosanoids and white blood cells in the beneficial effects of limited reperfusion after ischemia-reperfusion injury in skeletal muscle. Am J Surg. 1990;160:151-155.
2. Bast A, Haenen RMM, Doelman, CJA. Oxidants and Antioxidants: State of the Art. Am J Med. 1991;91:3c2s-3c13s.
3. Bengtson A, Holmberg P, Heideman M. The ischaemic leg as a source of complement activation. Br. J. Surg. 1987: 74; 697-700.
4. Bulkley GB. Free radical-mediated reperfusion injury: A selective review. Br. J. Cancer. 1987: 55, Suppl. VIII; 66-73.
5. Carden DL, Korthuis RJ. Mechanisms of postischemic vascular dysfunction in skeletal muscle: Implications for therapeutic intervention. Microcirc. Endoth. Lymphatics, 1989; 5: 277-298.
6. Haapaniemi T, Sirsjo A, Nylander G, Larsson J. Hyperbaric oxygen treatment attenuates glutathione depletion and improves metabolic restitution in postischemic skeletal muscle. Free Radical Research. 1995: 23(2); 91-101.
7. Kitani K, Fujita. The effects of Lipo-PGE1 and hyperbaric Oxygen in the treatment peripheral vascular diseases. Dept. of Anaesthesiology and Reanimatology, School of Medicine, Gumma University Hospital, Japan. In: Proceedings Joint Meeting Hyperbaric Medicine; International Congress on Hyperbaric Medicine. 1989.
8. Kleij van der AJ, Vink H, Henny ChP, Bakker DJ, Spaan JAE. Red blood cell velocity in nailfold capillaries during hyperbaric oxygenation. In: Advances in Experimental Medicine and Biology (vol.345); Oxygen transport to tissue. Eds. P. Vaupel, R. Zander. 1994: 175-180 (ISBN 0-306-44632-4).
9. Korthuis RJ, Granger DN, Townsley MI, Taylor AE. The role of oxygen-derived radicals in ischemia-induced increases in canine skeletal muscle vascular permeability. Circ Res. 1985: 57: 599.
10. Mink RB, Dutka AJ. Hyperbaric oxygen after global cerebral ischemia in rabbits reduces brain vascular permeability and blood flow. Stroke. 1995: 26(12); 2307-2312.
11. Malcolm OP, Fantini G. Ischemia: Profile of an enemy. J Vasc Surg. 1987; 6: 231-234.
12. Nelson KDO, Herndon B, Reisz G. Pulmonary effects of ischemic limb reperfusion: Evidence for a role for oxygen-derived radicals. Critical Care Medicine. 1992: 19(3); 360-363.
13. Parks DA, Granger DN. Contributions of ischemia and reperfusion to mucosal lesion formation. Am J Physiol. 1986;250:G749-G753.
14. Paterson IS, Klausner JM, Goldman G, Kobzik L, Melbourn VR, Shepro D, Hechtman HB. Thromboxane mediates the ischemia-induced neutrophil oxidative burst. Surgery 1989; 106(2): 224-229.
15. Sackett DL, Haynes RB, Guyatt GH, Tugwell P. Clinical Epidemiology. In: A basic science for clinical medicine. Second Edition 1991. Little, Brown and Company. Boston/Toronto/London. (ISBN 0-316-76599-6).
16. Sinclair AJ, Barnett AH, Lunee J. Free radicals and antioxidant systems in health and disease. Brit J Hosp Med. 1990: 43; 334-344.
17. Slagsvold CE, Rosén L, Stranden E. The relation between changes in capillary morphology induced by ischemia and postischemic transcutaneous pO2 response. Int. J. Microcirc: Clin. Exp. 1991; 10: 117.
18. Suval WD, Hobson RW, Boric MP, Ritter AB, Durán WN. Assessment of ischemic-reperfusion injury in skeletal muscle by macromolecular clearance. J Surg Res. 1987; 42: 550-559.
19. Walker PM, Linsay TF, Labbe R. Salvage of skeletal muscle with free radical scavengers. J Vasc Surg. 1987;5:68-75.
20. Zamboni WA, Roth AC, Russel RC, Graham B, Suchy H, Kucan JO. Morphologic analysis of the microcirculation during reperfusion of ischemic skeletal muscle and the effect of hyperbaric oxygen. Plast. Reconstr. Surg. 1993: 91; 1110-1123.

WHICH ROLE FOR HBO IN THE PREVENTION OF POST-TRAUMATIC SUPERIMPOSED INFECTIONS?

G. Vezzani[1], A. Pizzola[1], A. Guerrini[1], M. Mordacci[1], L. Cantadori[1], P. Menozzi[2]

The traumatic event has the inherent possibility of determining a local state of hypoxia, as a consequence of the muscular, nervous and, above all, vascular lesion, but it can also determine a grave state of systemic hypoxemia due to acute hypovolemia and to intense reflex vasoconstriction.

It is a well-established notion that hypoxic tissue is highly exposed to the risk of infection, firstly due to depression of specific immunity, thus facilitating bacterial proliferation, secondly due to the slowing-down of tissue repairing processes and thirdly, because of the possible interference between tissue hypoxia and certain antimicrobial agents.

The use of HBO in the prevention of post-traumatic superimposed infections is therefore to be considered in three distinct stages:

1) antibacterial action of HBO (bactericidal or bacteriostatic effect of HBO),
2) interaction of HBO with antimicrobial agents,
3) direct action of HBO on the eukaryotic cell, both as a reinforcement for the aspecific immune response and also as an indispensable substrate in tissue-repairing processes.

HBO can have bacteriostatic or bactericidal effects. Such mechanisms are related to the production of reactive oxygen species (ROS). ROS production has been shown also during clinical exposure to HBO.

In this report HBO treatment refers only to acute sepsis.

Valuation on the effects of HBO on bacteria: Inhibition of biosynthesis of amino acids and proteins.

The effect demonstrated in E. coli (1), with the oxygen at 4.2 ATA, is capable to inactivate the dihydroxyacid dehydratase which catalyzes the formation of ketoisovalerate, an intermediate in the synthesis of valine and leucine. The inhibition of aminoacids biosynthesis leads to increased levels of uncharged tRNA, which is responsible for inducing the stringent response. This response is characterized by increased levels guanosine and by inhibition of bacterial synthesis of carbohydrates, lipids, and nucleotides. Proteolysis is enhanced and bacterial growth is completely arrested.

Direct action of ROS on bacterial nucleic acids.

The exposition of P. aeruginosa at 100% O_2 at 2.9 ATA for 24 hours creates damages in bacterial nucleic acids and in ribosomal proteins, as documented in ultrastruc-

[1] Azienda USL Parma, Ospedale di Fidenza Servizio Anestesia-Rianimazione e Terapia Iperberica (Prim. Prof. G. Vezzani)
[2] 1 Division Medica, Oepedale di Fidenza

tural electronic microscopical studies (2). It is very interesting to note how in E. coli superoxide anion is mutagen both in "vivo" and in "vitro" (3) and independently of direct action, the alteration of bacterial protein synthesis enhances action of other antimicrobials.

ROS action will be mentioned later. At this moment it is impossible to determine whether clinical expositions of HBO can cause bacteriostasis or bactericidal effects. For example several strains of C. perfingens require an exposition of 3 ATA for 18 h. for a bactericidal effect (4), for P. aeruginosa, P. vulgaris and S. typhosa at 3 ATA for 24 h and E. coli 20 ATA for 6 h. (5). Nevertheless even the clinical exposition induces a defensive bacterial response which involves several well known genes, such as soxR and oxyR regulon. This regulons can codify for several proteins in reparative actions on nuclear acids and antioxidative action from which emerges a potential synergic activity of ROS with antimicrobial agents which inhibits protein synthesis.

HBO was also used alone in various biological sepsis models. In a first model (6) C. perfingens was implanted in mouse muscle by means of agar discs. HBO exposure was as follows: 4 treatments of 90 min. each at 3 ATA within the first 48 hours. At the end of these treatments, no vital C. perfingens were found, whereas bacterial proliferation persisted in the normobaric oxygen controls. In a second model, a known number of colony forming units (CFU) of C. perfingens was injected together with epinephrine in mouse muscle. A considerable reduction in mortality was obtained with a protocol of 3 treatments at 3 ATA for 90 min. within the first 24 hours, 2 treatments on day 2 and day 3.

A lower number of treatments did not modify mortality rate compared with the controls.

Others biological models were created by induction of polymicrobic sepsis by implantation of fecal matter enclosed in gelatine capsules in the peritoneal cavity of rats. According to the author (7), only HBO treatment is able to reduce mortality from 100% (controls) to 8% (HBO treated animals).In another biological model, a known number of CFU's of B. fragilis, E. coli and S. fecalis was introduced in the peritoneal cavity of rats with a significant cut in mortality (23% compared with 79% in the controls) (7). However, in more recent experiments, in abdominal sepsis induced in rats by means of E. coli and by B. fragilis there were no changes in mortality rates even in the presence of HBO treatment (8). In our experiment, polymicrobic sepsis induced in rats with double cecal puncture show no significant decrease in mortality in HBO treated rats compared with the controls. It is thus evident that it is impossible to draw clear-cut conclusions at this stage for the following reasons:

1) Totally different biological models were utilized in animals phylogenetically far removed from man,
2) Some biological models are completely artificial and therefore incomparable with the human pathologies they are intended to represent,
3) It is restrictive and conceptually erroneous to consider oxygen administered at higher pressures than atmospheric pressure to be antibiotic in itself, as has been sustained by some authors (9), given the highly complex and as yet unknown action of oxygen on the eukaryotic cell.

Apart from what has been specified in the introduction, one of the variants in the bacterium/HBO relationship is the possible interaction between the antimicrobial and

HBO. Such interaction depends essentially on 1) the chemical structure of the antimicrobial, 2) the place of action (intra- or extraphagocytic), 3) the mechanism of action.

As far as point 1 is concerned, there are antimicrobials containing a hydroquinone ring able to produce ROS once the ring is oxidized. The most notable of these is Rifamycin, whose mechanism of action, as far as we know, is likely to be totally unrelated to oxygen pressures. In actual fact Kono (10) has demonstrated a considerable reduction in the bactericidal action of the antibiotic on E. coli when its action is performed in anaerobic conditions. It is quite plausible that ROS formation by oxidation of the quinone group is a highly synergic mechanism in the case of Rifamicyn, making its mechanism of action oxygen-dependent, at least indirectly. However, the presence of a quinone ring is not always essential to justify the action of molecular oxygen on the structure of the antimicrobial.

In fact, Ampicillin can act as an electron donor and/or super-oxide generator in the presence of molecular oxygen. ROS production is in the case sufficient to obtain biological effects (11).

The interaction between ROS and antimicrobial agents is quite specific within the phagocytes. These cells, in particular the polymorphonuclear (PMN) microphages, are able to produce ROS by virtue of the phenomenon known as "Oxidative Burst" and so to produce a powerful endocellular bactericidal action. It is, however, a well-established fact that such a phenomenon occurs in strict relation to the oxygen pressures to which the PMN are subjected (12) (Table 1). Due to the fact that some antibiotics act within the phagocytes, it is necessary to evaluate the problem of possible endocellular synergy between ROS and antibiotics, bearing in mind that the bactericidal action of Quinolones, Macrolides and Rifampicines is also intraphagocytic.

In 1990, Van Resburg (13) found that the intra/extra-phagocytic relationship of Quinolones was not sufficiently elevated to justify the bactericidal action of the antibiotic. In fact, various quinolones (Difloxacine, Pefloxacine, Ciprofloxacine) possess an effective anti-bacterial action in the presence of normal PMN, but their action is markedly reduced in the presence of PMN in patients with chronic granulomatose disease. Similarly, the intraphagocytic bactericidal action of Amoxicillin, Clindamycin, Eritromiycin and Roxitromycin is significantly reduced when it takes place in phagocytes with deficient bacterial killing in superoxide anion production (14). Synergy between ROS and certain macrolides, in particular Josamycin, is so conspicuous that in a strain of S. aureus sensitive to the macrolide it was possible to identify such synergy in an acellular system, inducing oxidative stress in the bacterium by means of the Xantine/Xantine oxidase system. It is thus totally reasonable to assume that HBO, in bringing tissue PO_2 back to normal values, acts as a powerful stimulus in the antibiotic/phagocytic ROS synergy, at least as far as the above mentioned antibiotics are concerned, thus enhancing intraphagocytic bacterial killing.

The antimicrobial's mechanism of action remains one of the fundamental issues in its interaction with oxygen. It is profitable at this point to make a distinction between antimicrobials inhibiting protein synthesis and between antimicrobials inhibiting resynthesis of the bacterial membrane, (-lactams and glycopeptides. The first group notoriously includes, among others, aminoglycosides, quinolones, macrolides, lincosamides. In the case of these antimicrobials, penetration within the bacterium is essential in order to inhibit protein synthesis. It has been known for some time that the mechanism of penetration of aminoglycosides is oxygen-dependent and such a mechanism is not present in anaerobic bacteria, which are in fact regularly resistant to aminoglycosides, even if ribosomes isolated from the bacterial corpus of C. perfringens and B. fragilis are susceptible to the action of Streptomycin and Gentamycin (15). In the case of the other antimicrobials it is quite legitimate to suppose that during HBO treatment damage is done to the bacterial membrane by the ROS, which facilitates penetration of the antimicrobials. For many years (16) it had been known that removal of an antibiotic from a bacterial culture was followed by a period of stasis in proliferation. The interim period preceding continuation of bacterial multiplication is defined as the Post Antibiotic Effect (PAE). This varies according to the bacterial species and according to the type of antibiotic used.

Moreover, it may be prolonged by hyperoxic exposure. Park (17) has demonstrated an increase in the PAE if the culture undergoes hyperoxic or even normobaric exposure. Above all, antibiotics inhibiting protein synthesis present a more conspicuous PAE with Gram-germs, whereas in the case of bacterial membrane resynthesis, PAE is non-existent for Gram-germs, with the notable exception of Imipenem with P. aeruginosa; it is present with variable values for Gram+ germs. Thus PAE, the existence of which has also been demonstrated in vivo (18) represents a way of synergism between antibiotics and HBO; moreover, it must be considered that during the PAE phase the bacterium is much more sensitive to phagocyitosis, a phenomenon known as Post Antibiotic Leucocyte Enhancement (PALE) (19). The most difficult problem at present is the explanation of possible synergy between HBO on the one hand and (-lactams and glycopeptides on the other. As already specified, PAE in the case of these antimicrobials is almost non-existent for Gram- and variable for Gram+ bacteria. An experiment we carried out on rats with induced polymicrobic peritonitis (Table 2) demonstrates synergy between HBO and Piperacillin, HBO and Meropenem but not between HBO and Ceftizoxime. As a rule, the data reported in literature do not document synergy between (-lactams and oxygen, but the excellent work of Erdmann and Zamboni (20) points out the existence of considerable synergy between HBO and Penicillin in streptococcal myositis in the mouse. At present, it can be supposed that synergy between HBO and (-lactams is possible if PAE exists in the case of the bacterium taken into consideration. PAE variation in (-lactams and also within the bacterial species may be dependent on the different scission speed of the covalent bond between the (-lactam and the target site (Penicillin Binding Proteins) and consequently on the half-life of the (-lactam/PBP complex, considering that this half-life depends above all on the molecular weight of the PBP's (21). In fact, in the bacilli the PBP's are of law molecular weight and (-lactam/PBP complex has a half-life of approximately 10 min. (22). In this case, PAE proves to be of short duration, whereas in the round-shaped forms the half-life is more prolonged and thus we might expect a more prolonged PAE. In Table 2 we can see considerable synergy between HBO and Vancomycin. Vancomycin presents PAE for example in the case of S. aureus, although it notoriously does not bond with PBPs, thus its synergy with HBO is somewhat mysterious, even if (23) it has been demonstrated in vitro that the antibiotic penetrates the bacterium and inhibits ribonucleic acid synthesis and therefore in this case the alteration of the bacterial membrane permeability due to ROS could induce entry of the antibiotic into the bacterial corpus.

In a further experiment, using the same biological model described in Table 2, we evaluated possible synergy between HBO and a few antibiotics used in association. If indeed the existence of PAE is considered to be an important factor in the possible HBO-antimicrobial synergy, there is no clear evidence in literature that antibiotic combinations present PAE as the sum of the PAE of each single antibiotic forming part of the combination.

We investigated into the following combinations:
- Piperacilline/Netilmicine (P/N),
- Ceftizoxime/Netilmicine (C/N),
- Ciprofloxacine/Netilmicine(Ci/N).

The simultaneous administration of the antibiotic combination + HBO to a group of rats (n=12), in which polymicrobic peritonitis had been induced, produced a statistically significant increase (p<0.05) in average survival time (AST) compared with the control group treated only with the antibiotic combination, but only in the case of the (P/N) and (Ci/N) combinations. These data prove that synergy between HBO and an antibiotic combination can take place even when one of the components of the association is not synergyzed by HBO if used singly, as in the case of Ci (see Table 2).

The relationship between hyperoxia and (-lactamase synthesis in bacteria subjected to hyperoxic stress still requires examination; on the other hand, nothing is known about the activity of the (-lactamase inhibitors (Sulbactam, Tazobactam and Clavulanic acid) and HBO.

For some antimicrobials, the anti-bacterial action takes the form of an antimetabolic action on the bacterium; this is what appears in the case of sulphamides. Various authors such as Pakman 24 have found synergy between hyperbaric oxygen and some sulphamides, in particular: Sulphisoxazole, Sulphamethoxazole and Trimetoprim on C. difteriae, some strains of S. aureus and P. aeruginosa. Literature in this connection is fairly rich and authors, considering the mechanism of action of sulphamides, generally believe that synergy between HBO and sulphamides may be explained by enzyme oxidation or more probably by oxidation of intermediate substrates in the metabolic pathway of folates.

Neutrophils are the first immunity cells to appear in the wound, by demarcation, diapedesis and migration through connective tissue. These processes are not greatly influenced by hypoxia because neutrophils can obtain energy also from glycolysis anaerobia (25, 26). However, hypoxia significantly reduces oxidative killing of the bacteria engulfed in neutrophils. During respiratory burst oxygen consumption increases to 50 times the normal amount. This consumption is essential for the conversion of molecular oxygen into superoxide, catalyzed by a membrane-bound NADPH-linked oxygenase. This marks the beginning of a cycle leading to the formation of numerous antibacterial radicals including hypohalites, hydroxyl ions, active aldehydes and lipid peroxides. Oxidative killing is the principal mechanism whereby neutrophils kill many organisms, such as S. aureus, E. coli, Klebsiella, Proteus, Serratia, Candida, Aspergillus and anaerobes (27, 28).

If molecular oxygen is available, superoxide production is proportional to its concentration (25–27). The Km for oxygen of the NADPH-linked oxygenase has recently been estimated at 60 mmHg (29). In vivo, various experiments document the relation between tissue oxygen tension and wound healing. A well-known work is that of Knighton and co-workers (30), emphasizing the effects of oxygen and Ampicilline on lesion diameter after intradermal injection of bacteria into guinea pigs. Gottrub and associates (31), Chang (32) created skin flaps in dogs with the purpose of studying the combined effects of perfusion and local oxygen tension on bacterial clearance. The authors' conclusions are as follows: Invasive, necrotizing infections developed only in regions where tissue oxygen tension was less than about 40-50 mmHg at time of inoculation.

All types of wounds alter vascular supply as a result of vessel injury and thrombosis. The consequence is a rapid succession of events including platelet degranulation and the release of complement, kinins and chemotactic factors. At a later stage, neutrophils, lymphocytes and, later, macrophages and fibroblasts migrate to the site of injury (25). The combination of decreased vascular supply and increased cellularity are at the basis of the hypoxic state of wounds in comparison with surrounding healthy tissue (26). Hypoperfused areas become hypoxic (PO_2 0 to 10 mmHg), hypercarbic (PCO_2 50 to 60 mmHg), and acidotic (pH 6.5 to 6.9) with lactate levels of up to 15 mmol (27). These conditions can interfere with collagen deposition. However, macrophages in a hypoxic, high-lactate environment produce an angiogenic factor that stimulates angiogenesis in adjacent, better-oygenated tissue (25, 26, 27). It must be stressed, however, that lactate is a more important stimulus to angiogenesis than hypoxia (28). Wound macrophages produce lactate aerobically, so lactate levels are high even when the wound is normally oxygenated. Thus PO_2 increment within the wound does not negatively influence angiogenesis, when macrophages are present.

Many studies both in vivo and in vitro (29, 30) document that fibroblast is an oxygen-dependent function. In fact, collagen hydroxilation, cross-linking and deposition are proportional to the partial pressure of oxygen. Many of the factors that induce gene expression of collagen are also able to induce angiogenesis, including lactate (31). Transcription yields procollagen, which undergoes post-translational modification in the cytoplasm, with hydroxilation of the proline and lysine residues, allowing the cross-linking within and between collagen strands that provides tensile strength. The action of the hydroxylase enzyme that catalyzes this reaction depends on numerous co-factors: vitamin C, oxoglutarate, Fe 2+, and oxygen substrate (32). If oxygen is considered to be a substrate rather than a co-factor, then the kinetics of the reaction with regard to oxygen can be measured. The Km for oxygenation of prolyl hydroxylase has been variously estimated at 20, 25, and 100 mmHg (33, 34, 35). Experimental data demonstrate that proline hydroxylation depends on tissue PO_2 and that 90% of the effect is obtained with PO_2 of 90 mmHg.

In an experiment we carried out on rats using the biological model of double cecal puncture we witnessed a reduction in mortality from 100% in the controls after 5 days to 28.5% if cecal ligation was preceded by lengthy pre-exposure (8 hours) to 100% O_2 at 2.0 ATA- (36). In different experiments we obtained data that we consider to be relatively comparable. Hyperoxic pre-exposure reduce mortality significantly in subsequent toxic hyperoxia in a group of pre-treated rats compared with the controls; in the same way, reduction in mortality is seen in the case of pre-treatment with endotoxin (37); it was observed that heat-shock treatment protects the rat from hyperbaric oxygen toxicity (38). A possible key to the interpretation of these experiments may reside in recent research that has aimed at demonstrating not only a toxic role of the ROS but a role as messengers in cell activation (39). A fundamental piece of data is the role of ROS in gene expression and thus the mode of activation of the transcriptional factors. A transcriptional factor that has recently been the object of a great deal of study in its relation with ROS is NF-KB.

NF-KB is a transcriptional factor which is composed in its active form of two subunits P50 and P65 proteins. Normally in the cytoplasm the NF-KB is present in an inactive form, being associated with its inhibitory sub-unit IK-B is present. Various agents are able to stimulate the NF-KB complex, LPS, ionizing radiation, protein synthesis inhibitors, etc. In this case the IK-B sub-unit is phosphorylated and released from the complex and the NF-KB can then be translocated to the nucleus where it binds to DNA at specific NF-KB binding regions. It can activate genes as different as those coding for TNF, IL-6, (-Interferon, or cell surface receptors such as ICAM-1, IL-2 receptors or other proteins like angiotensinogen. In fact, the response mediated by the activation of NF-KB is part of the protective immune, inflammatory, and acute phase reactions. Recent data document that in various cells and tissues there exists inhibition by antioxidants of the expression of several genes under regulation of the NF-KB transcriptional factor.

The vascular cell adhesion molecule-1 (VCAM-1) gene expression is markedly attenuated by the antioxidant pyrrolidine dithicarbamate (PDTC) (40). The IL-6 secretion by human fibroblasts was also inhibited by PDTC, N-acetylcysteine, or vitamin E (41). These data document that activation of NF-KB is under the control of an oxidant/antioxidant regulatory mechanism in which ROS play a central role, since they are able to switch on the process of NF-K3 activation.

Experiments have been performed on the relation between ROS and the trascriptional factor activator protein-1 (AP-1) (37). Some experiments concern the activation of heat shock transcription factors by delta-12-prostaglandin-J2 which is inhibited by intracellular glutathione (42). On the contrary, Hsp-70 synthesis is enhanced in glutathione-depleted cells (43). During HBO treatment there is considered to be an increase in ROS production, and so that state referred to as "low oxidative stress" by J. Remacle and co-workers (39) is likely to be realized. The general concept raised by these hypotheses and many data is that transient levels of ROS must influence gene expression in some way. The fact that physiological activation of gene expression can be observed in cells under mild oxidative stress. These effects are mediated partly by ROS in concentrations higher than those found in resting cells but still within the physiological range determined by the antioxidant capacity of the cells.

Table 1.

PO_2 mmhg	CFU per leukocyte
345	11
155	10
140	10 *
39	7

Number of Colony-Forming Units (CFU) per leukocyte at different oxygen pressures. *The difference between 10 and 7 is statistically significant ($p < 0.0_2$).

Table 2.

Antimicrobials	Increase in AST
Clindamycin	100
Piperacilline	96.5
Netilmycin	89.2
Vancomycin	78.5
Meropenem	64.5
Ciprofloxacine	2.9
Ceftizoxime	0.96
Metronidazole	0.2

The previous antimicrobials were used on rats with polymicrobic peritonitis induced by the method of cecal ligation and double puncture. One group was given only the antibiotic (OA), a second group antibiotic + HBO (A+HBO). After 5 days mortality rate and average survival times (AST) were calculated. As Clindamycin had the highest increase in AST, comparing AST of the OA with AST of the A/HBO group, this increase was made equivalent to 100, and thus a scale of synergies between antibiotics and HBO with relation to AST increase was obtained. It clearly emerges that the last three antimicrobials have no synergy with HBO, at least as far as this biological model is concerned.

REFERENCES

1. Brown OR: Dihydroxidacid dehydratase: the site of hyperbaric oxygen poisoning in branched-chain amino acid biosynthesis. Biochem Biophys Res Commun 85:1219-1224, 1978.

2. Clark JM: Inhibition of P. aeruginosa by hyperbaric oxygen. Ultrastructural changes .Infect Immun 4:488-491, 1971.

3. Gifford GD: Mutation of an auxotrophic strain of E. coli by high pressure oxygen. Biochem Biophys Res Commun 33:294-298, 1968.

4. Hill GB: Experimental effects of hyperbaric oxygen on selected Clostridial species.I. In-vitro studies. J Infect Dis 125.17-25, 1972.

5. Bornside GH: Inhibition of pathogenic enteric bacteria by hyperbaric oxygen: enhanced antibacterial activity in the absence of carbon dioxide. Antimicrob Agents Chemoter 7:682-687, 1975.

6. Hill GB: Experimental effects of hyperbaric oxygen on selected Clostridial species.II. In vivo studies in mice. J Infect Dis 125:26-35, 1972.

7. Thom SR: Intermittent hyperbaric oxygen therapy for reduction of mortality in experimental polymicrobial sepsis. J Infect Dis 154:504-510, 1986.

8. Muhuvich KH: Effect of hyperbaric oxygenation, combined with antimicrobial agents and surgery, in a rat model of intra-abdominal infection. J Infect Dis 157:1058-1061, 1988.

9. Knighton RD: Oxygen as an Antibiotic Arch Surg 125:97-100, 1990.

10. Kono Y: Oxygen enhancement of bactericidal activity of Rifamycin SV on E.coli and aerobic Oxydation Rifamicyn SV to Rifamicin S catalyzed by Manganous ions: the role of Superoxide. J Biochem 91: 381-395, 1982.

11. Umeki S: Ampicillin serves an electron donor. Int J Biochem 22:1291-1293, 1990.

12. Moelleken B: An adverse wound environment activates leukocytes prematurely. Arch Surg 126(11):225-231, 1991.

13. Van Rensburg C: Interactions of the oxygen-dependent antimicrobial system of the human neutrofil with difloxacin, ciprofloxacin, pefloxacin and flerexacin in the intraphagocitic eradication of S. aureus. J Med Microbiol 32:15-17, 1990.

14. Anderson T: An in vitro investigation of the intracellular bioactivity of Amoxycillin, Clindamycin and Erytromicin for S. aureus. J Infect Dis 153:593-600, 1986.

15. Bryan LE: Mechanism of aminoglycoside resistance in anaerobic bacteria: Cl perfringens and B. fragilis. Antimicrobic Agents Chemoter 15:7-13, 1979.

15. Bigger JM: The bactericidal action of penicillin on S. pyogenes. Ir J Med Set 227: 533-568, 1944.

17. Park MK: Hyperoxia prolongs the Aminoglycoside-induced Post-antibiotic effect in P. aeruginosa. Antimicrob Agents Chemoter 35: 691-695, 1991.

18. Craig WA:The Post-Antibiotic Effect in V. Lorian, Antibiotics in laboratory medicine 2nd ed. Williams and Wilkins, Baltimore, MD, 1986.

19. Pruul H: Enhancement of leucocyte activity against E. coli after brief exposure to Chloroamphenicol. Antimicrob Agents Chemoter 19: 945-951, 1979.

20. Erdmann D: HBO improves outcome of Streptococcal myositis in mice. Undersea & Hyperbaric Medicine vol 22, 13, 1995.

21. Fuad N: Mode of interaction between -lactam antibiotics and the exocellular DD-carboxypeptidase-transpeptidase from Streptomyces R 39 Biochem J 155:623-629, 1976.

22. Georgopapadoku NH: Penicillin-binding proteins in bacteria. Antimicrob Agents Chemoter 28: 148-157, 1980.

23. Grassi GG: Vancomicina e Teicoplanina in: Chemio antibioticoterapia, Masson, 287, 1989.

24. Pakman LM: Inhibition of P. aeruginosa by hyperbaric oxygen. I.Sulfonamide activity enhancement and reversal. Infect Immun 4:479-487, 1971.

25. Knighton DR: The defenses of the wound. In Howard, RJ and Simmons, RL (eds): Surgical infectious diseases, ed 2. Norwalk, CT, Appleton & Lange, 1988, 188-193.

26. Niinikoski J, et al: Radical mastectomy wound as a model for studies of human wound metabolism. Am J Surg 126:53, 1973.

27. Hunt KT: Physiology of wound healing In Cloves, GHA, Jr: Trauma, sepsis and shock: the physiological basis of therapy. Marcel Dekker, New-York, 1988, 443-471.

28. Jensen JA et al: Lactate regulates the expression of angiogenesis factor by macrophages. Fed Proc 43:587, 1984.

29. Niinikoski J: Oxygen and wound healing. Clin Plast Surg 4 (3): 361, 1977.

30. Forrester JC, et al: Tape-closed and sutured wounds: A comparison by tensiometry and scanning electron microscopy. Br J Surg 57:729, 1970.

31. Hussain MZ: Metabolic regulation of prolyl hydroxylase activation. In Barbul A, et al (eds): Growth factors and other aspects of wound healing: Biological and clinical implications, Progress in Clinical and Biological Research, Vol 226. Alan R Liss, New York, 1988, 229-235.

32. Prockop DJ, et al: The biosynthesis of collagen and its disorders, Part I N Engl J Med 301 (1):13, 1979.

33. Hutton JJ, et al: Cofactor and substrate requirements of collagen proline hydroxylase. Arch Biochem Biophys 118:231, 1967.

34. Myllyla R, et al: Mechanism of the prolylhydroxylase reaction. Kinetic analysis of the reaction sequence. Eur J Biochem 80:349, 1997.

35. De Jong L: Stoichiometry and kinetics of the prolyl 3-hydroxylase partial reaction. Biochim Biophys Acta 787:105, 1984.

36. Cantadori L, et al: Lunga esposizione ad ossigeno iperbarico a bassa pressione in sepsi sperimentali. Proceedings of International Symposium "Update of Hyperbaric Oxygen Therapy", Bologna, 1995.

37. Conference Report: Regulation of gene expression by O2 tension. Bethesda 1992. American Physiological Society.

38. Niu AKC: Heat-shock treatment protects rat from hyperbaric oxygen toxicity. Undersea & Hyperbaric Medicine, vol 21,55, 1994.

39. Remacle J et al: Low levels of reactive oxygen species as modulators of cell function. Mutation Research 316 (1995) 103-122.

40. Marui N, et al: Vascular cell adhesion molecul-1 (VCAM-1) gene transcription and expression are regulated through an antioxidant-sensitive mechanism in human vascular endothelial cells. J Clin Invest 92, 1886-1874, 1993.

41. Raes M, et al: effects of antioxidants on IL-6 secretion induced by IL-1 in human cultured lung fibrobalts. Involvement of NF-KB, In : Oxidative stress, Cell activation and Viral infection, C. Pasquier et al. Eds., Birkhauser Verlag, Basel, 77-90, 1994.

42. Koizumi T, et al: Activation of heat shock transcription factors by delta-12-prostaglandin-J2 and its inhibition by intracellular glutathione. Biochem Pharmacol 45, 2457-1464, 1993.

43. Freeman ML: Synthesis of hsp-70 is enhanced in glutathione-depleted Hep G2 Cells. Radiat Res, 135, 387-393, 1993.

WHICH ROLE FOR HBOT TO IMPROVE TISSUE SALVAGE AFTER ACUTE MUSCULO-SKELETAL TRAUMA?

J. Niinikoski

Department of Surgery, University of Turk, Turku, Finland

According to definition, both muscle and bone must be involved in acute musculo-skeletal trauma, but injury to other tissues such as skin, major blood vessels, connective and nerve tissues can also be involved. The injury may be so severe that either the viability of the tissue is in question, or, if the tissue survives, functional deficit is possible. Like in crush injuries the injury gradient is important in acute severe musculo-skeletal trauma (24, 25). In these cases a transition of tissue-injury severity from irreversibly damaged to minimally traumatized to normal exists. A "gray zone" between the irreversibly damaged and minimally traumatized tissues may or may not survive. Improving survival of this gray-zone tissue is crucial in the management of acute musculo-skeletal trauma (27). This also serves a target for hyperbaric oxygen therapy (HBOT).

Physical damage and ischemia may contribute to each other in such a way that a vicious circle effect results (8, 25). Physically damaged tissues are contused or in discontinuity. The leakage of fluid through injured capillaries and cell walls results in tissue edema while disruption in cell activities causes loss of function. Edema results in progressive ischemia and hypoxia since the diffusion distance from the capillary to the cell is increased. Local tissue oxygen tensions should be 30–60 mmHg for effective wound repair and leukocyte oxidative killing mechanisms to occur (11, 18, 22). If critical ischemia is not corrected but continues, the tissues die. In closed injuries of the extremities increasing intracompartmental pressure becomes greater than the capillary perfusion pressure. Tissues within compartment become ischemic, cease to function, and die.

In soft tissue trauma, at the site where microcirculation is disrupted, plasma will leak into the injured tissue and cause further edema. At this level, oxygen supply to the cells will be only that resulting from the physically dissolved oxygen in the plasma. Under ordinary circumstances, this fraction of oxygen is insufficient for tissue needs.

TREATMENT OF ACUTE MUSCULO-SKELETAL TRAUMA

Acute musculo-skeletal trauma must be recognized without a delay and treated aggressively to prevent or minimize irreversible damage to injured tissues. Appropriate interventions must be started at the scene of the accident and continued until the problem is resolved (27). Splinting, control of bleeding, application of compression dressings to open wounds, and prevention of dependent edema are directed at preventing additional injury. Most important, however, is to employ basic and advanced life-support measures if required to keep the patient alive.

The emergency department physician is expected to perform a thorough physical examination, ascertain the severity of the injury, initiate appropriate x-ray and laboratory studies, and contact the specialists required for definitive care of the injury. When an open wound is a component of the musculo-skeletal trauma it must be inspected, cultured, irrigated, and covered with sterile dressings. Tetanus prophylaxis is taken care of. Antibiotics are administered intravenously. Broad spectrum antibiotic coverage is recommended. Attention to maintain blood volume is crucial.

Definitive treatment and follow-up care will be given by the specialist surgeon. The classification system for musculo-skeletal trauma should be used as a guideline (7). Additional studies such as intracompartmental tissue pressure measurements and angiography may be carried out to help the specialist determine the definitive treatment. Surgical intervention such as debridement, fasciotomy, and stabilization of fractures is required. Vascular reconstructive surgery can deal effectively with large vessel trauma. Further, attention to the patient's hemodynamics and nutritional status is essential. The volume and oxygen carrying capacity of the circulating blood must be maintained normal. Hyperbaric oxygen therapy should be employed to optimize tissue repair and achieve maximal tissue salvage (25, 27).

THE ROLE OF HBOT IN ACUTE MUSCULO-SKELETAL TRAUMA

Hyperbaric oxygen therapy can be used as an adjunct for the treatment of acute ischemic musculo-skeletal trauma. Hyperbaric oxygen is administered in either a multiplace or monoplace hyperbaric chamber. The multiplace chamber is pressurized with air and the patient breathes oxygen through a mask or intubation tube. The monoplace chamber is pressurized with oxygen and the patient breathes pure oxygen directly. Normally, pressures of 2-2.5 ATA are used.

Under HBO hemoglobin in the circulating blood becomes fully oxygenated and in addition, oxygen physically dissolves in plasma in direct proportion to the partial pressure of oxygen. Under HBO, enough oxygen can become physically dissolved in plasma to meet tissue oxygen requirements without support from hemoglobin-borne oxygen (3). At 2-2.5 ATA oxygen pressure physically dissolved oxygen in plasma increases over tenfold. This primary effect of HBO generates a favorable gradient for oxygen diffusion from functioning capillaries to ischemic tissue sites. This increment in oxygen supply may be the factor that allows the compromised tissues to survive, and so tissue viability and function are maintained (27).

Vasoconstriction is the second fundamental effect of HBO in the treatment of acute musculo-skeletal trauma (25). Vasoconstriction as such would appear to be undesirable in ischemic conditions because it reduces blood flow. However, the hyperoxygenation effect of HBO adequately compensates for the decreased flow so that the net effect is no reduction in tissue oxygenation. Inhibition of edema also has a beneficial effect on blood flow in the microcirculation (19).

The third effect of HBOT important in acute musculo-skeletal trauma is its role in wound and bone healing and prevention of infection in compromised tissues. In soft tissue wounds the most important effects of HBOT are the stimulation of fibroblast proliferation and differentiation, increased collagen deposition, neovascularization of ischemic tissue as well as enhanced leukocyte microbial killing (1, 16, 17). On the other hand, the supply of oxygen is a fundamental and, to a great extent, limiting factor in the healing of fractures[5] and recovery from osteomyelitis (13, 14). Variations in oxygen supply could determine the type of tissue that differentiated in a culture of multipotent mesenchymal cells. Hyperoxia caused the differentiation to osseous tissue, whereas hypoxia resulted in cartilage formation (2). In animal experiments HBOT has been found to stimulate the healing of fractures (21, 30).

HBO has direct effects on microorganisms. This is an additional mechanism that has relevance to the treatment of acute musculo-skeletal trauma and prevention of post-traumatic sequealae (10). In controlled studies in animal models HBO alone could erad-icate Staphylococcus aureus in infected bone (12).

Hyperbaric oxygen also seems to protect tissues from reperfusion injury often involved in acute musculo-skeletal trauma (20, 23, 28, 29, 31). The mechanism of action is not known at present. However, the key to successful outcome with HBOT in the reperfusion injury appears to be its timely application (25).

Theoretically, the beneficial effect of HBOT in acute ischemic musculo-skeletal trauma is manyfold. HBOT improves the survivability of injured limbs and tissues. It accelerates the demarcation process and reduces the chances of infection developing in the transition zone between the injured and nonviable tissues. Further, HBOT enhances and supports repair mechanisms of soft and hard tissue lesions involved in acute mus-culo-skeletal trauma.

THE CLINICAL USE OF HBOT IN ACUTE MUSCULO-SKELETAL TRAUMA

Clinical experience with hyperbaric oxygen in acute musculo-skeletal trauma is rel-atively limited. The complexity and diversity of these injuries make double-blind con-trolled clinical trials nearly impossible. Most clinical reports describe the benefits of HBOT in very subjective terms. In reports dealing with crush injuries, the authors state that HBOT is beneficial because an injury of similar magnitude treated without HBO would have resulted in amputation (25). Recent reviews indicate that the more frequent the HBO treatments the higher the likelihood of success. HBOT has also reduced edema and congestion, especially in its applications for reimplantations (4, 6) and the skeletal muscle compartment syndrome (25).

In cases with severe ischemia HBO therapy should be instituted as soon as possible, because anoxic tissues quickly die. Muscle and peripheral nerve tissues die after four to six hours of ischemia while bone cells die after 12 to 18 hours. There is a question of whether debridement of the wounds and stabilization of the fractures should be insti-tuted before the first hyperbaric oxygen treatment. It is recommended that surgical intervention takes place before the first hyperbaric oxygen treatment. However, if the operating room is not immediately available, the patient should receive hyperbaric oxy-gen at pressures of 2.0 to 2.5 ATA for 60–90 minutes. If the operating room becomes available, the HBOT is interrupted and resumed after surgery is completed (25).

Hyperbaric oxygen treatment schedules for acute musculo-skeletal trauma vary according to what the desired effect of HBO is. If HBOT is used to promote healing of injured tissues, pulses of HBO once or twice a day appear to be sufficient. However, if tissue viability is threatened due to acute ischemia, HBOT should be given frequently enough to maintain oxygenation adequate for tissue survival. Serial measurements of local oxygen tension in injured tissues give a guideline to the frequency of hyperbaric oxygen treatments. Hyperoxia of muscle, bone, and subcutaneous tissues may persist significant periods of time after a 60–90 minute exposure to oxygen at 2.0–2.5 ATA. It is recommended that hyperbaric oxygen should be given at four to six hour intervals until the ischemic condition is resolved, usually in 24 to 48 hours. If improvement occurs, the frequency of the HBO treatments is decreased over four to six days. By that time the ischemic tissue should have stabilized, that is, tissue perfusion is restored and edema reduced. When treating patients under HBO with accelerated protocols, the possibility of toxic effects of oxygen should be minimized (25, 27).

In the future, the use of hyperbaric oxygen therapy in the acute musculo-skeletal trauma will be based on objective criteria rather than clinical diagnoses. Methods are now available to assess tissue oxygenation during HBO exposures. For instance, those injured tissues which increase their transcutaneous oxygen tensions significantly during an HBO exposure are highly likely to heal and survive (9, 15). Further, the measurement of interstitial fluid pressure in the compartment syndrome provides an objective parameter for starting and quantifying the benefits of HBOT (26).

CONCLUSION

Hyperbaric oxygen therapy is an ideal adjunct in the treatment of acute musculo-skeletal trauma in which tissue ischemia is involved. The immediate beneficial action site of hyperbaric oxygen therapy is the "gray zone" in the gradient of tissue injury. The primary goal of HBOT in this area is maintenance of tissue viability and function during the initial ischemia and hypoxia. A secondary goal is promotion of healing of both soft and bone tissues. Although HBOT will not revitalize dead tissue, it speeds up demarcation and prevents infection of the injured tissue.

REFERENCES

1. Bakker DJ, Niinikoski J (1994) Chronic hyperbaric oxygen therapy indications. Final Report. In: Wattel F, Mathieu D (eds), 1st European Consensus Conference on Hyperbaric Medicine. Lille, France, September 19-21, 1994. Reports and Recommendations. European Committee for Hyperbaric Medicine, pp 71-86.

2. Basset AC, Herrmann I (1961) Influence of oxygen concentration and mechanical factors on differentiation of connective tissue in vitro. Nature 190:460.

3. Boerema I, Meijne NG, Brummelkamp WK, Bouma S, Mensch MH, Kamermans F, Stern Hanf M, Van Aalderen W (1960) Life without blood. A study of the influence of high atmospheric pressure and hypothermia on dilution of the blood. J Cardiovasc Surg 1:133.

4. Buncke HJ, Alpert BS, Johnson-Giebink R (1981) Digital replantation. Surg Clin N Am 61:383.

5. Coulson DB, Ferguson AB, Diehl RC (1966) Effect of hyperbaric oxygen on the healing femur of the rat. Surg Forum 17:449.

6. Edwards RJ, Im MJ, Hoopes JE (1991) Effects of hyperbaric oxygen preservation on rat limb replantation: a preliminary report. Ann Plast Surg 27:31.

7. Gustilo RB, Mendoza RM, Williams DN (1984) Problems in the management of type III (severe) open fractures: A new classification of type III open fractures. J Trauma 24:742.

8. Hargens AR, Akeson WH (1981) Pathophysiology of the compartment syndrome. In: Mubarak SJ, Hargens AR (eds), Compartment Syndromes and Volkmann's Contracture. WB Saunders Co, Philadelphia, pp 47-70.

9. Hart GB, Meyer GW, Strauss MB, Messina VJ (1990) Transcutaneous partial pressure of oxygen measured in a monoplace hyperbaric chamber at 1, 1.5 and 2 ATM Abs oxygen. J Hyperbaric Med 5:223.

10. Hunt TK, Halliday B (1980) Inflammation in wounds: from "laudable pus" to primary repair and beyond. In: Hunt TK (ed), Wound Healing and Wound Infection: Theory and Surgical Practice, Appleton-Century-Crofts, New York, pp 281-293.

11. Knighton DR, Halliday B, Hunt TK (1984) Oxygen as an antibiotic: The effect of inspired oxygen on infection. Arch Surg 119:199.

12 . Mader JT, Brown GL, Guckian JC, Wells CH, Reinarz JA (1980) A mechanism for the ameliorization by hyperbaric oxygen of experimental Staphylococcal osteomyelitis in rabbits. J Infec Dis 142:915.

13. Mainous EG (1977) Hyperbaric oxygen in maxillofacial osteomyelitis, osteoradionecrosis, and osteogenesis enhancement. In: Davis JC, Hunt TK (eds), Hyperbaric Oxygen Therapy. Undersea Medical Society, Bethesda, Maryland, pp 191-203.

14. Marx RE, Johnson RP (1988) Problem wounds in oral and maxillofacial surgery: The role of hyperbaric oxygen. In: Davis JC, Hunt TK (eds), Problem Wounds. The Role of Oxygen. Elsevier Science Publishing, New York, pp 65-123.

15. Mathieu D, Wattel F, Bouachour G, Billard V, Defoin JF (1990) Post-traumatic limb ischemia: prediction of final outcome by transcutaneous oxygen measurements in hyperbaric oxygen. J Trauma 30:307.

16. Niinikoski J (1994) Chronic hyperbaric oxygen therapy indications. Introductory Report. Hyperbaric oxygenation and healing disorders. In: Wattel F, Mathieu D (eds), 1st European Consensus Conference on Hyperbaric Medicine. Lille, France, September 19-21, 1994. Reports and Recommendations. European Committee for Hyperbaric Medicine, pp 58-70.

17. Niinikoski J, Hunt TK (1996) Oxygen and healing wounds: tissue-bone repair enhancement. In: Oriani G, Marroni A, Wattel F (eds), Handbook on Hyperbaric Medicine, Springer-Verlag, Berlin, pp 475-497.

18. Niinikoski J, Hunt TK, Dunphy JE (1972) Oxygen supply in healing tissue. Am J Surg 123:247.

19. Nylander G, Lewis D, Nordström H, Larsson J (1985) Reduction of postischemic edema with hyperbaric oxygen. Plast Reconstr Surg 76:596.

20. Nylander G, Nordström H, Lewis D, Larsson J (1987) Metabolic effects of hyperbaric oxygen in postischemic muscle. Plast Reconstr Surg 79:91.

21. Penttinen R, Niinikoski J, Kulonen E (1972) Hyperbaric oxygenation and fracture healing. A biochemical study with rats. Acta Chir Scand 138:39.

22. Silver IA (1969) The measurement of oxygen tension in healing tissue. Progr Resp Res 3:124.

23. Sirsjo A, Lehr HA, Nolte D, Haapaniemi T, Lewis DH, Nylander G, Messmer K (1993) Hyperbaric oxygen treatment enhances the recovery of blood flow and functional capillary density in postischemic striated muscle. Circ Shock 40:9.

24. Strauss MB (1981) Role of hyperbaric oxygen therapy in acute ischemias and crush injuries - an orthopedic perspective. HBO Rev 2:87.

25. Strauss MB (1994) Crush injury and other traumatic peripheral ischemias. In: Kindwall EP (ed), Hyperbaric Medicine Practice. Best Publishing Company, Flagstaff, Arizona, pp. 525-549.

26. Strauss MB, Hargens AR, Gershuni DH, Greenberg DA, Grenshaw AG, Hart GB, Akeson WH (1983) Reduction of skeletal muscle necrosis using intermittent hyperbaric oxygen in model compartment syndrome. J Bone Joint Surg 65A:656.

27. Strauss MB, Hart GB (1984) Crush injury and the role of hyperbaric oxygen. Topics in Emergency Medicine 6:9.

28. Thom SR (1990) Antagonism of CO-mediated brain lipid peroxidation by hyperbaric oxygen. Toxicol Appl Pharmacol 105:340.

29. Thomas MP, Brown LA, Sponseller DR, Williamson SE, Diaz JA, Guyton DP (1991) Myocardial infarct size reduction by synergistic effect of hyperbaric oxygen and recombinant tissue plasminogen activator. Am Heart J 120:791.

30. Yablon IG, Cruess RL (1968) The effect of hyperbaric oxygen on fracture healing in rats. J Trauma 8:186.

31. Zamboni WA, Roth AC, Russell RC, Graham B, Suchy H, Kucan JO (1993) Morphologic analysis of the microcirculation during reperfusion of ischemic skeletal muscle and the effect of hyperbaric oxygen. Plast Reconstr Surg 91:1110.

NOTES

WHICH IS THE ROLE OF HBOT IN THE TREATMENT OF CHRONIC MUSCULO-SKELETAL POST-TRAUMATIC SEQUELAE?

E.M. Camporesi

Professor and Chair, Department of Anesthesiology, Research Professor of Physiology, Medical Director, Hyperbaric Center SUNY HSC @ Syracuse, NY 13210

INTRODUCTION

The use of hyperbaric oxygen therapy after crush injury and acute traumatic ischemia has been demonstrated to be beneficial in a relatively small number of patients, but it is gaining wider acceptance after the publication of the Hyperbaric Oxygen Committee Report of 1992, updated in 1996 by the Undersea and Hyperbaric Medical Society. The rationale and specific application of hyperbaric oxygen in this acute syndrome will be reviewed in this paper to obtain parameters defining the duration of the acute period. It is possible, in fact, to identify a transition toward a chronic syndrome, after traumatic involvement of muscle, tendon, and bone. The use of hyperbaric oxygen therapy for chronic syndromes derived from complex musculoskeletal post-traumatic sequelae is much less clear, and will be discussed later in this report. We will comment on observations from the literature in two specific conditions: acute muscular post-ischemic salvage, also with utilization of HBO for treatment of compartment syndrome, as well as more recently published reports, on ligament healing following trauma.

This last area of research has attracted significant attention in the world of sports medicine in the past few years. since several major professional sport teams have promulgated the unsubstantiated use of hyperbaric therapy, at relatively low oxygen pressure, to speed up the healing time following sport injuries after major athletic events. Aside from the visibility of sport injuries, and the broad financial implication in the world of sport, should such improvement in healing be demonstrated, a large group of patients undergo post-traumatic muscular-ligamentous rehabilitation after suffering from sequelae. In this group, perhaps, healing could be hastened by the appropriate use of hyperbaric oxygen therapy. The following review is based on acute crush injury and the literature published on the early phase of chronic post-traumatic sequelae.

HBO AND ACUTE CRUSH INJURY

Acute traumatic ischemia (ATI) occurs when an injury compromises the circulation to an extremity. This compromise may place portions of the extremity or the entire extremity at risk of necrosis or amputation. Secondary complications such as infection, nonhealing wounds, and non-union in fractures may develop. Ischemia can result either from injury to large vessels, as in open fractures with interruption of major arteries, or at the microcirculation level, as in severe crush injuries and in skeletal muscle compartment syndromes, or from combinations of the two.

The rationale for using HBO in ATI is based on the pathophysiology of these conditions and how the mechanisms of HBO influence them. The immediate threat to the limb is whether perfusion is sufficient to maintain viability of the tissues. Post-traumatic edema, which is associated with traumatic injuries and ischemia, further reduces oxygen availability to tissues. When tissue oxygen tensions fall below 30 mmHg, the host responses to infection and ischemia are compromised (1, 2). Specifically, white blood cell killing becomes defective or nonexistent and the host experiences depletion of radical scavengers at the reperfusion site (3–10).

It has been suggested whenever hyperbaric oxygen (HBO) is used for an ATI, that the injury should be classified by a Standard Classification Method such as the Gustilo Grading System or the Mangled Extremity Severity Score (MESS) (see Tables 1 & 2) (1, 2). For skeletal muscle-compartment syndromes, the use of HBO should be based on clinical findings coupled, when available, with interstitial fluid pressure measurements of the compartment (Table 3).

Ninety-three cases using HBO in crush injuries have been reported in the English language literature, as for example in refs. 11 and 12. Although none were controlled studies, all showed benefits from HBO for traumatic ischemias. In addition, Strauss summarized the reports of over 600 cases from the Eastern European literature (13). An extension on the use of HBO in acute traumatic injuries has been defined for treatment of compartment syndromes (14) and in complicated fractures (15).

Table 1. Use of HBO for open fractures, (Gustilo Classification)[1] and crush injuries.

TYPE	MECHANISM	EXPECTED OUTCOME	HBO INDICATIONS
I	Small (< 1 cm) laceration from inside to outside	Usually no different than a closed fracture	None
II	Large laceration, but minimal soft tissue damage	Usually no different than a closed fracture	Compromised hosts such as diabetics, advanced peripheral vascular disease, collagen to vascular diseases, etc. where concern is raised about primary healing of flaps
III	Crush Tissue		
	A. Sufficient soft tissue to close wound (primarily or delayed)	Infections and/or nonunion rates < 10%	Same as for Type II fractures
	B. Flaps or grafts required to obtain soft tissue coverage	About 50% incidence of complications (infection, nonunion)	All injuries
	C. Major (macrovascular) vessel injury	About 50% incidence of complications (infection, nonunion)	All injuries

Table 2. Use of HBO for mangled extremities (Mess Score, Johansen)[2].

	(Points)
A. Skeletal/Soft-Tissue Injury	
Low energy (stab, simple fracture- low velocity gunshot wound)	1
Medium energy (open or multiple fractures, dislocation)	2
High energy (close-range shotgun or high velocity GSW, crush injury)	3
Very high energy (above plus gross contamination, soft tissue avulsion)	4
B. Limb Ischemia	
Pulse reduced or absent, but perfusion present	1*
Pulselessness, paresthesias, diminished capillary refill	2*
Cool, paralyzed, insensate, numb	3*
*Double score if ischemia time >6 hours	
C. Shock	
Systolic BP-Always >90 mmHg	0
Hypotension transiently	1
Persistent hypotension	2
D. Age	
> 30	0
30-50	1
> 50	2

The recommended treatment schedule is three 90-min treatments per day during the first 48 hrs, followed by two 90-min treatments daily during the subsequent 48 hrs and one 90-min treatment daily during the third period of 48 hrs. By the sixth day, restored perfusion, edema reduction and demarcation or recovery should be sufficient to discontinue HBO therapy. Early application of HBO, preferably within 4 to 6 hours of the injury, is essential for efficacy. If surgery must be delayed, HBO therapy should be started before surgery.

Although Johansen et al. recommended primary amputation if MESS Score is seven (7) or greater, HBO should be used in the following situations, as shown below:

MESS SCORE	HBO INDICATIONS
7 (possibly 8)	Uncompromised host where age, hypotension and mild-to-moderate ischemia significantly contribute to the score
5, 6	Compromised hosts with diabetes, peripheral vascular disease, collagen vascular disease, etc.
3, 4	Severely compromised hosts with advanced levels of the above conditions

Table 3. Use of HBO for the Skeletal Muscle Compartment Syndrome.

I. Clinical Findings
    1. Severe pain in muscle compartment
    2. Marked increase in pain with passive stretch of muscles in the compartment
    3. Marked swelling of the compartment
    4. Marked tenseness of the muscle compartment
    5. Neuropathy, myelopathy and/or encephalopathy

II. Skeletal-Muscle compartment pressure measurements:
    1. Greater than 40 mmHg in the uncompromised host
    2. Rising <u>serial</u> compartment pressure measurements as values approach 35 mmHg.
    3. 30-40 mmHg in mildly compromised host (diabetic, peripheral vascular disease, collagen vascular disease, etc.).
    4. 20-30 mmHg in hypotensive patients where systolic blood pressure is 33 to 50% lower than is expected.

HBO INDICATIONS: Either or both of the following exist:

A.   3 (or more) clinical findings (from Section I of the above table).

B.   Any one of the above permutations for skeletal-muscle compartment pressure measurements (from Section II of the above table).

HBO AND SUB-ACUTE SKELETAL MUSCLE INJURY

The deleterious effects of ischemia and reperfusion of skeletal muscle can be ameliorated by intermittent hyperbaric oxygenation. A recent article (16) in Plastic and Reconstructive Surgery reviews the effects of HBO on early and late ischemia-induced skeletal muscle injury. This carefully designed study verifies how repeated bouts of hyperbaric oxygen therapy could reduce the ischemia-induced damage to skeletal muscle in an experimental rat model. The skeletal muscle injury was assessed from uptake of a radio-labeled marker (^{99m}technetium-pyrophosphate) and by analysis of muscle energy metabolites.

In this model of ischemia a tourniquet was applied around the left thigh for three hours, in half the rats, and for four hours in the remaining half. Rats were randomly allocated to four groups, two treated with HBO following release of the tourniquet, and two untreated. Muscle biopsies were taken from the postischemic and the nonischemic leg 48 hours after reperfusion. Treatment of animals was with anesthesia during the ischemia and during the biopsies. Hyperbaric oxygen treatment was delivered at 2.2 atm for 45 minutes of 100% O_2 at different times: starting immediately after the release of ischemia (time 0), and at 4, 8, 16, 24, 32, and 40 hours following tourniquet release. This treatment regimen is about twice more frequent than common clinical applications. Control rats were handled similarly to treatment rats.

Uptake of the radio-labeled metabolite is an index of more advanced cellular muscle damage, and was significantly lower in hyperbaric oxygen treated rats versus untreated rats with both three or four hours of ischemia. At the measurement time of 45 hours, 4 hrs of ischemia resulted in significant changes in levels of intracellular muscle compounds: adenosine triphosphate (ATP) and phosphocreatine (PC) were higher and lactate levels (Lac) were less in the hyperbaric oxygen-treated rats than in the untreated animals. More dramatically, both untreated groups after three and four hours of ischemia had nearly 50% spontaneous mortality at 48 hours, while the mortality in the two groups treated with HBO was approximately 10%. The difference in mortality is significant.

In this study, skeletal muscle injury following ischemia and reperfusion was significantly less in hyperbaric oxygen treated and untreated rats. Mortality was also significantly reduced in the hyperbaric oxygen groups. The results indicate favorable effects of HBO on postischemic muscle cells, both after the early reperfusion phase (between 5 and 12 hours) and at a longer time limit, 48 hours after reperfusion. The model shows a significant mortality in HBO untreated animals, underlining the gravity of the clinical syndrome of an albeit minor ischemia and reperfusion injury. The use of the radio-labeling agent to assess skeletal muscle damage verifies that this test can assess non-invasively the extent of damage in a post traumatic situation. In the discussion the authors conclude that uptake of his label is not indicative of muscle necrosis, but rather signals an early stage of muscle damage, reversible in some fibers, but leading to necrosis in others (17).

Finally, regarding the lower mortality observed, the release of lactate during reperfusion is known to result in acidosis and increased potassium release. The reduction of lactate levels and of skeletal muscle injury produced by hyperbaric oxygen probably diminishes the systemic effects of these factors, but it is not clear yet if those are key factors in the causation of mortality. The study concludes that hyperbaric oxygen therapy provided in this intensive manner during the reperfusion period restores the energy content in the muscle cell and optimizes the possibility of preserving an intact cell structure.

A canine model for compartment syndrome with ischemia and external pressure has been previously reported (14) to compare the tolerance of skeletal muscle to tourniquet compression (ischemia only) and to acute compartment syndrome (ischemia and increased interstitial pressure), with evaluation of the damage through metabolite studies and with electron microscopy. In this study elevated tissue pressure as in compartment syndrome was concluded to act synergistically with ischemia to produce more severe cellular deterioration than the ischemia alone.

In an interesting accompanying discussion (18) Zamboni reviews the rationale of utilization of the use of hyperbaric oxygen for ischemia-reperfusion injury; in fact, until recently, a concern had been expressed that additional oxygen availability during the time of reperfusion would increase free radical production and increase tissue damage. Several lines of research, instead, have actually shown that hyperbaric oxygen antagonizes the ill effects of reperfusion injury. This was borne out in axial skin flaps studied in rats, demonstrating that HBO significantly improves skin flap survival in microvascular perfusion after 8 hours of global ischemia (19, 20). Subsequent models of ischemia-reperfusion injury also demonstrated improved blood flow in capillary density with hyperbaric oxygen treatment (21). Kaelin et al. (22) have shown that hyperbaric oxygen treatment during reperfusion significantly improves survival of free skin flaps following microvascular reattachment and ischemia times of up to 24 hours.

Several studies (23, 24, 25) enabled the extension of the beneficial effect of HBO in reperfusion injury to skeletal muscle; HBO administered during and up to one hour following four hours of global ischemia significantly reduced neutrophil adherence in venules and also blocked the **progressive vasoconstriction in nearby arterioles**. The mechanism of action is the prevention of neutrophil adhesion, and the subsequent free-radical liberation and consequent arteriole vasoconstriction, a situation which precedes the end point of ischemia-reperfusion injury, vessel thrombosis, and tissue death.

The fact that neutrophil endothelial adherence is dependent on an intact CD18 function in this model provides indirect evidence that hyperbaric oxygen is affecting the neutrophil CD18 adhesion molecule. A similar mechanism has been demonstrated by Thom (5) using a rat model of brain ischemia-reperfusion injury after carbon monoxide intoxication. Hyperbaric oxygen does not alter other important neutrophil functions such as the oxidative burst or neutrophil chemotaxis and migration. This finding is very important because HBO can block adhesion of neutrophils which is associated with ischemia-reperfusion injury, **without increasing the risk of infectious complications**, because the other neutrophil functions are not altered. This stands in sharp contrast to the use of monoclonal antibodies, which can block many important anti-inflammatory neutrophil functions, resulting in increased infection.

Zamboni concludes that his positive experience of HBO utilization in muscle survival in revascularized extremities in human flaps, with ischemia times of up to 14 hours, supports that the timing of initiation of hyperbaric oxygen treatment is critical to a successful outcome; a 100% salvage rate was found with hyperbaric oxygen within 24 hours of surgery while a 0% is found when treatment begins over 72 hours after surgery. With these observations, and the mounting evidence that neutrophil mediation is producing intermediate products deleterious to reperfusion injury, we are able to extend within a 24 hour period the useful adjunct of hyperbaric oxygen.

LIGAMENT REPAIR

Very recently, an abstract (27) studied the effect of hyperbaric oxygen on ligament healing, in a rat model, by comparing the result of the effect on mechanical strength and rate healing of a standardized injury to medial collateral ligament (MCL) in rats treated with HBO. After standardized surgical laceration of MCL in the right knee, the left knee was utilized as internal control. Two groups of animals were studied; Group A recovered without HBO, while Group B received HBO treatment at 2.8 atm for 1.5 hours per day for five days immediately after wound closure. Different cohorts of animals of both groups were sacrificed at 2, 4, and 6 weeks after MCL, although HBO treatment was limited to the first week after injury.

A mechanical study was conducted on the amputated hind limbs after various times. The femur and tibia were mounted on a material testing machine and distracted at a constant rate of 10 mm/min, measuring the force to failure and stiffness of the ligament. The result showed that at two weeks, in both groups, the force to failure and stiffness were less in the injured side compared to the control side. The differences decreased at four weeks and were completely obliterated at six and eight weeks. These preliminary data indicate that early recovery was hastened and improved with hyperbaric oxygen one hour weekly for five days after acute ligament injury.

DISCUSSION

This review of recent experimental data supports that acutely initiated injury and one to two days old ischemia-reperfusion injuries in muscle and skin are largely improved with additional utilization of hyperbaric oxygen therapy. This observation extends the beneficial effect of HBO previously noted in the literature on acute crush injury, limb reattachment, and traumatic ischemia. It is speculative at this moment to extend further validation of HBO therapy to a longer time base, as certainly it needs to be proven that beneficial effects would persist when initiated more than one week after injury. It is possible to hypothesize that if hyperbaric oxygen therapy is initiated early after the injury and <u>continued</u> in a chronic phase of rehabilitation (past the first week), continuing beneficial effects might be observed, dependent upon revascularization and better nutritional blood flow phenomena. However, it is not clear at this moment that this might be the case, although some tantalizing observations have been made in patients with chronic flow limitation due to peripheral vascular disease (28).

METHODS OF HBO APPLICATIONS

The data reviewed support that more elevated atmospheric pressure of oxygen should be utilized acutely within the first 24–48 hours, between 2.2 and 2.8 ata. An analogy with chronic wound-healing treatments, support that treatments extending past one week of time should be limited to lower pressures, between 2 and 1.8 ata. The duration of each treatment usually is up to two treatments per day for 60–90 min in the early recovery phases, and is usually 60 min when treatments are applied after one week.

We suggest it would be important to support such working hypothesis with observations on patients undergoing rehabilitation therapy for one to four week periods, and after significant immobilization, as post fractures in limbs. Such controlled studies are fraught with difficulties, because of the difficulty of assuring similar levels of impairment and the possible superimposed complication of immobilization-mediated atrophy in the muscular skeletal system under study. This area deserves attentive collection of human results and possibly the development of an animal model for rehabilitation therapy. It is my opinion that at this stage the evidence of the utility of HBO in long term post traumatic sequelae is not yet available, certainly for observation extending past two weeks after injury.

REFERENCES

1. Gustilo RB, Williams DN: The use of antibiotics in the management of open fractures. Orthopaedics 1984; 7:1617-1619.
2. Johansen K, Daines M, Howey T, Helfet D, Hansen ST Jr.: Objective criteria accurately predict amputation following lower extremity trauma. J Trauma 1990; 30:568-573.
3. Bolli R: Oxygen-derived free radicals and postischemic myocardial dysfunction ("stunned myocardium"). J Am Coll Cardiol 1988; 12:239-249.
4. Stewart RJ, Mason SW, Taira MT, Hasson GE, Naito MS, Yamaguchi KT: Effect of radical scavengers and hyperbaric oxygen on smoke-induced pulmonary edema. Undersea & Hyperbaric Medicine 1994: 21:21-30.
5. Thom SR: Functional inhibition of Leukocyte B2 integrins by hyperbaric oxygen in carbon monoxide-mediated brain injury in rats. Toxicol Appl Pharmacol 1993; 123:248-256.
6. Thom SR: Dehydrogenase conversion to oxidate and lipid peroxidation in brain after CO poisoning. J Appl Physiol 1992; 73:1584-1589.
7. Thom SR, Elbuken ME: Oxygen-dependent antagonism of lipid peroxidation. Free Radic Biol Med 1991; 10:413-426.
8. Zamboni WA, Roth AC, Russell RC, Graham B, Suchy H, Kucan JO: Morphological analysis of the micro-circulation during reperfusion of ischemic skeletal muscle and the effect of hyperbaric oxygen. Plast Reconstr Surg 1993; 91:1110-1123.
9. Zamboni WA, Roth AC, Russell RC, Nemiroff PM, Casas L, Smoot EC: The effect of acute hyperbaric oxygen therapy on axial pattern skin flap survival when administered during and after total ischemia. J Reconstr Microsurg 1989; 5:343-347.
10. Zamboni WA, Roth AC, Russell RC, Smoot EC: The effect of hyperbaric oxygen on reperfusion of ischemic axial skin flaps: a laser Doppler analysis. Ann Plast Surg 1992; 28:339-341.
11. Barthelemy L, Bellet M, Michaud A, Cabon P: The value of thermography in the appreciation of the effectiveness of hyperbaric oxygen therapy in the treatment of acute arteritis of the lower limbs. Bord Med 1976; 9:1095-1100.
12. Szekely O, Szanto G, Takats A: Hyperbaric oxygen therapy in injured subjects. Injury 1973; 4:294-300.
13. Strauss MB: Role of hyperbaric oxygen therapy in acute ischemias and crush injuries - an orthopedic perspective. HBO Review 1981; 2:87-106.
14. Strauss MB, Hart GB: Hyperbaric oxygen and the skeletal-muscle compartment syndrome. Contemporary Orthopedics 1989; 18-167-174.
15. Strauss MB: Editorial. Cost-effective issues in HBO therapy: complicated fractures. J Hyperbaric Medicine 1988; 3:199-205.
16. Haapaniemi T, Nylander G, Sirsjo A, Larsson J: Hyperbaric oxygen reduces ischemia-induced skeletal muscle injury. Plast Reconstr Surg 97:3, 602-607, 1996.
17. Crenshaw AG, Friden J, Hargens AR, Lang GH, Thornell LE: Increased technetium uptake is not equivalent to muscle necrosis: Scintigraphic, morphological and intramuscular pressure analyses of sore muscles after exercise. Acta Physiol Scand 148:187, 1993.
18. Zamboni WA: Discussion, "Hyperbaric oxygen reduces ischemia-induced skeletal muscle injury" by Haapaniemi, T, et al, Plast Reconstr Surg 97:3, 608-609, 1996.
19. Zamboni WA, Roth AC, Russell RC, et al: The effect of acute hyperbaric oxygen therapy on axial-pattern skin flap survival when administered during and after total ischemia. J Reconstr Microsurg 5:343, 1989.
20. Zamboni WA, Roth AC, Russell RC, et al: Effect of hyperbaric oxygen on reperfusion of ischemic axial skin flaps: A laster Doppler analysis. Ann Plast Surg 28:339, 1992.
21. Sirsjo A, Lehr HA, Nolte D, et al: Hyperbaric oxygen treatment enhances the recovery of blood flow and functional capillary density in postischemic striated muscle. Circ Shock 40:9, 1993.
22. Kaelin CM, Im MJ, Myers RAM, et al: The effects of hyperbaric oxygen on free flaps in rats. Arch Surg 125:607, 1990.
23. Nylander G, Lewis D, Nordstrom H, et al: Reduction of postischemic edema with hyperbaric oxygen. Plast Reconstr Surg 76:596, 1985.
24. Strauss MB, Hargens AR, Gershuni DH, et al: Reduction of skeletal muscle necrosis using intermittent hyperbaric oxygen in a model compartment syndrome. J Bone Joint Surg 65A: 65, 1983.
25. Zamboni WA, Roth AC, Russell RC, et al: Morphological analysis of the microcirculation during reperfusion of ischemic skeletal muscle and the effect of hyperbaric oxygen. Plast Reconstr Surg. 91: 110, 1993.
26. Mileski WJ, Sikes P, Atiles L, et al: Inhibition of leukocyte adherence and susceptibility to infection. J Surg Res 54:349, 1993.
27. Horn DA, Webster HM, Amin HM, Weissbrich O, Mascia MF, Werner FW: Effect of hyperbaric oxygen on ligament healing in a rat model in: UHMS Annual Scientific Meeting, Anchorage, Alaska, 23, S 13, 1996.
28. Fischer B, Jain KK, Jacob St, Schnaiter A: Increase in exercise capacity in patients with ischemic leg pain by treadmill ergometry under hyperbaric oxygenation. In: Hyperbaric Medicine, Proceedings of the Joint Meeting, 2nd European Conference on Hyperbaric Medicine, Basel 1988, D.J. Bakker, ed., Foundation for Hyperbaric Medicine, Basel, 1990, pp 337-340.

ROLE OF HYPERBARIC OXYGEN THERAPY FOR IMPROVING FINAL CLINICAL OUTCOME IN ACUTE MUSCULO-SKELETAL TRAUMA

D. Mathieu, R. Neviere, N. Lefebvre-Lebleu, F. Wattel

Aside the life threatening consequences of severe limb trauma (shock, hemorraghe, fat embolism, etc.) in which prehospital management and intensive care have decreased mortality, final outcome of severely injured patients is primarily determined by the extent of musculo-skeletal injury and especially of the vascular supply. Occurrence of secondary infection, non-healing wound and non-union of bones is also mainly determined by the presence of an hypoxic component in the wound.

Clinical series report a total amputation rate of 13 to 23 percent and up to 60 percent when an arterial trauma is associated with musculo-skeletal damage (1–5). Acute wound ischemia may result from a direct damage to blood vessels but, even if an adequate first surgical repair has been done, a secondary amputation may be necessary because of a persistent ischemia, a secondary vascular thrombosis, an infection, or a compartment syndrome (5–8). These complications may, by themselves, lead to life threatening consequences if amputation is too long delayed (9).

In this situation, hyperbaric oxygen proves to be useful for three main reasons :
- as an adjunctive treatment to surgical and medical therapy
- as a condition allowing transcutaneous oxygen measurements to get higher predictive and monitoring value
- as a cost-saving measure when associated to conventional treatment

HBO AS AN ADJUNCTIVE TREATMENT TO SURGICAL AND MEDICAL THERAPY

Severe limb injury combines in multiple different ways fractures, vascular and nervous injuries and soft tissue (cutaneous and/or muscular) lesions. After the initial surgical procedures allowing osteosynthesis, vascular and nervous repairs, fasciotomie and debridement, patient and limb survival may still be in jeopardy because secondary complications such as persisting ischemia or Occurrence of a compartment syndrome. This is thought to be due to the capillary bed damage induced by acute ischemia, resulting in an increased permeability of capillary endothelium to water, electrolytes, and organic substances (10, 11). Increased blood flow through the damaged capillaries causes diapedesis of blood cells and leakage of intravascular fluids with interstitial edema, and consequently increases the diffusion distance for oxygen from the intact circulation to the injured area (12, 13). The pressure generated by swollen tissues enclosed within unyielding fascial compartments further compromises perfusion, and results in a vicious circle leading to compartment syndrome (14). Finally, infection of the wound and/or bones, favored by local hypoxia, may occur and further compromise final outcome (15).

Hyperbaric oxygen therapy has been advocated as an adjunctive treatment to surgery and wound care because of its effects on peripheral oxygen delivery, edema reduction, cutaneous and muscular necrosis (16–19), and infection prevention (20, 21). Detailed presentation of both experimental and clinical data are exposed by others experts and are beyond the scope of this report. We shall focus here on final outcome.

Published clinical experience with HBO as an adjunct to surgical measures in acute limb ischemia is limited. Smith et al. (22) were the first to report good results from HBO in traumatic ischemic lesions of the lower extremities. Slack et al. (23) treated a group of 22 patients of whom 13 (59 %) "did well." Szekely et al. (24) administered HBO therapy to 19 patients with severe injury to limb, vascular damage, extensive skin loss, and anaerobic infection associated with open fractures. In 13 patients (68 %), the procedure was "beneficial." Monies-Chas et al. (25) treated 7 patients in whom ischemia of a lower limb persisted despite apparently successful arterial repair. Complete limb salvage was accomplished in 6 patients, and amputation of toes only was carried out in the 7th. Shupak (26) reported a series of 13 patients with severe limb trauma associated with acute schemia. Most of the cases had an association of open fracture with injury to major blood vessels and significant soft tissue damage. The average delay from the moment of injury to definitive surgical treatment was 12 hours. HBO was indicated where aggravation of peripheral ischemia was noted despite maximal surgical treatment. Complete limb salvage was accomplished in 8 cases (61.5 %). In 4 cases (30.7 %), lowering of ischemia level distally was observed. One case (7.7 %) showed no improvement. When estimating the final outcome, the authors stressed that HBO has been used as a last resort where the surgeons clinical impression beforehand was that high amputation was apparently unavoidable in all cases.

The only prospective randomized study in the field was done by Bouachour et al. (19). A total of 31 patients with crush injuries were assigned in a blinded randomized fashion within 24 h following surgery to hyperbaric oxygen treatment (session of 100 % O_2 at 2.5 ATA for 90 min; twice daily sessions for 6 days) or placebo (session of 21 % O_2 at 1.1 ATA for 90 min; twice daily sessions for 6 days). All patients received the same standard therapies (anticoagulants, antibiotics, and wound dressings). The two study groups (treatment group, n = 16; placebo group, n = 15) were similar in terms of risk factors (diabetes mellitus, previous neurological deficit, peripheral vascular disease); number, type, or location of vascular injuries, neurological injuries, and fractures; injury Severity Score; type, location, or timing of surgical procedures. Complete healing was obtained in 15 patients in the treatment group vs 7 patients in the placebo group (p < 0.005). A new surgical procedure (amputation, vascular surgery, skin flaps, and grafts) was performed in 1 patient in the treatment group compared with 6 patients in the placebo group (p < 0.025). No significant differences were found between the two groups considering the length of hospital stay and the number of wound dressings (Table 1).

In summary, it can be concluded from the literature that HBO has been shown to be effective as an adjunctive therapy to surgery and intensive care in the management of crush injuries of the limb. Studies show the effectiveness of HBO in improving wound healing, reducing amputation rate or lowering amputation level, and reducing repetitive surgical procedures. Effects on hospital length of stay, complete healing time, or wound dressing number are less evident.

Table 1 : Results of Bouachour's study comparing in a prospective randomized design the effects of HBO versus placebo in 31 patients with crush injuries of the limb (19)

Injury	Placebo (n = 15)	HBO (n = 16)	P
Arterial Injury	0	2	n.s.
Neurological Injury	0	2	n.s.
Fractures	11	12	n.s.
Open Fractures (Type III)	6	7	n.s.
Soft Tissue Injury (Grade II)	5	3	n.s.
Soft Tissue Injury (Grade III)	10	13	n.s.
Injury Severity Score	9.3 ± 1	9.5 ± 1.4	n.s.
Length of Hospitalization	23.3 ± 16.8	22.4 ± 12.4	n.s.
Complete Healing	7	15	0.004
Tissue Necrosis	8	1	
New Surgical Procedures	3 (6 patients)	2 (1 patient)	0.015
Skin Flaps and Grafts	6	1	
Vascular Surgery	0	1	
Amputation	2	0	
Wound Dressing	16.8 ± 9.5	16.9 ± 13.2	n.s.
Time of Healing (days)	58.7 ± 19.1	49.3 ± 21.6	n.s.

n.s.: non-statistically different

HBO AS A TEST FOR FINAL OUTCOME PREDICTION

As reported previously, in limb injury, once adequate surgical repair and intensive care have been done, final outcome is mainly determined by the persistence or the reappearance of tissue ischemia.

It is well established that transcutaneous oxygen pressure is linked to oxygen delivery, i.e., the result of oxygen content and blood flow (27, 28). If oxygen content is normal, regional transcutaneous tension can be used as a measure of tissue perfusion (29). Every limitation of regional blood flow, arterial narrowing, occlusion from thrombosis, intramural dissection, or external compression leads to a reduction in transcutaneous oxygen pressure. Based on these facts, $PTCO_2$ measurement has been proposed to predict final outcome in major limb trauma (30). Kram and Shoemaker showed that transcutaneous oxygen tensions can be used to detect the Occurrence of an arterial injury, but did not correlate values to outcome (31). White et al. (32) reported that $PTCO_2$ higher than 50 torr is associated with good outcome whereas values lower than 40 torr are associated with amputation.

Unfortunately, in normal atmospheric conditions, we found these values not sufficiently discriminative and tried to improve this test by an oxygen challenge both in normobaric and hyperbaric conditions (33). For this, 23 patients with major vascular trauma of the limb were evaluated by clinical examination and transcutaneous oxygen pressure measurements. Sixteen had arterial repair and 7 had clinical evidence of peripheral ischemia without an arterial lesion. In normal air, the transcutaneous oxygen values in the traumatized limb of these 23 patients were significantly lower than in the nontraumatized limb. But neither the absolute $PTCO_2$ value, nor the ratio between the traumatized limb's $PTCO_2$ and that of the nontraumatized one, can predict the final outcome (amputation). In hyperbaric oxygen (2.5 ATA), this ratio is significantly higher in the group where the surgery will succeed than in the group where final amputation will be needed (81.2 26.0 vs. 15.2 13.1; p < 0.01). The overall sensitivity and specificity of prediction of the limb's final outcome when the bilateral $PTCO_2$ ratio in 2.5 ATA pure oxygen is less than 0.40, are 100 % and 94 %, respectively. But what is perhaps more interesting is that, when considering a ratio value of less than 0.20, amputation can be predicted with a 100 % true predictive value.

The reason why HBO condition improve $PTCO_2$ predictive value is that a low level of $PTCO_2$ can be produced either by a low limb blood flow or by a low oxygen content. In limb ischemia, the fall in the limb blood flow leads to a skin vasoconstriction and an increase in tissue oxygen extraction. As a result, the oxygen quantity available for diffusion through the skin—which is the true value measured by the transcutaneous electrode—is decreased to a level far lower than the level usually related to the actual limb oxygen delivery. When the arterial oxygen content is increased, by increasing, for instance, the oxygen pressure inhaled by the patient, either a significant blood flow remains, with the oxygen delivery to the limb increasing, the skin vasoconstriction decreasing, and the $PTCO_2$ increasing to a level reflecting again the true limb oxygen delivery, or the remaining blood flow is too low and the oxygen delivery does not increase, the skin vasoconstriction remains unchanged, and the $PTCO_2$ remains low. In brief, the change in $PTCO_2$ following an increase in the inhaled amount of oxygen may be a way to measure more accurately the remaining blood flow in limb ischemia.

Table 2. Classification of open fractures (from 37) and place for HBO as determined by the first European Consensus Conference on Hyperbaric Medicine (38)

Type	Injury	Complication Rate	Comment	HBO
I	small (< 1 cm) laceration from inside to outside	less than 1 %	often managed without formal surgical debridement	No HBO
II	laceration more than 1 cm long without or with minimal soft tissue injury	less than 5 %	excellent results with immediate surgical debridement and later delayed primary closure	No HBO
III Subtype A	crush injury component; adequate soft tissue coverage	infection 4 % amputation 0 %	complication rates little different from types I and II fractures	No HBO
Subtype B	Inadequate (loss of sufficient) soft tissue to cover bone and close wound	infection 52 % amputation 16 %	external skeletal fixation and free grafts have greatly advanced the management of these fractures; complication rates remain high	HBO (type 2 recommend-ation)
Subtype C	arterial injury	infection 42 % amputation 42 %	these complication rates exist after arterial repair	HBO (type 2 recommend-ation)

When comparing the usefulness of transcutaneous oxygen measurement to the common clinical signs, such a clear cut-off between the two groups does not appear for any of the clinical signs more commonly used.

These results show that transcutaneous oxygen measurements at 2.5 ATA pure oxygen are a valuable, non-invasive adjunctive method for prediction of the final outcome of major vascular trauma of the limbs.

After the first $PTCO_2$ evaluation to predict final outcome, repetition of $PTCO_2$ measurement may be useful to follow evolution. It allows early detection of any vascular complication occurring during treatment that might require medical or surgical intervention. This is of particular interest in this acute condition. In this case, a sudden fall in $PTCO_2$ must lead to suspicion of an arterial or venous thrombosis or an extrinsic compression by edema requiring urgent surgery to remove obstruction or to decompress. (34)

HBO AS A COST-SAVING MEASURE WHEN ASSOCIATED TO CONVENTIONAL TREATMENT

In limb injury, HBO is used as an adjunctive therapy to surgery and intensive care. Beside its effects on healing and its predictive value, HBO is also interesting by its cost-saving effect.

In a cost-saving analysis, Strauss (35) established, considering that a primary amputation with 18 months follow-up costs 41,000 US dollars and that adding HBO to the medico-surgical cost of a patient with acute limb trauma adds approximately 4,800 U.S. dollars, that a reduction of only 12 percent of the amputation rate will cover all the extra cost of HBO.

Considering the complicated refractory soft tissue and bone lesions, Marroni et al. (36) claimed that adjunctive HBO saves for a patient more than 13,000 ECU (European Currency Units) as compared with the 4,800 ECU extra cost for HBO session.

Using the results obtained by Bouachour et al. (19), considering an average cost of 120 ECU for a HBO session, 300 ECU for an hospitalization day, and 10,000 ECU for an orthopedic surgical procedure, the total saving may be estimated at 2,500 ECU by patient in favor of HBO use.

CONCLUSION

Adding HBO to conventional surgical and medical care of severe limb trauma is associated with an improvement in wound healing and functional outcome. It allows a closer monitoring of limb vitality by transcutaneous oxymetry. It has been shown to be cost-effective and should be used on a larger scale in integrated medico-surgical protocols.

REFERENCES

1. Bizer L. Peripheral vascular injuries in the Vietnam War. Arch Surg 1969 ; 98 : 165 -169.
2. Connolly GF, Whittaker D, Williams E. Femoral and tibial fractures combined with injuries to femoral and popliteal artery. J Bone Jt Surg Am Vol 1971 ; 53 - A : 56 - 58.
3. Gill SS, Eggleston FC, Singh CM, et al. Arterial injuries of the extremities. J Trauma 1976 ; 16 : 766 - 772.
4. Gorman JA. Combat arterial trauma. Analysis of 106 limb-threatening injuries. Arch Surg 1969 ; 98 : 160 - 164.
5. Keeley SB, Sydner WH, Weigelt JA. Arterial injuries below the knee : Fifty-one patients with eighty-two injuries. J Trauma 1983 ; 23 : 285 - 292.
6. Drapanas T, Hewitt RL, Weichert RT, et al. Civilian vascular injuries. A critical appraisal of three decades of management. Ann Surg 1970 ; 172 : 351 - 360.
7. Rich NM, Baugh JH, Hughes CW. Acute arterial injuries in Vietnam, 1000 cases. J Trauma 1970 ; 10 : 359 - 369
8. Lange RH, Bach AW, Hansen ST, et al. Open tibial fractures with associated vascular injuries : Prognosis for limb salvage. J Trauma 1985 ; 25 : 203 - 208.
9. Miller HH, Welch CS. Quantitative studies of the time factor in arterial injuries. Ann Surg 1949 ; 130 : 428 - 438.
10. Scully, RW, Hughes CW. The pathology of ischemia of skeletal muscle in man. Am J Pathol 1956 ; 32 : 805 - 830.
11. Landis EM. Microinjection studies of capillary permeability. III. The effects of local oxygen on the permeability of the capillary wall to fluid and to plasma protein. Am J Physiol 1928 ; 83 : 528 - 540.
12. Haimovici H. Myopathic-nephrotic-metabolic syndrome associated with massive acute arterial occlusions. J Cardiovasc Surg 1973 ; 14 : 589 - 600.
13. Winniger AC. Biopathological disturbances in the revascularization stage of ischemic limbs. J Cardiovasc Surg 1973 ; 14 : 640 - 648.
14. Hargens AR, Akeson WH. Pathophysiology of the compartment syndrome. In : Mubarak SJ, Hargens AR, eds. Compartment syndrome and Volkman's contracture. W.B. Saunders, Philadelphia (USA) ; 1981, pp. 47 - 70.
15. Hunt TK, Lissey M, Grislis G, et al. The effect of different ambient oxygen tensions on wound infection. Ann Surg 1975 ; 181 : 35 - 39.
16. Strauss MB. Crush injury. In : Camporesi EM, Barker AC eds : hyperbaric oxygen therapy ; a critical review , UHMS, Bethesda, USA, 1991, pp. 121 - 125.
17. Strauss MB. Crush injury and other acute traumatic peripheral ischemias. In : Kindwall EP eds : Hyperbaric Medicine Practice, Best Publishing Company Flagstaff (USA), 1994 ; pp 525 - 549.
18. Malerba F, Oriani G, Farnetti A. HBO in orthopedic disorders. In : Oriani G, Marroni A, Wattel F eds : Handbook on Hyperbaric Medicine. Springer, Berlin, 1996 ; pp 409 - 427.
19. Bouachour G, Cronier P. Hyperbaric oxygen therapy in crush injuries. In : Oriani G, Marroni A, Wattel F eds : Handbook on Hyperbaric Medicine. Springer, Berlin, 1996 ; pp 428 - 442.
20. Hohn DC, MacKay RD, Holliday B, et al. The effects of oxygen tension on the microbicidal function of leucocytes in wounds and in vitro. Surg Forum 1976 ; 27 : 18 - 20.
21. Mandell GL. Bactericidal activity of aerobic and anaerobic polymorphonuclear neutrophils. Infect Immun 1974 ; 9 : 337 - 341.
22. Smith G, Stevens J, Griffiths JC, et al. Near avulsion of foot treated by replacement and subsequent prolonged exposure of patients to oxygen at two atmospheres pressure. Lancet 1961 ; 2 : 1122 - 1123.
23. Slack WK, Thomas DA, De Jode LRJ. Treatment of trauma, ischemic disease of limbs and varicose ulceration. In Brown IW Jr, Cox BG, eds. Proceedings of the third international congress on hyperbaric oxygen medicine. National Academy of Sciences, National Research Council Washington (USA); 1966, pp. 621 - 624.
24. Szekely O, Szanto G, Takats A. Hyperbaric oxygen therapy in injured subjects. Injury 1973 ; 4 : 294 - 300.
25. Monies-Chas I, Hashmonai M, Hoerer D, et al. Hyperbaric oxygen treatment as an adjunct to reconstructive vascular surgery in trauma. Injury 1977 ; 8 : 274 - 277.
26. Shupack A, Gozal D, Ariel A, Melamed Y, Katz A. Hyperbaric oxygenation in acute peripheral post-traumatic ischemia. J Hyper Med, 1987, 2 : 7 -14.
27. Shoemaker WC, Vidyssagar D. Physiological and clinical significance of PTCO2 and PTCO2 measurements. Crit Care Med, 1981, 9 : 689 - 690.
28. Tremper KK, Shoemaker WC. Transcutaneous oxygen monitoring of critically ill adults, with and without low flow shock. Crit Care Med 1981, 9 : 706 - 709.
29. Hauser CJ, Shoemaker WC. Use of a transcutaneous PO2 regional perfusion index to quantify tissue perfusion in peripheral vascular disease. Ann. Surg. 1983, 197 : 337 - 343.
30. Kram HB, Shoemaker WC. Use of transcutaneous O2 monitoring in the intraoperative management of severe peripheral vascular disease. Crit. Care Med 1983, 11 : 482 - 483.
31. Kram HB, Shoemaker WC. Diagnosis of major peripheral arterial trauma by transcutaneous oxygen monitoring. Am. J. Surg 1984, 147 : 776 - 780
32. White RA, Nolan L, Harley D, et al. Noninvasive evaluation of peripheral vascular disease using transcutaneous oxygen tension. Am. J. Surg., 1982, 144 : 68 - 75.
33. Mathieu D, Wattel F, Bouachour G, et al. Post-traumatic limb ischemia. Prediction of final outcome by transcutaneous oxygen measurements in hyperbaric oxygen. J Trauma 1990, 20 : 307 - 314.
34. Mathieu D, Neviere R, Wattel F. Transcutaneous oxymetric in hyperbaric medicine. In : Oriani G, Marroni A, Wattel F eds : Handbook on Hyperbaric Medicine. Springer, Berlin, 1996, pp 686 - 698.
35. Strauss MB. Cost-effective issues in HBO therapy : complicated fractures J. Hyper. Med. 1988 ; 3 : 199 - 205.

36.   Marroni A, Oriani G, Wattel F. Cost benefit and cost efficiency evaluation of hyperbaric oxygen therapy. In :
        Oriani G, Marroni A, Wattel F eds : Handbook on Hyperbaric Medicine. Springer, Berlin, 1996, pp 879 - 886.
37.   Gustillo RB, Mendoza RM, Williams DN. Problems in the management of type III (severe) open fractures : a
        new classification of type III open fractures. J Trauma 1984 ; 24 : 742 - 746.
38.   Wattel F, Mathieu D. Proceedings of the 1st European Consensus Conference on Hyperbaric Medicine, CRAM,
        Lille, 1994.

SECTION I – PART 4

The 4th European Consensus
Conference on Hyperbaric Medicine

The 4th European Consensus Conference on

Hyperbaric Oxygen in the Treatment of Foot Lesions in Diabetic Patients

Section I – Part 4

December 4 and 5, 1998—London, England

ORGANIZED BY EUROPEAN COMMITTEE FOR HYPERBARIC MEDICINE

CONTENTS

Scientific Committee
>   Daniel Mathieu (France)
>   Martin R.Hamilton-Farrell (United Kingdom)
>   Giorgio Oriani (Italy)

Organising Committee
>   Martin R.Hamilton-Farrell
>   Stephen Brearley
>   Catherine Condon
>   David Levy

THE QUESTIONS

1. What is the rationale for hyperbaric oxygen in the treatment of foot lesions in diabetic patients?
2. Which diabetic patients may benefit from hyperbaric oxygen for the treatment of foot lesions?
3. What is the place of hyperbaric oxygen in the multidisciplinary team approach to these lesions?
4. How can the efficacy of hyperbaric oxygen for these lesions be evaluated?
5. Is hyperbaric oxygen cost effective in the treatment of these lesions?

THE JURY

Andrew J.M. Boulton, President (United Kingdom)
Gérard Cathelinau (France)
Ernst Chantelau (Germany)
Ezio Faglia (Italy)
Dinis da Gama (Portugal)
Alberto de Leiva (Spain)
Francesco Malerba (Italy)
John Ross (United Kingdom)
Pascal Priollet (France)
Stephen Thom (United States of America)

LITERATURE REVIEWERS

Bruno Martini (France)
Jörg Schmutz (Switzerland)

THE CONFERENCE IS SUPPORTED BY

Undersea and Hyperbaric Medical Society
European Underwater and Baromedical Society
International Congress on Hyperbaric Medicine
Société de Physiologie et de Médecine Sub-Aquatiques et Hyperbares de Langue
    Françaises (France)
Société Nationale Française de Médecine Interne (France)
Association de Langue Française pour l'Etude du Diabète et des Maladies Métaboliques
    "ALFEDIAM" (France)
Société Suisse de Médecine Sub-Aquatique et Hyperbare (Switzerland)
Societa Italiana di Medicine Subacquea e Iperbarica (Italy)
Societa di Anestesia Analgesia Rianimazione e Terapia Intensiva (Italy)
British Medical Association (United Kingdom)
University of Manchester Department of Medicine (United Kingdom)
University of Sheffield School of Health and Related Research (United Kingdom)
Kings Healthcare NHS Trust (United Kingdom)
National Hyperbaric Centre, Aberdeen (United Kingdom)
Japanese Society for Hyperbaric Medicine (Japan)
Geselschafft für Tauch und Uberdruckmedizin (Germany)
Verband Deutscher Druckkammerzentren e.V. (Germany)
Foundation Platform Hyperbare Zuurstof (Netherlands)
Academic Medical Center, Amsterdam (Netherlands)
Comite Coordinator de Centros de Medicina Hiperbarica (Spain)

THE CONFERENCE HAS BEEN ASSISTED FINANCIALLY BY

British Hyperbaric Association (United Kingdom)
Forest Healthcare NHS Trust (United Kingdom)
North West Emergency Recompression Unit (United Kingdom)
Diving Diseases Research Centre (United Kingdom)
Verband Deutscher Druckkammerzentren (Germany)

THE CONFERENCE IS SPONSORED BY

- Sechrist Industries Inc.
- Smith & Nephew Healthcare Ltd.
- Musgrave Systems Ltd.
- Environmental Tectonics Corporation.
- Haux Life Support.
- Hemocue.
- Hytech Hyperbaric and Diving Systems.
- Jane Saunders and Manning Ltd.
- Mara Engineering Ltd.
- Radiometer Ltd.
- RDG Medical.
- Sat Medical.
- Sayers Hyperbaric and Dicing Systems GmbH.

NOTES

Methodology of ECHM Consensus Conferences

Consensus Conferences aim to create an objective and complete review of current literature and knowledge on a particular topic or field. This method has the advantage of involving a diverse group of experts, thus increasing objectivity. Participants in consensus conferences are selected from a broad range of relevant background to provide consideration of all aspects of the chosen topic and maximum objectivity. The opportunity to meet with other experts in the same field and share comments and information is also a valuable aspect of consensus meetings.

In a Consensus Conference, experts present their review of the literature relating to a specific topic before a jury and an audience. Thereafter, the jury gathers in a secluded place to discuss the presentations, and presents its finding in a consensus statement that includes recommendations for clinical practice based on the evidence that was presented. These recommendations are published in one or more medical journal.

The application of Evidence-Based Medicine methodology to the consensus conference process help the jury members to reach a consensus and strengthens the recommendation made. Thus, it is proposed each jury members assess the literature and the evidences presented by the experts and grade those according to their quality.

We propose each jury members use the same grading scale which has been extensively validated.

BASIC STUDIES (TISSULAR, CELLULAR OR SUBCELLULAR LEVEL)
1. strong evidence of beneficial action
2. evidence of beneficial action
3. weak evidence of beneficial action
4. no evidence of beneficial action or methodological or interpretation bias preclude any conclusion

ANIMAL STUDIES WITH CONTROL GROUP
1. strong evidence of beneficial action
2. evidence of beneficial action
3. weak evidence of beneficial action
4. no evidence of beneficial action or methodological or interpretation bias preclude any conclusion

HUMAN STUDIES
1. strong evidence of beneficial action based on at least 2 concordant, large, double-blind, controlled randomized studies with no or only weak methodological bias
2. evidence of beneficial action based on double-blind controlled, randomized studies but with methodological bias, or concerning only small sample, or only a single study

3. weak evidence of beneficial action based only on uncontrolled studies: (historic control group, cohort study)
4. no evidence of beneficial action (Case report only) or methodological or interpretation bias preclude any conclusion

We recommend jury conclusions are made according to the level of supporting evidence.

Type I recommendation or Standards are supported by level 1 evidence. Type II recommendation or guidelines are supported by level 2 evidence and type III or options by levels 3.

In using such a methodology, we expect every individual reading the jury conclusions can immediately assess the strength of evidence supporting each statement and how he has to apply it in his own practice.

LITERATURE REVIEW
Role of HBO in the treatment of diabetic foot lesion

Jacques Martini

CHU Toulouse Rangueil—Toulouse, France

The diabetic foot ulcer is one of the most common and devastating complication of diabetes mellitus and is associated with high morbidity and mortality. These ulcers represent a common precursor of amputations. Although the pathogenesis of foot ulceration is well known, the treatment remains difficult and requires a multidisciplinary approach including prevention, education, and aggressive treatment. The main goal is the reduction of amputation rate.

This management requires surgical therapy (radical debridement, vascular surgery) medical cares (metabolic control, appropriate antibiotics, dressing) and non-weight-bearing. Adjunctive therapy like hyperbaric oxygen may be helpful.

EPIDEMIOLOGY

Diabetic foot ulcers affect 4 to 10% of the diabetic population (1–2) and the prevalence increased with age (3). Twenty percent of hospital admissions of diabetics are because foot problems with high risk of amputations (4). Incidence of amputation is 15 fold higher in this population and diabetic accurated for 50 % to 70 % of the non traumatic amputations (7). The risk of reamputation is therefore very important; contralateral amputation occurs at a rate of approximately 10 % per year. The morbidity and mortality associated with amputation are significant. Except this human cost, economic cost is very high; it is caused by amputation cost and the length of hospital stay estimated between 14 and 45 days (8) Recently, the cost of this pathology, evaluated in Netherlands, is estimated at 10531 pounds per patient for a length of hospitalisation stay about 41,8 days (9).

PATHOGENESIS OF DIABETIC FOOT

Diabetic foot ulcers are consequences of three problems; neuropathy, vascular disease, and infection.

Neuropathy is the most common of the complications of diabetes, affects 30% of diabetic patients (10) and is present in 80% of patients with foot ulceration (1-11). Neuropathy is characterized by loss of sensation, motor and autonomic dysfunctions.

Ulcer can be caused by loss of sensation with painless trauma caused generally by footwear. Motor neuropathy may lead to deformations with alteration of pressure distribution, new high pressure points and repetitive stress. In these sites, callus occurs. Autonomic neuropathy may cause alteration in blood flow, diversion of nutritic flow and cutaneous ischemia (12).

Ulceration is the consequence of microtraumatisms caused by callus associated to cutaneous ischemia.

Peripherical vascular disease is more frequent and sooner in diabetic population. This is characterized by atheroschlerosis in large vessel, with stenosis and thrombosis (13), and is associated to microangiopathy (14). The cumulative incidence of lower extremity arterial disease (LEAD) rises with age and duration of diabetes to reach 45 % by 20 years diabetes duration. LEAD is associated to an increase in hospital mortality and higher amputation rates (15).

The main locations of atheroma are the deep femoral, anterior, and posterior tibial arteries. Arterial wall is characterized by mediacalcosis that causes reduction of compliance and calcifications (16).

Clinically, in many patients, claudication is not present; the prevalence is 0.2 % to 10.9 % (16). LEAD is detected therefore by ischemic ulcer.

The detection and follow up of LEAD is based at first on clinical exam with a search for signs of critical ischemia (claudication, palpation of peripherical pulses, skin changes, and femoral bruits). This exam is completed by ankle-brachial index (ABI) measurement, except in presence of madialcalcose. In this case, ABI is surestimated (13-17).

When ischemic lesion is present, the likelihood of healing may be assessed by the measurement of tissue PO_2 levels (18). A level above 30 mm Hg is correlated with good prognosis. If level below 30 mm Hg, revascularization must be discussed with results of Doppler and arteriography (15).

Infection decreases the prognosis of chronic wound and is the main cause of hospitalization.

Infection is facilitated by poor metabolic control and local ischemia. Leukocytes functions and cellular immunity are altered by hyperglycemia and low PO_2 level (19). Evolution of infection is marked by extension to the deep tissues with cellulitis and osteomyelitis. Bone culture is the gold standard to detect the pathogen (20). In third of cases there is a single pathogen (Staphylococcus or Streptococcus). The remaining to third are polymicrobial with aerobic or anaerobic pathogens.

TREATMENT

Treatment requires multidisciplinary approach including revascularization, antibiotics, metabolic control, surgical treatment, and footwear. Decrease of major amputation rate can be obtained (21).

Management of the treatment is guided by the depth of ulceration, the presence of osteitis, ischemia and infection (11). Classifications of severity of wound, like Wagner classification, is very helpful (22). Without ischemia, infection control is the first step including antibiotics, surgical debridement, and dressing. The goal is to restore granulation tissue and improved healing. For plantar ulcer, the discharge is obtained with off-loading shoes or casting. Metabolic control must be improved to restore good leukocytes functions (19) and is based in intensification of treatment of diabetes with insulinotherapy and self-monitoring of blood glucose.

ROLE OF OXYGEN IN HEALING

After injury, most of events for healing can proceed in very low oxygen tension, but several important steps need a good O_2 level to be achieve. It was shown that:

- Polymerization and secretion of collagen by fibroblast can be accomplished only when oxygen is present at rather high partial pressure. The mechanism of oxygen effect is the hydroxylation of proline and lysine residues in pro-collagen (23)
- Cell replication also requires oxygen
- Poor O_2 level increases susceptibility to infection and inversely raising PO_2 levels enhances resistance
- Angiogenesis occurs most rapidly when it proceeds from high oxygen tension

HBO therapy is an intermittent administration of 100 % oxygen inhaled at pressure greater, than sea level. All indication of HBO therapy are characterized by local hypoperfusion, hypoxia or both.

With HBO therapy elevation of tissue oxygen tension is very helpful for fibroblast replication, development of a collagen matrix. Diffusion of oxygen away of functional capillaries is important to preserve marginally viable tissue, to enhance collagen deposition angiogenesis and bacterial killing in wounds (24-25).

Vasoconstriction induced by increase O_2 pressure may have favorable effect on the neurologenic oedema. This oedema is explained by high blood flow with compression of capillaries. Moreover, HBO therapy has been shown to improve RBC deformability (26-27).

In summary, HBO therapy have very interesting effects in diabetic foot ulcers, especially ischemics and infected ulcers

INDICATIONS OF HBO THERAPY IN DIABETIC FOOT ULCERS

In diabetic ulcers, HBO therapy must be associated to optimal conventional treatment. The main indication seems to be limb salvage and reduction of amputation. Several groups have reported increased limbs salvage. BARONI in 1987 has reported a statistically significant reduction of amputation with HBO therapy (28). In the treated group, the amputation rate was 12.5% vs 40% in control group (p<0.001). Healing was obtained in 16/18 patients in treated group with a length of hospitalisation of 62 days. Only 1/10 patients treated in control group and 9 patients did not heal 82 days later. ORIANI in 1990 has obtained 95% salvage rate in HBO treated group with only an amputation rated of 4.8 % vs 33 % in control group (29). CIANCI reported in 1988, in a series of 19 diabetic patients, a salvage rate of 89%. Forty-two percent of these patients were referred because of infection or non-healing wounds with an average stay of 35 days (30).

CIANCI, in another series of 41 patients with very severe lesions (97 % were believed to have limb-threatening lesions and average Wagner score was 4), obtained a salvage rate of 78% with an average length of stay of 27 days. Twenty-six of thirty-one salvage patients have been followed for an average of 30 months and 92% of them remain ambulatory without further lesions. Two patients (8 %) have suffered below knee amputations (31).

Recently FAGLIA has evaluated HBO therapy in addition to comprehensive protocol in decreasing major amputation rate in a 70 diabetic patients. Thirty-five underwent HBO therapy and 33 received conventional treatment. In the treated group, three required major amputation (8.6 %) and 11 (33.3 %) in the non-treated group (p=0.016). The relative risk for the treated group was 0.26 (95 %) ci 0.08-0.94. The transcutaneous oxygen tension increased significantly in subjects treated with HBO. FAGLIA concluded to the protective role of HBO therapy (adds ratio 0.084) (32).

But in less severe wounds, HBO therapy seem to be effective. In 1997, ZAMBONI, in a prospective study, reported a significant improvement of healing. Ten insulin-dependent diabetic patients were referred for HBO therapy because of chronic lower extremity wounds and were compared to five-control patients during 7 weeks. At the end, significantly greater reduction in wound surface area was obtained (p<0.05) (33). Previously WEISZ in 1993 (34) could obtain complete healing with HBO therapy in 11/14 patients who presented chronic non-healing wounds without response to treatement for at least 3 months. Assessment of effectiveness included transcutaneous measurements of tissue PO_2 with elevation from 20 ± 10 mmHg during air breathing to 643 ± 242 mm Hg while breathing pure oxygen at 2.5 ATA (35). They were treated with HBO in 56 ± 10 consecutive HBO sessions. In 1990, WATTEL reported 75 % of healing rate if transcutaneous PO_2 values was 100 mm Hg in pure oxygen at 2.5 ATA. This data were confirmed by HART (36).

The impact of HBO therapy on infection is well know. DOCTOR in 1992 showed a quicker control of infection spread with 4 sessions of HBO therapy (37). Positive cultures decreased from initial 19 to 3 in study group as against from 16 to 12 in the control group (p<0.05) and amputation rate was significantly less; 2 against 7 in controls.

About economic aspect, the impact of HBO therapy is not negligible. Reduction of amputation rates, acceleration of healing may lead to reductive of length hospitalization stay. CIANCI reported that cost of wound required HBO therapy was less than primary amputations. But this data must be discussed if patients benefit from ambulatory treatment (30).

INDICATION OF HBO THERAPY IN DIABETIC FOOT ULCER

All diabetic foot ulcers do not need to be referred to HBO therapy (38). Previously, assessment of blood flow must be effected and transcutaneous PO_2 seems to be helpful.

At first, $TCPO_2$ level may select patients to HBO therapy or revascularization and detected patients who have elevation of $TCPO_2$ level with hyperbaric oxygen. If transcutaneous O_2 levels are low and unresponsive and revascularization not possible, the prognosis is very guarded.

For diabetic patients, foot ulcers are very often associated to chronic complications like coronary heart diseases, renal insufficiency, and retinopathy. These pathologies could be contra-indications to HBO therapy and must be evaluated before treatment.

CONCLUSION

Although multidisciplinary approach of diabetic foot ulcers impairs prognosis and reduces amputation rates, this strategy is inadequate for some patients. In diabetic foot ulcers, the causes of non-healing (ischemia, infection) may be corrected by hyperbaric oxygen. HBO therapy seems to be helpful in diabetic foot ulcers. Limb salvage, infection seem to be the main indications. If the cost is high, reduction of duration of healing and hospitalization stay are favorable compared to primary amputation cost. A good selection of patients by transcutaneous PO_2 measurement is absolutely necessary.

REFERENCES

1. Boulton AJM. The pathway to ulceration: aetiopathogenesis. In A. J. M. Boulton, H. Connor, P. R. Cavanagh. The foot in diabetes (second edition). Chichester, John Wiley and Sons: 1995: 37-48.
2. Reiber GE. The epidemiology of diabetic foot problems. Diabetic Med 1996; 13: S6 - s11.
3. Plummer ES., Albert SG. Focused assessment of foot care in older adults. J. Am. Geriatr. Soc. 1996; 44: 310 - 313.
4. Block P. The diabetic foot ulcer : a complex problem with a simple treatment approach. Milit, Med. 1981; 146 - 644.
5. Bild DE., Selby JV. Sinnock P., Browner WS., Braveman P., Showstack JA. Lower extremity amputation in people with diabetes. Epidemiology and prevention. Diabetes Care 1989; 13: 24- 31.
6. Fylling CP., Knighton DR. Amputation in the diabetic population: incidence, causes, cost treatment, and prevention. J. enterostom Ther. 1989; 16: 247 - 255.
7. Vaucher JP., Assal JP. Le pied diabétique et son traitement. Med Hyg 1981; 39: 1341 - 1346.
8. Halimi S., Benhamou PY., Charras H. Le coût du pied diabétique. Diabete Metab. 1993; 19: 518 - 522.
9. Van Houtum WH., Lavery LA., Harkless LB. The costs of diabetes-related lower extremity amputations in the Netherlands. Diabetic Med. 1995; 12: 777 - 781.
10. Ziegler- D. Diagnosis and management of peripheral neuropathy. Diabetic Med 1996; 13: S34-S38.
11. Caputo GM., Cavanagh PR., Ulbrecht JS., Gibbons GW., Karchmer AW. Assessment and management of foot disease in patients with diabetes. N Engl. J. Med. 1994; 331: 854 - 860.
12. Gilmore JE., Allen JA., Hayes JR. Autonomic function in neuropathic diabetic patients with foot ulceration. Diabetes Care. 1993; 16: 61 - 67.
13. Murray HJ., Boulton AJM. The pathophysiology of diabetic foot ulceration. The diabetic foot. Clinics in Podiat. Med. and Surg. 1995 ; 12, 1 : 1 - 17.
14. Tooke JE., Brash PD. Microvascular aspects of diabetic foot disease. Diabetic med. 1996 ; 13 : S26-S29.
15. Orchard TJ., Strandness DE. Assessment of peripherical vascular disease in diabetes ; report and recommendations of an international workshop sponsored by the American Heart Association and the American Diabetes Association. Diabetes Care. 1993 ; 16 : 1199-1209.
16. Matsuda A. Gangrene and ulcer of the lower extremities in diabetic patients. Diabetes Res. Clin. Pract. 1994 ; (supp 24) : 209 - 213.
17. Mc Nelly MJ., Boyko EJ., Ahroni JH., Stensel VL., Reiber GE., Smith DG. et al. The independent contributions of diabetic neuropathy and vasculopathy in foot ulceration. Diabetes care. 1995 ; 18 ; 2 : 216 - 219.
18. Ballard JL., Eke CC., Bunt TJ., Killeen JD. A prospective evaluation of transcutaneous oxygen measurements in the management of diabetic foot problems. J. Vasc. Surg. 1995 ; 22 : 485 - 492.
19. Gallacher SJ., Thomson G., Fraser WD., Fisher BM., Gemmell CG., Mac Cuish AC. Neutrophil Bactericidical Function in Diabetes Mellittus : evidence for association with blood glucose control. Diabetic Med. 1995 ; 12: 916 - 920.
20. Warren SJ. Treatment of lower extremity infections in diabetics. Drugs 1991 ; 42 : 984 - 996.
21. Larsson J., Apelqvist J., Agardh CD., Stentröm A. Decreasing incidence of major amputation in diabetic patients : a consequence of a multidisciplinary foot care team approach ? Diabetic Med. 1995 ; 12 : 770 - 776.
22. Wagner. The diabetic foot. Orthopedics. 1987 ; 10 : 163 - 172.
23. Levene CI., and al. The activation of protocollagen proline hdroxylation by ascorbic acid in cultured 3T6 fibroblasts. biochem biophys Acta. 1974 ; 338 - 29.
24. Davis JC. The use of adjuvant hyperbaric oxygen in treatment of the diabetic foot. Clin Podiatr Med Surg. 1987 ; 4 : 429 - 437.
25. Mader JT. and al. A mechanism for the amelioration by hyperbaric oxygen of experimental staphylococcal osteomyelitis in rabbits. J Infect Dis. 1980; 142: 915 - 922.
26. Mathieu D. and al. Erythrocyte filterability and hyperbaric oxygen therapy. Med Sub Hyperbar. 1984; 3: 100 - 104.
27. Nemiroff PM. Synergistic effects of pentoxifylline and hyperbaric oxygen on skin flaps. Arch. Otolaryngol. Head Neck Surg. 198 ; 114 977 - 981.
28. Baroni G. and al. Hyperbaric oxygen in diabetic gangrene treatment. Diabetes Care. 1987; 10: 81 - 86.
29. Oriani G. and al. Hyperbaric oxygen therapy in diabetic gangrene. J Hyperbar. Med. 1990; 5: 171 - 175.
30. Cianci P. and al. Salvage of the problem wound and potential amputation with wound care and adjunctive hyperbaric oxygen therapy ; an economic analysis. J Hyperbar. Med. 1988; 3: 97 - 101.
31. Cianci P. and al. Adjunctive hyperbaric oxygen in the salvage of the diabetic foot. Undersea Baromedical Res. 1991; 18(suppl): 109.
32. Faglia E. and al. Adjunctive systemic hyperbaric oxygen therapy in treatment of severe prevalently ischemic diabetic foot ulcer. A randomized study. Diabetes Care. 1996; 19: 1338 - 1343.
33. Zamboni WA. and al. Evaluation of hyperbaric oxygen for diabetic wounds: a prospective study. Undersea Hyperb Med. 1997; 24: 175 - 179.
34. Weisz G. and al. Treatment of the diabetic foot by hyperbaric oxygen. Harefuah. 1993; 124: 678 - 681 (abstract).
35. Wattel F., and al. Hyperbaric oxygen therapy in chronic vascular wound management. Angiology. 1990; 41: 59 - 65.
36. Hart GB. and al. Transcutaneous partial pressure of oxygen measured in a monoplace hyperbaric chamber at 1, 1.5, 2 atm abs oxygen. J Hyperbar. Med. 1990; 5: 223 - 229.
37. Doctor N and al. Hyperbaric oxygen therapy in diabetic foot. J Postgrad Med. 1992; 38: 112 - 114.
38. Williams RI. Hyperbaric oxygen therapy and the diabetic foot. J Am Podiatr. Med. Assoc. 1997; 87: 279 - 292.

ROLE OF HYPERBARIC OXYGEN IN THE TREATMENT OF DIABETIC FOOT LESIONS

Jörg Schmutz

Foundation for Hyperbaric Medicine, Kleinhüningerstrasse 177,

CH 4057 Basel-Switzerland

This paper is a review of the Medline® database on hyperbaric oxygenation (HBO), diabetic foot, and occlusive vascular disease.

When we review this literature it is obvious that amputation at any level is the most feared complication of the diabetic foot.

The concept of multidisciplinary approach to the diabetic foot has dramatically reduced the incidence of amputations in diabetic foot. Once the diabetic foot becomes ischemic, necrotic, and infected, the use of vascular procedures, surgery, or angioplasty with and without tissue transfer has improved treatment throughout the world. Our presentation, after a short explanation of the rationale existing for the use of HBO, is aimed to compare these results with those of HBO. We will also examine the outcome of the non-ischemic diabetic foot with and without HBO.

For this purpose, considering that this presentation should mainly serve as a review of the literature, we will largely rely on data shown in tables with only few comments.

RATIONALE FOR THE USE OF HBO

Chronic non-healing diabetic wounds are to some extent always hypoxic. The grade of hypoxia is further dependent on the status of the regional perfusion and the grade of infection. Hypoxic wounds are more susceptible to infection since the bacterial killing of macrophages is insufficient in the hypoxic environment. This is true for animals and humans so that many of the existing data rely on animal studies.

Several studies have shown that HBO is in the position to increase the tissue PO_2. Ackermann (1966) showed that HBO at 2 ATA increases the muscular PO_2 by a factor of 5.6. Hunt (1964) showed that the PO_2 of an infected non-ischemic wound is hypoxic and that it can be raised by a factor of more than 10 through HBO at 2 ATA.

The correction of tissue hypoxia is beneficial for wound infection and wound healing. Hohn (1976) showed that the killing ability of macrophages is increased twice when PO_2 is raised from hypoxic values to 150 mm Hg. Mader (1980), Mendel (1990), Knighton (1984, 1986) have confirmed these data. In a more complex ischemic hind model, Hall et al. (1966) produced full thickness foot wounds. On a total of 32 wounds, 84% of HBO treated versus 56% control healed, 6 control animals died, none of the HBO did. Diabetics have an increased susceptibility to infections which in part related to neutrophil dysfunction. Borer et al. (1997) found that after 2 weeks of HBO treatment the neutrophil adhesion and superoxide anion release capacity is restored for patients with diabetic foot.

There are many experimental data published between 1965 and 1985 showing that a PO_2 around 30-40 mm Hg is necessary to promote angiogenesis. Uhl et al. (1994) has reconfirmed all these data in an ischemic wound model. More recently, Angeles et al. (1997) have experimentally shown that there is an optimal oxygen dose for which endothelial cells begin to initiate wound healing. This value is located between 2.0 and 2.5 ATA at the tissue level. Renstra et al. (1998) showed that HBO stimulates the production of dermal fibroblast through an increase in the number of growth factor receptors. It seems to be true for young and old fibroblasts. This new insight into the mechanism of action of HBO could explain the synergistic effect found on wound healing when growth factors are applied together with HBO (Zhao et al., 1994; Wu et al., 1995). These results have been recently confirmed in an animal model of myocutaneous flap transplantation. In this study by Bayati-S. et al. (1998) the success of the transplants were best when growth factors were applied together with HBO. Finally Hammarlund et al. (1994), Zamboni et al. (1997) could clinically confirm the wound healing effect in one double-blind and one prospective study.

Besides its effect on infection control and wound healing, HBO also has valuable effects in the perioperative setting. There is a marked anti-edematous effect which has been mostly investigated in situations of reperfusion injuries and compartment syndrome. Zamboni (1993) showed that there is a leukocyte sludging in traumatized reperfused tissue which is responsible for tissular reperfusion injury. This mechanism, which is mediated by the expression of CD18 adhesion sites on the surface of the neutrophils is antagonized by HBO. This has been confirmed by Thom et al. (1993) using the reperfusion situation of CO poisoning.

This anti-edematous effect of HBO which can be of direct, practical interest to the surgeon dealing with diabetic foot, has been confirmed experimentally and clinically several times (Nylander et al., 1985; Strauss et al., 1983; Bartlett et al., 1998,; Bouachour et al., 1996).

TREATMENT OF THE ISCHEMIC DIABETIC FOOT

We will not discuss here the different types of wound care, dressing, systemic antibiotics, types of debridements. Our main purpose was to compare HBO with vascular procedures. The results of our survey are indicated in Table 1 and 2.

It is difficult to compare the studies within each table as well as between both tables. It can roughly be said that the surgical approach of the diabetic ischemic foot is fraught with a major amputation rate of roughly 9% to 23%. For the same category of patients, the adjunctive use of HBO produces a major amputation rate of 9% to 30% (The study by Davis having been published 11 years ago).

Up to this point, both treatment modalities seem to be equivalent with a slight advantage to surgery. This picture must however be put into perspective by the publication of four comparative studies. The first one, by Oriani et al. (1990) is a prospective, not randomized, controlled study which shows a statistically significant limb salvage with the adjunctive use of HBO. The second one, by Faglia et al. (1997), is a true prospective randomized study comparing the treatment of patients with severely ischemic diabetic gangrene with and without hyperbaric oxygen. This study shows a statistically highly significant advantage for HBO, independently of the amount of previous vascular procedures which were equally distributed among both study groups.

Another prospective, not randomized, comparative study (Zamboni, 1997) shows that HBO allows a faster healing of diabetic wounds, again independently of the amount of vascular surgeries or osteomyelitis.

The fourth study by Stone et al. (1995) is a retrospective one, and shows in a single major referral wound care center that limb salvage is clearly augmented by the adjunctive use of HBO, this despite a clinical presentation which was worse in the HBO group.

Patency of the operated vessels diminishes over time with values somewhere around 75% at 2 years and less than 50% at 3 years. On the other hand, Cianci (1993) showed a limb salvaging effect for HBO treated patients during 30 months. At this point, it can be said that HBO seems able to maintain its effects for a duration which compares with the expected duration of a vascular intervention.

A study by Reifsnyder et al. (1997) gives some better insight into the etiology of major amputation after vascular surgery. These authors analyzed 53 patients which had a major amputation after having had vascular reconstruction. Forty-nine percent of the bypasses were thrombosed, 34% had to be amputated despite of a patent bypass, and 8% had to be amputated because of a graft infection, while another 9% had a technical intra-operative problem.

All in all, our review shows that HBO is a potent adjunct in the treatment of the ischemic diabetic foot, and that it is able at least to complete the vascular approach of the ischemic diabetic foot patient. In case of wound healing failure after successful vascular surgery as well as in cases where vascular procedures are not feasible, HBO should also be considered before amputation is performed.

TREATMENT OF THE ISCHEMIC NON-DIABETIC FOOT

Here again, following the same procedures, we have listed the publications dealing with the treatment of this pathology in two tables (Table 3 and 4). One reason for this is the existing controversial issue regarding the concept of microangiopathy in diabetic foot. On the other hand, problems encountered in the treatment of a critical leg ischemia in non-diabetic patients are similar to those encountered in the ischemic diabetic foot. Treatment strategies are also aimed to a restoration of blood flow to the extremities. These strategies are completed with wound dressings, antibiotics, debridements, minor. As a consequence of this, some of the studies mentioned above like the one by Chang et al. (1996), Albereksten (1997), and Panayiotopoulos (1997) approach both patient categories in a similar way.

The data showed here especially for the HBO treated patients are less homogenous and less abundant compared to the ischemic diabetic foot. The amputation rate without HBO lies between 10% and 38% compared with 20% to 25% with HBO. Except for the study by Wattel et al. (1990), who recommend the strict integration of HBO in a comprehensive treatment scheme, data with HBO are older and not adjunctive to vascular surgery.

Patency of the grafts in Table 3 are similar to those of the diabetic foot and lie between 52% and 55% after 2 years. So again the benefit of vascular surgery is lost with time.

As a conclusion, our literature review seems to support the adjunctive use of HBO in the treatment of ischemic foot lesions if HBO is integrated in a multidisciplinary approach. Data are better for the ischemic diabetic foot than for the ischemic non-diabetic foot.

We will now examine the treatment of the osteomyelitic, non-ischemic diabetic foot. The results are presented in Table 5. We have no comparative data with HBO.

The treatment of diabetic foot without HBO, with and without conservative surgery allows a limb salvage rate of 13% to 25%. This is slightly more than the salvage rate achieved in the ischemic foot. Neuropathic pressure sores seem to heal only with strict pressure relief.

Many publications argue that the aggressive amputation of a toe or of a metatarsal bone with or without vascular intervention allows a fast, efficient, and cheap management of the problem. However, recent publications have shown that this idealized picture is far from perfect. The slightest resection of a single toe or part of a toe changes radically the status of the patient (Lavery, 1995), leading later to increased risk for more and more resections (Murdoch, 1997). There is a need for more conservative surgery in order to keep the patient's foot as intact as possible. In this setting HBO may prove to be a most valuable adjunct.

There is still an amputation burden on the non-infected diabetic foot. Controlled studies with the adjuvant use of HBO with or without growth factors seem warranted on the base of the sound experimental data as well as on the good clinical results achieved in the ischemic foot.

ECONOMICS OF THE DIABETIC FOOT

We have summarized here the financial results of our literature survey in Table 6 and 7. We have changed all data into US $ in order to allow an easier reading.

As a first remark it seems obvious that any real savings does not have to be studied in the context of hospital and/or treatment costs but rather in the context of percentage in limb salvage. Any treatment which would cost a little more than the actual state of the art but which would allow a better limb salvage is cheap and competitive.

When one tries to extrapolate the cost savings through HBO using the comparative data presented by Faglia et al. (1997) with the costs of Apelquist et al. (1995), we obtain an additional expense of US $266,000 (average of 38 HBO sessions for 35 patients). The total cost for the major and minor amputations would have been of US $1,088,000. In the group of patients which were not treated with HBO, the total cost for the major and minor amputations would have been of US $1,211,200.

The total costs would have been US $1,354,000 for the HBO patients and US $1,211,200 for the patients treated without HBO. Related to the number of patients in each group, the cost per patient were US $31,085 in the HBO group and US $36,703 in the group without HBO.

Our calculation should be completed by the hospital costs for both groups. In Faglia's study, though data are statistically not different, they have a definite financial impact. The average hospital stay in the group of patients not treated with HBO was seven days longer (16%) than for those treated with HBO. There are no data in the study of Apelquist et al. (1995) to quantify these extra costs.

SUMMARY

Our review shows that HBO is a valuable adjunct to the actual multidisciplinary treatment of the ischemic diabetic foot. It completes quite favorably the comprehensive treatment of the patient in allowing a statistically significant savings in major amputations and in social costs in th European setting.

There is a further potential for similar outcome improvement in the non-ischemic diabetic foot. Further research with the use of other new technologies like growths factors should be stimulated (Williams et al., 1998).

Table 1: Outcome of ischemic diabetic foot without HBO

Author	Patients	Selection	Aim of Study	Treatment	Methodology	Patency bypass	Amputation	Follow-up	Remarks
Bunt/96 USA	14 90	14 TcPO$_2$>30 90 TcPO$_2$>30	Assess prognostic value of TcPO$_2$	amputation 22 no revascular. 67 revascularization	Prospective		9% healing failure 50% healing failure 9% healing failure		TcPO$_2$ helps direct therapy
Serletti/95 USA	30	Documented PVD	Assess revasc + free tissue transfer	revasc + free tissue transfer	Retrospective		8 (27%) amputated	22 months	
Alberektsen/97 Denmark	46 PVD 43 PVD+ diabetes	Gangrene	Assess healing	Revasc: open Revasc: failed (?)	Retrospective		1 major amp. 4 (80%) major amp.		
Panayiotopoulos /97 UK	71 PVD 38 PVD+ diabetes	Ischemic limbs	Assess cost and outcome of PVD with/without diabetes	Revascularization	Prospective	38% 47%	24% BK amp. 55% limb amp. 28% BK amp. 44% limb amp.	36 months	No statistical difference between diabetics and non diabetics
Chang/96 USA	849 PVD 125 PVD + infection + diabetes	Ischemic limbs	Assess expeditious management	Revascularization	Retrospective		111 (11%) partial foot		
Mohan/96 USA	32	Non-healing, gangrene	Assess revascularization	Revascularization	Prospective	75%	3 occlusion 2 major amp. (9%) 3 major amp. (9%) with patent bypass 2 late major amp. (7%)	24 months	Chronic renal failure, poor foot circulation = poor outcome
Ballard/95 USA	55 (66 limbs)	TcPO$_2$ > 30 TcPO$_2$< 30	Assess treatment	Debridement, minor amp. Revascularization	Prospective		24% failure 17% failure	Wound healing or no rest pain	

Table 1: Outcome of ischemic diabetic foot without HBO (continued)

Author	Patients	Selection	Aim of Study	Treatment	Methodology	Patency bypass	Amputation	Follow-up	Remarks
Weaver/96 USA	35	Extensive forefoot ischemia	Assess Syme amputation	Revascularization Syme amputation	Prospective		14% healing failure after revascularization 23% healing failure without revascularization	42 months	
Faglia/96 Italy	26	PVD	Assess effect angioplasty	As indicated			15% failure	12 months	
Larsson/95 Sweden	187 (171 PVD)	Amputees	Assess clinical characteristics in relation to amputation	As needed	Prospective		25 (13%) no healing of stump 88 (47%) above ankle 74 (39%) below ankle	Until healing or death	
Castronuovo/97 USA	53 PVD	Limb ischemia	Assess skin perfusion pressure as therapeutic and outcome predictor	Revascularization No revascularization					
Barbano/95 Italy	89	80 PVD, 68 Wagner 4	Assess vasc. reconstruction	17 fem-dist bypass 13 ileo-femor PTA Overall	Retrospective		4 (23%) major amp 3 (23%) major amp 55 toes 12 transmetatarsal 12 legs 5 thigh 5 atypical	Healing or amputation	
Mills/91 USA	55	Localized gangrene/ forefoot infection	Assess delayed treatment	As indicated/33 Bypass	Retrospective		29% amputations	24 months	Delay in 16 patients (29%) worse amp. In 6 (11%) patients

Table 2: Outcome of ischemic diabetic foot with HBO

Author	Patients	Selection	Aim of Study	Treatment	Methodology	HBO	Amputation	Follow-up
Strauss/98 USA	144	Problem wound	TcPO$_2$ as outcome predictor	As needed	Retrospective	2.0 ATA Mono	12.5%	Healing/ Amputation
Mathieu/97 France	29	Critical limb ischemia	TcPO$_2$ and laser Doppler flowmetry as outcome predicters	As needed	Prospective	2.4 ATA	20%	Healing/ Amputation
Faglia/97 Italy	35 + HBO 33 no HBO	Critical limb ischemia	Assess HBO	As needed vascular procedures	Prospective, randomized	2.4-2.8 ATA	8.6% major 33.3% major	
Cianci/88 USA	13	Critical limb ischemia	Assess HBO	As needed	Retrospective	2.0 ATA Mono	15% major	One year
Wattel/91 France	59	None	TcPO$_2$ as outcome predictor	As needed	Prospective	2.4 ATA	11% major	
Oriani/90 Italy	62+ HBO 18 no HBO	None	Assess HBO	As needed	Retrospective	2.4 2.8 ATA	5% major 33% major	
Baroni/87 Italy	18+ HBO 10 no HBO	None	Assess HBO	As needed	Retrospective	2.4-2.8 ATA	11% major 40% major	

Table 2: Outcome of ischemic diabetic foot with HBO (continued)

Author	Country	Patients	Selection	Aim of study	Treatment	HBO	Methods	Amputation	Follow-up
Davis/87	USA	168	None	Assess HBO	As needed, no vascular procedure	2.4 ATA	Retrospective	30% major, most old pat. with periph. Vasc. Dis.	
Zamboni/97	USA	10	Wound ischemia	Assess HBO	As needed, no vascular procedure	2.0 ATA	Prospective	Significant better wound healing	4-6 months
Cianci/93	USA	40	Wound ischemia Wagner 4	Assess HBO	As needed, 50% had vascular procedure	40, 2.0 ATA	Retrospective	7 (22%)	30 (12-84) months
Stone/95	USA	87 with HBO 382 no HBO	Consecutive patients	Assess HBO	As needed	19 ± 13	Retrospective	28% with HBO 53% w/out HBO	Unknown
Watel/95	France	40 HBO 50 lesions	No healing > 6 weeks, no surgery possible	Assess TcPO2 as outcome predictor	As needed	2.5 ATA BID, 90'	Prospective	10% in patients, 72% in wounds	Unknown

Table 3: Outcome of ischemic foot without HBO

Author	Patients (limbs)	Selection	Aim of Study	Treatment	Methodology	Amputation	Amputation	Follow-up	Remarks
Leseche/97 France	25	Critical ischemia	Assess allografts	Bypass	Prospective	22%	52%	2 years	Risk of postanastomotic stenosis
Konradsen/00 Denmark	39 (34)	Csystolic blood pressure < 30	Assess revascularization	Arterial reconstruction	Retrospective	10% amputation, 70% ulcer healing	90%	1 year	Without surgery 70% amputation
Eckstein/96 Germany	56	Limb threatening ischemia	Assess pedal revascularization	Auto/allograft	Restrospective	37% amputations	55%	0-112 months (median 25)	
Lofberg/96 Sweden	82 (86)	Chronic critical limb ischemia	Assess b-k percutaneous transluminal angioplasty	Angioplasty	Prospective	38% amputations	?	36 months	

Table 4: Outcome of ischemic foot with HBO

Author	Patients	Selection	Aim of Study	Treatment	Methodology	HBO	Amputation	Follow-up
Uryama/87 Japan	10+HBO+PGE+ sympathectomy 21+ PGE+ sympathectomy	Ischemic ulcers	Assess combined treatment HBO	Vascular surgery not indicated	Retrospective	3 ATA	80% complete or partial healing: 52% complete or partial healing	Unkown
Sakakibara/84 Japan	106 TAO 43 PVD	Ischemic ulcers with failure of previous vascular surgery	Assess HBO	As needed	Retrospective	30 times 2 ATA, 50, 75', QID	79% complete or partial healing 81% complete or partial healing	Unknown, Long!
Wattel/90 France	20 (9 PVD 11 diabetes)	Non healing wound	Assess TcPO$_2$ as outcome predictor	As needed	Retrospective	46 times 2.5 ATA, 90' QID-BID	75% healing	Unknown

Table 5: Treatment of the non-ischemic diabetic wound without HBO

Author	Patients (limbs)	Selection	Aim of Study	Treatment	Methodology	Amputation	Follow-up	Remarks
Ha-Van/96 France	64	No ischemia, osteomyelitis	Compare surgery and medical treatment	32 medical treatment 32 conservative surgery	Retrospective	18 (57%) healing 25 (78%) healing	?	
Venkatesan/97 UK	22	No ischemia	Assess conservative treatment	12 weeks antibiotics (5-72)	Retrospective	4 (18%) amputation 1 recurrence	27 months	surgery not needed
Lipsky/97 USA	108	88 soft tissue infection 20 osteomyelitis	Compare two antibiotics	ofloxacin versus ampicillin/ sulbactam	Prospective, multicentric	14 amputations at unkown level (13%)	unknown	infected bone had to be removed
Chantelau/96 Germany	39	Neuropathic, Wagner 1-2	Assess effect of antibiotics	Dressings with or without antibiotics	Double-blind	50% placebo healed 31% antibiotics healed	20 days	
Steed/96 USA	118	No ischemia	Assess topical growth factors	Debridements growth factors placebo	Double-blind	better healing with frequent debridements 48% healed 25% healed		
Murdoch/97 USA	90	Great-toe and 1st ray amputees	Assess reamputation history	As needed	Retrospective	60% 2nd amp 21% 3rd amp 7% 4th amp 17% b-k amp	5-15 years	Average time to 2nd amputation is 10 months

Table 6: Cost of diabetic foot without HBO

Author	Land	Patients	Criteria					Method	Follow-up
Apelqvist/95	Sweden	274	Healing no ischemia	Healing ischemia	Min. amp	Maj. amp.	social costs	retro	3 years
			16'100 $	26'700 $	43'100 $	63'100 $	Included		
Bouter/93	Netherlands	6'497	No criteria				social costs	retro	2 years
			10'152 ECU (US $ 11'100)				excluded		
Thompson/93	New Zealand	357	Hospital	Hospital + out patient			social costs	retro	Annual/?
			12'500 $	600'000 $			excluded		
Apelqvist/93	Sweden	314	Primary healing	Amputation			social costs	retro	Healing/ death
			51'000 SEK (3'000-808'000) or 6362 US $ (374-127'004)	344'000 SEK (27'000-992'000) or 42915 US $ (3'368-123'754)			excluded		
Panayiotopoulos/97	UK	104	33 Diabetics	71 Non diabetics			social costs	prosp	Healing/ death
			£ 9181 (US $ 15'209)	£ 6'350 (US $ 10'519)			excluded		
Halimi/93	France	60'000	No criteria				social costs		Statistical estimation
			11'667 $				?		

Table 7: Cost of diabetic foot with HBO

Author	Land	Patients	Criteria		Method	Follow-up
Cianci/93	USA	39	Ischemia Wagner 4 hospital cost 32'300 $	Ischemia Wagner 4 HBO cost 16'000 $	Retrospective	30 (12-84) months

REFERENCES

1.   Ackerman NB et al. Oxygen tensions in normal and ischemic tissues during hyperbaric therapy. Studies in rabbit. JAMA. 1966; 198: 1280-3.
2.   Albrektsen-SB et al. Minor amputations on the feet after revascularization for gangrene. A consecutive series of 95 limbs. Acta-Orthop-Scand. 1997; 68 : 291-3.
3.   Angeles A et al. Hyperbaric oxygen and angiogenesis. Undersea & Hyperbaric Medicine, 1997; 24: Supp. 31.
4.   Apelqvist et al. Long-term costs for foot ulcers in diabetic patients in a multidisciplinary setting. Foot-Ankle-Int. 1995; 16 : 388-94 ISSN: 1071-1007.
5.   Apelqvist-J et al. Diabetic foot ulcers in a multidisciplinary setting. An economic analysis of primary healing and healing with amputation. J-Intern-Med. 1994; 235 : 463-71.
6.   Ballard-JL et al. A prospective evaluation of transcutaneous oxygen measurements in the management of diabetic foot problems. J-Vasc-Surg. 1995; 22 : 485-90; discussion 490-2.
7.   Barbano-PR et al. Risultati della rivascolarizzazione ed amputazione nella gangrena diabetica del piede. Importanza dell'approccio multidisciplinare. [Results of revascularization and amputation of the gangrenous diabetic foot. Importance of a multidisciplinary approach]. Minerva-Cardioangiol. 1995; 43 : 97-104.
8.   Baroni et al. Hyperbaric oxygen treatment in diabetic gangrene. Diabetes care. 1987. 10 : 81-6.
9.   Bartlett et al. Rabbit model of the use of fasciotomy and hyperbaric oxygenation in the treatment of compartment syndrome. Undersea & Hyperbaric Medicine. 1998, 25 Suppl. 77.
10. Bayati-S et al. Stimulation of angiogenesis to improve the viability of prefabricated flaps. Plast-Reconstr-Surg. 1998; 101 : 1290-5.
11. Borer RC et al. Neutrophil adhesion and superoxide anion release in diabetic patients treated with hyperbaric oxygen. Undersea & Hyperbaric Medicine. 1997; 24 : 15.
12. Bouachour G et al. Hyperbaric oxygen Therapy in the management of crush injuries: a double-blind placebo-controlled clinical trial. J. Trauma. 1996; 41 : 333-9.
13. Bouter KP et al. The diabetic foot in Dutch hospitals: epidemiological features and clinical outcome. Eur J Med. 1993; 2 : 215-8.
14. Bunt-TJ & Holloway-GA. TcPO2 as an accurate predictor of therapy in limb salvage. Ann-Vasc-Surg. 1996 May; 10 : 224-7.
15. Castronuovo-JJ et al. Skin perfusion pressure measurement is valuable in the diagnosis of critical limb ischemia. J-Vasc-Surg. 1997 ; 26 : 629-37.
16. Chang-BB et al. Expeditious management of ischemic invasive foot infections. Cardiovasc-Surg. 1996; 4 : 792-5.
17. Chantelau E et al. Antibiotic treatment for uncomplicated neuropathic forefoot ulcers in diabetes: a controlled trial. Diabet Med. 1996; 13: 156-9.
18. Cianci P et al. Salvage of the difficult wound/potential amputation in the diabetic patient. In DJ Bakker & J. Schmutz. Proceedings 2. European Conf. Hyp. Med. 1988. 77-87.
19. Davis-JC. The use of adjuvant hyperbaric oxygen in treatment of the diabetic foot. Clin-Podiatr-Med-Surg. 1987 Apr; 4 : 429-37.
20. Eckstein HH et al. Pedal bypass for limb threatening ischaemia an 11 year review. Br J Surg. 1996; 83 : 1554-7.
21. Faglia-E et al. Adjunctive systemic hyperbaric oxygen therapy in treatment of severe prevalently ischemic diabetic foot ulcer. A randomized study. Diabetes-Care. 1996 Dec; 19 : 1338-43.
22. Halimi-S et al. [Cost of the diabetic foot]. Le cout du pied diabetique. Diabete-Metab. 1993 Dec; 19 : 518-22.
23. Hammarlund et al. Hyperbaric oxygen reduced size of chronic leg ulcers: a randomized double-blind study. Plast Reconstr Surg. 1994; 93 : 829-33.
24. Hart GB & M Strauss. Responses of ischemic ulcerative conditions to OHP. In Smith Ed. 1st Int. Congress on Hyperbaric Medicine. Aberdeen Univ. Press. Aberdeen. 1979, 312-4.
25. Ha van G et al. Treatment of osteomyelitis in the diabetic foot. Contribution of conservative surgery. Diabetes care. 1996; 19 : 157-60.
26. Hohn DC et al. Effect of O2 tension on microbicidal function of leucocytes in wounds and in vitro. Surg Forum. 1976; 27: 18-20.
27. Hunt TK. A new method of determining tissue oxygen tensions, Lancet. 1964; 2 : 1370-1.
28. Knighton DR et al. Oxygen as an antibiotic: the effect of inspired oxygen on infection. Arch Surg. 1984; 119: 199-204.
29. Knighton DR et al. Oxygen as an antibiotic: a comparison of the effects of inspired oxygen concentration and antibiotic administration on in-vivo bacterial clearance. Arch Surg. 1986; 121: 191-5.
30. Konradsen L et al. Chronic critical limb ischemia must include leg ulcers. Eur J Vasc Endovasc Surg. 1996; 11 : 74-7.
31. Lavery LA et al. Increased foot pressures after great toe amputation in diabetes. Diabetes care. 1995, 18 : 1460-2.
32. Lee-SS et al. Hyperbaric oxygen in the treatment of diabetic foot infection. Chang-Keng-I-Hsueh. 1997 Mar; 20 : 17-22.
33. Leseche G et al. Femorodistal bypass using cryopreserved venous allografts for limb salvage. Ann Vasc Surg. 1997 : 11 : 260-6.
34. Lipsky BA et al. Antibiotic therapy for diabetic foot infections: comparison of two parenteral to oral regimens. Clin Infect Dis. 1997; 24 : 643.8.
35. Lofberg AM et al. The use of below-knee percutaneous transluminal angioplasty in arterial occlusive disease causing chronic critical limb ischemia. Cardiovasc Intervent Radiol. 1996; 19 : 317-22.

36. Mathieu et al. Comparison of laser doppler flowmetry and transcutaneous oxygen pressure for prediction of healing in diabetic foot lesions treated by HBO2. Undersea & Hyperbaric Medicine. 1997; 24 : 15.

37. Mendel V et al. Hyperbaric oxygenation- its effect on experimental chronic osteomyelitis in rats. Proc. 2nd Europ. conf. clinical Medicine. Ed. D. D Bakker, J. Schmutz. 1988. 77-85. ISBN: 3-908229-01-4.

38. Mills-JL et al. The diabetic foot: consequences of delayed treatment and referral. South-Med-J. 1991; 84 : 970-4.

39. Mohan-CR et al. Revascularization of the ischemic diabetic foot using popliteal artery inflow. Int-Angiol. 1996; 15.

40. Murdoch DP et al. The natural history of great toe amputation. J Foot Ankle Surg. 1997 36, 204-8, discussion 256.

41. Nylander G et al. Reduction of post-ischemic edema with hyperbaric oxygen. Plast Reconstr Surg. 1985; 76: 596-601.

42. Oriani G et al. Hyperbaric oxygen therapy in diabetic gangrene. J Hyperbaric Medicine. 1990; 5. 171-5.

43. Oriani G et al. Oxygen Therapy and diabetic gangrene: A review of 10 year's experience. 1992. Proc. XVIIIth annual meeting. European Undersea Baromedical Society. Ed. J. Schmutz & J. Wendling. 178-81.

44. Panayiotopoulos-Yp et al. Results and cost analysis of distal [crural/pedal] arterial revascularization for limb salvage in diabetic and non-diabetic patients. Diabet-Med. 1997 Mar; 14 : 214-20.

45. Pinzur-Mset al. Benchmark analysis on diabetics at high risk for lower extremity amputation. Foot-Ankle-Int. 1996 Nov; 17 : 695-700.

46. Reenstra et al. Hyperbaric oxygen increases human dermal fibroblast expression of EGF-receptors. Undersea & Hyperbaric Medicine. 1998; 25 : 166.

47. Reifsnyder T et al. Limb loss after lower extremity bypass. Am J Surg. 1997; 174 : 149-51.

48. Sakakibara K et al. The role of hyperbaric oxygen therapy in the salvage of ischemic limbs from inevitable amputation in chronic peripheral vascular disease - with particular reference to those having had unsuccessful surgery. Proc 8th Int Cong. Hyperbaric Medicine. Ed. EP. Kindwall. Best Pub. 1984, 223-8.

49. Serletti-JM et al. Atherosclerosis of the lower extremity and free-tissue reconstruction for limb salvage. Plast-Reconstr-Surg. 1995; 96 : 1136-44.

50. Steed DL et al. Effect of extensive debridement and treatment on the healing of diabetic foot ulcers. Diabetic Ulcer Study Group. J Am Coll Surg. 1996; 183 : 61-4.

51. Stone J et al. Diabetes, 1995, 44, 1.

52. Strauss MB et al. Reduction of skeletal muscle necrosis using intermittent hyperbaric oxygen in a model compartment syndrome. J Bone Joint Surg. 1983; 65-A: 656-62.

53. Strauss MB et al. The predictability of transcutaneous oxygen measurements for wound healing. Undersea & Hyperbaric Medicine. 1998; 25 : 24.

54. Urayama H et al. Hyperbaric oxygenation to ischemic ulcers in combination with sympathetic denervation and PGE1 Infusion. Proc. 9th Int. Symposium Underwater Hyperbaric Physiol. Ed. Undersea Hyperbaric Medical Soc. Bethesda. 1987, 839-45.

55. Thom SR. Functional inhibition of leukocyte B2 integrins by hyperbaric oxygen in carbon monoxide-mediated brain injury. Tox Applied Pharmacol. 1993; 123: 248-56.

56. Thompson C et al. Importance of diabetic foot admissions at Middlemore hospital. N Z Med J. 1993; 106(995): 178-80.

57. Venkatesan P. Conservative management of osteomyelitis in the feet of diabetic patients. Diabet Med. 1997; 16 : 487-90.

58. Vezzani-G et al. [Non-surgical treatment of peripheral vascular diseases: diabetic foot and hyperbaric oxygenation]. Trattamento non chirurgico delle vasculopatie periferiche: piede diabetico ed ossigenoterapia iperbarica. Minerva-Anestesiol. 1992 Oct; 58 : 1119-20.

59. Wattel F et al. Hyperbaric oxygen in chronic vascular wound management. Angiology. 1990; 42: 59-65.

60. Wattel F et al. Hyperbaric oxygen in the treatment of diabetic foot lesions. Search for healing predictive factors. J Hyperbaric Medicine. 1991; 6 : 263-8.

61. Weisz-G et al. [Treatment of the diabetic foot by hyperbaric oxygen] Harefuah. 1993 Jun 1; 124 : 678-81, 740.

62. Williams-RL et al. Wound healing. New modalities for a new millennium. Clin-Podiatr-Med-Surg. 1998 Jan; 15 : 117-28.

63. Wu-L et al. Effects of oxygen on wound responses to growth factors: Kaposi's FGF, but not basic FGF stimulates repair in ischemic wounds. Growth-Factors. 1995; 12 : 29-35.

64. Zamboni-WA et al. Evaluation of hyperbaric oxygen for diabetic wounds: a prospective study. Undersea-Hyperb-Med. 1997 Sep; 24 : 175-9.

65. Zamboni et al. Morphological analysis of the microcirculation during reperfusion of ischemic skeletal muscle and the effect of hyperbaric oxygen. Plast Reconstr Surg. 1993; 91 : 1110-23.

66. Zhao-LL et al. Effect of hyperbaric oxygen and growth factors on rabbit ear ischemic ulcers. Arch-Surg. 1994 Oct; 129 : 1043-9.

NOTES

EXPERT REPORTS
Incidence and cost of foot lesions in diabetic patients

Jan Apelqvist

Department of Internal Medicine—University Hospital, Lund, Sweden

The diabetic foot can be defined as conditions including infection, ulceration, and destruction of deep tissues associated with neurological abnormalities and peripheral vascular disease in the lower limb. Approximately 40–60 % of all amputations in the lower leg are performed in patients with diabetes. The number of population-based studies is limited. In most studies the incidence is reported as the number of amputations per 100 000 inhabitants per year and has been estimated to be 7–206. The best way to describe the incidence of amputation regarding diabetes would be to describe the number of primary amputations per 1000 diabetic patients/year. This is usually not possible since the true prevalence of diabetes is not known. The difference in incidence is in many cases explained by design, demographic factors, prevalence of diabetes, variations in registration system, and different reimbursement of various procedures. Considering these factors the most common incidence of diabetes related amputations is between 5–24/100 000 inhabitants/year or 6–8/1000 diabetic subjects a year.

In most reports, both the number of amputations and the diagnosis of diabetes are underestimated. In a study in southern Sweden, a continuous registration of all amputation was performed and compared with official inpatient register during the period 1982–1993. Sixty-three percent of all amputation procedures performed in the lower extremity were found in official register. Only 36% of the diabetes-related amputations were noted in the official register. This finding is in agreement with other reports. In western countries 15–19% of all diabetic patients undergoing amputation are diagnosed only at the time of amputation. Diabetic patients more frequently have below-ankle amputations than non-diabetic patients. As a consequence, studies that primarily focus on above ankle amputations do underestimate the total number of diabetes-related amputations.

Of the diabetic-related amputations, 70–90% are preceded with a foot ulcer. Foot ulcers in diabetes are related to delayed healing, infection, and gangrene. In most cases amputation has to be performed because of deep infection and/or ischemia alone or in combination. The most common indications described in the literature have been gangrene, infection, and a non-healing ulcer. Although frequently reported, a non-healing ulcer should not be considered an indication for amputation.

The prevalence of foot ulcer in developed countries has been estimated to approximately 4–10% of diabetic individuals. A corresponding incidence of 2,2–5,9% has been reported. It has to be recognised that most of these data are based on cross-sectional studies of selected patient populations mainly of diabetic subjects below 50 years of age. In a study focused on younger diabetic subjects of type I or type II diabetes, the prevalence of foot ulcer has been estimated to 1,7–3,3%, compared to 5–10% where a majority of patients are older or of type II diabetes. It is reasonable to believe that a substantial underestimation of the prevalence of foot ulcer exists. This was verified in a population-based study including 90% of all diabetic subjects about 25 years of age in 6 primary health-care districts in southern Sweden, where 47% of all foot ulcers were not known to either foot care team or physician. The importance of that finding is further emphasised by the reality that only 25–50% of diabetic subjects do get regular foot inspections.

Numerous factors have been suggested to be related to the development of foot ulcer. There is a general agreement that the most important risk factor for development of foot ulcer is presence of peripheral sensimotor neuropathy. The estimated prevalence of peripheral neuropathy varies from 20–70%, depending on studied population, definitions and diagnostic criteria. Of foot ulcers described in cross-sectional studies, 80–90% were precipitated by external trauma, usually improper shoes. However it has to be recognised that foot ulcers in diabetes are a heterogeneous composition of different kinds of ulcer with different type and site with regard to predisposing cause. A strong relation has been established between abnormal foot pressure and incidence of plantar ulcerations, i.e., stress ulcer. This pressure causes tissue damages, initially as blister, haemorragia, minor skin injury, and later callus formation. If this condition continues without proper protection, an ulcer develops with a high probability for foot infection. In the above mentioned cross-sectional studies the proportion purely in neuropathic lesion, neuro-ischemic lesions, and purely ischemic lesions varied extensively. Approximately 70–100% of ulcers had signs of peripheral neuropathy with various degree of peripheral vascular disease. Healing rates of foot ulcers are unknown with exception of excellence where it is between 80–90%. However the outcome is strongly related to type, site and cause of ulcer. Key factors being infection ischemia, pressure relief, and wound management. There is a complexity of factors related to outcome of foot ulcer in patients with diabetes, and the importance of evaluating these factors is well recognised. A multidisciplinary approach that includes prevention, patient and staff education, and a multifactorial treatment of foot ulcer has been reported to reduce amputation rates by 49–85%.

The diabetic foot is related to high cost to the society due to delayed healing, high risk for lower extremity amputations, and disability. The recent year several reports have focused on the economic impact of prevention and treatment of diabetic foot. There are, however, few studies in which an evaluation and a comparison of cost effectiveness of different alternatives have been considered. Different measures to prevent foot ulcers and amputations have been discussed such as use of protective footwear, patient and staff education, and preventive foot care. The cost effectiveness of these strategies has been studied but convincing results for each type of prevention has not yet been shown. It has been claimed that prevention will reduce cost due to a decrease in amputation rates, but to show cost effectiveness of reduction in cost for amputation must be compared with relation to the additional cost for prevention. The difficulty regarding this kind of cost-effectiveness studies regarding prevention is probably related to difficulties of isolating one specific strategy in relation to other preventive measures, lack of population based data and adequate follow-up time, and problems regarding the recurrence rate of ulcer and patient compliance. The cost effectiveness of a screening and foot protection program, including chiropody services and prescription of protective foot wear for diabetic patients who were judged to be at high risk for foot ulceration and treatment of established lesions, has recently been shown (McCabe 1998). In that study the total additional cost for the prevention program were lower than the estimated cost for those major amputations that averted to the program.

Another type of strategy to avoid amputations in high-risk individuals such as a patient with a foot ulcer is a multidisciplinary treatment. Such secondary prevention is the establishment of diabetic foot-care teams for management of foot ulcer. The cost for treatment of diabetic foot ulcers are high both in patients where primary healing is achieved and when amputations are performed. Costs are high both in the short run, defined as the time until healing has been obtained, and in a long term when cost for prevention and treatment of new and recurrent ulcers are included, as well as costs associated with disability from previous amputations. The long-term disability cost concerns changes in living conditions, home care, and social service. Comparisons between results from different reports must be interpreted with caution because these studies have been performed using different methodology, variation in settings and patient selection, in countries with different organisation and financing of health care, and with different policies regarding prevention and treatment. In many cases not all authors have mentioned from what year the costs have been calculated. The variation regarding which costs are included in the evaluation is also large.

The total cost for healing of a foot ulcer is strongly linked to the type of lesion. In a study examining cost of primary healing compared with those of amputation, the average total cost for patients whose ulcer healed primarily was SEK 51 000 (GB£ 5100) in 1990 currency, corresponding to 61 000 in 1996. The average total cost for patients who underwent an amputation was SEK 344 000 (1990) corresponding to 418 000 (1996). Since this was not a randomised study the patients in the two groups were not completely comparable regarding background variables, such as type of lesions. In estimating the cost for ulcer healing it is important to reflect on the severity of the ulcer.

Several reports have focused on the high cost of amputation. Amputation in these studies has been considered costly as a result of its consequences rather than the cost of the surgical procedure itself. This is one of the reasons why it is essential to follow the patient with regard to the use of resources until a specific point, such as complete healing, or defined time period should be equally long for all patients. One of the most important actions to reduce costs and achieve cost effectiveness in the management of the diabetic foot is to avoid amputations. Apart from the monetary cost the consequences on the quality of life also has to be considered.

An attempt to estimate and describe the expected economic consequences of an optimal preventable foot ulcer in the diabetic population in Sweden has recently been presented. The yearly cost of prevention was estimated to approximately SEK 500 million in 1996 prices. This prevention included inspection of feet and footwear, foot care and protective shoes for high-risk cases. The cost for this and multidisciplinary foot care teams for patients with foot ulcer were estimated. The total cost for management of the diabetic foot were estimated to SEK 1,200 000 000–2,400 000 000 (based on a foot ulcer prevalence of 3 vs. 8 %). If the number of amputations in diabetic patients could be reduced by 50% with these secondary and primary preventive measures the cost for amputation could be lowered with about SEK 400 millions annually. In Sweden the annual diabetes-related amputations are estimated at 1400, compared to the USA with 54 000.

A reason why reports mainly are concentrated on investigating the cost only for treatment of diabetic foot ulcers, without a complete health economic evaluation, is that the cost for many therapies and treatment strategies are still unknown. Due to the complexity of treating these patients, the resource use and costs associated with different options some times have to be examined before controlled comparative studies for health economic evaluation can be designed. In many cases randomisations are not ethically feasible.

One of these controversies is the cost for treatment of patients with diabetes mellitus and critical ischemia with regard to vascular surgery vs. primary major amputation. Some studies have reported that successful revascularisation results in lower short-term hospitalisation cost than primary amputation. Conflicting results has been reported by other authors, who argue that costs might possibly be saved by performing a primary amputation and thus avoiding long and fruitless courses of reconstructive surgery. Other studies have reported that the cost of an amputation was similar to that of vascular reconstruction, but that high cost after surgery in patients undergoing major amputation was related to an increased need for home-care and social service support. Therefore, in an economic analysis long-term follow up of patients who have undergone vascular surgery or amputation, it is required to evaluate the total costs of repeated vascular surgery, amputation, home care, social service, support, and death. The current controversy regarding costs concerns the number of unsuccessful reconstructive procedures after which patients have to undergo an amputation, whereas it is feasible to claim that a successful vascular reconstruction will be related to lower costs due to decreased need of home-care and social service. The conclusion regarding choice between revascularisation and primary amputation should not be cost, but the possibility to save a leg from major amputation.

Another controversy is the choice between aggressive systematic anti-microbial treatment of foot infections combined with incision and drainage vs. an early amputation. The discrepancies between different studies in that area are that the studies are performed from different perspectives. Most authors who argue for an early amputation because of its association with decreased costs do not seem to consider the consequences after surgery and the need for the patient for further treatment until healing is achieved, often in other clinics, which also implies further costs. A cost-effective analysis of different treatment alternatives for foot infections in patients with diabetes mellitus who did not have systemic infection showed that the least expensive strategy was a long course of oral antibacterial therapy following initial hospitalisation for surgical debridement. The most expensive strategy was immediate amputation. Other authors have argued that an early major amputation in patients with foot infections were and who unlikely candidates for arterial reconstruction, would prevent delay in rehabilitation, resulting in decreased long term morbidity and reduced health-care costs. An argument for early digit amputation in the case of deep infection has been that the cost would be reduced. The choice between immediate amputation or conservative treatment should not be based on the cost of antibacterial treatment, since in a Swedish study the costs for antibacterial agents in relation to total costs varied between 1–2% depending of type of ulcer. In the case of infection the choice between anti-microbial treatment combined with incision and drainage or early amputation should be based on the possibility of saving the limb and avoiding a major amputation. The cost effectiveness and the importance of non-invasive investigations in patients with suspected osteomyelitis is controversial.

Both regarding discussion of vascular surgery and treatment of deep infections, the influence of patient quality of life has to be considered.

The number of health-economic evaluations of topical treatment of foot ulcers is limited. One reason is probably due to difficulties in comparing treatment alternatives until a defined endpoint such as complete healing. Another reason is likely due to the long healing time for foot ulcer and problems in registering the resource used during that time. Some of these problems are previously described and discussed. The cost of topical treatment has gotten increasing interest, especially after the introduction of new topical agents such as growth factors and a tissue engineering products. In most cases material cost for traditionally used ulcer dressings are lower in relation to total cost for topical treatment. In a comparison of 8 treatment alternatives, material cost for one treatment week varied between 6 and 51% of total cost depending on type of dressing. The highest cost was related to cost for staff and travelling. The key factor in that evaluation was the frequency of dressing changes and velocity of healing in treatment weeks.

When evaluating cost effective management of diabetic foot ulcer the long-term perspective has to be considered. In a report of long-term prognosis for patients with diabetes mellitus after healing of an initial ulcer, 34%, 61%, and 70% had developed a new foot ulcer after 1, 3, and 5 years of follow-up, respectively. The long-term cost of foot ulcers in patients with diabetes mellitus were estimated during 3 years after healing of initial ulcer with or without amputation. The highest costs were reported for inpatient care, social service support and home care. The annual extra cost for social service support and home care were highest for patients who required a major amputation, approximately US $15 200–US $16 700 (1990 values) compared with US $1200–2200 for patients without critical ischemia and initial ulcer that was primary healed.

It can be concluded that cost effective management of diabetic foot ulcers/lesions is a complex matter and should not only focus on short-term cost until healing, but also on long-term cost. The diabetic foot is a major economic problem, and the management

---

TABLE 1 : FACTORS ASSOCIATED WITH FOOT ULCER

- Age
- Socio-economic status
    Low social position
    Access to health care
    Compliance/Neglect
    Education
- Neuropathy
    Sensorimotor dysfuntion
    autonomic neuropathy
- Peripheral vascular disease
    Metabolic control
- Extrinsic Factors
    Poor footwear
    Walking barefoot
    Fall/Accidents
    Objects inside shoes
- Intrinsic factors
    Limited joint mobility
    Bony prominences
    Foot deformity/osteoarthropathy
    Callus

of the resultant ulcers has not always been conducted in a most cost-effective way. Early amputation may seem less expensive in the short perspective, but amputations cause high costs to society because of prolonged hospitalisation, rehabilitation, and the need for home care and social service. More support concludes that foot ulcer and subsequent amputations lead to high cost for society. For the individual patient an amputation results in lifelong disability, decreased quality of life, and often premature death.

TABLE 2 : FACTORS ASSOCIATED WITH OUTCOME

- Age, sex, race
- Duration and type of diabetes
- Peripheral vascular disease
- Infection
- Microangiopathy
- Type, site, cause of ulcer
- Limited joint mobility, foot deformity
- Oedema
- Multiple cardiovascular disease
- Smoking
- Metabolic factors

TABLE 3: REDUCTION OF MAJOR AMPUTATION IN DIABETES MELLITUS

Area	Author (yr)	Reduction %
Memphis**, USA	Runyan (1975)	68
Atlanta, USA	Davidson et al (1981)	49
Umeå*, Sweden	Lindegård et al (1984)	68
Geneve, Switzerland	Assal (1985)	85
Kings College, UK	Edmonds et al. (1986)	50
Tucson, USA	Malone et al (1989)	66
Kisa*, Sweden	Falkenberg (1990)	78
Manchester, GB	Fernando (1991)	39
Louisville, USA	Griffiths och Wiemen (1992)	53
Boston, USA	LoGerfo et al. (1992)	56
Lund*, Sweden	Larsson et al. (1995)	78

* Population based study ** Reduction in in-hospital stay

Table 4. Costs associated with foot ulcers and non-traumatic lower extremity amputations in diabetic patients.

Authors	Country	Costs transformed To $US 1996 prices
Primary healing		
Apelqvist et al, 1994	Sweden	12 437
Healing with amputation		
Apelqvist et al, 1994	Sweden	83 999
Bild et al, 1989	USA	15 920 – 23 880
Eckman et al, 1995	USA	31 964 – 32 993
Gibbons et al, 1993	USA	25 494
Gupta et al, 1988	USA	81 947
van Houtum et al, 1995	Netherlands	18 959
Mackey et al, 1986	USA	85 588
Panayiotopoulus et al, 1997	UK	24 752
Raviola et al, 1988	USA	40 596 – 80 794

Table 5. Costs associated with vascular surgery and lower extremity
amputations in diabetic patients with foot ulcers and critical ischemia.

Authors	Country	Vascular surgery	Amputation to year	Costs corresponding
Gibbons	USA	$US 15796 *1	$US 18341	1990
Gupta	USA	$US 26194 *2	$US 27225 (3 years follow-up)	1978-1981
Johnson	UK	£ 6016 *1 £ 15975 *3	£12476 (6 months treatment)	1991-1992
Mackey	USA	$US 28374 *1 $US 56809 *3	$US 40563	1984
Panayiotopoulus	UK	£ 9161 £ 4611 *1 £ 18063 *3	£ 15500	1994-1995
Raviola	USA	$US 20300	$US 20400	1985
Raviola	USA	$US 28700 *5 $US 42200 *3	$US 40600	1985

*1 = Successful

*2 = 3 years follow up

*3 = failed

*4 = 6 months treatment

*5 = complicated

REFERENCES

1. Aguila MA, Reiber GA, Koepsell TD. How does provider and patient awareness of high-risk status for lower-extremity amputation influence foot-care practice? Diabetic Care, 1994, 17, 9: 1050.

2. Andreassen TT, Oxlund H. The influence of experimental diabetes and insulin treatments on the biomechanical properties of rat skin incisional wounds. Acta Chir Scand; 1987, 153: 405.

3. Apelqvist J, Larsson J, Agardh C-D. Long-term prognosis for diabetic patients with foot ulcers. J Int Med; \ 1993, 233: 485.

4. Apelqvist J. Den Diabetiska Foten, The State of the Art. Socialstyrelsen mars 1995.

5. Apelqvist J. The Wound healing in Diabetes. Outcome and costs. In Healing the Diabetic Foot Wound. Harkless L, Armstrong G (eds). Clinics in Podiatric Medicine and Surgery. 1998; 15: 21-39.

6. Apelqvist J, Larsson J, Agardh C-D. The influence of external precipitating factors and peripheral neuropathy on the development and outcome of diabetic foot ulcers. J Diabetes Complications, 1990,4: 21.

7. Apelqvist J, Stenström A. Fotinfektioner i den Diabetiska Foten. Lundberg, Södertälje 1995, ISBN 91-86326-83-6.

8. Apelqvist J, Agardh C-D. The association between clinical factors and outcome of diabetic foot ulcers. Diabetes Res Clin Pract, 1992: 18: 43.

9. Apelqvist J, Castenfors J, Larsson J, et al. Prognostic value of systolic ankle and toe blood pressure levels in outcome of diabetic foot ulcer. Diabetes Care 1989, 12: 373.

10. Apelqvist J, Castenfors J, Larsson J, Stenström A, Agardh C-D. Wound classification is more important than site of ulceration in the outcome of diabetic foot ulcers. Diabetic Medicine, 1989, 6: 526.

11. Apelqvist J, Larsson J, Agardh C-D. The importance of peripheral pulses, peripheral oedema and local pain in the outcome of diabetic foot ulcers. Diabetic Med; 1990, 7: 590.

12. Apelqvist J, Larsson J, Agardh C-D. Medical risk factors in diabetic patients with foot ulcers and severe peripher al vascular disease and their influence on outcome. J Diabetic Compl, 1992, 6: 167.

13. Apelqvist J, Larsson J, Agardh C-D. Long-term prognosis for diabetic patients with foot ulcers. J Int Med; 1993, 233: 485.

14. Apelqvist J, Ragnarson Tennvall G, Larsson J. Topical treatment of diabetic foot ulcers: an economic analysis of treatment alternatives and strategies. Diabet Med, 1994;12 :123-128.

15. Apelqvist J, Ragnarson Tennvall G, Persson J, et al. Diabetic foot ulcers in a multidisciplinary setting. An economic analysis of primary healing and healing with amputation. J Intern Med, 1994, 235 : 463-471.

16. Apelqvist J, Ragnarson Tennvall G, Larsson J, et al. Long-term costs for foot ulcers in diabetic patients in a multi disciplinary setting. Foot Ankle Int, 1995; 16 : 388-394.

17. Apelqvist J, Ragnarson Tennvall G. Cavity foot ulcers in diabetic patients: a comparative study of cadexomer iodine ointment and standard treatment. Acta Derm Venereol, 1996 ; 76:231-235.

18. Assal JP, et al. Patient education as the basis for diabetes care in clinical practice. Diabetologia, 1985, 28 : 602.

19. Arkkila P, Kantola I, Viikari J. Limited Joint Mobility in Non-Insulin-Dependent Diabetic (NIDDM) Patients: Correlation to Control of Diabetes, Artherosclerotic Vascular Disease, and Other Diabetic Complications. J Diab Comp, 1997; 11:208-217.

20. Armstrong DG, Todd WF, Lavery LA, et al. The Natural History of Acute Chartcot's Arthropathy in a Diabetic Foot Specialty Clinic. Diabetic Medicine, 1996,14 : 357-363.

21. Assal JP. Cost-effectiveness of diabetes education. PharmacoEconomis, 1995; 1: 68-71.

22. Barnett S, Shield J, Potter M, et al. Foot pathology in insulin dependent diabetes. Archives of Disease in Childhood 1995; 73 : 151-153.

23. Barth R, Campbell L, Allen S, et al. Intensive education improves knowledge compliance and foot problems in type II diabetes. Diabetic Med; 1991, 8 :117-9.

24. Bild DE, Selby JV, Sinnock P, et al. Lower-Extremity amputation in people with diabetes. Diabetes Care, 1989, 12 no 1.

25. Bentcover JD, Champion AH. Economic evaluation of alternative methods of treatment for diabetic foot ulcer patients: cost-effectiveness of platelet release and wound care clinics. Wounds, 1993; 5 : 207-215.

26. Bild DE, Selby JV, Sinnock P, et al. Lower-Extremity amputation in people with diabetes. Diabetes Care, 1989, 12 no 1.

27. Birke J, Rolfsen R. Evaluation of a Self-Administered Sensory Testing Tool to Identify Patients at Risk of Diabetes-Related Foot Problems. Diabetes Care, 1998, 21, no 1.

28. Bloomgarden Z, Karamally W, Metzeger J, et al. Randomised, controlled trial of effects of diabetes patient education. Diabetes Care 1987;10 : 263-272.

29. Borssén B, Bergenheim T, Lithner F. The epidemiology of foot lesions in diabetic patients aged 15-50 years. Diabetic Med 1990, 7 : 438-444.

30. Boulton A. The Pathogenesis of Diabetic Foot Problems: an Overview. Diabetic Medicine, 1996, 13 : 12-16.

31. Boulton AJM. The pathway to ulceration: Aetiopathogenesis. p 37. In The foot in diabetes. Boulton AJM, Connor H, Cavanagh PR. (ed) 2nd ed. Wiley New York, 1994.

32. Boyko E, Ahroni J, Davignon D, et al. Diagnostic Utility of the History and Physical Examination for Peripheral Vascular Disease among Patients with Diabetes Mellitus. J Clin Epidemiol, 1997, 50, 6 : 659-668.

33. Boyko E, Ahroni J, Smith D, et al. Increased Mortality Associated with Diabetic Foot Ulcer. Diab Med, 1996, 13 : 967-972.

34. Cavanagh PR, Simonean G, Ulbrecht J. Ulceration, unsteadiness and uncertainty: The biomechanic consequences of diabetes mellitus. J Biomech, 1993, 26, 1 : 23-40.
35. Consensus meeting regarding foot problems in diabetic patients. Stockholm: Spri, 1998. (in Swedish)
36. Criado E, et al. The Course of Severe Foot Infection in Patients with Diabetes. Surg Gynecol & Obstet, 1992, 175: 135.
37. Da Silva AF, Desgranges P, Holdsworth J, et al. The management and outcome of critical limb ischaemia in diabetic patients: Results of a National Survey. Diabetic Medicine, 1996, 13 : 726-728.
38. Davidson JK, Alogna M, et al. Assessment of program effectiveness at Grady Memorial Hospital - Atlanta. p. 329-48. In: Educating diabetic patients. (Eds. Steiner G, Lawrence P). Springer-Verlag, New York, 1981.
39. Deerochanawong C, et al. A survey of lower-limb amputation in diabetic patients. Diabetic Med 1992; 9 : 942-46.
40. Diabetes Vital Statistics 1996. American Diabetes Association.
41. Drummond MF, O'Brien B, Stoddart GL, Torrance GW. Methods of the economic evaluation of health care programmes. Oxford: Oxford Medical Publications, 1997.
42. Eckman MH, Greenfield S, Mackey WC, et al. Foot infections in diabetic patients. Decision and cost-effective ness analyses. JAMA, 1995 ; 273 : 712-720.
43. Edelman D, Hough D, Glazebrook K, et al. Prognostic Value of the Clinical Examination of the Diabetic Foot Ulcer. J Gen Intern Med, 1997, 12 : 537-543.
44. Edelman D, Matchar D, Oddone E. Clinical and Radiographic Findings That Lead to Intervention in Diabetic Patients With Foot Ulcers. Diab Care, 1996, 19, 7.
45. Edmonds ME, Walters H: Angioplasty and the diabetic foot. Vascular Medicine Review, 1995, 6 : 205-214.
46. Edmonds ME, Blundell MP, Morris ME, et al. Improved survival of the diabetic foot: the role of a specialized foot clinic. Quart J Med. New Series, 1986, 60(232) : 763.
47. El-Shazly M, Abdel-Fattah M, Scorpiglione N, et al. Risk Factors for Lower Limb Complications in Diabetic Patients. J Diab Comp, 1998: 12:10-17.
48. Eneroth M, Apelqvist J, Stenström A. Clinical Characteristics and Outcome in 223 Diabetic Patients With Deep Foot Infections. Foot and Ankle. 1997, 18 : 716-722.
49. Falkenberg M. Metabolic control and amputations among diabetics in primary health care - a population-based intensified programme governed by patient education. Scand J Prim Health Care, 1990, 8 : 25-29.
50. Fedele D, Comi G, Coscelli C, et al. A Multicenter Study on the Prevalence of Diabetic Neuropathy in Italy. Diabetes Care, 1997, 20 no 5.
51. Ferguson MWJ, Herrick SE, Spencer MJ, et al. The histology of diabetic foot ulcers. Diabetic Medicine, 1995, 12 : 1-4.
52. Fernando DJS, Hutchison A. Risk factors for non-ischaemic foot ulceration in diabetic nephropathy. Diabetic Med, 1991, 8, 3 : 223-225.
53. Fernando DJ , Masson EA, Veves A, et al. Relationship of limited joint mobility to abnormal foot pressures an diabetic foot ulceration. Diabetes care, 1991, 14, 1: 8-11.
54. Fletcher F, Michael A, Jacobs R: Healing of foot ulcers in immunosuppressed renal transplant patients. Clinical Orthopaedics and Related Research, 1993, 296 : 37-42.
55. Fletcher E, MacFarlane R, Jeffcoate J. Can foot ulcers be prevented by education? Diabetic Med, 1992, 9, 2 : 41.
56. Frykberg R G (ed): The High Risk Foot in Diabetes Mellitus. New York. Churchill Livingstone 1991.
57. Frykberg R, Piaggesea, Donaghoue V et al. Difference in Treatment of Foot Ulcerations in Boston, USA and Piza, Italy. Diabetes Research and Clinical Practice, 1997, 35 : 21-26.
58. Frykberg RG. Team approach toward lower extremity amputation prevention in diabetes. J Am Podiatr Med Assoc, 1997; 87 : 305-312.
59. Fylling CP, Knighton DR. Amputation in the diabetic population: Incidence, causes, cost, treatment and prevention. J Enterostom Ther, 1989, 16 : 247.
60. Giacalone VF, Krych SM, Harkless LB: The university of Texas health science center at San Antonio: Experience with foot surgery in diabetics. J of Foot and Ankle Surg., 1994, 33 : 6.
61. Gibbons GW, Marcaccio Jr, Burgess AM, et al. Improved quality of diabetic foot care. 1984 vs 1990. Reduced length of stay and costs, insufficient reimbursement. Arch Surg, 1993, 128: 576.
62. Goodson WH, Hunt TK. Wound healing in experimental diabetes mellitus. J Surg Res, 1977, 22: 221.
63. Gough A, Clapperton M, Rolando N, et al. Randomised Placebo-controlled trial of granulocyte-colony stimulating factor in diabetic foot infection. Lancet, 1997;350 : 855-859.
64. Griffiths G D, Wiemen T J. Meticulous attention to foot care improves the prognosis in diabetic ulceration of the foot. Surg Gyn Obstet, 1992, 174, 1: 49.
65. Gupta SK, Veith FJ, Ascer E, et al. Cost factors in limb-threatening ischaemia due to infrainguinal arteriosclero sis. Eur J vasc Surg, 1988 ; 2:151-154.
66. Harkless L, Armstrong D, Fish S. (Eds) Healing The Diabetic Wound Clinics in Podiatric Medicine and Surgery, 1998, 15 : 21-39.
67. van Houtum WH, Lavery LA, Harkless LB. The cost of diabetes-related lower extremity amputations in the Netherlands. Diabet Med, 1995, 12 : 777-781.
68. van Houtum WH, Lavery LA. Outcomes associated with diabetes-related amputations in the Netherlands and in the State of California, USA. J Int Med, 1996, 240 : 227-231.
69. Humphrey LL, Palumbo PJ, Butters MA, et al. The contribution of non-insulin-dependent diabetes to lower-extremity amputation in the community. Arch Intern Med, 1994, 154, 25: 885.
70. Jeffcoate WJ, MacFarlane RM, Fletcher EM: The description and classification of diabetic foot lesions. Diabetic Medicine, 1993, 10 : 676-679.

71.   Johnson BF, Evans L, Drury R, et al. Surgery for limb threatening ischemia: A reappraisal of the costs and bene
      fits. Eur J Endovasc Surg, 1995; 9 : 181-188.
72.   Jones R B, Gregory R, Jones E W, et al. The Quality and Relevance of Perpheral Neuropathy Data on a Diabetic
      Clinical Information System. Diabetic Medcine, 1992; 9 : 934-937.
73.   Jörneskog G. Functional microangiopathy in the digital skin of patients with diabetes mellitus. Department of
      Internal medicin, Karolinska Hospital and the Department of Medicine, Danderyds Hospital, Karolinska
      Institute, Stockholm 1995.(Thesis).
74.   Knighton D, Fiegel VD. Growth factors and repair of diabetic wounds. In the Diabetic Foot. 5th edition. Levin,
      M. O'Neal, L. Bowker, J. (eds). Moss Yearbook London, 1993 : 247-257.
75.   Kobelt G. Health economics. An introduction to economic evaluation. London OHE, Office of Health
      Economics, 1996.
76.   Kumar S, Ashe HA, Parnell LN, et al. The prevalence of foot ulceration and its correlates in type 2 diabetic
      patients: A population based study. Diabetic Med., 1994, 11, 480.
77.   Larsson J, Apelqvist J. Towards less amputations in diabetic patients. Acta Orthop Scand, 1995, 66 (2) : 181-192.
78.   Larsson J, Apelqvist J, Agardh CD, Stenström A. Decreasing incidence of major amputation in diabetic patients: a
      consequence of a multidisciplinary foot care team approach? Diabetic Med. 1995, 12 : 770.
79.   Lavery L, Ashry H, Houtum W, et al. Variation in the Incidence and Proportion of Diabetes-Related
      Amputations in Minorities. Diab Care, 1996, 19, no 1.
80.   Lavery L, Armstrong D, Walker S. Healing Rates of Diabetic Foot Ulcers Associated with Midfoot Fracture Due
      to Charcot's Arthropathy. Diab Med, 1997, 14 : 46-49.
81.   Lavery L, Armstrong D, Harkless L. Classification of Diabetic Foot Wounds. The Journal of Foot and Ankle
      Surgery, 1996, 35(6) : 528-531.
82.   Lavery L, Armstrong D, Vela S, et al: Practical Criteria for Screening Patients at High Risk for Diabetic Foot
      Ulceration. Arch Intern Med. 1998, 158 : 25.
83.   Lehto S, Rönnemaa T, Pyörälä K, et al. Risk Factors Predicting Lower Extremity Amputations in Patients
      With NIDDM. Diabetes Care, 1996, 19 no 6.
84.   Levin M E , O'Neal L W and Bowker J H. (eds). The Diabetic Foot. 5th ed. St. Louis, Mosby Year Book, 1993.
85.   Levy LA: Survey of socioeconomic and medical implications of diabetes and the lower limb. J of the American
      Podiatric Med Ass, 1993, 83 no 5.
86.   Lindegård P, et al: Amputations in diabetic patients in Gotland and Umeå counties 1971-1980. Acta Med Scand,
      1984, 687 : 89-93.
87.   Lithner F, Törnblom N. Gangrene localized to the feet in diabetic patients. Acta Med Scand; 1984, 215: 75.
88.   Lithner F, Bergenheim T, Borssén B. Extensor digitorum brevis in diabetic neuropathy: a controlled evaluation in
      diabetic patients aged 15 - 50 years. J Int Med, 1991; 230 : 449-453.
89.   Litzelman D, Marriott D, Vinicor F. Independent Physiological Predictors of Foot Lesions in Patients With
      NIDDM. Diab Care, 1997, 20, no 8.
90.   Litzelman DK, Slemenda CW, Langefeld CD et al. Reduction of lower extremity clinical abnormalities in patients
      with non-insulin-dependent diabetes mellitus. Annals of Internal Med; 1993, 119, 36.
91.   LoGerfo FW, Gibbons GW, et al. Trends in the care of the diabetic foot. Expanded role of arterial reconstruction.
      Arch Surg, 1992, 127(5) : 617-20.
92.   Mackey WC, McCullough JL, Conlon TP, et al. The cost of surgery for limb-threatening ischemia. Surgery, 1986,
      99 : 26-35.
93.   Malone JM, Snyder M, Anderson G. Prevention of amputation by diabetic education. Am J Surg; 1989,
      158 : 520.
94.   Mayfield J, Reiber G, Nelson R, et al. A Foot Risk Classification System to Predict Diabetic Amputation in Pima
      Indians, Diabetes Care, 1996, 19, 7 : 704-709.
95.   Mayfield J, Reiber G, Sanders L, et al. American Diabetes Association. Technical Review of Preventive Foot Care
      in Patients with Diabetes Mellitus 1998. In manuscript.
96.   Mazzotta MY. Nutrition and wound healing. Journal of the American Medical Association. 1994, 84 n∞9 sep.
97.   McCabe CJ, Stevenson RC, Dolan AM. Evaluation of a diabetic foot screening and protection programme.
      Diabet Med, 1998; 15 : 80-84.
98.   McIntyre Bridges Jr, R. Deitch, EA. Diabetic Foot Infections. Pathophysiology and Treatment. Surg. Clinics of
      North America, 1994, 74 (3) : 537.
99.   McNeely M, Boyko E, Ahroni J, et al. The Independent Contributions of Diabetic Neuropathy and Vasculopathy
      in Foot Ulceration. Diab Care, 1995, 18, nc 2.
100. Mills JL, Beckett WC, Taylor SM. The diabetic foot: consequences of delayed treatment and referral. South. Med
      J. 1991, 84 : 970-974.
101. Morrison WB, Schweitzer ME, Wapner KL, et al. Osteomyelitis in feet of diabetics: clinical accuracy, surgical
      utility, and cost-effectiveness of MR imaging. Radiology,1995;196 : 557-564.
102. Moss SE, et al. The prevalence and incidence of lower-extremity amputations in a diabetic population. Arch
      Intern Med, 1992, 152 : 610.
103. Murray H, Young M, Hollis S, et al. The Association Between Callus Formation, High Pressures and Neuropathy
      in Diabetic Foot Ulceration. Diab Med, 1996; 13 : 979-982.
104. Naughton G, Mansbridge J, Gentzkow G. A metabolically active human dermal replacement for the treatment of
      diabetic foot ulcers. Artificial Organs, 1997; 21 : 1203-1210.
105. Nelson RG, et al. Lower-extremity amputations in NIDDM. 12-yr follow-up study in Pima indians. Diabetes
      Care; 1988, 11(1): 8.

106.   Panayiotopoulos YP, Tyrrell MR, Arnold FJL, et al. Results and cost analysis of distal (crural/pedal) arterial revascularisation for limb salvage in diabetic and non-diabetic patients. Diabet Med, 1997;14 : 214-220.

107.   Pecoraro RE, Reiber GE, Burgess, et al. Pathways to diabetic limb amputations. Diabetes Care, 1990, 13, 5 : 513,

108.   Pecoraro RE, Ahroni JH, Boyko EJ, et al. Chronology and determinants of tissue repair in diabetic lower-extremity ulcers. Diabetes, 1991, 40 : 1305.

109.   Pedersen A, Bornefeldt-Olsen B, Krasnik M, Ebskov L, Leicht B, Sager P, Helgstrand U, Holstein P. Halving the number of leg amputations: The Influence of Infrapopliteal Bypass. Eur J Vasc Surg, 1994, 8 : 26-30.

110.   Perler BA. Cost-efficacy issues in the treatment of peripheral vascular disease: primary amputation or revascularization for limb-threatening ischemia. J Vasc Interv Radiol, 1995 ; 6:111S-115S.

111.   Ragnarson Tennvall G, Apelqvist J. Cost-effective management of diabetic foot ulcers. A review. Pharmaco Economics, 1997;12 : 42-53.

112.   Raviola CA, Nichter LS, Baker JD, et al. Cost of treating advanced leg ischemia. Bypass graft vs primary amputation. Arch Surg, 1988;123 : 495-496.

113.   Reiber GE, et al. Risk factors for amputations in patients with diabetes melllitus. A case-control study. Ann Int Med; 1992, 117(2) : 97.

114.   Reiber GE. The Epidemiology of Diabetic Foot Problems. Diab Med, 1996, 13 : 6-11.

115.   Reiber GE. Who is at risk of limb loss and what to do about it? J of Rehabilitation Research and Development, 1994, 31, 4 : 357.

116.   Reiber GE, Pecoraro R, Koepsell T. Risk Factors for Amputation in Patients with Diabetes Mellitus. Annals of Internal Med. 1992, 117, 2.

117.   Reiber GE. Diabetes foot care. Guidlines and financial implications. Diabetes Care; 1992, 14, 1 : 29-13.

118.   Reiber G, Boykoe, Smith D. Lower Extremity Foot Ulcers and Amputations in Diabetes. In: Harrys M, Cowie C, Stern M, et al. (eds). Diabetes in America 2nd Ed. NIH publication, 1995, 95-1468.

119.   Retting B, Shrunger D, Recker R, et al. A randomised study of the effects of a home diabetes education program. Diabetes Care,1986; 6 : 256-61.

120.   Rosenquist U. An epidemiological survey of diabetic foot problems in the Stockholm county 1982. Acta Med, 1984, 187: 55.

121.   Runyan JW. The Memphis Chronic Disease Program. JAMA, 1975, 231: 264-67.

122.   Sing S, Evans L, Datta P, et al. The costs of managing lower limb-threatening ischemia. Eur J Vasc Surg 1996; 12 : 359-362.

123.   Silhi N. Diabetes and wound healing. Journal of Wound Care, 1998, 7, 1.

124.   Sonnaville J, Colly L, Wijkel D. The prevalence and determinants of foot ulceration in type II diabetic patients in a primary health care setting. Diab Research and Clinical Practice, 1997, 35 : 149-156.

125.   Susman KE, Reiber G, Albert SF. The diabetic foot problem - a failed system of health care? Diabetes Research and Clinical Practice, 1992, 17: 1.

126.   Taylor Jr LM, Porter JM. The clinical course of diabetics who require emergent foot surgery because of infection of ischemia. J Vasc Surg, 1987; 6 : 454-459.

127.   Thomson F, Masson E, Boulton A. The Clinical Diagnosis of Sensory Neuropathy in Elderly People. Diab Med, 1993, 10: 843-846.

128.   Thompson C, McWilliams T, Scott D, Simmons D. Importance of diabetic foot admissions at Middlemore. New Zealand Med Journ. 1993, 12 : 178.

129.   Uccioli L, Faglia E, Monticone G, et al. Manufactured shoes in the prevention of diabetic foot ulcers. Diabetic Care, 1995, 18, 10: 1374.

130.   Walsh CH. A healed ulcer: what now? Diabetic Med. 1996, 13: S58.

131.   Walters DP, Gatling W, Mullee MA, et al. The distribution and severity of diabetic foot disease: A community study with comparison to a non-diabetic group. Diabet Med, 1992, 9: 354.

132.   Warram JH, Kopczynski J, Janka HU, et al. Epidemiology of non-insulin dependent diabetes mellitus and its macrovascular complications. A basis for the development of cost-effective programs. Epidemiology and clinical decision making 1997;26 : 165-188.

133.   Williams DRR. The size of the problem: epidemiological and economic aspects of foot problems in diabetes. p 15. In The foot in diabetes. Boulton AJM, Connor H, Cavanagh P. (ed) 2nd ed. Wiley, New York, 1994.

134.   Wyle Rosett J, Walker EA, Shamoon, et al. Assessment of Documented Foot Examinations for Patients with Diabetes in Inner-city Primary Care Clinics. Arch. Fam. Med., 1995, 4 : 46-50.

135.   Young M, Boulton A, Macleod A, et al. A multicentre study of the prevalence of diabetic peripheral neuropathy in the United Kingdom hospital clinic population. Diabetologia, 1993, 36:150-154.

PATHOPHYSIOLOGY AND MANAGEMENT OF THE DIABETIC FOOT

Nicolaas Christiaan Schaper
Department of Internal Medicine
Academic Hospital, Maastricht-Netherlands

THE PROBLEM OF THE DIABETIC FOOT

Diabetes mellitus is characterised by various complications, like retinopathy, nephropathy, neuropathy, and premature atherosclerosis, but foot complications are one of the most serious and costly. Amputation of (a part of) a lower extremity is usually preceded by a foot ulcer (1). As shown in several studies, a strategy including prevention, patient and staff education, multifactorial treatment of foot ulcers, and close monitoring can reduce amputation rates by 49–85% (1,2). In this review the epidemiology, pathophysiology, and the management of diabetic foot problems will be described.

The scope of the problem

Several population-based studies have reported a prevalence of foot ulcers between 3% to 10% in diabetic patients (2). These ulcers occur particularly in older type 1 or type 2 patients (>45 years). It has been estimated that 15% of all diabetic patients during their lifetimes will have a diabetic foot ulcer (3). The majority of these ulcers are treated on an out-patient basis and heal after appropriate therapy. However, in a substantial number of patients long term hospitalization will be required, frequently because of concurrent infection or progressive gangrene. Based upon several studies performed in the Netherlands one can estimate that presently in this country, at least, 12.000 diabetic patients have a foot ulcer and (in 1989) almost 4.000 hospital admissions were due to a diabetic foot ulcer (4). In 1992 one or more lower extremity amputations were performed in 1585 patients; the costs related to these amputations were 10% of all the costs spent on health care for diabetic patients (5). In the USA more than 50,000 diabetic-related amputations are performed yearly and corresponding figures have been shown in other developed and non-developed countries (1). Of all lower extremity amputations, 40% to 60% are related to diabetes mellitus. Almost all (>80%) of these amputations are preceded by a foot ulcer, with uncontrolled infection or progressive gangrene as the major indications for amputation. Mortality after these amputation is high; 5-year mortality is less than 30–50%, probably due to the poor physical condition of the patients (1).

Pathophysiology

The spectrum of foot lesions varies in different regions of the world, but, the pathways to ulceration are probably identical in most patients. Diabetic foot lesions frequently result from a combination of two or more risk factors occurring together (6).

Major factors are distal symmetric diabetic polyneuropathy (neuropathy), altered biomechanical loading of the foot (biomechanical stress), impaired tissue perfusion due to macrovascular disease, and secondary infection of an ulcer (6). In contrast to what is sometimes believed, diabetic microvascular disease does not seem to be an important factor in the occurrence of diabetic foot lesions (7).

Neuropathy

In the majority of patients diabetic peripheral neuropathy plays a central role and up to 50% of type 2 diabetic patients have significant neuropathy and at-risk feet (8). This neuropathy is characterised by chronic senserimotor loss and sympathetic denervation, which usually progresses slowly and insidiously, from the toes to more distal regions of both feet and legs (9). Somatic neuropathy leads to a foot with impaired sensation for noxious stimuli, like pain or temperature. Typical symptoms are burning, numbness, pareshesiae, and pain, which is not related to ambulation. However, many patients do not have any complaint, limiting the value of history. Motor neuropathy leads to wasting of the small intrinsic muscles of the foot, and, probably due to imbalance of the flexors and extensors, various deformities can develop, like clawing of the toes or prominent metatarsal heads (10). The sympathetic denervation results in a warm (due to increased shunt blood flow) and dry skin, prone to cracks and fissures. These various changes result in a deformed, insensitive, and warm foot, which is abnormally loaded during standing and walking (1,6,10).

Biomechanical stress

Prospective studies have shown that in many patients the combination of loss of protective sensation and abnormal loading of the foot finally lead to a breakdown of the skin (10). This abnormal loading of the foot, due to foot deformities and abnormal walking pattern, is aggravated by a loss of mobility of the joints (Limited Joint Mobility), which is believed to be caused by non-enzymatic glycation of the tissues surrounding the joints (10). In patients with, for instance, a plantar ulcer, these abnormalities can result in chronic repetitive stress on the skin covering the metatarsal heads. Due to loss of protective sensation the repeated mechanical trauma is not perceived by the patient and the patient continues walking in footwear not adapted to the altered loading of the foot (11). As a normal physiological response, a callus is formed. Unfortunately, this callus acts as an "foreign body," further increasing the already elevated plantar pressures (and presumably shear forces); finally the skin breaks down and a chronic non-healing ulcer is formed. In other neuropathic patients an acute external trauma precipitates a chronic ulcer. Whatever the primary cause, the patient continues walking on the insensitive foot, which will impair subsequent healing.

Impaired tissue perfusion

Macrovascular disease is one of the major complications of both type 1 and type 2 diabetes mellitus (12). While the abnormalities of the microcirculation are rather specific for diabetes, macrovascular disease is characterised by premature atherosclerosis which is histologically not different from non-diabetic patients. However, in the legs there are some marked clinical differences. Obstructive atherosclerotic vascular disease is frequently bilateral, more frequent below the knee, and has a more progressive course (7). Many patients have no or relatively mild complaints, despite severe ischemia or gangrene, probably due to co-existent sensor neuropathy. Clinical examination of these neuro-ischemic ulcers is, in our experience, also unreliable, as for instance loss of temperature or color do not occur in many patients, probably due sympathetic denervation. The diagnosis of peripheral vascular disease is, however, of paramount importance, as adequate perfusion is essential for healing. In neuro-ischemic ulcers it is likely that both increased biomechanical stress and impaired tissue perfusion play a role. Plantar pressures during standing and walking are sufficient to occlude microcirculatory blood flow, and it is likely that when perfusion pressure is already reduced increased plantar pressures can severely impair tissue perfusion (10).

DIAGNOSIS OF THE ULCERATED FOOT

On examination the following items must be addressed.

The type
Most ulcers can be classified as neuropathic, ischemic, or neuro-ischemic, which will guide further therapy. Furthermore, signs of increased biomechanical stress (deformities, callus) and secondary infection must be sought.

The site and depth
Neuropathic ulcers frequently occur on the plantar surface of the foot, tips of the toes or in areas overlying a bony deformity. Ischemic ulcers are more common on the tips of the toes or the lateral border of the foot. Due to overlying callus or necrosis the depth of an ulcer can be difficult to determine. Therefore, all ulcers should be debrided as soon as possible, except ischemic ulcers without signs of infection. In neuropathic ulcers this debridement can usually be performed without (general) anesthesia. When bone is probed before initial debridement, the risk of osteomyelitis is increased (13).

The principles of clinical examination are depicted in Table 1. It should be noted that history is of limited value, given the absence of symptoms in many neuropathic patients or patients with neuro-ischemia. Clinical examination should always be performed both supine and standing, as foot deformities are frequently only observed during standing.

Several classification systems have been proposed for the diagnosis of diabetic polyneuropathy. In daily practise, history is taken, several sensory modalities (pain, light touch, vibration, position) are tested, muscle strength is determined, and Achilles tendon reflexes are examined (14). With the Semmes-Weinstein monofilaments light touch (and possibly deep pressure) can be assessed in a semi-quantitative fashion and the inability to sense a 10 gram monofilament is associated with an increased risk of ulceration. It should be noted that Achilles tendon reflexes are of limited value, as these reflexes may be absent in an older population. Clinical assessment of the vascular status is difficult and frequently unreliable (15). Palpation of pulses is affected by room temperature, biological variation, and skill of the examiner. If all foot pulses are detected, severe peripheral ischemia is less likely, but not excluded. Preferably, also the systolic Doppler ankle pressure should be measured, as described below. With the use of a computerised pressure platform, plantar pressures can be assessed reliably and these pressures have been shown to predict future ulceration. Unfortunately, these systems are too expensive for daily practise and these systems measure pressure (and not shear forces), only on the plantar aspect of the foot. However, increased biomechanical stress can be inferred from callus, bony prominences, and close shoe inspection (15).

MANAGEMENT OF THE ULCERATED FOOT

Treatment is based on the following principles, and healing rates of 80–90% can be attained. The best wound care cannot compensate for continued injury, ischemia, or infection. Patients with an ulcer deeper than subcutis should be treated aggressively and, depending on local resources and infrastructure, hospitalization must be considered.

Relief of pressure

Mechanical unloading is the cornerstone in the treatment of neuropathic or neuro-ischemic foot ulcers (10). Total contact casting is an effective therapy for plantar neuropathic ulcers. The plaster must be applied with great skill and must be changed each 2 weeks. Also temporary footwear and customized insoles, which unload the ulcer, have been used effectively. Ulcers between toes can be unloaded with gauzes or orotheses. Patients must be instructed to limit standing and walking.

Restoration of skin perfusion

If severely impaired, restoration of skin perfusion is essential for healing. As described above, the diagnosis of impaired peripheral ischemia can be difficult in diabetic patients, given the poor reliability of clinical examination. Therefore, in many patients more objective information must be obtained, like measurements of systolic ankle and toe pressures or transcutaneous pressure of oxygen ($TcpO_2$) (16). As an initial screening ankle brachial indexes (Doppler systolic ankle pressure/systolic brachial artery pressure) are useful; when the index is < 0.9 , further non-invasive vascular evaluation is indicated. However, it should be noted that Doppler systolic ankle pressures can fail to detect peripheral vascular disease in diabetic patients.

Decreased compressibility of the foot arteries due to media calcification can result in falsely elevated systolic pressures (16). Therefore, in our experience any patient with signs of peripheral ischemia, with an index < 0.9 or with an ulcer, which does not improve despite optimal therapy in 2–3 weeks, should be evaluated further. Healing is likely, either primary or after minor amputation when systolic ankle pressure is > 90 mmHg, toe pressure is > 55 Hg and $TcpO_2$ is > 40 mmHg (16).

In diabetic patients obstructive lesions seem to be localised, in particular, in the vessels below the knee, with relative sparing of the foot arteries (7). Therefore, distal bypass surgery is frequently needed and although these procedures can be technically difficult and time-consuming, excellent results have been obtained. As the results of arterial revascularisation are not different between diabetic and non-diabetic patients, these procedures should always be considered in case of severe vascular disease (12). At present, pharmacological treatment is of little value in patients with (severe) peripheral ischemia.

Aggressive treatment of infection

In a superficial ulcer (not deeper that skin) with extensive cellulitis antibiotics are probably indicated. Treatment, preferrably oral, should be aimed primarily at Staphylococcus aureus and at Streptococci (e.g., flucloxacilline) (17). There is no place for topical antibiotic treatment. A deep infection is a limb-threatening condition. Probably due to neuropathy, signs and symptoms can be mild or absent; sometimes edema and metabolic dysregulation are the only signs (18). The patient should be referred immediately to a footcare specialist for a drainage procedure, irrespective of the vascular status (12). The infected compartment should be opened adequately, with removal of necrotic or poorly vascularised tissue, including infected bone. If necessary, a revascularisation procedure can be performed after control of infection. Deep infections are usually polymicrobial and intravenous broad spectrum antibiotic treatment should be started immediately, aimed at gram positive and negative microorganisms, including anaerobes (17). This empiric antibiotic therapy must adjusted based upon the results of the gram stain and when the results of the culture are known. Several methods can be used to obtain a reliable specimen for microbiological examination. Superficial swabs have been shown to be inferior, because of contamination with colonizing microflora and the difficulty of recovering anaerobes. Curretement of the ulcer base or needle aspiration seems to be preferable (19). To exclude osteomyelitis, a foot radiograph should be taken when an ulcer is deeper than the subcutis or when the patients presents with a chronic ulcer (e.g., 1 month). In one (small) study, favourable results have been reported on granulocyte-colony stimulating factor (G-CSF) in diabetic patients with deep foot infections; this interesting therapy needs further study (20).

Optimal metabolic control and treatment of co-morbidity

Optimal diabetes control (blood glucose levels below 10 mmol/l) should be attained as soon as possible, given the deleterious effects of hyperglycemia on control of infection and wound healing. If necessary, intravenous insulin treatment should be started with frequent blood glucose monitoring. Both edema, which is often multifactorial, and malnutrition should be treated.

Local wound care

In the acute phase wound debris must be removed repeatedly by mechanical debridement or irrigation. The wound is inspected daily, except when total contact casting is prescribed. At present, there are insufficient data for the use of occlusive dressings in diabetic foot ulcers. Therefore, an absorbent, non-adhesive, non-occlusive dressing is advised. Promising results have been reported on various topical agents (including growth factors) and hyperbaric oxygen treatment (21,22). However, further studies are needed before these treatments can be advised. Footbaths are contraindicated as they induce maceration of the skin.

Determination of the cause and prevention of recurrence

Diabetic foot ulcers are a recurrent disease; in one specialised centre the recurrency rate after 5 years was 80% (23). Therefore, as soon as possible the patient must be included in a comprehensive foot care program, which should include life long observation, proper protective footwear, and foot care practices (2). Insufficient footwear is the major cause of ulceration in both neuropathic and neuro-ischemic ulcers and appropriate footwear (adapted to the altered biomechanics and deformities) is essential in prevention. Finally, attention should be given to the contralateral foot. In our experience, hospitalized patients have a high incidence of heel necrosis, and special measures should be taken to prevent decubitus in this region.

ORGANISATION OF FOOT CARE

As described above, the diabetic foot is a multifactorial disease, with a high recurrency rate. Management of the diabetic foot should be coordinated by a multi-disciplinary foot care team, which has shown to be effective in reducing amputation rate. The team should be responsible for the management of diabetic foot ulcers and usually includes at least an internist, a surgeon (preferably both a vascular and orthopedic surgeon), a shoemaker, a chiropedist, and a diabetic nurse. Facilities for out-patient treatment should be present; in several countries a chiropodist plays a central role in such a diabetic foot clinic. This foot clinic must be part of a comprehensive foot care program, which aims to identify the high risk patient, to provide the appropriate preventive measures, to treat lesions as early as possible, and to educate not only the patient, but also the health care providers involved with diabetic patients (2).

TABLE 1 : EXAMINATION

1. History	Previous ulcer/amputation, previous foot education, social connectedness, cause of ulcer

2. Neuropathy	Symptoms
	Loss of protective sensation
	    Semmes-Weinstein monofilaments
	    Vibration perception (tuning fork)
	    Tactile sensation (cotton wool)
	    Achilles tendon reflexes

3. Vascular status	Claudication, pedal pulses Discoloration (rubor) on dependency
4. Skin	Edema, redness, crepitations Callus, dryness, cracks
5. Bone/joint	Previous amputation Deformities (e.g., claw toes, hammer toes) or bony prominences Loss of mobility
6. Footwear	Assessment of both inside and outside
7. Ulcer	Site, dimensions/depth, exposed bone or tendons, probing of bone, pain, pus
8. General symptoms of infection	Fever, elevated blood glucose levels, elevated ESR, leucocytosis

REFERENCES

1. Reiber GE. The epidemiology of diabetic foot problems. Diabet Med, 1996;13, 1 : S6-S11.
2. Edmonds ME, van Acker K. Education and the diabetic foot. Diabet Med, 1996; 13, 1 :S61-S64.
3. Moss SE, Klein R, Klein B. The prevalence and incidence of lower extremity amputation in a diabetic population. Arch Intern Med, 1992 ; 152 : 610-615.
4. Bouter KP, Storm AJ, de Groot RRM, Uitslager R, Erkelens DW, Diepersloot RJA. The diabetic foot in dutch hospitals: epidemiological features and clinical outcome. Eur J Med, 1993 ; 2 : 215-218.
5. Van Houtum WH, Lavery LA, Harkless LB. The cost of diabetes related lower extremity amputations in the Netherlands. Diabet Med, 1995 ; 12 : 777-781.
6. Boulton AJM The pathogenesis of diabetic foot problems: an Overview. Diabet Med, 1996; 13, 1 :S12-S16.
7. LoGerfo FW, Coffman JD. Vascular and microvascular disease of the foot in diabetes. Implications for foot care. New Eng J Med, 1984 ; 25 : 1615-1619.
8. Young MJ, ALM Boulton, Macleod AF, Williams DRR, Sonksen PH. A multicentre study of the prevalence of diabetic peripheral neuropathy in the United Kingdom hospital clinic population. Diabetologia, 1993 ; 36 : 150-154.
9. Ziegler D. Diagnosis and management of diabetic peripheral neuropathy. Diabet Med, 13, 1 : S34-S38.
10. Cavanagh PR, Ulbrecht JS, Caputo GM. Biomechanical aspects of diabetic foot disease : aetiology, treatment and prevention. Diabet Med, 1996 ; 13, 1 : S17-S27.
11. Apelqvist J, Larsson J, Agardh CD. The influence of external precipitating factors and peripheral neuropathy on the development and outcome of diabetic foot ulcers. J Diabet Complications 1990 ; 4 : 21-25.
12. Caputo GM, Cavanagh PR, Ulbrecht JS, Gibbons GW, Karchmer AW. Assessment and management of foot disease in patients with diabetes mellitus. N Eng J Med, 1994 ; 331 : 854-860.
13. Grayson ML, Gibbons GW, Balogh K, Levin E, Karchmer AW. Probing the bone in infected pedal ulcers. A clinical sign of underlying osteomyelitis in diabetic patients. JAMA, 1995 ; 273 : 271-723.
14. International guidelines on the out-patient management of diabetic peripheral neuropathy. Diabet Med : in press.
15. De Heus-van Putten MA, Schaper NC, Bakker K. The clinical examination of the diabetic foot in daily practise. Diabet Med, 1996 ; 13, 1 : S55-S57.
16. Tacolander R, Rauwerda JA. The use of non-invasive vascular assessment in diabetic patients with foot lesions. Diabet Med, 1996 ; 13, 1 :S39-S42.
17. Lipsky BA, Pecoraro RE, Larson SA, Hanley ME, Ahroni JH. Outpatient management of uncomplicated lower extremity infections in diabetic patients. Arch Int Med, 1990 ; 150 : 790-797.
18. Eneroth M, Apelqvist J, Sendström A. Clinical characteristics and outcome in 223 diabetic patients with deep foot infections. Foot and Ankle Int, 1997 ; 11 : 716-722.
19. Grayson ML. Diabetic foot infections, antimicrobiological therapy. Inf Dis Clin North America, 1995 ; 9 : 143-161
20. Cough A, Clapperton M, Rolando N, Foster AJM, Philpott-Howard J, Edmonds ME. Randomised placebo-controlled trial of granulocyte-colony stimulating factor in diabetic foot infection. Lancet, 1997 ; 350 : 855-859.
21. Clinical evaluation of recombinant human platelet-derived growth factor for the treatment of lower extremity diabetic ulcers. Steed DL and the Diabetic Ulcer Study Group. J Vasc Surg, 1995 ; 21 : 71-81.
22. Naughton G, Mansbridge J, Gentzkow G. A metabolically active human dermal replacement for the treatment of diabetic foot ulcers. Artifical Organs, 1997 ; 21 : 1-7.
23. Apelqvist J, Larsson, Agardh CD. Longterm prognosis for diabetic patients with foot ulcers. J Intern Med 1993 ; 233 : 485-491.

NOTES

THE DIABETIC FOOT
Medical and podiatric aspects

Michaël Edmonds and Alethea Foster
Kings Diabetes Centre—Denmark Hill, London

Foot ulceration is a leading cause of hospital admission for patients with diabetes and an extremely expensive complication of diabetes. The prevalence of foot ulceration in two-community based surveys in the United Kingdom was 5% in Oxford (1), and 7.4% in Poole (2), whereas the incidence of foot ulceration in a four year follow up study of 469 consecutive diabetic patients in Manchester, UK, without previous history of foot ulceration, was 10.2% (3). In a cohort of 2990 individuals with diabetes in Wisconsin, USA, the four year incidence of foot ulceration was 9.5% in subjects who were on insulin and whose diabetes began before the age of 30 years (1210 individuals), and in the remainder was 10.5% (4).

A recent, comprehensive summary of the direct costs of diabetic foot disorders in the USA has shown that the treatment of ulceration in non-insulin dependent diabetes accounted (in 1986) for $150 million—1.3 % of the £ 11.6 billion estimated direct cost for diabetes as a whole for that year—and that the average health care cost for a diabetic patient undergoing lower limb amputation (in 1985) was $24,700 (5). In the UK in 1986–87, in the North Western Region, admissions for diabetes with peripheral vascular disease and neuropathy accounted for 20.8% of the total bed days attributed to diabetes as principal cause (6). On the assumption that this reflects activity in the UK as a whole, around £ 12.9 million of the £ 1 billion devoted to the care of people with diabetes could be attributed to the care of people with these complications.

CLASSIFICATION AND DIAGNOSIS OF THE DIABETIC FOOT

The feet are the target of peripheral neuropathy leading chiefly to sensory deficit and autonomic dysfunction. Ischaemia results from atherosclerosis of the leg vessels which in the diabetic is often bilateral, multisegmental, and distal, involving arteries below the knee. Infection is rarely a sole factor but often complicates neuropathy and ischaemia. Nevertheless, it is responsible for considerable tissue necrosis in the diabetic foot. For practical purposes, the diabetic foot can be divided into two entities: the neuropathic foot in which neuropathy predominates and there is a good circulation, and the neuroischaemic foot where there is both neuropathy and absence of foot pulses. The purely ischaemic foot, with no concomitant neuropathy, is rarely seen in diabetic patients and its management is the same as for the neuroischaemic foot.

The neuropathic foot results in a warm, numb, dry, and usually painless foot in which the pulses are palpable. It leads to three complications—the neuropathic ulcer, which is found mainly on the sole of the foot, the neuropathic (Charcot) foot, and rarely, neuropathic oedema. In contrast, the neuroischaemic foot is cool and the pulses are absent. It is complicated by rest pain, ulceration on the margins of the foot from localised pressure necrosis, and gangrene.

Infection often complicates ulceration in both the neuropathic and neuroischaemic foot. The ulcers are portals of entry for bacteria and it is often a polymicrobial infection that spreads rapidly through the foot causing overwhelming tissue destruction (7). Such tissue destruction is the main reason for major amputation in the neuropathic foot.

Recent studies have indicated that approximately 50% of the diabetic feet presenting to dedicated foot clinics are neuropathic and 50% neuroischaemic (7,8).

However, amputation is not an inevitable consequence of vascular disease or neuropathy. Early recognition of the 'at risk' foot, the prompt institution of preventative measures, and the provision of rapid and intensive treatment of foot complications in multidisciplinary foot clinics has reduced the number of amputations in diabetic patients (7, 8).

The principal task in diagnosing the neuropathic or the rieuroischaemic foot is to ascertain the presence or absence of pulses. The most important manoeuvre is thus the palpation of foot pulses, an examination which is often undervalued. If either of the pulses in the foot can be felt, i.e., posterior tibial or dorsalis pedis, then it is highly unlikely that there is significant ischaemia. Absence of both pulses in the foot indicates a reduction in circulation. This can be confirmed by measuring the pressure index, which is the ratio of ankle systolic pressure to brachial systolic pressure. In normal subjects, the pressure index is usually >1, but in the presence of ischaemia is <1. Thus, absence of pulses and a pressure index of <1 confirms ischaemia. Conversely, the presence of pulses and a pressure index of >1 rules out ischaemia, and this has important implications for management, namely that macrovascular disease is not an important factor and arteriography is not indicated.

However, between 5–10% of the total diabetic population have non-compressible peripheral vessels giving an artificially elevated systolic pressure, even in the presence of ischaemia. It is thus difficult to assess the diabetic foot when the pulses are not palpable, but the pressure index is >1. There are two explanations. The examiner may have 'missed' the pulses, particularly in an oedematous foot, and should go back to palpate the foot after the vessels have been located by Doppler ultrasound. If the pulses remain impalpable, then ischaemia probably exists in the presence of medial wall calcification. In these circumstances, blood velocity waveforms obtained by Doppler ultrasound should be examined and toe pressures measured (see below).

The Doppler waveform becomes abnormal, distal to an obstructing lesion, with loss of normal rapid systolic upstroke and loss of diastolic flow. With diminishing flow, the waveform becomes flattened or 'damped' before it finally disappears. Several methods of signal analysis have been proposed to quantify changes in flow waveform and provide an index of severity of arterial disease (9).

Measurement of toe systolic pressure requires a toe cuff and a device for detecting toe blood flow, e.g., laser Doppler or a form of plethysmography. A toe pressure of 30mmHg or less is indicative of severe ischaemia and a very poor prognosis (10).

Similarly, a transcutaneous oxygen pressure measured on the dorsum of the foot of less than 30 mmHg is also evidence of severe ischaemia (11).

NEUROLOGICAL STATUS

Neurological status can be assessed by detecting sensation to pinprick and cotton wool, and vibration using a 128 cps tuning fork starting at the distal foot and moving proximally to confirm a symmetrical stocking distribution of peripheral neuropathy.

Knee and ankle jerks should be examined; their absence is evidence of peripheral neuropathy, although knee jerks are retained until surprisingly late. It is difficult to examine the autonomic nerves except to note a dry skin with marked fissuring as indicative of a sweating autonomic deficit.

Having diagnosed a neuropathy, it is important to ascertain whether the patient has lost protective pain sensation that would render him susceptible to foot ulceration.

Two clinical investigations are useful: vibrometry and nylon filaments. Vibration threshold can be measured using a hand-held Biothesiometer (Bio-medical instrument Company, 15764 Munn Road, Newbury, Ohio 44065, USA). The vibration threshold increases with age, and values must always be compared with age adjusted nomograms.

Nylon monofilaments test the threshold to pressure sensation. These are of various diameters and can be obtained from Hanson's Disease Foundation Inc., Carville, LA (12). The filament is applied to the foot until it buckles, when the patient is able to detect its presence. Buckling of the 5.07 monofilament occurs at 10g of linear pressure and is the limit used to detect protective pain sensation. If the patient does not detect the filament, then protective pain sensation is assumed to be lost.

Thus, the neuropathic foot is diagnosed in the presence of neuropathy and palpable pulses with a pressure index of >1, and the neuroischaemic foot in the presence of neuropathy and impalpable foot pulses.

NEUROPATHIC FOOT

Neuropathy

Peripheral neuropathy in the foot leads to both somatic and autonomic damage. Small fibre neuropathy may initially dominate, with associated loss of pain and heat sensation. A 'pseudosyringomyelic' pattern may result in which loss of heat sensation is distal and length related (13), and pain and thermal sensation is lost before sensations of light touch or vibration (14).

Sympathetic denervation which is characteristic of diabetic neuropathy is also a result of small fibre loss (15). A peripheral sympathetic defect has been documented by direct measurement of sympathetic activity in postganglionic C fibres in the diabetic neuropathic limb (16), and sympathetic nerve endings to small arterioles in the diabetic limb are either entirely absent or are found at a significantly greater distance from effector sites compared with controls (17).

Eventually a mixed fibre neuropathy develops in the diabetic foot involving both small and large sensory myelinated fibres with reduction in touch, vibration, and proprioception sense as well as pain and temperature. Motor fibres are also affected with slowed motor conduction velocities and reduced or absent action potentials of the intrinsic muscles of the feet. This can lead to wasting and weakness of intrinsic foot muscles and subsequent deformity including claw toes, resulting in abnormal distribution of weight bearing as well as friction from footwear, with subsequent ulceration (see below).

Blood flow

The neuropathic foot has an abnormally increased blood flow, as shown by Doppler (18, 19) and venous occlusion plethysmography (20). Blood flows on average five times higher than normal have been measured at the big toe and midfoot. These measurements confirm earlier observations of increased resting blood flow in patients with severe neuropathy of various aetiologies including diabetes. The spontaneous variations in resting flow which are secondary to sympathetic nerve activity are considerably reduced in the neuropathic foot.

Increase in blood flow is associated with arteriovenous shunting in the neuropathic limb, resulting in prominent turgid veins over the dorsum of the foot and lower part of the calf in the recumbent position (21). The concept of shunting is supported by evidence from Doppler sonograms which show a rapid forward flow of blood, highly suggestive of arteriovenous shunting that allows blood to proceed rapidly to the venous side of the circulation. Venous PO_2 is raised in the neuropathic limb approaching that of arterial blood (22) and venous pressure is raised in the neuropathic limb (23). The presence of substantial arteriovenous shunting might in theory jeopardise capillary nutritional blood flow. New methods of examination show that this is not the case. Measurement of capillary blood flow by laser Doppler flowmetry shows, overall, a higher flow than normal and this is further confirmed by direct visualisation of capillary blood flow velocity using television microscopy (24).

Despite the overperfusion under resting conditions, neuropathy leads an to impaired blood flow response to physical stimuli. Thus there are abnormalities of neurogenic vasodilation such as the flare response which occurs on stimulation of nociceptive C fibre, and this may be an important part of the response to foot trauma. A decreased flare response to iontophorectically applied acetylcholine has been demonstrated in the sole of the foot in patients with neuropathic ulcers and Charcot osteoarthropathy (25); similar abnormalities are present in the skin of the dorsum of the foot at an earlier stage of neuropathy, as defined by a raised vibration sensory threshold (26). Other vascular responses are also abnormal in the neuropathic foot, including a limitation of maximal blood flow in response to heating, and a marked diminution of vasoconstriction in response to the foot being placed dependent. The failure to vasoconstrict contributes to the excessive blood flow when upright, and to the oedema which to a greater or lesser extent often develops in severe neuropathy. Increased capillary permeability in long term diabetes must also contribute to this problem.

Sympathetic denervation of richly innervated capillaries also causes increased uptake by bone of technetium methylene diphosphonate, giving very striking isotopic scans of bones that appear normal on conventional radiography (28). It is likely that this causes a resorption of bone leading to osteopenia, as it does in other situations such as paraplegia.

There is evidence of cortical bone thinning in the feet and hands of severely neuropathic diabetic patients (29) and this might predispose to the extensive bony destruction which occurs in Charcot osteoarthropathy, and this is discussed below.

The properties of the vessel walls in the neuropathic limb may contribute to the haemodynamic abnormalities. The arterial walls are stiff, probably as a result of medial wall calcification. This increased stiffness has been inferred from raised ankle systolic pressures and shortened transit times of the pulse waveform. Diffuse atherosclerosis may give rise to increased pulse wave velocity but, in the neuropathic limb, medial wall calcification may also be responsible. An association between diabetic neuropathy and medial wall calcification has been demonstrated (30). Eleven out of 13 patients who underwent unilateral sympathectomy developed Monckeberg's sclerosis on the operated side, having had normal radiographs before the procedure. Bilateral sympathectomy was carried out in seven patients, all of whom showed calcification on both sides later. Thus, sympathetic denervation may be responsible for medial wall calcification.

Sweating

Diminished or absent sweating in the feet and legs commonly occurs in patients with diabetic neuropathy as a manifestation of peripheral sympathetic denervation. Indeed, anhidrosis of the feet may be responsible for cracking of the skin, resulting in a portal of entry for infections. The sweating loss normally occurs in a stocking distribution, which can extend into the trunk, and above which there may be excessive sweating. Patchy sweating loss sometimes occurs.

Except for sweat glands located in the palm and soles, most human sweat glands do not secrete appreciable amounts of water under basal conditions. It is thus necessary to activate sweat glands to detect all functioning glands (31) and this may be done either locally by iontophoresis or intradermal injection, or by physiological activation, such as whole body heating or by stimulating the sympathetic nervous system by extraneous stimuli such as coughing.

Local stimulation of sweat glands can be achieved by application of cholinergic agents either by intradermal injection or iontophoresis. The sweat responses induced by acetylcholine has two components. The first or direct response is due to stimulation of muscarinic sweat gland receptors. The second response is via the local axon reflex which is mediated by sympathetic post ganglionic axons. This response can be recorded using the quantitated sudomotor axon reflex test (QSART) (32).

Direct stimulation of sweat glands can also be achieved by iontophoresis of pilocarpine which binds to the muscarinic receptors. The secretion of sweat can be recorded by the silastic imprint method in which a silasti impression material is spread over the relevant area and when this hardens, each sweat droplet leaves an impression so that both its size can be measured and total droplets from sweat glands be counted. Sweat glands will only be activated if they have an intact sympathetic nervous system and they do not respond when denervated (31).

In the thermoregulatory sweat test stimulation of sweating is achieved by total body warming in which the oral temperature must rise to 38°C or increase by 1.0°C (33). Areas of sweating are identified by an indicator powder mixture. Finally, sympathetic activation of sweat glands by stimuli such as a loud noise or a cough causes the skin potential to change and this is detected by recording electrodes placed in pairs on the dorsal and vertical surfaces of the foot (34).

Sweating defects assessed by QSART and silastic imprint methods show a relationship with abnormalities of autonomic function, assessed by heart rate variability and the Valsalva manoeuvre. Most patients with postural hypotension have absent foot sweating, indicative of their common cause, namely, sympathetic denervation; 75% of those with neuropathic foot ulcers and 36% with Charcot joints also show absence of sweating in their feet (35). Loss of pain sensation is correlated with diminished sweating.

Pressure

The presence of excessive pressure is a prerequisite for the development of a neuropathic ulcer. Cross sectional studies have shown that foot pressures in neuropathic diabetic subjects are higher compared to non-neuropathic subjects, and foot ulcers develop predominantly in a areas of high pressure (36). Recently, a prospective study has shown that high foot pressures are predictive of subsequent foot ulceration (37).

Plantar pressure can be measured with a number of commercially available systems. However, progress has not yet been reached to the point of positive identification of a threshold pressure at which ulceration would be likely to occur in an individual with loss of protective sensation. Furthermore, different systems for measuring pressure distribution yield different results in the same patient (38). Elevated foot pressures are more likely to be present when the foot is deformed.

The presence of neuropathy, even in its very earliest form with relatively mild sensory defects, may itself predispose to elevated foot pressures. Patients with foot ulcers tend to be heavier than others, although weight does not itself necessarily cause high foot pressure. Although vertical forces are obviously important, horizontal or shear forces must also be instrumental in damaging the neuropathic foot, and the sites of healed ulcers have been shown to correspond to the sites of maximal shear forces.

Shear forces are difficult to measure, and there are no commercially available instruments to measure shear force. However, recent interest has resulted in several groups attempting to measure this. The underlying principle is to use magneto-resistive elements attached to the sole and by this means horizontal shear forces can be measured. Tappin et al. (39) were the first to describe the use of this technique for measuring discrete plantar stresses with a uniaxial shear transducer. Laing et al. (40) have further developed Tappin's device by making it smaller in diameter and thickness. A triaxial transducer incorporating a biaxial shear stress section has been described by Lord et al. (41) and this measures shear in two orthogonal directions. The transducer is mounted in an inlay which can directly replace the normal deep inlay of an extra depth shoe.

Deformity

Deformities of the feet are more likely to be associated with abnormal pressures. Abnormalities are congenital or acquired as a result of neuropathy. Congenital abnormalities may be more common, although this has not been systematically investigated. Neuropathy causes weakness of the small muscles of the foot with clawing of the toes and prominence of the metatarsal heads, and this may be one reason for reduced toe loading in neuropathic patients. Some patients have congenitally clawed toes, and the distinction from those with a neuropathic basis may be impossible by the time of foot ulceration. Other deformities that predispose to abnormal pressures include hallux rigidus, hammer toes, and bunions (7). The most severe abnormalities are those of the Charcot foot: they are very liable to ulceration, especially when there is a 'rocker bottom' sole.

Limitation of joint motion secondary to glycation of connective tissues can lead to deformity and high plantar pressures. The normal foot has been described as a mobile adapter, and when mobility is impaired, elevated plantar pressure during walking results. Limitation of the ankle joint results in a fixed plantar flexion deformity (equinus) which leads to high mechanical loads under the forefoot (42). Callus formation is common in the diabetic foot and also causes elevated plantar pressure. In a study of 17 patients, peak plantar pressures were reduced after sharp debridement of callus by an average of 26% (43).

In addition, gait pattern is disturbed in patients with diabetic neuropathy and this may alter the foot pressure distribution, making the foot more prone to the effects of high pressure (44).

Oedema

The presence of foot oedema may not only underlie the development of foot ulcers when the shoes become too tight, but also (in theory at least) could impede healing of established ulcers. Oedema is common in elderly patients, but in diabetic patients there are additional reasons for its occurrence, either from neuropathy or less commonly from fluid retention or nephrotic syndrome in patients with diabetic nephropathy.

Oedema is a complication of severe diabetic neuropathy. It has long been recognised and was observed in 35 of 125 patients with neuropathy described by Martin (45). It is therefore not a rare phenomenon, although severe intractable oedema resulting from neuropathy is exceptional. This form of oedema probably results from the major haemodynamic abnormalities associated with neuropathy. Thus, the high blood flow, vasodilatation, and arteriovenous shunting resulting from sympathetic denervation lead to abnormal venous pooling and recently high venous pressures have been demonstrated in the neuropathic foot (23).

Oedema probably occurs because of loss of the venivasomotor reflex, which normally occurs on standing and results in an increase in precapillary resistance; the inability of the foot to compensate for the rise in venous pressure would thus predispose to oedema formation. Relief of oedema by administration of the sympathomimetic agent ephedrine (46) lends further strength to the argument that sympathetic failure is the cause of oedema, and is discussed in greater detail below.

COMPLICATIONS OF THE NEUROPATHIC FOOT

Neuropathic Ulcer
Presentation
The most frequent complication of the neuropathic foot is the neuropathic ulcer. Its classical position is under the metatarsal heads, but it is more frequently found on the tips of the toes and occasionally on the dorsum of the toe, between the toes, and on the heel. The neuropathic ulcer is usually surrounded by callous tissue and is generally painless. The ulcers on the plantar surface of the feet are usually circular, with a punched out appearance often penetrating to involve deep tissues including bone.

Neuropathic ulcers result from mechanical, thermal, or chemical injuries that are unperceived by the patient because of loss of pain sensation. Loss of sensation, especially awareness of pain, is obviously a vital predisposing factor, although autonomic neuropathy is also important. Motor neuropathy also plays a role with paralysis of the small muscles contributing to structural deformities such as claw toes. This leads to prominence of the metatarsal heads in the ulcerated foot.

Direct mechanical injuries may result from treading on nails and other sharp objects, but the most frequent cause of ulceration from mechanical factors is neglected callosity. This results from excess friction at the tips of the toes and from high vertical and shear forces under the plantar surface of the metatarsal heads on walking. The repetitive mechanical forces of gait eventually result in callosity formation, inflammatory autolysis, and subkeratotic haematomas. The callosities are painless and are neglected by the patient. The presence of haemorrhage into a callus is a sign of early ulcer formation, with a 50% chance of finding an ulcer when it is removed (47). Tissue necrosis occurs below the plaque of callus, resulting in a small cavity filled with serous fluid which eventually breaks through to the surface with ulcer formation.

At this stage, infection usually supervenes, caused by organisms from the surrounding skin which are usually Staphylococcus aureus or Streptococci. If drainage is inadequate, cellulitis develops with spread of sepsis to infect underlying tendons and bones and joints. Occasionally Staphylococci and Streptococci are present together and these can combine to produce a rampant cellulitis that extends rapidly through the foot, producing marked necrosis within only a few hours. Streptococci secrete hyaluronidase which facilitates widespread distribution of necrotising toxins from Staphylococci. Enzymes from these bacteria are also angiotoxic and cause in situ thrombosis of vessels. If both vessels are thrombosed in the toe, then it becomes necrotic and gangrenous and this is probably the basis of so-called 'diabetic' gangrene in which tissue necrosis is seen only a few centimetres away from a bounding dorsalls pedis pulse. Aerobic gram negative organisms as well as anaerobic organisms flourish in deep seated infections. Both aerobic and anaerobic organisms can rapidly infect the bloodstream and occasionally result in life-threatening bacteraemia.

Severe sepsis in the diabetic foot is often associated with gas in the soft tissues. Subcutaneous gas may be detected by direct palpation of the foot and the diagnosis is confirmed by the appearance of gas in the soft tissue on the radiograph. Although Clostridial organisms have previously been held responsible for this presentation, non-Clostridial organisms are more frequently the offending pathogens. These include Bacteroides, Escherichia and anaerobic Streptococci.

Fungal infections also occur but usually do not cause systemic upset. However, infections of toe nails (tinea unguirn) and interdigital spaces (tinea pedis) by such fungi as Trichophyton and Candida albicans can serve as portals of entry for bacteria.

In addition to mechanical injury, ulceration can also result from thermal or chemical injury. Thermal injuries cause direct trauma and damage to the epithelium. This often results from bathing feet in excessively hot water, the injudicious use of hot water bottles, from resting the feet too close to a fire or radiator, or from walking bare-foot on hot sand during holidays in warm climates.

Chemical trauma can result from the use of keratolytic agents such as 'corn plasters.' They often contain salicylic acid which causes ulceration in the diabetic foot.

Management of Neuropathic Ulceration
The management of ulceration in the purely neuropathic foot falls into three parts:

1. removal of callus and local treatment
2. eradication of infection and
3. reduction of weight bearing forces

1. Removal of callus
The callus which surrounds the ulcer must be removed by expert chiropody. Excess keratin should be 'pared' away with a scalpel blade to expose the floor of the ulcer and allow efficient drainage of the lesion and re-epithelialisation from the edges of the ulcer. A simple non-adhesive dressing should be applied, after cleaning the ulcer and surrounding tissue with saline. Use of wound healing factors is being explored and recent studies have shown that it may speed healing in the neuropathic foot (48).

2. Eradication of infection
A bacterial swab should be taken from the floor of the ulcer after the callus has been removed. A superficial ulcer may be treated on an outpatient basis and oral antibiotics prescribed, according to the organism isolated, until the ulcer has healed. The patient should be instructed to carry out daily dressings of the ulcer.

If cellulitis or skin discolouration is present, the limb is threatened and urgent hospital admission should be arranged. The limb should be rested, and the ulcer irrigated with 2% Milton (sodium hypochlorite) solution. After blood cultures have been taken, intravenous antibiotics are administered to treat possible Staphylococci, Streptococci, gram negative bacteria, and anaerobes (flucloxacillin 500 mg 6 hourly, amoxycillin 500 mg IV 8 hourly, ceftazidine 1 g 8 hourly and metronidazole 1 g per rectum 8 hourly). This antibiotic regimen may need revision after the results of bacterial cultures are available. Blood glucose may need to be controlled with an intravenous insulin pump.

In the neuropathic foot, it is important that all necrotic tissue be removed and abscess cavities drained surgically. If gangrene has developed in a digit, a ray amputation to remove that toe and part of its associated metatarsal is necessary and is usually very successful in the neuropathic foot (7).

3. Reduction of weight bearing forces

Bed rest in the acute stages of ulceration is ideal and will obviously remove the weight bearing forces to promote healing. Proper care should be taken of the heels and foam wedges used to protect them from pressure in bed. However, bed rest is not always possible. In the short term, a total contact plaster cast (with minimum of padding) can be applied to 'unload' the ulcer and reduce shear forces (49). Other forms of cast have become popular, especially removable casts, such as the Scotch cast (50). Padded hosiery may also help to relieve pressure. With regular rotation, these padded socks have been shown to reduce plantar pressures for at least 6 months (51). In the long term, redistribution of weight bearing forces can be achieved by special footwear, which is fashioned from casts of the patient's foot. Insoles made of closed cell polyethylene foams such as Plastazote have energy absorbing properties. These can be heated and moulded to the shape of the foot to cushion the plantar surface of the foot and to spread the forces of weight bearing evenly (Fig 1). When subject to wear and tear, Plastazote insoles can 'bottom out,' and it is now possible to use more durable materials such as Poron. Indeed, composite insoles are often made with an upper layer of polyethylene foam for total contact and a lower layer of microcell rubber for resilience (52) (Fig 2). When there has been previous ulceration, a rigid weight distributing cradle is required, as well as cushioning, to relieve weight from high pressure areas and to transfer it to other less vulnerable areas. Traditionally, cork cradles have been used, but recently Plastazote cradles have been manufactured often with 'windows' cut out (and filled in with cushioning material such as Neoprene) for weight relief at these sites.

Moulded insoles must be accommodated in extra depth shoes. When the foot is not deformed, shoes fashioned from commercial lasts and available 'off the shelf' can be used. If the patient has a foot deformity with healed neuropathic ulcers, it is necessary to make individual lasts from casts of the patient's foot. In either case, the heels must be low, and slipping is prevented by using lace-ups. The forefoot should be broad and square and the uppers of high quality leather which will adapt to toe pressure (53). When pressure points are not adequately relieved by cushioned insoles, it is necessary to modify the soles of the shoe. When the ulcer is under the plantar surface of the first toe, a rigid rocker sole allows the shoe to rock like a see saw on a pivot under the centre of the shoe, minimising contact between the forefoot and floor during gait.

If the ulcer is under the metatarsal heads, a metatarsal bar placed just proximal to the heads can re-apportion weight bearing forces along the shafts.

Charcot Foot
Presentation

The most frequent location of the neuropathic joint is the tarsal-metatarsal region, followed by the metatarsophalangeal joints and then the ankle and subtalar joints (54). The initial presentation is often a hot, swollen foot which can be uncomfortable in up to one third of cases and is often misdiagnosed as cellulitis or gout. The precipitating event is usually a minor traumatic episode such as tripping.

If the patient presents within a few days, radiographs are often normal, although isotope bone scans may be grossly abnormal with localised areas of high uptake representing excessive osteoblastic activity and heralding eventual radiological abnormalities. A common early radiological abnormality is fracture, which is followed by osteolysis, bony fragmentation, and finally joint subluxation and disorganisation. In addition to fracture, erosions, periosteal new bone formation, and sclerosis are also prominent bony findings in the development of the Charcot joint. Sclerosis is usually associated with lucency in the heads of the metatarsals, the final appearance being similar to the Frieberg's infraction lesion associated with osteonecrosis of the epiphysis of the metatarsal head. These initial bony abnormalities eventually lead to secondary joint destruction with subluxation of the metatarsophalangeal joints, dislocation of the tarsal, subtalar and ankle joints, and fragmentation of bone and soft tissue calcification (55).

The process of destruction takes place over a few months only and leads to two classic deformities: the rocker bottom deformity, in which there is displacement and subluxation of the tarsus downwards, and the medial convexity, which results from displacement of the talonavicular joint or from tarsometatarsal dislocation. If these deformities are not accommodated in properly fitting footwear, ulceration at vulnerable pressure points often develops (Fig 3).

Pathogenesis

The development of Charcot osteoarthropathy depends on both peripheral autonomic and somatic defects. Recent studies have indicated a specific deficit of small fibre function (56). Furthermore, an adequate blood supply is necessary, and notably the development of the Charcot foot has been described in the foot after successful arterial bypass surgery (57). It is suggested that the evolution is as follows. Sympathetic denervation of arterioles causes an increase of blood flow which in turn causes rarefaction of bone, making it prone to damage even after minor trauma. Bone formation and structure are closely linked with vascular changes. Large venules containing rapid linear velocities of blood flow cause resorption of bone spicules (58). In animals, the site of maximum bone calcium loss after paraplegia corresponds to areas of maximum blood flow, which may lead to increased resorption of bone (59). Histological studies of Charcot joints have shown marked increase in vascularity with vessel dilatation and trabecula resorption by large numbers of osteociasts (60). Thus, increased bony blood flow can lead to bony resorption and susceptibility to fracture (see above). Loss of sensation from somatic neuropathy permits abnormal mechanical stresses to occur, normally prevented by pain. Relatively minor trauma can then cause major destructive changes in susceptible bone.

Management

It is essential to make the diagnosis early, before extreme joint destruction has taken place. The initial presentation of unilateral warmth and swelling in a neuropathic foot after an episode of minor trauma is suggestive of a developing Charcot joint.

There is no definite treatment that halts the progression of the disease, but immobilisation may help. Treatment comprises rest (ideally bed rest), or the avoidance of weight bearing by the use of crutches until the oedema and local warmth have resolved. Alternatively, the foot can be put in a well-moulded rion walking plaster cast.

Immobilisation is continued until bony repair is complete, usually a period of 2–3 months. Recently, bisphosphonates have been used to inhibit osteoclastic activity leading to a reduction in foot temperature and resolution of symptoms (61).

Neuropathic Oedema

Pathogenesis

This has been discussed earlier in this chapter.

Management

The use of a sympathomimetic agent, by stimulating vasoconstriction, might be expected to reduce this form of oedema and, indeed, ephedrine has a rapid and substantial effect on relieving neuropathic oedema (46). It results in a rapid decrease of weight, a reduction in peripheral diastolic flow, and an increase in sodium excretion, all associated with rapid diminution of oedema over a few days. The effect of ephedrine is possibly complex, and as well as its peripheral effects, it may have central effects on the control of salt and water homeostasis. The usual dosage of ephedrine is 15–30 mg thrice daily, although it may be necessary to increase this to 60 mg thrice daily.

The Neuroischaemic Foot

Presentation

The clinical features of ischaemia are intermittent claudication, rest pain, ulceration, and gangrene. However, the most frequent symptom is ulceration. The ulcers present as areas of necrosis often surrounded by a rim of erythema. In contrast to ulceration in the neuropathic foot, callus tissue is usually absent. Furthermore, ulceration in the ischaemic foot is often painful, although this varies from patient to patient according to the coexistence of a peripheral neuropathy. In the ischaemic foot, the most frequent sites of ulceration are the great toe, medial surface of the head of the first metatarsal, the lateral surface of the fifth metatarsal head (Fig 4), and the heel.

Pathogenesis

The main factor responsible for a reduction in blood supply to the foot is atherosclerosis of the large vessels of the leg. In the diabetic subject, atherosclerosis is often multisegmental, bilateral, and distal, involving tibial and peroneal vessels (62). In the end stages, occlusion can be particularly extensive in the foot vessels (63). Conversely, involvement of the aorto-iliac vessels is twice as common in non-diabetics as in diabetics. The predilection to atherosclerosis for the vessels below the knee in diabetes is unexplained.

The actual histo-pathology of the large vessel wall is similar to that in non-diabetics. Fatty deposits occur in plaques within the intima. The plaques are most commonly localised at bifurcations, on the posterior walls of arteries, and where the arteries are compressed by muscle fascia as in the adductor canal (64).

So called small vessel disease involving capillaries and arterioles had been thought to contribute substantially to impaired circulation in the feet. However, the significance of obliterative lesions of arterioles and capillaries with endothelial proliferation and basement membrane thickening is not known, and the role, if any, in the development of ischaemic foot lesions remains to be elucidated. Although there is little evidence of an occlusive microvascular disease, functional abnormalities of the capillaries such as increased leaking of albumin from the capillaries to the interstitium may be important (65). However, previous emphasis on small vessel disease in the diabetic foot has led to therapeutic nihilism and inappropriate care.

Tissue necrosis in the ischaemic limb is usually associated with minor trauma often complicated by infection. The traumas include direct pressure from tight shoes or socks, thermal and chemical injuries, and injudicious cutting of the nails. When external pressures on localised areas of skin exceed capillary pressure, tissue necrosis follows. Initial incidents are often trivial and lead to trivial injuries. However, they are frequently neglected and rapidly lead to ulceration.

Minor trauma is often followed by infection. Ulcers serve as portals of entry for bacteria, and sepsis can rapidly spread through the foot. In the non-ischaemic foot, there is a good collateral circulation which can counteract major infection. In the diabetic ischaemic foot, obstructive disease is common in the metatarsal arteries (63), and this reduces communication in and between the plantar and dorsal arterial arches. The digital arteries are thus converted into 'end arteries' (66). Many bacteria can elaborate angiotoxic substances which cause a septic thrombosis.

Advancing infection can thus obliterate digital arteries and the tissue perfused by that artery becomes necrotic, followed by rapid advancement of sepsis through the foot.

Management

Management can be divided into two parts: medical treatment and revascularisation either by angioplasty or arterial reconstruction.

Medical

Medical management is indicated if the ulcer is small and shallow and is of recent onset within the previous month. Furthermore, it is the mainstay of treatment for those patients in whom reconstructive surgery is not feasible or possible because of widespread cardiovascular or cerebrovascular disease. Ischaemic ulcers may be painful and it may be necessary to prescribe opiates. It is the role of the podiatrist to remove necrotic tissue from the ulcers and, in the case of subunqual ulcers, to cut back the nail to allow drainage of the ulcer. Ulcer swabs are taken as with the neuropathic foot and the ulcers are cleaned with normal saline and dressed with a sterile non-adherent dressing. It is important for the diabetologist to eradicate infection with prompt and specific antibiotic therapy after consultation with the microbiologist. However, severe sepsis in the ischaemic foot is an indication for emergency admission, first to control sepsis by intravenous antibiotics and surgical drainage, and secondly to assess the possibility of revascularisation either by angioplasty or reconstruction. Footwear should be supplied to accommodate the foot and in most cases an extra depth, ready-made shoe to protect the borders of the foot is adequate, unless there is severe deformity, when bespoke shoes will be needed. If any lesion, however small and apparently trivial, in the pulseless foot has not responded to conservative treatment within four weeks, then the patient should be considered for arteriography and revascularisation, and in many cases, where there is severe ischaemia, referral will need to be initiated at a much earlier stage.

Revascularisation

There has been much interest in the optimal management of peripheral vascular disease in both diabetic and non-diabetic patients with recommendations published in the first and second European Consensus Documents on Critical Leg Ischaemia (67,68). One of the most important advances in diabetic foot care has been the development of new techniques of revascularisation of the ischaemic foot which has led to a reduction in the number of major amputations in diabetic patients. The economic cost of reconstruction is less than that of amputation (69), and successful revascularisation has been associated with excellent mobility (70).

A modern vascular service is necessary to treat such arterial disease effectively, and this includes an imaging service to support complimentary interventional radiology and surgical vascular management. The vascular service should carry out percutaneous catheter procedures, including angioplasty and thrombolysis, and bypass surgery including distal revascularisation.

Modern vascular imaging includes conventional non-invasive Doppler ultrasound to assess the pressure index and blood velocity pattern of the leg arteries, and Duplex ultrasound to give both anatomical and functional images. This is particularly useful in the assessment of the tibial and foot vessels. However, the gold standard is arteriography complimented by digital subtraction arteriography (DSA) which allows excellent views of the tibial and foot vessels.

Angioplasty

Recently, great advances have been made in percutaneous catheter techniques. Angioplasty balloons have been incorporated into guide wires and this has enabled lesions in the distal calf to be accessible to angioplasty (71). Percutaneous catheter procedures including angioplasty have thus become established methods of treating peripheral vascular disease. Angioplasty is minimally invasive with a low mortality, low morbidity, needing short hospital stay, and the techniques are repeatable. Given the same lesion, a diabetic patient will do equally well as a non-diabetic following femoral popliteal angioplasty, assuming equality of other factors, such as inflow or outflow (72). There is a growing body of literature advocating angioplasty as the initial management of vascular disease where appropriate The second report of the European Consensus on Critical Ischaemia recommends that, if angiography shows a technically suitable lesion and an experienced radiologist is available, a percutaneous catheter procedure should be tried as the first option, even though surgery may eventually be needed. Furthermore, important adjunctive techniques to percutaneous balloon angioplasty have recently been developed, including thrombolytic therapy, which can be used to treat occlusions of up to one month's duration (73).

These can be used in diabetic patients, although the presence of proliferative retinopathy increases the risk of haemorrhage, and therefore a thorough ophthalmic assessment is necessary before this treatment.

Overall, it is important that early referral is made for catheter procedures before extensive tissue deficit as occurred. In these circumstances, experience has shown that a restoration of pulsatile blood flow is necessary from distal bypass surgery. Throughout such percutaneous procedures, it is extremely important to supervise the medical care of diabetic patients, who are often old and frail with impaired cardiac and cerebovascular function. It is important that they do not get dehydrated, and if the serum creatinine is raised, renal function is protected by appropriate measures such as intravenous dopamine infusion (renal dose) during the procedures.

Arterial bypass

Recent advances in vascular surgery have led to the reappraisal of the optimum management of critical leg ischaemia, resulting in an expanded and successful role of arterial reconstruction in diabetic patients (74). There has been an improved understanding of the pattern of atherosclerotic occlusion with an emphasis on arteriographic delineation of the distal arteries, leading to success with distal arterial reconstruction. The microcirculation in the foot is not occluded in the diabetic patient (75), so that once the foot arteries are revascularised, excellent capillary perfusion results. Bypass grafting to infra-popliteal arteries for limb salvage is both technically feasible and durable with autogenous vein being superior to prosthetic grafts. In a group of unselected patients, including both diabetic and non-diabetic, patency rates were 72% in vein grafts and 51 % in prosthetic grafts at follow up after three years (70).

Recent reports have confirmed the value of the distal bypass in selected diabetic patients. Graft patency and limb salvage after 56 vein bypasses to the dorsal pedal artery resulted in actuarial graft patency and limb salvage of 92% and 98% respectively at 36 months (76). Similar results have come from a further study in 72 diabetic patients with tibial artery disease reporting one-and five year limb salvage rates of 81 and 72% respectively (77). Thus, distal vein graft reconstruction for limb threatening ischaemia produces excellent patency rates and contributes significantly to limb salvage in these patients. The mean cost of primary arterial reconstruction is substantially cheaper than the cost of amputation. Distal bypasses are the most expensive of bypass surgery, as further operations are sometimes needed during follow up of the primary procedure, yet still their mean cost remains less than major amputation (70). Whilst under the care of the vascular service, the patient will need close medical supervision from the diabetologist and there should be close collaboration between the vascular surgeon, radiologist, and diabetologist with a combined vascular x-ray conference providing an ideal forum for discussion and planning of treatment.

THE FOOT IN DIABETIC NEPHROPATHY

Foot ulcer, sepsis, and gangrene resulting from peripheral vascular disease, neuropathy, or both together, are common in patients with diabetic nephropathy and renal failure. These problems and their management are, in general, similar to those in diabetes uncomplicated by renal disease. The most striking difference in nephropathy patients is the presence of extensive digital arterial calcification, which occurs both in feet and hands (78,79). Digital gangrene of toes and fingers occurs predominantly in those with calcified vessels and is almost specific for patients with diabetic renal failure; it can occur in any of these patients, whether on dialysis or receiving transplantation. Of 80 patients with diabetic nephropathy who received a renal transplant, 11 developed digital gangrene; all had severe digital calcification. The pathophysiological changes that precipitate digital gangrene are not clearly understood.

ORGANIZATION OF DIABETIC FOOT CARE: THE DIABETIC FOOT CLINIC

It is vital that there is close liaison between chiropodist, shoe fitter, physician, and surgeon in the care of the diabetic foot; since 1981, diabetic foot problems have been treated within a special Diabetic Foot Clinic at King's College Hospital (25). It has provided intensive chiropody, close surveillance, prompt treatment of foot infection, and a footwear service by the attending shoe fitter.

It has achieved a 50% reduction in major amputations (7) by adhering to four main strategies:

1. Accurate diagnosis of the neuropathic and neuroischaemic syndromes of the diabetic foot.
2. Rapid and appropriate treatment of foot lesions including sepsis.
3. Intensive follow up of patients.
4. Prevention of foot lesions.

The ultimate treatment is, of course, prevention, and this therapeutic approach must be through education of the patient in foot care and regular examination of the feet. It has been shown that patients who develop foot lesions have significantly less knowledge of diabetes, including foot care (80). Moreover, it has been clearly shown that education reduces the number of major amputations in a diabetic clinic population (81). Routine examination of the feet in diabetic patients is an important part of management, in order to identify those at risk of ulceration and to prevent its occurrence. However, it is a commonly under-utilised preventive measure (82).

CONCLUSION

Ulceration of the non-ischaemic diabetic foot depends on the presence of neuropathy, and is especially likely to occur in areas of the foot where high pressure (often associated with foot deformities) leads to the development of excessive callus which eventually breaks down and ulcerates.

Damage to small nerve fibres is the essential element of the neuropathy, causing loss of thermal and pain sensation, and sympathetic defects leading to diminished sweating and grossly altered haemodynamics. The arteries in the feet of these patients are rigid, and blood flow greatly increased both in skin and bones, causing both oedema and osteopenia; nutritive capillary flow remains unimpaired. Ulceration in the neuro-ischaemic feet results from pressure necrosis, often unperceived because of co-existent neuropathy. The main reduction in blood supply to the foot is related to atherosclerosis of the large vessels of the leg which, in the diabetic patient, is often multisegmental, bilateral, and distal, involving tibial and peroneal vessels.

The feet of diabetic patients must be carefully examined for the presence of deformities, callus formation, evidence of ischaemia and neuropathy in order to institute effective measure.

Optimum care of the diabetic foot is provided in a diabetic foot clinic where the skills of chiropodist, shoe fitter and nurse receive full support from physician and surgeon. Many lesions of the diabetic foot are avoidable and thus patient education is of immense importance.

REFERENCES

1.   Neil HAW, Thompson AV, Thorogood M et al. Diabetes in the elderly: the Oxford community diabetes study. Diabetic Medicine 1989; 6: 608-613.
2.   Walters DP, Gatling W, Mullee et al. The distribution and severity of diabetic foot disease: a community study with a comparison to a non diabetic group. Diabetic Medicine. 1992; 9: 354-358.
3.   Young MJ, Bready JL, Veves A et al. The prediction of diabetic neuropathic foot ulceration using vibration perception thresholds: a prospective study. Diabetes Care 1994; in press.
4.   Moss SE, Klein R, Klein BEK. The prevalence and incidence of lower extremity amputation in diabetic population. Arch Intern Med 1992; 152: 610-616.
5.   Relber GE. Diabetes foot care: financial implications and practical guidelines. Diabetes Care. 1992; 15 suppl 1: 29-31.
6.   Williams DRR. The size of the problem epidemiological and economic aspects of foot problems in diabetes. In: The Foot in Diabetes 2nd edition., Boulton AJM, Connor H, Cavanagh P eds. John Wiley & Sons 1994, Chichester, England, p 15-24.
7.   Edmonds ME, Blundell MP, Morris HE et al. The diabetic foot: impact of a foot clinic. QJM 1986, 232: 763-771.
8.   Thomson FJ, Veves A, Ashe H et al. A team approach to diabetic foot care - the Manchester experience. The Foot 1991; 1: 75-82.
9.   Sidaway AN, Curry KM. Non invasive evolution of the lower extremity arterial system, In: Frykberg RG (ed), The High Risk Foot in Diabetes Mellitus. Churchill Livingstone, Edinburgh, 1991, pp 241-254.
10. European Working Group on Critical Leg Ischaemia. Second European Consensus Document on Chronic Critical Leg Ischaemia. Eur J Vasc Surg 1992; 6 (suppl. A).
11. Jacobs MJHM, Ubbink D. Th, Kitslaar PJEHM et al. Assessment of the microcirculation provides additional information in critical limb ischaemia. Eur J Vasc Surg. 1992; 6: 135-741.
12. Birke JA, Sims DS. Plantar sensory threshold in the ulcerative foot. Lepr Rev 1986; 57: 261-267.
13. Said B, Slama G, Selva J. Progressive centripetal degeneration of axons in small fibre type diabetic polyneuropathy. A clinical and pathological study. Brain 1983; 106: 791-807.
14. Guy RJC, Clark CA, Malcolm PN, Watkins PJ. Evaluation of thermal and vibration sensation in diabetic neuropathy. Diabetologia 1985; 28: 131-137.
15. Watkins PJ, Edmonds ME. Sympathetic nerve failure in diabetes. Diabetologia 1983; 25: 73-77.
16. Fagius J. Microneurographic findings in diabetic polyneuropathy with special reference to sympathetic nerve activity. Diabetologia 1982, 23: 415-520.
17. Imparato AM, Kim GE, Thomas PK. Abnormal innervation of the lower limb epineurial arterioles in human diabetes. Diabetologia 1981; 20: 31-38.
18. Scarpello JH, Martin TR, Ward JD. Ultrasound measurements of pulse wave velocity in the peripheral arteries of diabetic subjects. Clin Sci 1980, 58, 53-57.
19. Edmonds ME, Roberts VC, Watkins PJ. Blood flow in the diabetic neuropathic foot, Diabetologia 1982; 22: 9-15.
20. Archer AG, Roberts VC, Watkins PJ. Blood flow patterns in painful diabetic neuropathy. Diabetologia 1984; 27: 563-567.
21. Ward JD, Simms JM, Knight G, Boulton AJM, Sandler DA. Venous distension in the diabetic neuropathic foot (physical sign of arteriovenous shunting). J R Soc Med 1983; 76: 1011-1014.
22. Boulton AJM, Scarpello JHB, Ward JD. Venous oxygenation in the diabetic neuropathic foot: evidence for arteriovenous shunting? Diabetologia 1982; 22: 6-8.
23. Purewal TS, Goss DE, Edmonds ME, Watkins PJ. Venous pressure is raised in the diabetic neuropathic foot - a new observation from direct venous cannulation. Diabetic Medicine 1993; A24: 57.
24. Flynn MD, Tooke JE, Watkins PJ. Abnormal capillary blood flow in the diabetic neuropathic foot, assessed by direct television microscopy. Dia Med 1986; 3: 587A.
25. Parkhouse N, Le Quesne PM. Impaired neurogenic vascular response in patients with diabetes and neuropathic foot lesions. N Engl J Med 1988; 318: 1306-1309.
26. Walmsley D, Wiles PG. Early loss of neurogenic inflammation in the human diabetic foot. Clin Sci 1991; 80: 605-610.
27. Flynn MD, Tooke JE. Microcirculation and the diabetic foot. Vasc Med Rev 1990: 1: 121-138.
28. Edmonds ME, Clarke MD, Newton S, Barrett JJ, Watkins PJ. Increased uptake of bone radiopharmaceutical in diabetic neuropathy. Quart J Med 1985; 57: 843-855.
29. Cundy T, Edmonds ME, Watkins PJ. Osteopaenia and metatarsal fractures in diabetic neuropathy. Diab Med 1985; 2: 461-464.
30. Edmonds ME, Morrison N, Laws JW, Watkins PJ. Medial arterial calcification and diabetic neuropathy. BMJ 1982, 284, 928-930.
31. Kennedy WR, Navarro X. Evaluation of sudomotor function by sweat imprint methods. In: Low PA (ed) Clinical Autonomic Disorders: Evaluation and Management. Little, Brown and Company, Boston, 1993; p253-261.
32. Low PA, Kihara M, Cardione C. Pharmacology and morphometry of the eccrine sweat gland in vivo. In: Low PA (ed) Clinical Autonomic Disorders: Evaluation and Management. Little, Brown and Company, Boston, 1993; p 367-373.
33. Fealey RD. The thermoregulatory sweat test. In: Low PA (ed) Clinical Autonomic Disorders: Evaluation and Management. Little, Brown and Company, Boston, 1993 ; p 217-229.
34. Low PA. Laboratory evaluation of autonomic failure. In: Low PA (ed) Clinical Autonomic Disorders: Evaluation and Management. Little, Brown and Company, Boston, 1993; p 169-195.

35. Ahmed ME, Le Quesne P. Quantitative sweat test in diabetics with neuropathic foot ulceration. J Neurol Neurosurg Psychiatry 1986; 49(9): 1059-1062.

36. Cavanagh PR, Ulbrecht JS. Clinical plantar pressure measurement in diabetes: rationale and methodology. The Foot 1994 (in press).

37. Veves A, Murray HJ, Young MJ, Boulton AJM. The risk of foot ulceration in diabetic patients with high foot pressure: a prospective study. Diabetologia 1992; 35: 660-663.

38. Cavanagh PR, Ulbrecht JS. Plantar pressue in the diabetic foot. In: Sammarco GJ (Ed). The Foot in Diabetes. Lea and Febiger, Philadelphia, 1991, pp 54-70.

39. Tappin JW, Pollard J, Bechett EA. Method of measuring shear forces on the sole of the foot. Clin Phys Physiol Meas 1980; (1): 83-85.

40. Laing P, Deogan H, Cogley D et al. The development of the low profile Liverpool shear transducer. Clin Phys Physiol meas 1992; 13: 115-124.

41. Lord M, Hosein R, Williams RB. Method for in shoe shear stress measurement. J Biomed Eng 1992; 14: 181-186.

42. Cavanagh PR, Ulbrecht JS. Biomechanical aspects of foot problems in diabetes. In: eds. Boulton AJM, Connor H and Cavanagh PR. The Foot in Diabetes. John Wiley & Sons Ltd. Chichester, 1994; p25-35.

43. Young MJ, Cavanagh PR, Thomas G, Johnson MM, Murray H, Boulton AJM. The effect of callus removal on dynamic plantar foot pressures in diabetic patients. Diabetic Med 1992; 9: 55-57.

44. Cavanagh PR, Derr JA, Ulbrecht JS, Maser RE, Orchard TJ. Problems with gait and posture in neuropathic patients with insulin dependent diabetes mellitus. Diabetic Med 1992; 9; 469-474.

45. Martin MM. Diabetic neuropathy. Brain 1953; 76: 594-624.

46. Edmonds ME, Archer AG, Watkins FJ. Ephedrine: a new treatment for diabetic neuropathic oedema. Lancet 1983; i: 54-55.

47. Rosen RC, Davids MS, Bohanske LM. Haemorrhage into plantar callus and diabetes mellitus. Cutis 1985; 35: 339-341.

48. Krupski WC, Reilly LM, Perez S, Moss KM, Crombleholme PA, Rapp JH. A prospective randomized trial of autologous platelet derived would healing factors for the treatment of chronic non healing wounds: a preliminary report. J Vasc. Surg 1991; 14: 526-536.

49. Mueller MJ, Diamond JE, Sinacore DR et al. Total contact casting in treatment of diabetic plantar ulcers. Diabetes Care 1989; 12: 384-388.

50. Burden AC, Jones GR, Jones R, Blandford RL. Use of the 'Scotchcast boot' in treating diabetic foot ulcers. Br Med J 1983; 286: 1555-1557.

51. Veves A, Masson EA, Fernando DJS, Boulton AJM. Studies of experimental hosiery in diabetic neuropathic patients with high foot pressures. Diabetic med 1990; 7: 324-326.

52. Chantelau E, Leisch A. Footwear, uses and abuses. In: eds. Boulton AJM, Connor H and Cavanagh PR. The Foot in Diabetes. John Wiley & Sons Ltd. Chichester, 1994; p 99-108.

53. Tovey Fl. Establishing a diabetic shoe service. Practical Diabetes 1985; 2: 5-8.

54. Sanders LJ, Frykberg RG. Diabetic neuropathic osteoarthropathy: the Charcot foot. In: The High Risk Foot in Diabetes. Frykberg RG (ed). Churchill Livingstone, New York, 1991 p 227-238.

55. Sinha S, Munichoodappa CS, Kozak GP. Neuroarthropathy (Charcot joints) in diabetes mellitus. Medicine (Baltimore), 1972; 51: 191-210.

56. Stevens MJ, Edmonds ME, Foster AVM, Watkins PJ. Selective neuropathy and preserved vascular responses in the diabetic Charcot foot. Diabetologia 1992; 35, 148-154.

57. Edelman SV, Kosofsky EM, Paul RA, Kozak GP. Neuro-osteoarthropathy (Charcot's Joint) in diabetes mellitus following revascularisation surgery: three case reports and a review of the literature. Arch intern Med, 1987; 147: 1504-1508.

58. McClugage SG, McCuskey RS. Relationship of the microvascular system to bone resorption and growth in situ. Microvasc Res 1973; 6: 132-134.

59. Verhas M, Martinello Y, Mone M et al. Demineralisation and pathological physiology of the skeleton in paraplegic rats. Calcif Tissue Int 1980; 30: 83-90.

60. Brewer AC, Allman RM. Pathogenesis of the neurotrophic joint: neurotraumatic vs neurovascular. Radiology 1981; 139: 349-354.

61. Selby PL, Young MJ, Boulton AJM. Famidronate - a definitive treatment for diabetic Charcot neuroarthropathy? Diabetic Med 1992; 9 (suppi 2): A27

62. Strandness DE Jr., Priest RE, Gibbons GE. Combined clinical and pathologic study of diabetic and non diabetic peripheral arterial disease. Diabetes 1964; 13: 366-372.

63. Ferrier RM. Radiologically demonstrable arterial calcification in diabetes mellitus. Australian Annals of Medicine 1967; 13: 222-226.

64. Wheelock FC, Gibbons GW, Marble A. Surgery in diabetes. In: Marble A, Krall LP, Bradley RF, Christlieb AR, Soeldner JS eds. Joslin's Diabetes Mellitus. Lea and Febiger, Philadelphia 1985, p712-731.

65. Parving HH, Rasmussen SM. Transcapillary escape rate of albumin and plasma volume in short and long term juvenile diabetes. Scand J Clin Lab Invest 1973; 32, 81-87.

66. O'Neal LW. Surgical pathology of the foot and clinicopathologic correlations. In: Levin ME and O'Neal LW, Bowker JH (eds). The Diabetic Foot CV Mosby, St Louis 1993; p 457-491.

67. Dormandy J ed. European Consensus Document on Critical Limb Ischaemia. Berlin: Springer-Verlag; 1989.

68. Second European Consensus Document on Chronic Critical Leg Ishcaemia. Circulation 1991; 84 N∞5.

69. Cheshire NJW, Wolfe JHN, Noone MA. The economics of femorocrural reconstruction for critical leg ischaemia with and without autologous vein. Journal of Vascular Surgery 1992; 15: 167-175.

70. Cheshire NJW, Wolfe JHN. Critical leg ischaernia: amputation or reconstruction. Br Med J 1992; 304: 312-315.

71. Bakal C, Sprayregen S, Scheinbaum K et al. Percutaneous transluminal angioplasty of the infra popliteal arteries, results in 53 patients. Am J Radiol 1990; 1 54: 171-174.

72. Davies AH, Cole SE, Magee T et al. The effect of diabetes mellitus on the outcome of angioplasty for lower limb ischaemia. Diabetic Medicine 1992; 9: 480-481.

73. Traughber PD, Cook PS, Micklos TJ et al. Intra-arterial fibrinolytic therapy for popliteal and tibial artery obstruction. AJR 1987; 149: 453-456.

74. Logerfo FW, Gibbons GW, Pomposilli Jr B. Trends in the care of the diabetic foot. Arch Surg 1992; 127: 617-621.

75. Logerfo FW, Coffman JD. Vascular and microvascular disease of the foot in diabetes. New Eng Journal of Medicine 1984; 311: 1615-1619.

76. Tannenbaum G, Pomposelli GB, Maraccio EJ. Safety of vein bypass grafting to the dorsal pedal artery in diabetic patients with foot infection. J Vasc Surg 1992; 15: 982-990.

77. Woelfte KD et al. Distal vein graft reconstruction for isolated tibio-peroneal occlusive disease in diabetics with critical foot ishcaemia. How does it work? Eur J Vasc Surg 1993; 7: 409-413.

78. Grenfell A, Watkins PJ. Clinical diabetic nephropathy: natural history and complications. Clin Endocrinol Metab 1986; 15: 783-805.

79. Gonzalez-Carrillo M, Moloney A, Bewick M et al. Renal transplantation in diabetic nephropathy. Br Med J 1982; 285: 1713-1716.

80. Delbridge L, Appleberg M, Reeve TS. Factors associated with the development of foot lesions in the diabetic. Surgery 1983; 93: 78-82.

81. Assaf J-P, Gfeller R, Ekoe J-M. Patient education in diabetes. In: Bostrum H, Ljungstedt N (eds). Recent Trends in Diabetes Research. Stockholm: Almqvust & Wiksell 1981; pp 276-290.

82. Bailey TS, Yu HM, Rayfield EJ. Patterns of foot examination in a diabetes clinic. Am Journal of Medicine 1985; 78: 371-374.

TREATMENT OF DIABETIC FOOT PATIENTS:
Surgical aspects

Carlo Caravaggi and Sergio Dalla Noce
Diabetic Foot Centre, Abbiategrasso Hospital—Milan, Italy

With respect to the surgical approach to diabetic limbs, it is mandatory to remember that only with a correct settlement of diabetic foot pathology it is possible to apply a strategy of intervention that will allow for reducing the rate of amputations.

First of all it is necessary to remember that the diabetic foot can be characterised by neuropathy, vascular occlusive disease, or both conditions together.

The neuropathic foot is characterised by the loss of sensation and by the involvement of intrinsic muscles (1, 2) Once these small muscles lose the ability to function effectively digital contractures will begin to develop. The patients are then placed at risk of developing clavi and hammer toe deformities caused by dorsal contractures of the metatarsophalangeal joint. These buckling effects increase the pressure in the ball of the foot, potentially leading to hyperkeratosis followed by ulcerations.

The anterior or extensor compartment also appears to be the muscle group most commonly involved; the effect is that the normal antagonism between muscle groups is lost; that in turn favours the development of an ankle equinus. Obviously equinus increases the plantar pressure to the metatarsal heads compounding plantar keratosis.

In diabetes the involvement of sympathetic nerves is responsible for the development of the autonomic neuropathy. When the loss of control of vascular tone of arterioles and of the function of sweat glands is combined, the patients with autonomic neuropathy presents a warm, dry, and anhidrotic foot (3).

It must be remembered that the hyperaemia that occurs as a consequence of autonomic neuropathy does not selectively involve soft tissue. Since bones are highly innervated with sympathetic nerves the increase in blood flow, secondary to increasing of arterio-venous shunting, could be responsible of the osteopenia that characterises Charcot foot deformity (4).

Another aspect that is peculiar to diabetes is the vascular occlusive disease that presents a greater and more significant degree and a difference in pattern of obstruction involving the vessel more distally, and with progression in a distal-to-proximal fashion (5) compared to atherosclerotic patients.

As a result of this more distal origin of arteriolar sclerosis and the manner of progression, a less effective collateral circulation appears to develop. On the other hand, despite these findings, there is evidence that the changes that occur within the small vessels of the lower extremity do not result in a functional loss of perfusion to tissue.

ELECTIVE DIABETIC FOOT SURGERY

The acute phase

When facing a diabetic foot that presents an acute lesion we first have to answer this question: what about the status of peripheral blood supply?

The purpose of vascular evaluation is to determine whether adequate local circulation is present to support primary healing either with or without surgical intervention. Patients with palpable pulses are not at risk to develop non-healing wounds and ulcers and consequently the surgical approach can be done without restriction. When pulses are not palpable a careful vascular assessment is mandatory. Apart from Doppler ultrasound and transcutaneous oxygen tension that allow evaluation of tissue perfusion, we strongly recommend that any patient without palpable pulses be submitted to angiographic evaluation in order to state if vascular procedures (PTA and by-pass) are necessary and possible.

From a surgical point of view the acute phase of a diabetic foot lesion can be divided as follows:
1. abscess
2. necrotizing fasciitis
3. gangrene

1. Abscess

When facing an abscess in the diabetic foot, three basic issues must be considered. The first is the location and the extent of it in order to determine the best way to obtain adequate material for culture and sensitivity. The second is the surgical approach for drainage and debridement of the surrounding tissue, while the third is the determination of osseous structures and the most appropriate method for closure and foot salvage (6).

The incisions for drainage of abscess are made longitudinally or transversely depending on the location of pathology. Plantar abscess can involve the entire plantar fascia and deep compartments requiring consequently long, deep incisions. While performing drainage and debridement great attention must be taken in order to avoid damage of vascular-nervous structures. When we make plantar and dorsal drainage incisions we usually leave a rubber drainage that allows daily irrigation of the infected wound.

The debridement must be done as wide as possible' considering the degree of blood supply, making sure all infected and necrotic tissue is removed, including bones. Very often toe, ray, and minor amputations are necessary in order to reach healthy tissue. In this condition follow up of wounds will show which type of definitive surgical approach will be suitable for the solution of the problem.

2. Necrotizing fasciitis

Necrotizing fasciitis is a life-threatening infection that may arise spontaneously, especially in patients with diabetes and vascular peripheral disease (7). The most frequent anaerobic pathogen isolated is Peptostreptococcus; however S. Aureus or S. pyogen may be involved as well as the anaerobes Clostridium and Bacteroides.

The infection begins rapidly within 24 to 72 hours after surgery or injury with wide-spread dissemination through deep fascia planes and necrosis of subcutaneous tissue. Probing beneath the surface will demonstrate wide undermining of the skin with separation to the fascia overlying the muscles.

The subcutaneous fascia will appear grey and necrotic but muscles will not be involved.

The treatment of choice is represented by aggressive and wide debridement of the injured tissue as deep as necessary in order to reach healthy tissue that must be bleeding. Wide spectrum antibiotic therapy must be applied as soon as possible awaiting for the result of the swab; in this clinical situation we strongly suggest to start hyperbaric oxygen therapy as soon as possible in order to stop the infection.

3. Gangrene

Gangrene represents a very frequent complication of both neuropathic and vascular diabetic foot. In the neuropathic foot this pathology very often involves one or more toes without a tendency to compromise the whole foot. The loss of sensation that characterises the neuropathic diabetic foot is responsible for the presence of ulcers of the toes. Patients who sustain such injury and who are unaware of the problem can often convert a partial-thickness tissue loss to full-thickness loss by continuing ambulation on the foot with subsequent development of infection.

When the infection involves the digital arterioles of the toes gangrene will appear very rapidly (blue toe syndrome). In case of a widespread, untreated infection, the involvement of the vessel of the midfoot may precipitate the situation with the appearance of a gangrene that involves the whole foot and that may require a below-knee amputation. In case of a diabetic foot affected with occlusive vascular disease, the evolution of gangrene is generally more rapid with involvement of the whole foot.

The surgical approach in both situations consists of a debridement that must be as wide as possible in order to remove all non-vital tissues. In the case of an occlusive vascular process we recommend surgical removal of the infected and necrotic tissue (avoiding any definite surgical procedure) first, followed by an angiographic evaluation in order to submit the patients to any possible vascular procedures. Once the acute phase of the lesion is resolved, that is there are no more signs of tissue infection, the most suitable and definite surgical step has to be chosen considering the clinical status of the patient.

The Chronic Phase

Ulceration of the diabetic foot is the most common problem for which medical assistance is sought. As previously discussed, plantar ulcers, characteristic of diabetic neuropathy, are caused by weight-bearing pressure, while dorsal and side ulcers, characteristic of concomitant vascular disease, are usually caused by shoe pressure.

Taking neuropathic plantar ulceration into consideration we are convinced that, when there is normal blood supply, the healing of the lesion depends on only two factors: first the rapidity of the beginning of the treatment, and second the type of treatment. Very often the loss of the capacity of healing of the lesion is due to a concomitant deep infection (close to fascia or with the involvement of bone) that is secondary to a long period of inadequate treatment with a persist open wound. The first question that must be answered in treating an ulcer of a diabetic foot is to determine whether it is infected or not. Most of the ulcers are colonised and a superficial swab may document some bacterial growth (<10–5). Clinical signs as draining, deep, surrounding erythema and cellulitis, linphangitis, and odour characterise the infected status. In case of infection, depending on the degree, antibiotic therapy must be started in the hospital or at home taking clinical situation of the patient into account. The surgical debridement must be, as previously mentioned, as wide as possible in order to remove all tissue infected. As usual, a vascular evaluation will allow immediate estimation if the reason for the non-healing of the lesion is due to an inadequate blood supply and if there will be any opportunity to propose vascular procedures such PTA or by-pass.

Coming back to the question about the inadequate treatment, we believe that this problem is strongly correlated with the management of plantar neuropathic ulcers in particular. Since the principal condition that causes plantar ulceration is an abnormal peak of pressure on the plantar surface, the treatment of choice must be the relief of pressure that can be achieved both using total contact cast or different types of weight-relieving devices. We have recently demonstrated (data in course of publication) that the use of cast compared to rocker sole shoes with plastazote insoles will allow the complete healing of the plantar ulcer in a shorter time without any side effects.

We are therefore strongly convinced that almost all plantar ulcers can reach healing if placed in a cast. Obviously there are a few situations that contraindicate the use of a cast such as blindness, impaired blood supply (non-palpable pulses with $TcPo_2 < 30$ mmHg), walking instability, leg amputation, no home facilities.

The surgical debridement represents the first step, even in the treatment of plantar ulcers; the goal that we have to achieve is to transform a chronic wound, not able to heal, in an acute lesion removing all keratosis and necrotic tissues.

The second fundamental step is the wound care; the wound, once submitted to surgical debridement, must be dressed in order to maintain it moist and clean. In our experience we have reached good results using, after having performed wide debridement, hydrocolloids or semiocclusive dressings. Clinical trials are however necessary to demonstrate that in the treatment of neuropathic plantar ulcers these advanced medications are better than usual standard care (moist saline gauze).

The total contact cast is still considered the best and most widely used method for healing neuropathic plantar ulcers (8). This method is not unreasonably difficult but attention to details and principles is critical. Many authors have reported different percentages of side effects (from 5 to 20%); the most common is the production of superficial abrasions, blisters, new ulcerations due to pressure of the cast or movement within the cast. All these inconveniences have been observed in total contact casts constructed with plaster alone or together with fiberglass. In our centre we have applied a new technique in constructing off-bearing casts: first we have used only fiberglass material taking care to pad very carefully the leg and foot, employing pieces of foam in order to protect bony prominences. We have decided to always open a plantar window in order to allow daily dressing of the lesions. We have treated 120 patients in 3 years; we have first noticed a great acceptability of the cast by the patients since they are lightweight compared with plaster casts (10). As far as the results are concerned, we have reached the healing of the lesions in almost all patients with no important side effects.

NON-HEALING ULCERS

As mentioned before, when ulcers fail to heal or they recur after healing has been achieved, this is an indication of three major problems: excessive internal bony pressure that perpetuates the ulcer, infection of the bone below the ulceration, and inadequate vascular supply. In the past, corrective surgery in diabetic patients was avoided because of the assumption of inadequate blood supply to healing both in the neuropathic and ischaemic foot.

Since we have now understood that presumed prohibition is unwarranted, we are convinced that failure to remove the source of the lesion is more dangerous that the judicious use of surgery to correct a deformity and to relieve bony pressure. Obviously in case of inadequate vascular supply the patient should first be submitted to vascular surgery to obtain good tissue perfusion.

EXOSTECTOMY

Exostectomy has been typically performed in the midfoot area for plantar lesions very often associated with a Charcot foot deformity. As noted before, the healing of plantar lesions can be achieved by placing the ulcer in a cast if bony exposition is not present. Even in case of osteomyelitis, conservative treatment will allow for only a transient solution of the problem. In our experience we have always surgically treated all complicated plantar lesions, i.e., with bony exposition or infection of the bone.

There are three basic methods of performing an exostectomy in the presence of an open wound. The first technique, that we usually prefer to perform in our centre, is to excise the bone from an incision site removed from the ulcer to minimise contamination of the underlying bone. In the meantime we perform plantar ulcerectomy in order to obtain healthy tissue able to heal rapidly. An example would be the resection of a metatarsal head through a dorsal incision for plantar ulcer. The second approach (10) is to excise the ulcer (ulcerectomy) starting more or less two centimetres from the edges of the lesion and to perform exostectomy through the same incision prior to wound closure. Some authors support employing closed suction drainage, but we do not prefer this technique unless clear signs of infection are present. The advantage of excising the ulcer is that often the soft tissue are so fibrotic that it might be impossible for the wound to adequately granulate despite osseous resection. Ulcerectomy allows the healthy tissue to heal rapidly.

The final method of doing exostectomy consists in excising the ulcer to healthy wound margins and removing the involved bone. The wound is then left open and dressed daily; delayed primary closure is performed at a later time. We consider this approach in case of infected wounds when a second surgical step to remove additional bone may be necessary. Daily packing and irrigations may reduce the bacterial count.

This kind of surgical approach may certainly be an effective treatment for non-healing or recurrent plantar ulcers. However, isolated metatarsal heads resection are not free of later complication such as hyperkeratosis and consequent ulceration beneath the adjacent metatarsal heads due to secondary transfer of peak of pressure.

Moreover, this uneven metatarsal arch loses its characteristic to move weight-bearing from one metatarsal head to another, and can exacerbate pressure imposed upon adjacent metatarsal heads leading the foot to Charcot collapse. In order to avoid these problems we often prefer to perform the metatarsal head resection at the first episode of ulceration. In case of a new ulceration beneath the same metatarsal or involving other metatarsal heads, we perform the resection of the remaining heads to even the weight-parabola. Exostectomy may be applied also in case of chronic lesions involving the midfoot or rearfoot. This procedure seems to be of interest to chronic Charcot feet that have achieved suitable autoartrodesis of the joint.

OSTEOMYELITIS

Very often osteomyelitis complicates the presence of both neuropathic and ischaemic foot ulcers. While in the ischeamic ulceration the involvement of bone is principally due to the spread of infection in deep tissue secondary to inadequate vascular supply, in the neuropathic foot the infective bone involvement is mainly due to the failure of the healing of the plantar wound, very often due to incorrect treatment that is responsible for the presence of an open wound for a long period.

It is opportune to remember the increased frequency of clinically non-suspected osteomyelitis in the diabetic foot as stated by Newman et al. (11).

From a diagnostic point of view it is worth remembering that standard radiology is not very useful in this case since it doesn't allow to distinguish bone lesions due to neuropathic osteortropathy from those due to infection. Since microbiologic bone cultures obtained from a biopsy are not safe (12) due to the risk of skin lesion and spreading of infection, in our centre we prefer to submit patients to radionuclide imaging with autologous granulocyte labeled with Technetium-99 and to nuclear magnetic resonance.

SURGICAL TREATMENT OF OSTEOMYELITIS

As we know, osteomyelitis once established is seldom eradicated with medical treatment and therefore needs to be solved with surgery.

The main problem that the surgeon has to face when dealing with bone infection is to find a right balance between resecting sufficient bone to allow a definitive cure of the infection and saving as much as possible in order to maintain the stability of the residual foot. It is well understood that demolitive surgical intervention, as amputation of part of the foot, is very often followed by destabilisation and collapse of the whole foot, conducing to severe Charcot deformities.

Sometimes, when the midfoot is involved, in order to avoid amputation procedures and to save the whole foot, it is useful to start with antibiotic treatment that will last for almost three months. In case of failure with a medical approach appropriate surgical procedures will be applied. Many of the principles of surgical management of osteomyelitis in the diabetic foot are equally applicable to amputation surgery (see following chapter).

As mentioned before, the involvement of bone is very often due to a plantar wound that has been opened for a long time in a neuropathic foot. The metatarsal heads are one of the most common locations for the development of osteomyelitis due to the common presence of plantar ulcerations at the same place. In those cases in which only one metatarsal head is involved, we usually perform a resection of the involved head with a dorsal (13) incision followed by a wide plantar ulcerectomy. In case of recurrence of ulceration in the same place or beneath the adjacent metatarsal heads, we prefer to perform a panmetatarsal resection in order to even the metatarsal equilibrium.

When the first metatarsal head, is infected we remove sesamoids as well, and we stabilise the toe with K-wire. In case of osteomyelitis of the toes the treatment consists of an ablative procedure that transects or disarticulates all or part of the toe. It must be emphasised that not all toe amputations should be performed at the metatarsophalangeal joint level.

In case of infection of part of the bone of a toe it is possible to remove only the bone infected while preserving as much skin and subcutaneous tissue as possible, thus saving part of the toe. This technique permits ablation of the infected portion of the digit while preserving enough of the toe to serve as a spacer between the two adjacent toes. Charcot neuroatropathy very often is followed by non-healing midfoot ulceration complicated with osteomyelitis. The prominences involved are usually the navicular tuberosity medially and the base of the fifth metatarsal laterally. Since bone resection in this area may lead to later severe secondary deformities, before deciding for a demolishing surgical treatment it is better to start with an antibiotic therapy and follow the patient for at least three months.

Osteomyelitis involving the hindfoot is very difficult to treat because the skin is thin and there is very little subcutaneous tissue for coverage. The involvement of the heel often requires a very below-knee amputation. Only in case of osteomyelitis of the posterior portion of the tubercle of the calcaneus it is possible to perform a resection of the infected bone.

The procedure consists of posterior midline incision; exposure is obtained by splitting the Achilles tendon and reflecting it sharply off of the bone while preserving its attachments in the heel pad. An ulcerectomy is then performed, removing infected and necrotic tissue in order to allow healing of the lesion. The ablation of the bone must be generous in order to reach healthy bone tissue.

The wound is then closed either primarily or left open, waiting for delayed primary closure after periodic wound dressing. In our experience, in accordance with other authors (14), the rate of failure of this procedure is very low. However, if the clinical condition of the patients allows, we perform this procedure considering that the only alternative option possible would be a below-knee amputation.

RECONSTRUCTIVE SURGERY

As previously discussed, since many years ago a great complaint has been issued about the opportunity to submit diabetic foot to any elective and reconstructive surgical procedures (15). This has been signified to lose the opportunity to modify surgically most clinical situations at risk of ulceration; that in turn increases the risk of major amputation.

The understanding of the real vascular situation of the neuropathic foot has completely changed this approach. Anyway it must be noted that this kind of surgery is not free of risk caused by relative osteopenia that characterised the Charcot foot with great risk of post surgical destabilisation.

Digital Stabilisation

Contractures of the digit renders the patients at risk of formation of heloma; the concomitant presence of buckling of metatarsophalangeal joint shifts the fat pad anteriorly and enormously increases the pressure with subsequent creation of hyperkeratosis and ulceration. In our centre we apply the artrodesis of the proximal interfalangeal joint. The fusion serves to create a rectus digit through which the long flexor tendon will direct plantoflexory force at the metatarsophalangeal joint level eliminating retrograde buckling. Normally we prefer to stabilise the toes with a Kirschner wire (K-wire) (16).

Panmetatarsal Resection

In case of recalcitrant hyperkeratosis or ulceration the resection of the metatarsal head is widely used with good success as far as healing of the ulcer is concerned.

The major problem is connected with later deformities that often appear later and with the consequent transfer ulceration beneath adjacent metatarsal heads. In this situation a later panmetatarsal head resection is required.

Many authors have reported this procedure very successfully without any problem regarding the healing of the ulcer (17). In our experience we perform this procedure in case of recurrence of the ulcer after resection of metatarsal heads or directly in case of great deformity of the foot. When performing panmetatarsal resection sometimes we stabilise the metatatarsophalangeal joint space with K-wire for 6 weeks to enhance stability at this level.

Midfoot, Rearfoot, and Ankle Artrhodesis

Charcot deformity is the main indication for major arthrodesis procedure. The goal of this approach is to obtain stability of the affected joints reducing the risk of further ulceration and collapse of the whole foot. Banks and McGlamry (18) discussed the concept of Charcot joint reconstruction, particularly in diabetic patients. Reconstruction is considered in patients who have sufficient deformity or instability for whom an amputation will likely have to be done if surgery is not performed. In fact, arthrodesis in the Charcot foot was considered a form of limb salvage for many patients.

Harris and Brand (19) have demonstrated that artrhodesis was successful, provided that this procedure was performed early in the disease process or later in a quiescent state.

Warren and coll. (20) demonstrated a satisfactory result in a great percentage of diabetic patients submitted to arthrodesis of foot and ankle (81%). Failure to achieve arthrodesis was noted only in patients in whom external fixation has been employed or in those who had been immobilised for too short a time postoperatively.

In our centre we do not have great experience in this type of treatment. A careful analysis of the literature has pointed out that there are some principles of Charcot joint reconstruction that must be followed.

First the foot must be in a quiescent state without any signs of active inflammation. The acute phase, characterised by oedema, erythema, and warmth, indicating a state of instability of the bone involved, must be treated with absolute rest that can be achieved with bed rest, followed by a cast once the more active phase of swelling has passed. Our experience, confirmed by many other authors, strongly suggests that no weight must be borne by extremity until a quiescent state has been reached. Even when employing casts, we prefer to suggest the patient rest as much as possible or to use crutches or, if it is possible, a wheelchair.

Once the foot has entered the quiescent phase signed by dissipation of oedema, return of normal skin lines, and restoration of a symmetrical temperature gradient with the controlateral limb, surgical approaches can be considered.

Fixation should be of the most rigid form available that will render stability. Therefore, staple, K-wire and Steimann pins are used for many areas.

Lisranc's Joint

Lisranc joint is very often affected by Charcot process. The dislocation can be in a transverse plain deformity which lends itself to easier repair. In severe cases the metatarsal may be dislocated dorsally over the cuneiforms and cuboide; restoration of full length to the foot is almost impossible because of the adaptive contracture of the soft tissue. Arthrodesis of metatarsal directly to the navicular and cuboid to the talus and calcaneus with graft interposition is often necessary. In addition to resecting cartilage from the base of the metatarsal, care must be taken to also resect the intermetatarsal articulation; this procedure allows arthrodesis between the metatarsal and it further contributes to stability.

In order to obtain alignment at this joint level, which is important for an even distribution of weight across the ball of the foot postoperatively, all the metatarsals must be on the same plane with the forefoot in a slight valgus position. One way to obtain an appropriate parabola is to temporarily pin the first and fifth metatarsal base in position; this will create the wear-bearing plane for the forefoot. Next, working on the second metatarsal laterally, the intermediate metatarsals are aligned and temporally fixated in the same plane. Finally, the fifth metatarsal will usually require some adjustment for adequate juxtaposition to the fourth metatarsal. Permanent fixation may then be applied.

In case of severe disruption of the tarsus and midfoot, arthrodesis of the midfoot must be applied, requiring removal of the cuneiform and cuboid, leaving one with poor proximal references and irregular surface for arthrodesis. The relationship of the metatarsal may remain the most normal part of anatomy. This suggests fixing the metatarsal from side to side, creating an appropriate parabola before reconstructing the midfoot. The metatarsals are attached as a unit to the proximal portion of the foot. When the intercuneiform and naviculocuneiform joints are effected without gross displacement, then the more proximal joints are stabilised before one proceeds distally.

Triple and Plantar Arthrodesis

In many Charcot patients, multiple joint involvement is often the rule. Often the surgery will consist of fusing not only these joints but more distal segments as well. Many authors agree that it is preferable to avoid ankle arthrodesis if possible, since the rate of non-union is very high in neuropathic patients. Actually, Banks and coll. have not referred noticeable incidence of frank non-union; certainly they noted that talotibial and tiobiocalcaneal fusion do require a great period of time for adequate consolidation in these patients.

The finding is similar to that of Warren (20), who noted non-union only in those cases in which external fixation was used in lieu of internal fixation and in which the period of immobilisation was too short.

Tendon Achilles Lengthening

A main problem that must be faced when scheduling a surgical step on midfoot or ankle, or when deciding for midfoot amputation, is the equinus deformity that always follows these procedures. Equinus deformity will serve as a disruption force that instigates Charcot collapse in many neuropathic patients.

The loss of compensation for the equinus will be responsible for fractures and dislocation that involved the weakest point, i.e., tarso-metatarsal joint. Furthermore equinus will continue to exacerbate the rocker-bottom foot, increasing the risk of ulceration or additional deformity. In order to reduce the neuromuscular imbalance that exists in neuropathic diabetic patients we strongly recommend performing Achilles tendon lengthening in each patient submitted to midfoot and ankle surgery.

Two methods are available to lengthen Achilles tendon: open frontal plane approach and percutaneous technique. The approach that we prefer to perform in our centre is the percutaneous two-step method. Achilles tendon lengthening is usually performed as the last procedure once the final alignment of the foot is attained.

Each time we decide to perform an Achilles tendon lengthening we apply a permanent fiberglass cast, with a window to allow monitoring of the surgical procedure, that we change every seven days, taking care of the reduction of oedema and stabilisation of the wound status.

AMPUTATION IN DIABETIC FOOT

Amputation of part or all of the foot has been considered, consciously or not, as an admission of failure, a form of surgical defeat. This procedure should be instead considered in those patients who have a foot that is no longer either viable or functional, a positive procedure because it is the first step on the road to restored or renewed function.

As far as diabetic patients are concerned, the main problem in the past was correlated with the level of amputation. As mentioned many times, since diabetic vascular reconstructive procedures were considered useless, the amputation levels that proved to be optimal, in order to obtain a rapid and definite solution to the problem, was above or below knee amputation.

In the last few years we have learned from the literature first of all that distal vascular procedures of great interest in diabetic patients allow restoration of a good blood supply and tissue perfusion to foot and ankle (21). Moreover, we have learned that in diabetic patients the risk of controlateral amputation in the following five years from above or below knee amputation is greater than in non diabetic-patients.

Finally it must be remembered that in diabetics submitted to amputation, due to their older age and general conditions such as problems with ambulation, the possibility of success in dressing a leg prosthesis is lower that in non-diabetic patients, leading to bedrest, which in turn exposes patients to many complications that implicate reduction of life expectancy.

From an epidemiological point of view it is necessary to remember that the national Diabetes Advisory Board reports an estimated 5% to 15% of all diabetics will require an amputation at some time in their life. Moreover, the survival rate for diabetic amputees remains very low; survival rates are 50% for the first three years and 40% for the first five years after unilateral amputation.

Finally, actual data show that diabetic patients are 15 times more likely to undergo a lower extremity amputation than non-diabetic persons. Since, as reported before, the primary function of the lower extremity is locomotion, preservation of this function should be the goal of the surgeon who decides to submit diabetic patients to this surgical procedure.

Determination of the Amputation Level

The choice of the level of amputation must be done, taking into account the need to obtain rapid wound healing and to obtain a functional stump. Clinical features that may provide some indication of wound healing potential include palpable pulses, skin temperature, rubor, degree of sensory loss, capillary return, and more important bleeding of skin edges and tissue status at the time of surgery.

As far as palpable pulses are concerned, Burges and co-workers (22) reported satisfactory healing of below-knee amputation in 66% of diabetics and 72% of non-diabetics with absence of pedal pulses, concluding that the absence of palpable pulses does not reflect collateral circulation, which is the primary determinant of wound healing.

Mc Collogh (23) reported healing in 92% of 134 below-knee amputations when skin edges bled at the time of surgery, apart from the presence of pedal pulses. One of the most commonly used techniques applied to determine the level of amputation is Doppler ultrasonography; as far as diabetics are concerned this procedure is not suitable, since frequently it is possible to find artificially elevated systolic pressure due to arterial medial calcinosis. (Monckberg sclerosis) (24).

Transcutaneous oxygen tension (TcPO$_2$) has become a very popular non-invasive means of evaluating local cutaneous circulation in patients with peripheral vascular disease. To measure transcutaneous oxygen tension the skin is locally warmed to 448 C. A Clarck electrode applied to the extremity measures the oxygen emanating from the skin. We normally use this procedure in our centre and we have found, accordingly with international literature, that if pO$_2$ level is greater than 40 mmHg there is a great expectation for wound healing, while below 30 mmHg the risk of non-wound healing is very high.

Once vascular assessment has been made and vascular reconstructive procedure has been applied, we decide the amputation level, considering also other factors such as clinical signs and non-invasive procedures. It must be remembered that the general clinical condition of the patient remains the first and fundamental aspect that must be evaluated, since non-compliance and bedresting are clinical aspects that contraindicate conservative surgical amputation considering the loss of possibility to walk. Moreover, these patients will be exposed to post operative risk such as non-wound healing and infective complications.

PRINCIPLES OF TECHNIQUE IN AMPUTATION SURGERY

Regardless of specific amputation, the same basic principles must be considered when undergoing amputation procedure. Since skin is the critical tissue that could have problems in healing, great care must be taken in managing tissue to avoid damages. Incision always has to be carried directly from skin to bone with no attempt at additional soft tissue dissection in order to preserve deep circulation.

Skin flaps should be designed with as broad a base as possible and the length should be minimised. Care has to be taken to avoid dead space prior to skin closure, or else the area should be drained. It is very important to obtain skin closure without tension on the wound edges. We usually prefer not to apply sutures on deep tissue to avoid damage of deep circulation.

Since post-operative complications are very often a result for excessive bony prominences, it is necessary to round all bones that would be at risk of giving pressure ulceration before closure. Post-operative monitoring of the wound is of great importance for many reasons. Wound infection may be responsible for failure of the surgical step. We strongly recommend to maintain antibiotic therapy since healing. In case of signs of infection we periodically perform a swab in order to change antibiotic therapy if it is necessary.

In case of evidence of serious infection or hyschemia we promptly remove sutures, sometimes only partially, in order to permit drainage of liquid and reduce oedema. We also perform as soon as possible a wide debridement, removing all necrotic tissue, leaving the wound open. Follow up will show if a delayed primary closure will be possible or if a new surgical intervention would be required.

Digital Amputation

The indication for toe amputation, that is, the most frequently performed peripheral amputation, is a localised gangrenous or infection involving tissue and bone distal to proximal interfalangeal joint. In case of dry gangrenous process, it may be chosen to await spontaneous autoamputation (demarcation by alcohol dressing); in case of any signs of wet gangrene the surgical step should be expedited as soon as possible.

Once the level of amputation has been correctly identified, the classical technique consists of a dorsal transversal incision made on viable tissue over the involved phalanx. The incision is carried out across the dorsum to an equidistant point on the opposite side. A second horizontal incision is then placed around the tip of the toe, joining both ends of the previous dorsal incision. If it is necessary, osteotomy of the tuft can be carried out, using either power or manual bone cutting.

Finally the plantar skin flap is examined for any tendinous or other connective tissue debridement. If a tourniquet has been applied before it is then removed and if any free bleeders are found they must be clamped, coagulated or ligated. We prefer not to apply it but to perform hemostasis time by time.

Ray Resections

This procedure is applied in case infections or gangrene extend to the web space or involve the metatarsophalangeal joint. While this approach has been considered not as demolitive as transmetatarsal or Lisfranc's amputation, some consideration must be given to it. As far as walkable prostheses are concerned, we are strongly convinced that central ray resection may be useful, because it allows maintenance of medial and lateral foot columns that are very important for ambulation.

We instead strongly avoid performing first and second ray amputations because the left foot does not permit a better use of prosthesis devices compared to transmetatarsal amputation.

Moreover, from a surgical point of view, it is easier to perform a transmetatarsal amputation because of the plantar flap that it is generally wider and with a better blood supply, allowing healing in a shorter time period with less complications.

Finally we consider the amputation of fourth and fifth rays suitable when plantar skin is in good status, which allows us to prepare a suitable flap.

Technique

The procedure consists of removal of the toes as well as all or part of the metatarsals involved. We carry out a dorsal incision from skin to bone as usual in a distal direction to the metatarsophalangeal joint level when a teardrop skin incision is carried through the sulcus and web space plantarly.

In order to avoid destabilisation of Lisfranc's joint and consequent instability of remaining metatarsals, the metatarsals are generally transected at the flair of metatarsal base. Only amputation of fourth and fifth metatarsals may be done removing the ligamentous structures of metatarsophalangeal joint and excising the entire base. Since the base of the fifth metatarsal is the site of the insertion of the brevis peroneus, which is a very important muscle involved in dorsiflexion movement of the foot, we prefer, when the integrity of the skin allows, to perform transection to the flare of the base without removing the whole bone.

As previously mentioned we prefer not to apply a tourniquet but to perform hemostasis time by time. General attention must be kept while removing tendons and connective tissue, gentle management of the skin flap and sutures without tension; we do not apply, as usually, deep sutures in order to avoid damage to deep circulation.

As far as results are concerned we agree with the international literature (25) that states that a low success rate in ray resection is principally due to failure of the wound to heal and recurrence of transfer ulceration after resumption of ambulation.

Transmetatarsal Amputation

The indications for this procedure may be summarised as follows:

1. infection or gangrene of one or more toes, provided the gangrene has stabilised and does not involve the dorsal or plantar aspect of the foot causing loss of a great part of the skin of the plantar part of the foot.
2. stabilised infection or open wound of the distal portion of the foot.

The level of metatarsal amputation must be decided, providing the insertion of the tibialis anterior tendon is preserved in order to avoid loss of function that will result in an equinus deformity.

Technique

The technique consists of a dorsal incision at the level of the intended bone resection. At the plantar level the incision is made distal to the metatarsal heads and is extended transversely at the level of the flexor creases of the toes; the incision is made directly from skin to bone. Taking care while managing the skin, the plantar flap is reflected to the level of the intended bone resection. The metatarsals are then sectioned transversely in a slightly parabolic manner. All metatarsals are beveled on the plantar portion, with the first and fifth metatarsal being beveled on medial and lateral aspects, respectively.

Sesamoid bones are then removed, and nerves and tendon are identified and divided so that they can be removed and retracted proximally. The flap must be designed in order to cover the distal end of the bones, and the sutures that must be placed in a dorsal position have to be done without tension. We recommend not applying deep sutures, but we prefer to leave a small drain for 24–48 hours. Copious irrigation before closure is very important. We prefer, as already mentioned, not to use a tourniquet but to perform hemostasis time by time. We do not perform directly the lengthening of the Achilles tendon; that we prefer to postpone and apply in case of presence of equinus deformity. The wound is dressed and generally we place the foot in a posterior splint.

Results

We often decide to perform this kind of procedure, considering the high rate of success in primary healing and also considering the simple use of prosthesis which follows this type of surgical step.

The reasons for failure are connected with recurrence ulcerations at the stump site and inadequate healing of the wound.

These complications are generally due to abnormal pressure at the stump site and development of equinus deformity that can be modified, performing Achilles tendon lengthening.

Lisfranc and Chopart Amputation

Because of the invariable result in equinus this procedure was decried in the past and was substituted with below knee amputation. Since the need to apply a surgical step as conservative as possible and the need for the possibility to reduce the equinus risk performing percutaneous Achilles lengthening, this procedure has regained a new interest.

The indications for this level of amputation are conditions that are too advanced for transmetatarsal amputation or ray amputation.

Technique

A) Linsfranc amputation

First we start with an incision at the base of the fifth metatarsal which extends distally along the lateral edge of the metatarsal shaft to the neck of the metatarsal. We prolong the incision down and across the plantar surface, parallel to metatarsal heads, reaching medially the first metatarsalcuneiform joint. The dorsal incision, performed with a distal convexity, runs distally and parallel to the line of transverse metatarsal joints.

Once the flap is elevated at the periosteal level, exposing the tarsometatarsal joint, the lateral three metatarsal are disarticulated from cuboid and lateral cuneiform while first metatarsal is separated from the medial cuboid. Finally the second metatarsal is the last to be removed. Applying plantar flexion of the second metatarsal, it is possible to introduce a scalpel into the joint and remove the entire metatarsal from the cuneiform.

As usual the wound is copiously irrigated and a careful debridement is performed. Hemostasis must be done with great attention, and a rubber drainage is left for 24–48 hours. Very often, due to gangrene or infection involving part of the plantar skin, it is necessary to cut an unusual flap in order to obtain wound closure.

Sometimes we prefer to leave the wound partially opened and to reach healing by second intention instead of suturing the flap with tension. We generally apply a rigid dressing to avoid equinus deformity after two or three days of wound follow up. We prefer to use a removable posterior split since it allows periodic control of the skin status.

B) Chopart amputation

The incision is started just posterior to the navicular tuberosity and is carried distally along the medial border of the first metatarsal. Midway on the shaft of the metatarsal the incision is carried down across the plantar surface of the foot and a wide flap is designed.

Laterally the incision is made proximally along the shaft of the fifth metatarsal to a point midway between the lateral malleolus and the base of fifth metatarsal. Finally the dorsal incision is carried with a distal convexity parallel to the line of metatarsal heads; the plantar flap is then carefully elevated.

First the ligaments that hold the talonavicular joint are divided and the tibialis anterior tendon is firmly attached to the neck of the talus using a drill hole. The disarticulation is then completed, dividing the ligaments between calcaneus and cuboid.

After copious irrigation, careful debridement and hemostasis, the flaps are opposed without deep sutures and tension is avoided. As usual we leave a rubber drainage for 24 –48 hours and after that period we place the foot in a rigid dressing.

Results

Despite many concerns about the opportunity to perform such techniques due to problems connected with equinus deformity and consequent ulcerations, we agree with many authors who describe a good rate of success with Lisfranc and Chopart amputation (26).

We think that in order to obtain good success some precautions have to be taken: confirm the presence of a good blood supply, pay great attention to infection, take great care in the management of tissue during the surgical step, and great attention during the post-operative period to the wound.

Syme's Amputation

Many authors have discussed the usefulness of this procedure in diabetic patients. Provided there is a good blood supply and healthy condition of the skin of the heel, we prefer to perform a Syme's amputation rather that below-knee amputation because the first allows us to obtain:

1. a stump capable of transmitting the entire body weight
2. a stump with some leverage
3. easier use of prosthesis

Technique

A) One-stage

A plantar skin incision is made 2 cm proximal to the centre of malleolus, holding the foot at a right angle to the leg. It is then carried directly across the plantar surface of the foot to a point 2 cms proximal to the other malleolus.

Dorsally the incision is made from one malleolus to the other at a 458° angle to the sole of the foot and the long axis of the leg. Avoiding damage to the posterior tibial artery medially, the tibial and fibular collateral ligaments are divided from within the joint.

Talus is then dislocated plantarly from the ankle mortise and the Achilles tendon is divided, avoiding damage to the skin flap behind it. Afterward talus, calcaneous, and foot are removed. Great care has to be taken to separate the heel flap from the calcaneous because if during dissection the septa is opened, the heel fat pad will be decompressed, losing its function of hydraulic buffer

The removal of malleoli and subcondral portion of the distal tibia is performed with power equipment; the osteotomy must be made parallel to the ground. After copious irrigation and careful debridement the subcutaneous tissue and the skin of the heel flaps are sutured to the margin of the anterior incision across the front of the ankle.
Surgical drain must be used and left for 24–48 hours. It is paramount that the plantar fat pad of the heel be maintained directly beneath the tibial osteotomy.

B) Two-stage

In case of overt infection of the foot or if the plantar skin is heavily compromised, it is possible to perform this amputation in two steps. The technique is basically the same as for the one-stage procedure but it doesn't include the osteotomy of malleoli and distal tibial in the initial operating setting.

Once the infection is dominated by daily irrigation and antibiotic therapy, the patient is then returned to the operating room, and after a careful examination of the flap followed by debridement of infected and necrotic tissue, osteotomy is made and tissue closure is performed.

In case of loss of a great part of the plantar skin, we leave the wound open and we program a future autoskin graft in order to cover the loss of skin, or we dress periodically the lesion, awaiting a delayed primary healing.

Results

Data from the international literature show that by applying a correct surgical technique the rate of success as far as healing and prosthesis are concerned is fairly high (27).

SURGICAL VASCULAR APPROACH TO DIABETIC LESIONS

As mentioned before, one of the reasons that diabetic patients are prone to non-healing ulcers is an inadequate peripheral blood supply. The vascular approach to the diabetic patient has changed in the last few years; apart from proximal vascular reconstruction that has been routinely performed in diabetic patients, distal vascular procedure has gained great importance due to the understanding that small arterioles are not specifically involved in the atherosclerotic process in diabetes.

Thanks to the demonstration made by Dible and coll. in 1966 (28) that foot arteries from diabetic patients affected by critical ischaemia very often were not involved, it was possible to evaluate the opportunity to submit diabetic patients to distal vascular reconstructive procedures. The same author demonstrated that diabetic patients presented a typical pattern for the localisation of obstructive lesions: non-involvement of the iliac and femoral arteries but a considerable involvement of the tibial trunks, in contrast with the relative integrity of the vascular tree of the foot. Finally, many authors have even demonstrated that the aetiology of ischaemic lesions are not correlated to arterioles localisation of obstructive lesions but very often involve obstructive lesions placed below the popliteal artery.

All these considerations allow us to underline that both proximal and distal vascular procedures must be applied, when the anatomic situation is suitable, even in the diabetic foot, since very often this approach represents the only possibility to save the limb.

PERCUTANEOUS TRANSLUMINAL BALLOON ANGIOPLASTY

Angioplasty is a simple procedure performed under local anaesthesia that presents rare complications with virtually zero mortality rates. This technique has been the routine for the isolated stenosis and short occlusion in the iliac, femoral, and popliteal arteries while the value in the treatment of distal occlusion is still a matter of debate. Recently Caputo (29) and coll. have reported that PTA is suitable only for proximal arteries. In a recent paper Faglia and coll. (30) have demonstrated a good rate of success for this procedure applied to infra-inguinal arteries that has allowed an increase both in non-invasive vascular parameters and in healing rate of the ulcers. Despite the fact that the principle indication for distal PTA is short (< 10 cm) and single occlusive lesions, in our centre we have recently started to submit to this procedure even patients that present multiple obstructive lesions; according to other authors, we have noticed a significant increase in transcutaneous oxygen tension after distal PTA. We therefore consider angioplastic treatment the first vascular approach, considering its low rate of complications, leaving by-pass surgery as the last step in limb salvage. A great interest is growing up on new vascular endoscopic procedures such as rotablator and laser, which seem to be very useful, in particular when it is necessary to pass through a calcified stenosi allowing one to perform later PTA treatment.

DISTAL BY-PASS SURGERY

The vascular surgical approach to diabetic foot has been changed in the last ten years. Of great interest is the work made by LoGerfo et al. (21) who submitted to distal by-pass 104 patients, obtaining global perviousness and limb salvage results of 82% and 97% respectively at 18 months. As far as surgical distal by-pass techniques are concerned in diabetic patients, the proximal anastomosis may be the popliteal artery, due to the different distribution of occlusive lesions. Obviously, proximal anastomosis may be performed even on the common femoral artery, on the superficial femoral, or iliac artery. Since the short by-pass presents many advantages such as the need of minor entity of tissue dissection with lower incidence of infection and a low rate of failure caused by occlusion, we prefer to choose, as a proximal anastomosis, the more distal artery available, considering obviously the distribution of occlusive lesions. The ideal site for distal anastomosis, according to the literature, is the tibial artery. Very often due to distal occlusive lesions, it is necessary to perform this anastomosis on the foot arteries, which makes the risk of later failure greater. Once the artery has been reached, arteriotomy is performed in order to evaluate the run-off by instilling a heparin solution in the distal lumen; failure of this manoeuvre and the rise of flow resistance contraindicate continuing the operation. Sometimes a fogarty procedure may be applied to ameliorate the run-off. The prosthetic material of choice is usually the autologous veins (internal or external siphon or veins of the limbs). Using internal saphena a by-pass in situ is performed while with the external saphena a reverse technique is applied. In our centre we have recently applied a mini-invasive saphena vein harvesting (vasoview) which allows one, using endoscopic instruments, to isolate the greater saphena without the need of wide tissue incisions, but by means of two or three one-centimetre incisions made at inguinal, popliteal, and tibial sites. Finally we do not prefer to use artificial prosthetics, considering the high rate of later occlusion.

TISSUE ENGINEERING IN DIABETIC FOOT ULCERS

Open wounds which may result from neuropathic or ischaemic injuries or as a consequence of a surgical procedure need to be provided with coverage. There are ever-increasing numbers of coverage techniques available. Apart from direct closure, other approaches are available, such as skin graft, flaps, artificial skin and cultured cells. As far as skin flaps are concerned, data from literature are very poor and in our opinion unmistakable clinical trials are not available. In the last few years new technologies such as tissue engineering have offered the opportunity to create skin which can be used to treat patients with burns as well as chronic wounds. Tissue engineering human dermal replacements can be obtained either from eterologous newborn foreskin or directly from the patient's skin.

Few studies are available regarding both kinds of approaches. As far as eterologous skin graft is concerned, Richard A. (31) and coll. in 1997 treated 235 diabetic patients affected by full thickness ulcers of the plantar surface of the foot or of the heel in a randomised clinical trial. After a two week screening, during which the ulcer had to heal less than 50% and remain >1 cm^2, the patients in the treated group received one piece of graft weekly up to eight weeks. The control group was treated with conventional therapy such as moist wound dressing. Complete wound healing was defined as full epithelization of the wound with non-drainage. The result of the study indicated that at 12 weeks significantly more ulcers in the treated groups were healed compared to the control group (58% vs 31.7%). At week 32 there was a substantial improvement in healing compared to the control group (57.7 vs 42.4). Some considerations have to be made on the results of this study. As far as time of healing is concerned, our group has recently demonstrated in 50 patients affected by neuropathic foot ulcers (surface 471± 444 mm^2) treated by fiberglass casts a healing rate of 100% within 58.52±37.96 without important side effects (9). On the other hand the cost-effectiveness of this kind of approach, which consists of eight applications, must be emphasised, since the cost of the entire treatment seems to be very high. As mentioned before, autologous grafting represents the alternative approach made possible by tissue engineering technology. A small skin biopsy directly taken from the patient allows autologous keratinocytes and fibroblasts to be obtained, which are then separated and cultivated. The scaffold employed for the culture in both cases is a hyaluronic acid derivative. In our centre we have investigated, in an observational study, the value of the new advanced approach, treating 14 patients affected by neuropathic and ischaemic ulcers (7 plantar ulcers and 7 dorsal and marginal ulcers) (32). The treatment consisted of two consecutive applications of fibroblasts first and keratinocytes ten days later. The applications were performed on a clean and not contaminated wound bed. The median size of the ulcers was 149±162mm^2. All the plantar lesions were placed in a fiberglass cast while for the dorsal and marginal lesion a walkable tissue shoe with plastazote insole was employed. The results indicated a reduction of 73.8±18.4% of the ulcer surfaces in 70.7±24.3 days of follow up. In the same period, out of the 14 patients treated, five had reached complete healing of the ulcer. Moreover we have noticed that all patients with transcutaneous oxygen tension below 30 mmHg presented a slower healing time. Even this kind of approach, which seems to be effective and safe and less expensive, needs further clinical randomised trials to understand if the application of autolgous skin grafts will be able to significantly reduce the healing time in diabetic foot ulcers.

REFERENCES

1. Lippman HI. Must loss of limb be a consequence of diabetes mellitus? Diabetes Care, 1979, 2: 432.
2. Lippman HI. Prevention of amputation in diabetes. Angiology, 1979, 30 : 649.
3. Boulton AJM, Scarpello JHB, Ward JD. Venous oxygenation in the diabetic neuropathic foot : evidence of arteriovenous shuanting? Diabetes Care, 1982, 22 : 6-8.
4. Duncan Cp, Shim SS. The autonomic nerve supply of bone. J. Bone Joint Surgery, 1977, 59B : 323-330.
5. Conrad MC. Contributions of large and small vessel disease to severe ischemia of the lower extremities in diabetic and non diabetic, Vasc. Drug. Ther 1981, 2 : 17-28.
6. Livingston R. Plantar abscess of the diabetic patients. Foot and Ankle, 1985, 5 : 205-213.
7. Rea Wj. Necrotizing fascitiis. Am Surg, 1974, 108 : 552.
8. Boulton AJM. Use of plaster casts in the management of diabetic neuropathic foot ulcers. Diabetes Care, 1987, 9 :149-152.
9. Caravaggi C, Faglia E. Effectiveness and tolerabiliy of fiberglass total contact cast in the treatment of neuropathic foot ulcer. Abstract to ADA Congress Chicago 1998.
10. Leventen EO. Charcot foot : a technique for treatment of chronic plantar ulcer by saucerization and primary closure. Foot Ankle, 1986, 6: 295-299.
11. Newman LG, Waller J and coll. Unsuspected osteomyelitis in diabetic foot ulcers. JAMA, 1991, 266 : 1246.
12. Wheat J. Diagnostic strategies in osteomyelitis. Am J. Med, 1991, 218.
13. Harrelson JM. Management of diabetic foot. Orthop Clinical North Am. 1989, 20 : 605-619.
14. Crandal RC. Partial and total calcanectomy. J. Bone Joint Surg. (AM) 1981, 68 : 608-614.
15. O'Neal LW. Surgical pathology of the foot and clincopathology correlation. In Lewin ME O'Neal LW. The Diabetic Foot, 1988, 203-236.
16. Gudas CJ. Prophylactic surgery in diabetic foot. Clin. Pod. Med. Surgery, 1987, 4 : 445-458.
17. Jacobs RL. Hoffman procedure in ulcerated diabetic neuropathic foot. Foot and Ankle, 1982, 3: 142-149.
18. Banks AS, McGlamry ED. Charcot foot. J. Am.pod.Med Ass., 1989, 79 : 213-235.
19. Harris JR, Brand PW. Patterns of disintegration of the tarsus in the anaesthetics foot. J Bone Joint Surg., 1966, 484 : 4-16.
20. Warren AG. The surgical conservation of the neuropathic foot. Ann.R. Coll. Surg. Engl. 1989, 71 : 236-242.
21. LoGerfo FW, Goffman JD. Vascular and microvascular disease of the foot in diabetes. N. Eng.J Med., 1984, 311: 1615-1618.
22. Burges EM, Romano RL, Zenke JH. Amputation of the leg for peripheral vascular disease J. Bone Joint Surg. 1971, 53A : 874-890.
23. Mc Collough NC. Principle of amputation surgery in vascular disease In Evans CM: Surgery of the macrovascular System. New York, Churchill Livingstone 1983, 4 : 25-42.
24. Wagner WH, Keagy BA. Noninvasive determination of healing of major lower extremity amputation: the continued role of clinical judgement. J. Vasc. Surg., 1988, 703-709.
25. Gainfortune P, Fulla Rj. Ray resection in the insensitive disvascular foot: a critical review. J Foot Surg, 1985, 24 : 103-107.
26. Pinzur M, Kaminsky M. Amputation at the middle level of the foot: a retrospective and prospective review. J Bone Joint Surg. 1986 , 68a : 1061-1064.
27. Spittler AW. Syme amputation performed in two stages. J Bone Joint Surg. 1954, 36A :37-42.
28. Dible JH. The pathology of limb ischemia pathology monograph N.£ Edinburgh, Oliver and Boyd, 1966.
29. Caputo GM, Cavanagh PR, Ulbrecht JS, Gibbons GW, Karchmer AW. Assessment and management of foot disease in patients with diabetes. N. Eng. J. Med. 1994, 331 : 854.
30. Faglia E, Favales F, Quarantiello A, Cala P, Brambilla G, Rampoldi A, Morabito A. Feasibility and effectiveness of peripheral percutaneous transluminal ballon angioplasty in diabetic subjects with foot ulcers. Diabetes Care, 1996, 19: 1261.
31. Richard A, Pollak DPM. A human dermal replacement for the treatment of diabetic foot ulcers. Wounds, 1979, 1, 175-183.
32. Caravaggi C, Faglia E, Cavaiani P, Di Giglio R, Brunati S, Dalla Noce S, Sacchi G. Attecchimento e sicurezza degli innesti autologhi di fibroblasti e cheratinociti nel trattamento delle ulcere del piede diabetico Oral presentation AMD Congress Bologna, 1997.

NOTES

HYPERBARIC OXYGEN IN THE TREATMENT OF INFECTION OF THE DIABETIC FOOT

Jordi Desola

CRIS—Hyperbaric Therapy Unit—Barcelona, Spain

Chronic wounds often cause a hard interaction between microorganisms, wound healing, and tissue oxygen tension. Both aerobic and especially anaerobic germs need low oxidation-reduction potential levels to develop their activity; these hypoxic conditions make the development of tissue necrosis easier. Necrotic tissue is an optimal culture medium for many microorganisms; infection will enhance tissue hypoxia. This cycle also works in the opposite direction. Infection may cause necrosis, which will reduce oxygen tissue tension; and from that state comes optimal conditions for the development of infection.

FUNDAMENTALS

From a clinical point of view, an infectious disease is a compromise among three factors: the patient, the microorganism, and the therapeutic agent. Each component of this triangle produces both agonistic and antagonistic actions with and against the other two.

In the special case of the diabetic foot, a large series of factors will determine the outcome of the disease.

A.1.- Microorganism → Patient.

The microorganism acts against the diabetic patient, easily producing a chronic refractory infection; in that condition the oxygen tension of the wound will be very low. Some germs become optionally anaerobic as a mechanism of resistance.

B.1.- Antibiotic → Microorganism.

In the optimal situation the therapeutic agent will stop infection and will act at least in part bactericidally.

C.1.- Patient → Antibiotic.

The activity of the therapeutic agent is commonly limited in the diabetic patient, by means of a very reduced bioavailability of antibiotics, due to the local conditions inherent to the disease: associated microangiopathy, defects of posture and stability as a result of the diabetic neuropathy, and residual long-term trophic changes.

D.1.- Patient → Microorganism.

At the same time, the patient starts the natural host defence against infection, which is mainly based on leucocytic phagocytic killing. This leucodiapedic action, however, needs a normal tissue oxygen tension, without which it will be stopped (1–3).

On the other hand, the microorganism easily acquires resistance against the common antibiotics, and this therapeutic agent frequently becomes inefficient. The low antibiotic concentrations finally available to the wound, the frequent long duration of the treatments, and the polymicrobial condition of the disease make this mechanism easier yet.

F.1.- Antibiotic → Patient.

The patient also suffers the undesirable action of antibiotics in the form of side- or toxic effects. This is especially easy when long term treatments will be required due to the chronic refractory condition of the infection. Some of the most potentially effective antibiotics can not be used in long courses.

Alongside this, the infective profile of the diabetic foot is as a chronic refractory disease, frequently with multiresistant germs, low bioavailability of antibiotics, optimal local conditions for microorganism growth, reduced capability of starting effective phagocytic killing, and easy development of toxic effects of commonly used drugs.

MECHANISM OF HYPERBARIC OXYGENATION ON TISSUE INFECTION

The best treatment for this disease will be given by those therapies that will counteract all these conditions.

We will review now whether hyperbaric oxygenation (HBO) can accomplish some of these requirements. And we will follow the same steps as above. The triangle is now based on HBO, the patient and the wound, and the miroorganism. This is a clinical approach based in the real daily practice with these patients.

A.2.- Microorganism → Patient.

Patients sent to hyperbaric medical centres usually suffer from seriously advanced processes where wounds are refractory and infection acquires a very important role. Our patients are frequently highly compromised, and it is really difficult to manage with such advanced lesions, whose outcome would probably have been better if we had received them at an earlier stage. HBO can be the key factor to break the above vicious circle: infection-hypoxia-necrosis-more infection.

B.2.- Hyperbaric Oxygen → Microorganism.

a. Direct antimicrobial effect. HBO is bactericidal against spore-forming anaerobic microorganisms, which is widely known although sometimes disputed in spite of the existence of much experimental evidence (4,5) and consistent clinical data (6–9). Clostridium species need low oxidation/reduction potential in order to produce their haemolytic and necrotizing toxins, so HBO inhibits Clostridial toxin formation even before achieving the bactericidal effect (10–11). Much less widely known is that HBO is bacteriostatic against non-spore-forming anaerobic germs (12), like Bacteroides and others (13–14), is bacteriostatic against many fungus (15–21) and protozoa (22), and it can be also bacteriostatic against Staphylococcus (23,24), Escherichhia coli 5, Pseudomonas aeruginosa (26,27) and other germs with weak antioxidant defense (28,29).

The antimicrobial action is based in the production of free radicals, and other reactive oxygen-based molecules, which will produce oxidation of membrane lipids and proteins, degradation of DNA, and inhibition of metabolic functions of the microorganisms (30,31).

b. Antibiotic sinergic effect. HBO does not impair the action of antibiotics and/or chemotherapic agents. On the contrary, much of the time it has synergistic role (32,33). Some antibiotics suffer an important reduction of their action in anaerobic conditions (34), as happens with aminoglycosides (35–38), vancomycin (39), cotrimoxazole (trimethoprim/sulphamethoxazole) (40,41), fluorquinolones, nitrofurantoin (42), and rifamycins; this effect is extremely important in the case of fluorquinolones whose action is highly inhibited by low oxygen tension (43). Just the opposite happens with metronidazole (44), whose effect is higher in an anaerobic environment, which is the reason it is frequently used in the treatment of soft tissue necrotizing infections. There is no known effect of hypoxia on macrolides and tetracyclines, and it seems to be very weak on beta-lactam antibiotics.

An elevation of the tissue oxygen tension will make possible the restoration of the full activity of the antibiotic, as proved in some experimental in vitro studies (45). Other antibiotics experience not only this but a direct enhancement of their antimicrobial activity; this is the case of amykacin, tobramycin, and rifamycins. Experimental data has also proved an increase of effectivity of clindamycin and vancomycin when combined with HBO (46–47).

It can be summarized that HBO produces two different effects on antibiotics, either indirectly enhancing their natural activity when restoring normal tissue oxygen tension, or increasing their antimicrobial effect as a direct effect of HBO. However it is not a universal effect on antibiotics, because its effect varies between different antibiotics, and it only affects selected microorganisms (48–50).

C.2.- Patient → Hyperbaric Oxygen.

a. Enhanced bioavailability of antibiotics. HBO has a known angiogenetic action in compromised tissues, thus increasing tissue perfusion enhances antibiotics bioavailability.

b. Prolongation of post-antibiotic effect. After their administration, inhibition of growth of the germs is maintained during a period of time that varies depending of the kind of germ, conditions of the tissue, and type of antibiotic. This so-called Post-Antibiotic Effect (PAE) is enhanced by HBO by increasing duration and effectivity of antimicrobial effect (51–54). The PAE enhancement has been widely studied in relation to tobramycin and amykacin against Pseudomonas aeruginosa.

D.2.- Patient → Microorganism.

Recovery of leucocyte phagocytic killing. HBO strengthens natural defenses against infection thanks to the leucocytic phagocytic killing. Mader et al. proved in 1978 that HBO alone had the same effect in the treatment of chronic osteomyelitis as cephalothin (the best antibiotic for this disease at that time) but the mechanism for this beneficial effect was not clearly explained (55).

Some few years after this fundamental work, Mader proved in a very sophisticated experimental work published also in the Journal of Infectious Diseases, that HBO did not have a direct antimicrobial effect, but that it strengthened natural host defenses against the infection, by recovering the leucodiapedetic action of PMN when normal oxygen tension values were achieved, after some minutes of HBO (56). Many other works made this fundamental finding (57–62). It is well known today that the phago-cytic action of polymorphonuclear leucocytes is partially oxygen dependent, and that it is abolished when oxygen tissue is lower than 28 mmhg. Currently the clinical data on the treatment of osteomyelitis by means of adjunctive HBO is really valuable (63–65).

E.2.- Microorganism → Hyperbaric Oxygen.

Low microbial resistance. The action of HBO is based in free radical formation against which the bacteria can promote antioxidants. Anaerobic germs fail to produce these, and facultative anaerobics can do it in certain conditions, when they have the ability to produce more antioxidant enzymes (mainly superoxide dismutase, catalase, and glutathione peroxidase). Resistance of bacteria to HBO depends on their capacity to form these enzymes.

F.2.- Hyperbaric Oxygen → Patient.

Few toxic effects. HBO has few and well-defined side- and/or undesirable effects, which are easily controlled if it is applied in the correct way. That means whatever the indication for the therapy, maximal pressure, duration of any session, number of treatments given, and periodicity are adequate. Like all drugs HBO has direct effects, therapeutic effects, and of course undesirable effects.

However a wide experience confirms that the real incidence of these undesirable effects is very low. Some patients suffering from other diseases that require long treatments (chronic osteomyelitis, radiation induced injuries, and others) have shown in our experience an excellent tolerance to the long treatment periods they usually need. We perform some investigations prior to admitting a patient for HBO, among which is spirometry in order to detect pulmonary toxicity. In our experience, at the moment of finishing a long treatment, when spirometry is repeated, the majority of the patients not only have not suffered any deterioration of their respiratory function but many of them have even shown some improvement.

Many of the vascular surgeons who send us patients for HBO treatment are surprised by the significant improvement in the general condition of patients who have recovered physical activity and have extended their walking distance when previously limited by vascular disease, and in summary they have significantly enhanced their quality of lives.

CONCLUSION

In summary, the application of HBO to patients suffering from a DIABETIC FOOT, in relation to their cross-infection, will imply:

- Bactericidal effect against spore-forming anaerobic microorganisms, and bacteriostatic against non-spore-forming anaerobic germs, many fungus, some protozoa, and also some selected aerobic bacteria.
- Synergistic antimicrobial action with some antibiotics, either restoring their normal activity or increasing their direct activity and enlarging their post-antibiotic effect.
- Enhancement of drugs bioavailability.
- Recovery of oxygen-dependent phagocytic killing by means of increasing tissue oxygen tension.

- Restriction of microbial resistance.
- Low incidence of side effects.
- Amelioration of the general condition of patients, and of their vascular and functional capacity.
- Compatibility with the other treatments the patient is receiving.

My personal opinion is that no other therapeutic regime can offer such positive help to a diabetic patient who is suffering from a combination of pathological factors not, only in the foot but also throughout the body and its systems. The clinical data is very consistent (66–85).

The reason for this meeting is to discuss some relevant aspects of this therapy as applied to this compromising disease, which has been already described by the preceding papers, and which will be completed in the following presentations.

It is the role of the members of the Consensus Jury to decide and to consider the place of HBO in some of these steps and their possible strategic contribution in order to break the aforementioned pathological patient/microorganism/antibiotic triangle.

REFERENCES

1. Mandell GL. Bactericidal activity of aerobic and anaerobic polimorphonuclear neutrophils. Infect Immun, 1974; 9: 337-41.
2. Mandell GL, Hook EW. Leukocyte bactericidal activity in chronic granulomatous disease: correlation of bacterial hydrogen peroxide production and susceptibility to intracellular killing. J Bacteriol, 1969; 100:531-2.
3. Babior BM. Oxygen-dependent microbial killing by phagocytoses. New Engl J Med, 1978; 298:659-68.
4. Muhvich KH, Anderson LH, Mehm WJ. Evaluation of antimicrobials combined with hyperbaric oxygen in a mouse model of Clostridial myonecrosis (see comments). J Trauma, 1994; 36 (1) :7-10.
5. Holland JA, Hill GB, Wolfe WG, Osterhout S, Saltzman HA, Brown IW, JR. Experimental and clinical experience with hyperbaric oxygen in the treatment of Clostridial myonecrosis. Surgery, 1975; 77 (1) :75-85.
6. Desola J, Escola E, Moreno E, Munoz MA, Sanchez U, Murillo F. Tratamiento combinado de la gangrena gaseosa con oxigenoterapia hiperbarica, cirugía y antibióticos. Estudio colaborativo multicéntrico. (Combined treatment of gas gangrene with hyperbaric oxygenation, surgery and antibiotics. A multicentric collaborative study.) Med Clin (Barc), 1990; 94 (17):641-50.
7. Desola J, Escola E, Galofre M. Infecciones necrosantes de partes blandas. Perspectiva multidisciplinaria. (Soft Tissue Necrotizing Infections. A Multidisciplinary Approach). Med Clin (Barc), 1998; 110 (11):431-6.
8. Stevens DL, Bryant AE, Adams K, Mader JT. Evaluation of therapy with hyperbaric oxygen for experimental infection with Clostridium perfringens (see comments). Clin Infect Dis, 1993; 17 (2):231-7.
9. Thom SR. A role for hyperbaric oxygen in Clostridial myonecrosis (EDITORIAL). Clin Infect Dis, 1993; 17 (2) : 238.
10. Hill GB, Osterhout S. Experimental effects of Hyperbaric Oxygen on selected Clostridial species. I. In-vitro studies. J Infect Dis, 1972; 125 (1) :17-25.
11. Hill GB, Osterhout S. Experimental effects of Hyperbaric Oxygen on selected Clostridial species. II. In-vivo studies. J Infect Dis, 1972; 125 (1):26-35.
12. Hill GB. Hyperbaric oxygen exposures for intrahepatic abscesses produced in mice by nonspore forming anaerobic bacteria. Antimicrob Agents Chemother, 1976; 9:312-7.
13. Privalle CT, Gregory EM. Superoxide dismutase and O2 lethality in Bacteeroides fragilis. J Bacteriol, 1979; 138:139-45.
14. Schreiner A, Tonjum S, Digranes A. Hyperbaric oxygen therapy in bacteroides infections. Acta Chir Scand, 1974; 140(1):73-6.
15. Blaine DA, Frable MA. Mucormycosis. Adjunctive therapy with hydrogen peroxide. Va Med Q, 1996; 123(1):30-2.
16. Boelart JR. Mucormycosis (zygomycosis): Is there news for the clinician? J Infect, 1994; 28 (1):1-6.
17. Couch L, Theilen F, Mader JT. Rhinocerebral mucormycosis with cerebral extension successfully treated with adjunctive hyperbaric oxygen therapy. Arch Otolaryngol Head Neck Surg, 1988; 114 (7) :791-4.
18. Duplechain JK, White JA. Mucormycosis of the head and neck. J La State Med Soc, 1989; 141 (3) :9-13.
19. Ferguson BJ, Mitchell TG, Moon R, Camporesi EM, Farmer J. Adjunctive hyperbaric oxygen for treatment of rhinocerebral mucormycosis. Rev Infect Dis, 1988; 10(3):551-9.
20. Gamba JL, Woodruff W-W, Djang W-T, Yeates AE. Cranofacial mucormycosis: Assessment with CT. Radiology, 1986; 160:207-12.
21. Gudewicz TM, Mader JT, Davis CP. Combined effects of hyperbaric oxygen and antifungal agents on the growth of Candida albicans. Aviat Space Environ Med, 1987; 58(7):673-8.
22. Muhvich KH, Anderson LH, Criswell DW, Mehm WJ. Hyperbaric hyperoxia enhances the lethal effects of amphotericin B in Leishmania braziliensis panamensis. Undersea Hyperb Med, 1993; 20(4):321-8.
23. Barnwell P, Sopher S, Fleckinger RR, Rhoden CH, Smith IM. Treatment of Staphylococcus aureus infections in mice with oxygen at various pressures and concentrations. Am Rev Respir Dis, 1966; 94(5):756-60.
24. Irvin TT, Norman JN, Suwanagul A, Smith G. Hyperbaric oxygen therapy in experimental staphylococcal infection. Br J Surg, 1967; 54(7):595-7.
25. Brown OR. Mechanisms of hyperbaric-oxygen inhibition of growth and net biosynthesis of RNA, DNA, protein and lipids in Escherichia coli. Microbios, 1990; 64(260-261):135-51.
26. Pakman LM. Inhibition of Pseudomonas aeruginosa by hyperbaric oxygen. I. Sulfonamide activity enhancement and reversal. Infect Immun, 1971; 4(4):479-87.
27. Clark JM, Pakman LM. Inhibition of Pseudomonas aeruginosa by hyperbaric oxygen. II. Ultrastructural changes. Infect Immun, 1971; 4(4):488-91.
28. Baird RM. Postoperative infections from bacteroides. Am Surg, 1973; 39(8):459-64.
29. Desola J. Oxigenoterapia Hiperbárica en Patología infecciosa. Revisión y puesta al día. (Hyperbaric oxygen therapy in infection diseases. Review and update.) Enferm Infecc Microbiol Clin, 1986; 4(2):84-8.
30. Brown GL, Thomson PD, Mader JT, Hilton JG, Browne ME, Wells CH. Effects of hyperbaric oxygen upon S. aureus, Ps. aeruginosa and C. albicans. Aviat Space Environ Med, 1979; 50(7):717-20.
31. Park MK, Myers RA, Marzella L. Oxygen tensions and infections: Modulation of microbial growth, activity of antimicrobial agents, and immunologic responses. Clin Infect Dis, 1992; 14(3):720-40.
32. Knighton DR, Halliday P, Hunt TK. Oxygen as an antibiotic. A comparison of the effects of inspired oxygen concentration and antibiotic administration on in vivo clearance. Arch Surg, 1986; 121:191-5.
33. Knighton DR, Fiegel VD, Halverson T, Scheneider T, Brownn T, Wells CL. Oxygen as an antibiotic. The effect of inspired oxygen on bacterial clearance. Arch Surg, 1990; 125:97-100.
34. Verklin JR RM, Mandell GL. Alteration of effectiveness of antibiotics by anaerobiosis. J Lab Clin Med, 1977; 89:65-71.

35. Bayer AS, O'Brien T, Norman DC, Nast CC. Oxygen-dependent differences in exopolysaccharide production and aminoglycoside inhibitory-bactericidal interaction with Pseudomonas aeruginnnoa implications for endocarditis. J Antimicrob Chemother, 1989; 23:21-35.

36. Bryan LE, Kwan S. Mechanisms of aminoglycoside resistance or anaerobic bacteria and facultative bacteria grown anaerobically. J Antimicrob Chemother, 1981; 8 D:1-8.

37. Raval G, Park MK, Myers RAM, Marzella L. Hyperoxia modulates aminoglycoside activity in Gram-negative bacteria. Undersea Biomed Res, 1992; 19 : 25.

38. Reynolds AV, Hamilton-Miller JMT, Brumfitt W. Diminished effect of gentamycin under anaerobic or hypercapnic conditions. Lancet, 1976; 1:447 9.

39. Norden CW, Shaffer M. Treatment of experimental chronic osteomyelitis due to Staphylococcus aureus with vancomycin and rifampicin. J Infect Dis, 1998; 147:352-7.

40. Bastian FO, Jennings RA, Hoff CJ. Effect of trimethoprim/sulphamethoxazole and hyperbaric oxygen on experimental Spiroplasma mirum encephalitis. Res Microbiol, 1989; 140 (2) :151-8.

41. Virtanen S. Antibacterial activity of sulphamethoxazole and trimethoprim underdiminished oxygen tension. J Gen Microbiol, 1974; 84 : 145-8.

42. Seither RL Y, Brown OR. Paraquat and nitrofurantoin inhibit growth of Escherichia coli by inducing stringency. J Toxicol Environ Health, 1984; 14 (5-6) : 763-71.

43. Lesse AJ, Freer C. Oral ciprofloxacin therapy for Gram negative bacillary osteomyelitis. Am J Med, 1987; 82, IV : 247-53.

44. Tally FP, Sullivan CE. Metronidazole: Invitro activity, pharmacology and efficacy in anaerobic bacterial infections. Pharmacotherapy, 1981; 1:28-38.

45. Jonsson K, Hunt TK, Mathes SJ. Oxygen as an isolated variable influences resistance to infection. Ann Surg, 1988; 208 : 783-7.

46. Muhvich KH, Myers RA, Marzella L. Effect of hyperbaric oxygenation, combined with antimicrobial agents and surgery, in a rat model of intraabdominal infection. J Infect Dis, 1988; 157 (5) :1058-61.

47. Tack KJ, Sabath LD. Increased minimum inhibitory concentration with anaerobiasis for tobramycin, gentamicin, and amikacin, compared to latamoxef, piperacillin, chloramphenicol, and clindamycin. 1985 of therapy, 3198; (204) :210.

48. Thom SR, Lauermann MW, Hart GB. Intermittent hyperbaric oxygen therapy for reduction of mortality in experimental polymicrobial sepsis. J Infect Dis, 1986; 154(3):504-10.

49. Marzella L, Vezzani G. Effect of HYperbaric Oxygen on Activity of Antibacterial Agents. In : Oriani G, Marroni A, Wattel F., eds.Handbook on Hyperbaric Medicine. Berlin: Springer-Verlag, 1996; 699-713.

50. Park MK, Muhvich KH, Myers RAM, Marzella L. Effects of Hyperbaric oxygen in infectious diseases : basic mechanisms. In: Kindwall E., Ed. Hyperbaric Medicine Practice. Flagstaff, AZ : Best Publishing Company, 1994; 141-172.

51. Craig WA, Gudmundsson S. The postantibiotic effect. Antibiotics in laboratory medicine 1986; 515-36.6589.

52. Baquero F, Culebras E, Patron C, Perez-Diaz JC, Medrano JC, Viceente MF. Postantibiotic effect of imepenem on Gram-positive and Gram-negative micro-organisms. J Antimicrob Chemother, 1986; 18 E : 47-59.

53. Park MK, Muhvich KH, Myers RA, Marzella L. Hyperoxia prolongs the aminoglycoside-induced postantibiotic effect in Pseudomonas aeruginosa. Antimicrob Agents Chemother, 1991; 35 (4) :691-5.

54. Park MK, Myers RAM, Marzella L. Hyperoxia and prolongation of aminoglycoside induced postantibiotic effect in Pseudomonas aeruginosa : role of reactive oxygen species. Antimicrob Agents Chemother, 1993; 37 : 120-2.

55. Mader JT, Guckian JC, Glass DL, Reinarz JA. Therapy with hyperbaric oxygen for experimental osteomyelitis due to Staphylococcus aureus in rabbits. J Infect Dis, 1978; 138 (3) : 312-8.

56. Mader JT, Brown GL, Guckian JC, Wells CH, Reinarz JA. A mechanism for the amelioration by hyperbaric oxygen of experimental staphylococcal osteomyelitis in rabbits. J Infect Dis, 1980; 142 (6) :915-22.

57. Mader JT. Phagocitic killing and hyperbaric oxygen : antimicrobial mechanisms. HBO Review, 1981; 2 (1): 37-54.

58. Mader JT, Hicks CA, Calhoun J. Bacterial osteomyelitis. Adjunctive hyperbaric oxygen therapy. Orthop Rev, 1989; 18 (5) :581-5.

59. Mader JT, Adams KR, Wallace W-R, Calhoun JH. Hyperbaric oxygen as adjunctive therapy for osteomyelitis. Infect Dis Clin North Am, 1990; 4 (3) : 433-40.

60. Mader JT, Ortiz M, Calhoun JH. Update on the diagnosis and management of osteomyelitis. Clin Podiatr Med Surg, 1996; 13(4):701-24.

61. Mader JT, Shirtliff M, Calhoun JH. Staging and staging application in osteomyelitis. Clin Infect Dis, 1997; 25 (6) : 1303-9.

62. Sheftel TG, Mader JT, Penninck JJ, Cierny G, III. Methicillin-resistant Staphylococcus aureus osteomyelitis. Clin Orthop, 1985; (198) : 231-9.

63. Calhoun JH, Cobos JA, Mader JT. Does hyperbaric oxygen have a place in the treatment of osteomyelitis ? Orthop Clin North Am, 1991; 22 (3) :467-71.

64. Farnam J, Griffin JE, Schow CE, Mader JT, Grant JA. Recurrent diffuse osteomyelitis involving the mandible. Oral Surg Oral Med Oral Pathol, 1984; 57 (4) : 374-8.

65. Kerley TR, Mader JT, Hulet W-H, Schow CE. The effect of adjunctive hyperbaric oxygen on bone regeneration in mandibular osteomyelitis: report of case J Oral Surg, 1981; 39 : 619-23.

66. Bauer P, Larcan A. Oxygénotherapie hyperbare dans le traitement des ulcères ischemiques. Sang Thromb Vaiss, 1997; 9 (8) : 497-503.

67. Brakora MJ, Sheffield PJ. Hyperbaric oxygen therapy for diabetic wounds. Clin Podiatr Med Surg, 1995; 12(1):105-17.

68. Chantelau E. Hyperbaric oxygen therapy for diabetic foot ulcers (letter). Diabetes Care, 1997; 20 (7) :1207-8.

69.   Cianci P. Adjunctive hyperbaric oxygen therapy in the treatment of the diabetic foot. J Am Podiatr Med Assoc., 1994; 84 (9) :448-55.

70.   Cianci P, Hunt TK. Long-term results of aggressive management of diabetic foot ulcers suggest significant cost effectiveness. Wound Repair and Regeneration, 1997; 5 (2) : 141-6.

71.   Davis JC. The use of adjuvant hyperbaric oxygen in treatment of the diabetic foot. Clin Podiatr Med Surg, 1987; 4 (2) :429-37.

72.   Doctor N, Pandya S, Supe A. Hyperbaric oxygen therapy in diabetic foot. J Postgrad Med, 1992; 38 (3) : 112-4.

73.   Faglia E, Favales F, Aldeghi A, Calia P, Quarantiello A, Barbano P, Puttini M, et al. Change in major amputation rate in a center dedicated to diabetic foot care during the 1980s: Prognostic determinants for major amputation. J Diabetes Complications, 1998; 12 (2) :96-102.

74.   Faglia E, Favales F, Aldeghi A, Calia P, Quarantiello A, Oriani G, Michael M, et al. Adjunctive systemic hyperbaric oxygen therapy in treatment of severe prevalently ischemic diabetic foot ulcer. A randomized study. Diabetes Care, 1996; 19 (12) : 1338-43.

75.   Lee SS, Chen CY, Chan YS, Yen CY, Chao EK, Ueng SW. Hyperbaric oxygen in the treatment of diabetic foot infection. Chang Keng I Hsueh, 1997; 20 (1) : 17-22.

76.   Logerfo FW, Misare BD. Current management of the diabetic foot. Adv Surg, 1996; 30 : 417-26.

77.   Longoni C, Ferani R, Ghilardi G, Pecis C, Cugnasca M. Hyperbaric oxygen therapy and diabetic foot. Clinical and metabolic evaluations. Chir Piede, 1988; 12 (5) : 239-41.

78.   Mcdermott JE. The diabetic foot: evolving technologies. Instr Course Lect, 1993; 42 : 169-71.

79.   Norris T, Clarke D. Care of diabetic foot lesions (letter; comment). Am Fam Physician, 1996; 54 (1) :70-838X.

80.   Stone JA, Cianci P. The use of hyperbaric oxygen therapy in the treatment of diabetes-related lower extremity wounds. Clinical Diabetes, 1997; 15 (5) : 196-202.

81.   Unger HD, Lucca M. The role of hyperbaric oxygen therapy in the treatment of diabetic foot ulcers and refractory osteomyelitis. Clin Podiatr Med Surg, 1990; 7 (3) : 483-92.

82.   Vezzani G, Marziani L, Pizzola A, Guerrini A, Uleri G. Trattamento non chirurgico delle vasculopatie per iferiche: piede diabetico ed ossigenoterapia iperbarica. (Non-surgical treatment of peripheral vascular diseases: diabetic foot and hyperbaric oxygenation). Minerva Anestesiol, 1992; 58 (10) : 1119-20.

83.   Weisz G, Ramon Y, Melamed Y. Treatment of the diabetic foot by hyperbaric oxygen. Harefuah, 1993; 124 (11) :678-81.

84.   Williams RL. Hyperbaric oxygen therapy and the diabetic foot. J Am Podiatr Med Assoc, 1997; 87 (6) :279-92.

85.   Zamboni WA, Wong HP, Stepheson LL, Pfeifer MA. Evaluation of hyperbaric oxygen for diabetic wounds: a prospective study. Undersea Hyperb Med, 1997; 24 (3) : 175-9.

IS OXYGEN THERAPY A USEFUL THERAPY FOR CHRONIC WOUNDS IN DIABETES?
The Basics

Cheng Quah, Mark Rollins and Thomas K. Hunt
University of California, San Francisco—USA

Diabetics develop notoriously difficult foot problems that are associated with considerable morbidity and mortality. The major causes are ischemia/hypoxia and neuropathy, and they often coexist. When neuropathy and repeated injury are the sole problem, therapy is mechanical protection and "off-loading." When ischemia is the problem, however, the treatment is to enhance circulation/oxygenation. If large vessels are obstructed, surgical revascularization is the treatment of choice. However, even if palpable pulses are present, many diabetics have focal areas of low flow and hypoxia in their feet and ankles which may be the result of many pathophysiologic alterations, which include increased blood viscosity, platelet aggregation, trauma, and capillary endothelial thickening, vasospasm, etc. (1, 29). These microcirculatory problems seriously impair wound healing, and defective wound healing is, in the end, the single most frequent factor contributing to limb loss (36). Amputations remain unacceptably frequent and limb hypoxia/ischemia is the major feature in almost all cases.

Hypoxia is, in itself, a sufficient cause to delay or even prevent healing and is sufficient to explain much of the propensity of wounds in diabetics to infection. Even wounds in normal tissues are hypoxic when compared to non-wounded tissue. Ischemic foot wounds in diabetics are characteristically extremely hypoxic.

The question at hand in this conference is whether hyperbaric oxygen (HBO) can materially aid healing in the clinical context of diabetes by raising tissue oxygen concentrations. The answer that we will provide, by reviewing the basics of wound healing, is "yes it has that capability." However, basic considerations also make it entirely clear that HBO has limitations such that patients must be properly chosen, must be given appropriate wound care, and must be systemically as well as locally supported.

OXYGEN AND WOUND HEALING

Hopefully, the least contentious item to be discussed is the role of oxygen in healing. Oxygen clearly plays a large central role in wound healing. The effect of changing the O_2 tension in wounds has large consequences even in clinical terms. Strangely, while mechanisms of acceleration of wound healing by oxygen are well understood, credibility in terms of clinical therapy is still being established. We have long known that all the major components of wound healing, fibroplasia, collagen deposition, angiogenesis, epithelization, and bacterial killing, proceed in proportion to the amount of oxygen which is available to them. There can be no question that oxygen therapy is capable of delivering useful clinical results. Hopefully, the following review of the basic data will aid a consensus. We will develop these ideas and introduce the concept that the effects of oxygen therapy depend on the change which tissue hypoxia has developed.

THE NORMAL WOUND ENVIRONMENT

Injuries and infections, by interrupting local circulation and inciting inflammation, result in an environment of acute metabolic need that is characterized by low oxygen tension (40–60 mmHg), low pH (~7.3), high PCO_2, high lactate concentrations, and relatively rich in cytokines. This characteristic environment leads to phenotypic changes in local cells which then lead to healing (17, 34, 35).

COLLAGEN SYNTHESIS AND DEPOSITION

Although low tissue oxygen concentration (PO_2) can incite some aspects of repair, lactate is the dominant stimulus to the synthesis of collagen (Figure 1). Oxygen is best understood as a critical nutrient whose concentration governs the rate of collagen deposition once repair has been instigated by lactate (32).

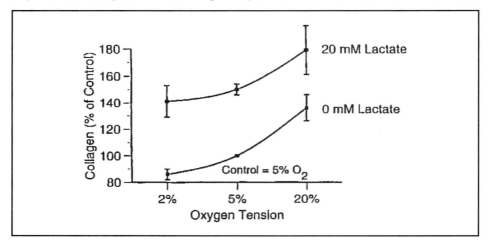

Figure 1. Effect of oxygen tension and lactate concentration on collagen synthesis. Fibroblasts incubated in various combinations of lactate concentrations and PO_2 were pulsed with tritiated proline. Secretion of hydroxylated collagen into the cell-conditioned medium was enhanced by both lactate and oxygen.

From: Skover GR. Cellular and biochemical dynamics of wound repair. Wound environment in collagen regeneration. Clinics in Podiatric Medicine and Surgery, 1991; 8:308. Reprinted with permission.

High lactate in the range of 5–15 mM, as found in wounds, is sufficient, by itself, to stimulate collagen synthesis (17, 18, 20). Hypoxia is not the reason that lactate concentrations rise so high in wounds. The operative reason is that leukocytes, macrophages, and fibroblasts (and tumor cells) normally produce large amounts of lactate through aerobic glycolysis (33). During aerobic glycosis, lactate is produced despite the presence of oxygen. Glycolytic cells, such as fibroblasts, have few mitochondria and little capacity to produce CO_2. Adding oxygen does not increase CO_2 production or decrease lactate significantly in wounds.

The high lactate levels shift the equilibrium ratio of NAD+/NADH toward NADH and reduces the NAD+ "pool." When this NAD+ "pool" is reduced for hours or days, affected cells undergo a phenotypic change and assume healing functions. The mechanism is complex.

Under normal life conditions, NAD+ is metabolized to adenosine diphosphoribose (ADPR). ADPRibose combines with various proteins, both nuclear and cytoplasmic, thus regulating their function. Among their many functions, ADPRibosylations suppress collagen gene transcription in the nucleus and prolyl hydroxylase activity in the cytoplasm (10, 43). Injuries change this normal equilibrium. In wounds, the elevated lactate levels reduce the NAD+ pool. ADPRibosylations diminish, thus releasing the normal repression of collagen synthesis. The collagen mRNA pool then rises (10, 43). As a result, procollagen is synthesized (10). The molecular mechanisms leading to increased mRNA are not known.

This explanation of control of collagen synthesis without reference to growth factors may be surprising. In fact, growth factors may exert their effects on collagen through ADPRibosylation mechanisms. IGF-1 and PDGF, for instance, markedly increase lactate production by fibroblasts. We have evidence that IGF-1 reduces ADPRibosylations and as a result increases collagen and VEGF in RNA. Other growth factors have not been tested in this light. We do know, however, that many cytokines are released by hypoxic cells. It is clear by now that excessive cytokine release is harmful. VEGF causes vascular permeability. Without its expression leading to angiogenesis, prolonged edema would be the expected result of hypoxia, and this is what we see in chronic wounds.

Once procollagen peptide is synthesized, PO_2 becomes critical to its future. Procollagen must be hydroxylated in order to gain exit from fibroblasts. The enzymes for this step, prolyl- and lysyl-hydroxylases, both require oxygen as a substrate. Prolyl-hydroxylase regulates export of collagen and lysyl-hydroxylase facilitates extra-cellular cross-linking. They insert oxygen atoms derived from molecular oxygen as hydroxyl groups into selected collagen prolines and lysines. ADPRibosylation regulates these enzymes and hence collagen export (18). The Km, that is the PO_2 at which this reaction proceeds at half maximal speed, is in the 20–30 mmHg range (32). A median PO_2 of 20 mmHg is often measured in chronic wounds in diabetics. In these circumstances the rate at which collagen can be deposited is less than half maximal.

As seen in Figure 2, collagen export (deposition) is proportional to arterial (and tissue) PO_2. The maximum rate of collagen deposition occurs at about 250 mmHg (tissue) which is far higher than the normal oxygen tension in wounds. Only during hyperbaric oxygen therapy would these reactions reach maximum velocity even in normal wounded tissues. As shown (Figure 2), the collagen deposited in animals kept in a hyperoxic atmosphere is three times (!) that of animals kept in a hypoxic one. If both hypoxemia and vasoconstriction are operative, collagen deposition ("healing") can rise tenfold upon their correction (12, 14, 17, 21).

The effect of oxygen on collagen synthesis, deposition, and crosslinking is known in far greater detail. Fibroblast replication is also known to be optimal at a PO_2 of 40–60 mmHg (16). The mechanism(s) are not known.

In summary, efficient fibroblast replication, collagen production, and crosslinking vary according to PO_2 and are optimized in an environment of high oxygen tensions and high lactate levels (Figure 1). High oxygen and high lactate are able to coexist because

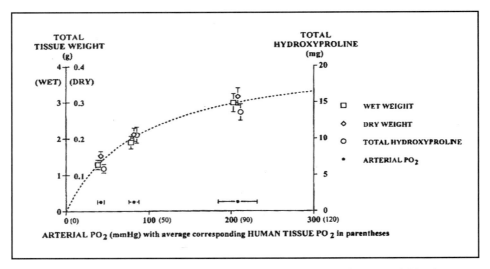

Figure 2. Wound tissue and hydroxyproline accumulation as a function of blood oxygen tension in rabbits. The shape of this curve is critical to understanding wound healing. It will be found in subsequent figures as well. It is typical of the family of curves which describe the rate of product formation, (vertical axis) from an enzyme reaction with respect to the concentration of a substrate (horizontal axis). In this case, it is the rate of collagen hydroxylation and tissue accumulation with respect to the concentration of oxygen. Oxygen is the substrate of prolyl hydroxylase governing the rate of collagen deposition. When oxygen is added, the rate at which collagen is hydroxylated and deposited rises dramatically but at a progressively slower rate with each increment of PO_2. In this illustration, the three product measurements have been fit to a generalized Michaelis-Menten curve with arterial PO_2 as the substrate. The Km, or half maximal reaction rate, estimated by this curve, and is consistent with other experimental data established for prolyl hydroxylase showing the Km of this process approaches normal wound oxygen tensions.

From: Hunt TK, Pai MP. The effect of varying ambient oxygen tension on wound metabolism and collagen synthesis. Surg Gynecol Obstet 1972; 135:561.

lactate is produced by glycolytic leukocytes, macrophages, endothelial cells, and fibroblasts whether or not they are oxygenated.

ANGIOGENESIS

Angiogenesis is also critical to healing. The common belief today is that hypoxia stimulates angiogenesis. This is a misstatement of fact. Hypoxia stimulates VEGF release from macrophages among many other cells, but angiogenesis is impaired in chronically hypoxic animals (2, 7, 9, 24, 39, 42).

Endothelial cells must synthesize and deposit collagen for basement membrane synthesis to provide structural support for budding vessels (7). It is not surprising, therefore, that the same intracellular signaling mechanism incites both collagen and VEGF release. Both are regulated by lactate and oxygen concentrations, etc., via ADPRibosylation mechanisms.

The effect of oxygen on angiogenesis is mediated through vascular endothelial growth factor. VEGF is the most important stimulator of angiogenesis in wounds. VEGF is unique; its receptors are exclusively located on endothelial cells (9). As in the case of collagen, lactate stimulates release of VEGF from wound macrophages even in the presence of oxygen. In fact, angiogenesis requires oxygen (7, 8, 11, 39).

Jensen et al. showed in 1986 that as in collagen synthesis, lactate also stimulates release of an angiogenic factor into the wound environment (20). This factor is now identified as VEGF (Constant, unpublished data). Lactate is particularly significant in stimulating angiogenesis because its presence, as noted, is compatible with a high oxygen tension, being the result of accumulated lactate due to aerobic glycolysis. Hence, lactate stimulates the release of VEGF while allowing angiogenesis and collagen deposition to flourish in a well-oxygenated environment. The mechanism by which lactate stimulates VEGF production also involves reduction of NAD^+ and therefore ADPRibosylation. However, it is not as clearly understood as in collagen, for it involves a more complex series of events.

Paradoxically, hyperoxia also leads to active VEGF. Feng (abstract) has exposed macrophages to various oxygen atmospheres. VEGF production is high at 2% and 5% oxygen, low at 10% to 40%, and high over 40% oxygen. Nitric oxide (NO) production is probably a part of the mechanism. Oxygen also stimulates the growth of endothelial cells as it does to fibroblasts and seems to be essential to tube formation in cultures. The mechanisms seem to involve oxidants, and NO appears to be particularly important.

VEGF, like collagen, is subject to post translational modification. In this case, ADPR is the modifying agent. The VEGF that is produced during normoxia and low lactate is ADP ribosylated and inactive (43). That is, when NAD^+ and ADPRibosylation are high, VEGF tends to be inactive. On the other hand, given reducing conditions like high lactate, in which ADPRibosylation is depressed, VEGF tends to be released in the un-ribosylated, i.e., active state (43).

The "bottom line" is that the rate of VEGF release and activity is proportional to lactate, while the rate of angiogenesis is directly proportional to wound PO_2 (24, 25). Knighton et al. showed that the rate and density of capillary growth in wounds is optimized in a hyperoxic environment (25). Gibson has confirmed that this effect increases even into hyperbaric levels (11). In addition, Siddiqui et al. found an increase in tissue oxygen capacitance following HBO exposure in the rabbit ischemic ear model (39). Sheffield also demonstrated an increase in baseline tissue PO_2, and response to an HBO challenge in diabetic patients with chronic foot wounds after HBO therapy (37). The increase was noted after approximately 2 weeks of therapy and improved with each additional week of HBO. Marx et al. reported similar changes in ischemic irradiated human tissues (28).

In summary, angiogenesis, in addition to collagen, is proportional to PO_2 over a wide range both above and below the normal physiologic range of oxygen tensions. The precise mechanism by which hyperoxia enhances angiogenesis is complex. Lactate stimulates VEGF synthesis even in the presence of oxygen. Oxygen is essential for angiogenesis. VEGF is inactivated by ADPRibosylation when oxygen is normal and lactate is low.

EPITHELIZATION

Epithelization is also promoted by oxygen exposure (30, 40). However the difference between epithelization and the former two events is that skin epithelium utilizes oxygen from the ambient air as well as from blood (2). The relative proportion of oxygen contribution from either is clearly variable. Uhl reported an increase in epithelization with HBO treatment at 100% O_2 under 2 atm. Reepithelization time (wound repair) was reduced by 2 days (p < 0.01) in normal tissue and 4.4 days in ischemic tissue (p < 0.001). This was demonstrated, by laser Doppler imaging, to be unaffected by changes in microvascular perfusion. Therefore increased epithelization was found to be due to high arteriolar oxygen in animals held at 50% O_2 at 1 atm for 20 days (42). Epidermal cells replicate best at 700 mmHg by one estimate (29). The literature, however, is conflicting.

OXYGEN AND WOUND INFECTION

Tissue oxygen tension has a major influence on the development of wound infection (22, 23). The mechanism lies in the production of bactericidal oxidants by leukocytes, and is the basis of the single most important bactericidal mechanism in wounds (3).

Immune defenses against wound infecting organisms are surprisingly few. For instance, there is no known specific antibody defense against the most common wound infecting organism, Staphylococcus aureus. A premium is thus placed on phagocytic killing. Diabetes interferes with migration and phagocytosis, but little is known about removing these obstacles except for close control of blood glucose. Following phagocytosis by leukocytes, two bactericidal mechanisms come into play (Figure 3). The first, a non-oxidative mechanism, involves exposing organisms to proteolytic enzymes which are contributed by lysosomal degranulation. The second, the oxidative burst, depends upon generation of oxidants derived from molecular oxygen.

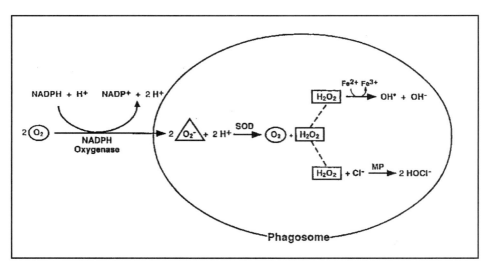

Figure 3. Schematic of superoxide and other oxidant production within the phagosome. NADPH indicates nicotinamide adenine dinucleotide phosphate; NADP+ is the oxidized form of NADPH; SOD, superoxide dismutase; and MP, myeloperoxidase

From: Allen DB, Maguire JJ, Mani M, Wicke C, Marcocci L et al. Wound hypoxia and acidosis limit neutrophil bacterial killing mechanisms. Arch Surg 1997;132:991-6. Reprinted with permission.

An NADPH-linked oxidase of leukocytes, the initial enzyme in the oxidative killing process, is activated by phagocytosis and converts molecular oxygen to superoxide (3, 16). Activation of this enzyme coincides with an enormous, often 50-fold, increase in oxygen consumption, hence the term "oxidative burst." A number of other oxidants are generated from superoxide within the phagosome, and bacterial killing is a result of oxidation of bacterial cell wall proteins (Figure 3).

The Km for oxygen of the reaction, $O_2 \rightleftarrows O_2^-$ is in the range of 40 to 80 mmHg (Figure 4)(3). Clearly, therefore, bacterial killing is extremely sensitive to local tissue PO_2. During air breathing at 1 atm, the PO_2 in the wound space in normal animals or humans is rarely above 50 mmHg, the oxygen concentration that corresponds to half the maximal rate of oxidant production (Figure 4). Leukocytes lose all oxidative bactericidal activity as PO_2 nears zero (13). Thus "normal" bacterial killing capacity is at or below half the potential maximum even in normal wound conditions and diminishes rapidly in the instance of poor perfusion and oxygenation (3). In a study of human postoperative patients by Hopf, wound PO_2 was the most sensitive predictor of wound infection, even more than the degree of contamination (14).

Warmth tends to vasodilate and increase local PO_2. A study in which operative patients were merely kept normothermic by use of a warm air blanket showed 60% lower infections than in controls who were not deliberately warmed to maintain normothermia. This study was stimulated by the observation that surface warmth

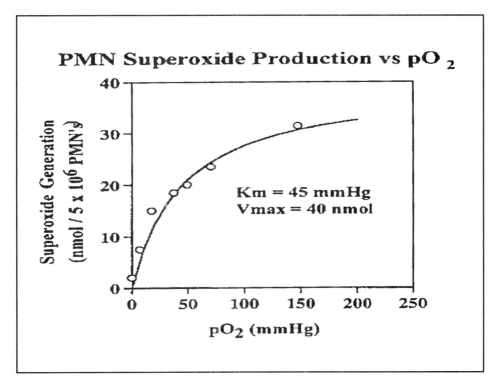

Figure 4. Relationship between oxygen tension and superoxide production by leukocytes. The experimental data have been mathematically fit to a Michelis-Menten curve. The calculated Km (half maximal reaction rate) of 45 mmHg s consistent with other experimental data.

elevates skin and subcutaneous PO_2 (27). Keeping patient's body temperature normal and skin temperature close to body temperature raises PO_2 in abdominal wounds by about 50% (Kurtz, unpublished). This suggests that chronic wounds should not be allowed to cool.

A study which compared the effects of blood glucose concentration, PO_2, pH, and temperature on bactericidal production by human leukocytes showed that PO_2 was the most important by far (3). Of interest is that the energy for the process comes from glucose, and lactate is released (i.e., aerobic glycolysis).

Wound infection produces a special case for hyperbaric oxygen. Not only are infections potentiated by hypoxia but infections further impair wound healing by consuming oxygen and thus decreasing the PO_2. Significant amounts of oxygen are consumed, creating an oxygen demand which often outstrips supply. The more leukocytes and bacteria there are in a wound, the higher the oxygen consumption, the lower the local PO_2, and the less collagen that can be produced. When infections become more severe, an unstable equilibrium is reached, resulting in a severely hypoxic environment. If oxygen tensions fall further, infection begins to dominate. Leukocyte bacterial killing becomes further impaired. This downward spiral may be interrupted in several ways, including warmth (to enhance perfusion), debridement (to remove infected tissue), drainage of abscesses to reduce oxygen demands, antibiotics, etc. Each of these interventions either increases supply of or decreases demand for oxygen so that the oxidative killing can be increased. HBO is a useful adjunct therapy when, for any reason, the blood/oxygen supply is impaired.

HYPERBARIC OXYGEN THERAPY

If hypoxia is the cause of failure to heal, provision of oxygen is the antidote. In chronic wounds, oxygen tensions are usually low on the kinetics curves for collagen and bactericidal oxidant production. At that point, provision of more oxygen is likely to make a major change (11, 35) (Figure 5). Indeed, in well oxygenated wounds (high on curve, Figure 5) HBO makes a relatively minor change in healing.

Transport of oxygen to tissue is fraught with many obstacles, however. Even under hyperbaric conditions, and even with normal vascular anatomy, oxygen is not necessarily successfully transported to tissue. It is vital, therefore, that one understands the fundamental concepts of oxygen delivery so that conditions can be made optimal for oxygen delivery. Many of the usual obstacles can be overcome.

Oxygen Transport
A. Perfusion
Wound/tissue PO_2 is highly dependent on perfusion. Perfusion is in turn dependent on the caliber of the local blood vessels and the blood pressure. Vessels are often occluded for various reasons in diabetics. However, vasoconstriction which follows sympathetic stimuli, that is, pain, cold, fear, exogenous catecholamines, and vasoconstrictive drugs can be an equally great obstacle. Each can independently cause a large drop in tissue perfusion, and all together can profoundly depress it (14, 15, 16). Therefore, for optimal perfusion and oxygenation, patients should be warm, pain-free, well-hydrated, and free of vasoconstrictive drugs (this includes beta adrenergic blockers). Tissue oxygen tension can be influenced by inspired oxygen only if perfusion is adequate (16). Although these caveats are elegantly simple, they are extremely important.

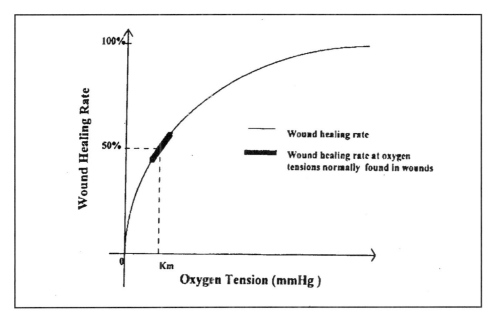

Figure 5. Wound healing is the result of many enzymes, the most critical of which are oxygenases. This figure demonstrates a generalized kinetics curve for production of a given product, with respect to PO_2. Starting from the normal point, it is clear that increasing PO_2 will be less valuable at higher oxygen tensions compared with therapy given at lower oxygen tensions. Although increasing oxygen is most advantageous in patients with initial tissue oxygen levels below normal, in order for hyperbaric oxygen therapy to be effective, reasonable blood flow must be present in order to deliver oxygen to the tissue. HBO therapy raises the arterial PO_2, increasing the arterial/tissue oxygen gradient and allowing more oxygen to be delivered to tissue.

B. Diffusion

Oxygen delivery to wound cells also depends on diffusion along a partial pressure gradient (16). The rate of delivery is inversely proportional to the square of the diffusion distance and directly proportional to the PO_2 at the initial point. Transport across long distances may, therefore, be achieved only with HBO therapy (5, 6, 40). Silver showed that diffusion distances are increased in wounds. In his hands, PO_2 at these distant sites often failed to change after increases in arterial oxygen tension at ground-level oxygen (40). Krogh calculated that hyperbaric conditions of 3 atm theoretically produces a threefold increase in diffusion distance from the capillary (26). Thus, HBO can overcome the large diffusion distances in wounds (see below).

C. Local Consumption

The driving force for collagen, angiogenesis, etc., is PO_2. Local PO_2 depends on a balance between supply and consumption. Wounds consume ~0.7 ml/100 ml of oxygen from the blood which passes through uninfected wounds (16). The plasma content of blood at 100 mmHg is ~0.3 ml/100 ml. Therefore, increasing blood oxygen tension only to 275 mmHg will increase the dissolved oxygen to 0.8 ml (100 ml) and provide sufficient oxygen from plasma alone (0.6 ml/100 ml O_2) for normal wound healing to occur, provided that perfusion is adequate (15, 19, 21). Since a small percentage of hemoglobin-bound oxygen is used by wounds, anemia is not deleterious to healing until hematocrit falls below about 15% (15, 16, 19, 21). In the instance of anemia plus poor perfusion, HBO may be the only way to maintain tissue PO_2 at levels consistent with repair.

Wound PO_2 depends heavily on the presence of wound infection or inflammation as discussed above. HBO, by increasing partial pressure, can lead to a higher arterial-cellular gradient and increase the tissue oxygen tension. This allows increased formation of oxygen radicals, and enables neutrophils to mount their "oxidative burst" in a normally hypoxic, infected wound. Numerous human and animal studies have demon-strated that an elevated wound PO_2 increases the clearance of bacteria, decreases infection rates and improves the rate of collagen deposition (14, 22, 23, 34). The magnitude of antibacterial potential of added oxygen is just now being realized.

In summary, HBO is capable of significantly enhancing repair. The real problem is assessing that it gets there. This is why, in our opinion, that results of HBO will now improve. Patients who do not need it and those who cannot transport it need not now be treated.

CYCLING

Several studies have shown the efficacy of HBO in promoting wound healing, particularly ischemic wounds and including "diabetic wounds" (4, 6, 34). However, the question still arises as to how such short exposures could influence an ongoing process. We know, of course that tissue hyperoxia actually lasts longer than the actual exposure, as a general rule about 90 minutes longer than the actual exposure (Figure 6) (Rollins, Hopf, Hunt, unpublished data). Secondly, the effects on bacterial killing, angiogenesis, collagen deposition are cumulative and will also last beyond the exposure time. For instance, since bacteria are killed during exposure, the bacterial count cannot bounce back to pre-treatment levels immediately. How quickly the bacteria counts rise again is not known. Nitric oxide production also rises temporarily, leading to increased perfusion. Though oxygen can produce vasoconstriction in many organ systems, we have found no evidence that it does so in either acute or chronic wounds. HBO also reduces leukocyte sticking to the previously hypoxic endothelium and promotes blood flow. This, too, will persist beyond the actual hyperoxic time.

By this "cycling," it is possible to accumulate the beneficial effects of HBO without toxicity. In another sense, "cycling" may have its own advantages. Hypoxia, as noted, is a signal (albeit brief) for collagen and VEGF synthesis. Since uninterrupted hypoxia is deleterious, it follows that cycled low/high PO_2 may be enough to allow wounds to take advantage of the intense hypoxic signals by turning them into enhanced responses during oxygen therapy.

THOUGHTS FOR THE FUTURE

Our assignment has been to assemble the basics on oxygen and healing. The basics not only defend the use of HBO under current rules, but also predict that those rules may change and expand its use.

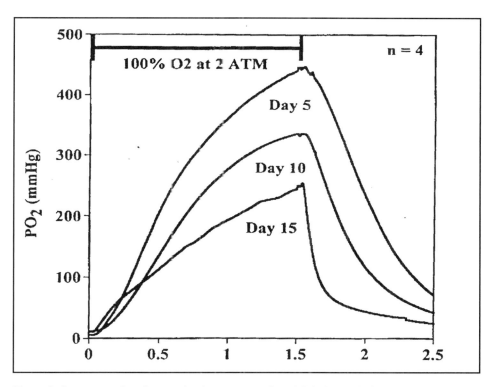

Figure 6. Oxygen tensions in a rat dead space wound model during and after a 90 minute 2 ATM HBO treatment. Rats (n=4) received HBO treatment twice daily for 90 minutes during 15 days and the wound oxygen tension was measured during and immediately after a single treatment on days 5, 10, and 15. On all days the measured PO_2 remained significantly elevated above baseline for more than an hour after treatment ended. The differences in the curves between days likely represent changes in not only oxygen delivery, but also consumption. These differences illustrate combined effects from changes in vascularity, capsular thickness, wound geometry, and total cellularity.

Almost unnoted today is the question of when hyperbaric oxygen should be used in the course of a given disease. The hostility in the medical community has forced many ethical providers to assume a defensive posture and relegate hyperbaric oxygen to a last ditch position, and then only as an adjunct.

In 1998 this may not be the best strategy. Basic studies show that hyperbaric oxygen is a powerful angiogenic agent. Angiogenesis appears to require wound inflammatory cells, which, as we all know, are very often present in the feet of diabetics well before ischemia leads to ulceration. This data suggests that properly timed hyperbaric therapy might prevent problem wounds. In this sense, the use of HBO may be quite analogous to its now sanctioned use to prepare impaired wound sites for skin grafting.

Similarly, more use of HBO as an adjunct to corrective vascular surgery may be useful. Clearly, HBO can lead to diminished peripheral resistance in ischemic limbs. The increased flow following treatment may make the difference between the success of a distal bypass and a failure.

CONCLUSION

There is no longer any doubt that the important constituents of wound healing are profoundly dependent upon the local concentration of oxygen, and this dependence persists through a wide range of oxygen concentrations from $PO_2=0$ to perhaps PO_2 @ 600 mmHg (Figure 5). Hypoxia in or near wounds in the feet of diabetics who have vascular disease is commonly observed. The conclusion which follows is that enhancing the partial pressure of oxygen in the wounded tissues of diabetics will be important to a significant segment of the diabetic population. The kinetics of the enzymes involved in the use of oxygen in wounds shows clearly that the major benefit of enhanced oxygen delivery will be obtained in patients whose tissue PO_2 is low, but responds markedly to oxygen breathing.

However, elevating PO_2 in these wounded tissues is in many cases difficult. Since HBO can clearly make a difference especially in hypoxic wounds, the question the practitioner should be asking is, "How can I maximize the delivery of O_2 to the wounded tissue?" Perfusion is critical. In addition to the usual clinical therapies for ischemic diabetic lesions, enhancement of perfusion by warmth, relief of pain, vasodilators, and occasional chemical sympathectomy enhance the delivery of oxygen and may potentiate the results of HBO. On the other hand, correction of mild to moderate anemia is unlikely to help, unless by this means local perfusion is enhanced.

The follow-up of patients with aggressive HBO therapy indicates that the results are durable (4). This indicates that HBO has wrought fundamental changes which sustain wound healing and maintain tissue integrity following the cessation of HBO treatments. One of these fundamental changes appears to be construction of a new vasculature. Clearly, HBO can make a difference, but in order to be effective it must be used in accordance with the basic principles.

REFERENCES

1. Aagenaes O, et al. Light and electron microscope study of skin capillaries of the diabetic. Diabetes, 1961; 10: 253.
2. Ahn ST, Mustoe TA. Effects of ischemia on ulcer wound healing: a new model in the rabbit ear. Ann Plast Surg, 1990; 24(1): 17-23.
3. Allen DB, Maguire JJ, Mani M, Wicke C, Marcocci L, et al. Wound hypoxia and acidosis limit neutrophil bacterial killing mechanisms. Arch Surg, 1997; 132: 991-6.
4. Cianci P, Hunt TK. "Adjunctive hyperbaric oxygen therapy in the treatment of diabetic wounds of the foot" in The Diabetic Foot, 5th Ed, ed by ME Levin, LW O' Neal, JH Bowker, Mosby Year Book, St Louis, 1993.
5. Davis JC. The use of adjuvant hyperbaric oxygen in the treatment of the diabetic foot. Clin Podiatr Med Surg, 1987; 4: 429.
6. Faglia E, Favales F, Aldeghi A, et al. Adjunctive systemic hyperbaric oxygen therapy in treatment of severe prevalently ischemic diabetic foot ulcer. Diabetes Care, 1994; 19 (12):1338.
7. Feng JJ, Hussain MZ, Constant J, Hunt TK. Angiogenesis in wound healing. J Surg Pathol, 1998; 3: 1-8.
8. Feng JJ, Gibson JJ, Constant JS, Hussain LZ, Hunt TK. Hypoxia stimulates macrophage vascular endothelial growth factor production. Abstract: Wound Healing Society, July, 1998.
9. Ferrara N, Davis-Smyth T. The biology of vascular endothelial growth factor. Endocr Rev, 1997; 18: 4-25.
10. Ghani QP, Hussain MZ, Hunt TK. Control of procollagen gene transcription and prolyl hydroxylase activity by poly (ADP-ribose). In: ADP-Ribosylation Reactions, G. Poirier and A. Moreaer (Eds) New York: Springer-Verlag, 1992, 111.
11. Gibson JJ, Angeles A, Hunt TK. Increased oxygen tension potentiates angiogenesis. Surg Forum, 1997; 48: 696.
12. Hartmann M, Jonsson K, Zederfeldt B. Effect of tissue perfusion and oxygenation on accumulation of collagen in healing wounds. Randomized study in patients after major abdominal operations. Eur J Surg, 1992; 158 (10): 521-6.
13. Hohn DC, Mackay RD, Halliday B, et al. Effect of O2 tension on microbicidal function of leukocytes in wounds and in vitro. Surgical Forum 1976; 27: 18.
14. Hopf HW, Hunt TK, West JM, Blomquist P, Goodson III WH, Jensen JA, et al. Wound tissue oxygen tension predicts the risk of wound infection in surgical patients. Arch Surg, 1997; 132: 997 -1004.
15. Hunt TK, Feng JJ. The role of perfusion and oxygenation in wound healing. Textbook of Wound Care (in press) 1998.
16. Hunt TK, Hopf HW. Wound healing and wound infection. What surgeons and anesthesiologists can do. Surg Clin N Amer, 1997; 77: 587.
17. Hunt TK, Pai MP. The effect of varying ambient oxygen tension on wound metabolism and collagen synthesis, Surg Gynecol Obstet, 1972; 135: 561.
18. Hussain MZ, Ghani QP, Hunt TK. Inhibition of prolyl hydroxylase by poly (ADP-ribose) and phosphoribosyl-AMP. J Biol Chem, 1989; 264: 7850-55.
19. Jensen JA, Goodson WH, Vasconez LO, et al. Wound healing in anemia, 1986; 144: 465.
20. Jensen JA, Hunt TK, Scheuenstuhl H, et al. Effect of lactate, pyruvate, and pH on secretion of angiogenesis and mitogenesis factors by macrophages. Lab Invest, 1986; 54: 574-8.
21. Jonsson K, Jensen SA, Goodson WH, et al. Tissue oxygenation, anemia and perfusion in relation to wound healing in surgical patients. Ann Surg, 1991; 214: 605.
22. Knighton DR, Halliday BJ, Hunt TK. Oxygen as an antibiotic: a comparison of the effects of inspired oxygen concentration and antibiotic administration on in vivo bacterial clearance. Arch Surg, 1986; 121 (2): 191.
23. Knighton DR, Halliday BJ, Hunt TK. Oxygen as an antibiotic: the effect of inspired oxygen on infection. Arch Surg, 1986; 119: 199-204.
24. Knighton DR, Hunt TK, Scheuenstuhl H, et al. Oxygen regulates the expression of angiogenesis factor by macrophages. Science, 1983; 221: 1233.
25. Knighton Dr, Silver IA, Hunt TK. Regulation of wound-healing angiogenesis-effect of oxygen gradients and inspired oxygen concentration. Surgery, 1981; 90 (2): 262.
26. Krogh A. The number and distribution of capillaries in muscle with calculations of the oxygen pressure head necessary for supplying the tissue. J Physiol, 1919; 52: 409.
27. Kurtz A, Sessler D, Lenhardt R, et al. Perioperative normothermia to reduce the incidence of surgical-wound infection and shorten hospitalization. N Engl J Med., 1996; 334: 1209-1215.
28. Marx, et al. Relationship of oxygen dose to angiogenesis induction in irradiated tissue. Am J Surg, 1990; 160: 519.
29. Mc Millian DE, et al. Forearm skin capillaries of diabetic, potential diabetic and non-diabetic subjects: changes seen by light microscopy. Diabetes, 1966; 15: 251.
30. Medawar PB. The cultivation of adult mammalian skin epithelium. Q J Microbiol Sci, 1948; 89: 187.
31. Moelleken B, Mathes S, Amerhauser A, et al. An adverse wound environment activates leukocytes prematurely. Arch Surg, 1991; 126: 225.
32. Myalla R, Ruderman LL, Kiviriko KI. Kinetic analysis of the reaction sequences. Mechanism of prolyl hydroxylase. Eur J Biochem, 1977; 80: 349-57.
33. Newsholme P, Costa Rosa LFP, Newsholme E, Curi R. The importance of fuel metabolism to macrophage function. Cell Biochem and Function, 1996; 14: 1-10.
34. Niinikoski J. Oxygen and wound healing. Clin Plast Surg, 1977; 4: 361-374.
35. Niinikoski J, Hunt TK, Dunphy JE. Oxygen supply in healing tissue. Am J Surg, 1972; 123 (3): 247-52.
36. Pecoraro RE. The nonhealing diabetic ulcer-a major cause for limb loss. Prog Clin Biol Res, 1991; 12: 161.

37.   Sheffield, PJ. Tissue oxygenation measurements, in Davis JC, Hunt TK, editors : Problem wounds: the role of oxygen, Elsevier, New York. 1988.

38.   Shima DT, Adamis AP, Ferrara N, et al. Hypoxic induction of endothelial cell growth factor in retinal cells: identification and characterization of vascular endothelial growth factor(VEGF) as the mitogen. Mol Med, 1995; 1: 182-93.

39.   Siddiqui A, Davidson JD, Mustoe TA. Ischemic tissue oxygen capacitance after hyperbaric oxygen therapy: a new physiologic concept. Plast Reconstr Surg, 1997; 99: 931.

40.   Silver IA. The measurement of oxygen tension in healing tissue. Progr Resp Res, 1969; 3: 124.

41.   Sunderkotter C, Goebeler M, Schulze-Osthoff K, et al. Macrophage-derived angiogenesis factor. Pharmacol Ther, 1991; 51: 195-216.

42.   Uhl E, Sirsjo A, Haapaniemi T, et al. Hyperbaric oxygen improves wound healing in normal and ischemic skin tissue. Plast Reconst Surg, 1994; 93: 835.

43.   Xiong M, Elson G, Legarda D, Leibovich SJ. Production of vascular endothelial growth factor by murine macrophages. Am J Path, 1998; 153: 1-12.

44.   Zabel DD, Feng JJ, Scheuenstuhl H, et al. Lactate stimulation of macrophage-derived angiogenic activity is associated with inhibition of poly (ADP-ribose) synthesis. Lab Invest, 1996; 74: 644-9.

CLINICAL TRIALS EVALUATING HBO IN THE TREATMENT OF FOOT LESIONS IN DIABETIC PATIENTS

Dirk Jan Bakker

Academic Medical Center, University of Amsterdam—Netherlands

There was a time when physicians received their patients, heard their complaints, and determined the best cause of action and therapy. Not everyone could be cured, but everyone could be confident that what was done was the best possible. Every physician was free, trusted, and determined what was in the best interest of his or her individual patient.

Times have changed, however, and medicine with it. Eddy explains that there is good reason to challenge the assumption that every individual practioner's decision is necessarily correct. There are too many variables in the whole decision making process to leave it to the individual physician. This variability occurs because physicians must make decisions about immensely complex problems, under difficult circumstances with very little support. Besides this there are many other factors: expectations of patients and their relatives, variability in individual patients reactions, incomplete information, politics, money, etc. We, as physicians, lack in many instances the information necessary for decision-making and what is needed to process this information. However, we have to act!

So we have to improve the decision-making power, to improve the capacity of physicians to take better decisions, not to remove the decision-making power from physicians. Eddy states: "We must give physicians the information they need; we must institutionalize the skills to use that information, and we must build processes that support, not dictate decisions"(22).

One way to do this is to learn from clinical trials that have been done and see if what they state is correct and if we can help our patients in incorporating this knowledge into our practice.

THE PROBLEM

Problem wounds are those which fail to respond to established medical and surgical management in the expected time frame. These wounds usually occur in compromised hosts with multiple local and systemic factors that inhibit tissue repair. This causes a significant morbidity and mortality. Many of these risk factors are well known. It is of course very important to identify and correct the underlying etiologic and risk factors which inhibit the healing process.

Problem wounds are most frequently located in the lower extremities. Regardless of the etiology, the basic mechanism of non-healing wounds is the interplay between varying degrees of tissue hypoperfusion and infection (47). The presence of diabetes mellitus is recognized as an important risk factor for a defective or non-healing of lower extremity wounds (11).

DIABETIC WOUNDS

The most common etiologic factors in non-healing diabetic wounds are ischaemia and infection. Ischaemia is caused by hypoperfusion. In diabetes mellitus two principal mechanisms adversely affect wound healing: a. Atherosclerosis and b. Defective cellular and humoral immunity.

There is decreased chemotaxis, decreased phagocytosis, and a decrease in chemotactic response, which reduces the inflammatory reaction. There is also an abnormal lymphocytic function (30, 48, 61). Cruse showed a synergistic effect of ischaemia and impaired immune response on wound infection (as is the case in diabetic patients) (18).

The diabetic foot is characterized by sensory, motor, and autonomic neuropathies that lead to alteration of pressure distribution, foot deformities, ulcerations, and infection.

The foot has been altered by diabetic vasculopathy and neuropathy. In most cases we find a mixed clinical picture of both vasculopathy and neuropathy.

The classical "mal perforans" ulcer is caused by loss of sensation and painless trauma. One must remember that this can also occur in the absence of ischaemia and frequently heals with conservative measures such as aggressive wound management and unweighting.

Vasculopathy in diabetes is not only sustained by macroangiopathy but also by impairment in flow in the small vessels and in the innervation of the vascular bed. Autonomic neuropathy may lead to islands of cutaneous ischaemia caused by alterations in blood flow (23, 24).

An excellent description of both macroangiopathic and microangiopathic changes in diabetes is given by Faglia et al. (26).

Even in the presence of palpable arterial pulses, many patients can have areas of low flow and hypoxia in feet and ankles. Contributing factors are:

- increased blood viscosity
- decreased red blood cell deformability
- platelet aggregation
- accelerated capillary endothelial growth
- hypoperfusion is a possible mechanism of injury to the subendothelial area of vessels
- capillary wall hyalinization leading to capillary obstruction

In some cases even a restored circulation fails to cause wound healing. Diabetic patients respond to local tissue stress with thrombosis and necrosis, as opposed to an inflammatory response in the non-diabetic population (15). Non-healing ulcers are a major cause for amputation and limb loss in diabetic patients (12, 55).

Classification of diabetic wounds is usually done by the grading system first described by Wagner (69). This was later adapted by Boulton (7). Foot and ankle ulcers in this system are graded by their severity, from 0, with no obvious ulcer in a foot at risk, until the most severe situation, grade 5, being gangrene of the whole foot.

In general, ulcers grading 1–3 tend to be predominantly neuropathic, whereas grades 4 and 5 are mainly vascular (7).

THE USE OF OXYGEN AND HYPERBARIC OXYGEN IN WOUND HEALING

The critical and fundamental role of oxygen in the physiology of wound healing is well documented (36, 37). A review of the wound healing effects of oxygen are given by Brakora and Sheffield (8). Hypoxia not only may impair or halt wound healing, but can also seriously impair leucocyte bacterial killing function (40, 58).

The most direct determinant of wound healing and control of infection is tissue oxygen tension. Perfusion, however, is the fundamental determinant of delivery of oxygen to the wound area. When arrived at the wound site, diffusion of oxygen occurs along a partial pressure gradient, so the partial pressure is an important factor.

Many factors cause an impaired oxygenation in the diabetic foot (74, 75). Measurements of tissue oxygen tensions ($TcpO_2$) in non-healing diabetic wounds showed values far below those where wound healing could be expected. Even breathing 100 % O_2 did not raise the $TcpO_2$ enough.

Sheffield (62) and Wattel and Mathieu (70, 71) showed that hyperbaric oxygen therapy resulted in elevation of tissue O_2 tension in diabetic patients with chronic wounds. A direct response and a response over time was demonstrated. After HBO therapy O_2 tissue levels remain above baseline levels for another 3–4 hours.

The rationale for using HBO in diabetic nonhealing wounds can be summarized as follows:

- Diabetic wounds are polymicrobial with a high incidence of anaerobic organisms. HBO increases the killing ability of leucocytes (42, 43, 44), is lethal to certain anaerobic bacteria, and inhibits toxin formation by certain anaerobes (1, 2, 3).

HBO:
- increases the flexibility of red blood cells and acts synergistically on blood flow with pentoxifylline (38, 45, 49).
- reduces tissue edema (50).
- preserves intracellular adenosine triphosphate (63).
- maintains tissue oxygenation in the absence of hemoglobin (6).
- stimulates fibroblast growth, increases collagen formation and deposition, promotes more rapid growth of capillaries (5, 39, 40, 58).
- terminates lipid peroxidation (66, 67).

HBO can not substitute for surgical revascularization in advanced arterial insufficiency and can not reverse an inadequate microvascular circulation. In judging clinical trials where the author(s) state that no vascular reconstruction was possible in his/her patients, one must know for sure that the vascular surgeons in that center were able to accomplish all known operative techniques, including pedal bypasses, etc.

There seems to be no reason to fear that HBO might increase tissue damage as a result of generation of oxygen free radicals (67, 68, 77). A vasoconstrictive effect of HBO has not been demonstrated in ischemic or hypoxic tissue (62).

WHEN TO CONSIDER HBO IN DIABETIC FOOT ULCERS?

HBO therapy is usually looked for when diabetic wounds are unsuccessfully treated for weeks or months with local wound care, surgical debridements, and antibiotics. Sometimes, even after successful reconstructive vascular surgery, wounds fail to heal. When amputation seems unavoidable, then HBO is considered as an "ultimum remedium."

There must, of course, be an adequate metabolic control of the diabetes mellitus and control of infection. The patient must have had a full vascular evaluation, both non-invasively and by angiography. A determination has to be done to judge the adequacy of the peripheral perfusion. If possible, arterial reconstructive surgery must have been performed.

This can be followed by transcutaneous oxygen mapping in a systematic, predetermined, and standardized way.

In general, foot and ankle ulcers with a Wagner grading 3, 4, or 5 will be candidates for HBO treatment. Grade 1 and 2 can usually be treated without supplemental oxygen.

In the literature, patient selection by measuring $TcpO_2$ while breathing normoxic air, 100% normobaric O_2, and 100% hyperbaric O_2 is advocated. This so-called "oxygen challenge test" has been found to have a predictive value for the outcome of the treatment (70).

Wyss found in a group of 188 patients with diabetic leg or foot ulcers that when the $TcpO_2$ was below 20 mm Hg, there were significantly more ulcers, rest pain, and necessary amputations, than when the $TcpO_2$ was above 20 mm Hg (76). White and Klein did a review of the literature and found that a $TcpO_2 \geq 40$ mm Hg was required for successful wound healing after an amputation (73).

Wattel and Mathieu found that when the $TcpO_2$ at 2,5 ATA 100% O_2 breathing was ≥ 100 mm Hg then all wounds healed. When tissue PO_2 was than lower 100 mm Hg, then there was no improvement or even aggravation of the wounds (71).

Campagnoli et al. found that a $TcpO_2 \geq 400$ mm Hg with HBO predicted healing. They also found that the faster the rise in tissue oxygen in patients, when initially exposed to HBO, the greater the likelihood of a favorable outcome (10).

Calhoun and Mader found that a $TcpO_2 \pounds 5$ mm Hg meant amputation. When the tissue PO_2 was ≥ 20 mm Hg, the chances of healing were 20%; when tissue PO_2 was ≥ 35 mm Hg, then chances of healing were 80% (9).

On the Lille Consensus meeting in 1994 it was concluded that an indication for HBO treatment was present when:

- $TcpO_2 \geq 200$ mm Hg at 2,5 ATA, 100 % O_2 breathing
- Toe pressure ≥ 30 mm Hg
- Ankle pressure ≥ 75 mm Hg (17).

Selection criteria in the Jefferson C. Davis Wound Care and Hyperbaric Medicine Center in San Antonio, TX, are as follows: When $TcpO_2$ on normoxic air breathing is ≥ 40 mm Hg, then HBO is not indicated. When the $TcpO_2$ on normoxic air breathing is between 10–40 mm Hg, then a test with 100% O_2 breathing is done at 1 ATA. If there is a significant rise in tissue PO_2 (≥ 50 %) then HBO treatment is indicated. When $TcpO_2$ $\pounds 20$ mm Hg and there is no rise with the above mentioned test, then HBO is considered useless and not given. Amputation is then unavoidable (8).

A review of recent literature on the value of TcpO$_2$ in predicting outcome is given by Matos and Nuñez. The total number of patients was ± 350 and TcpO$_2$ was also compared with values in 161 healthy volunteers (47).

The conclusion (or the hypothesis?) can be that we have now developed an objective criterium when or when not to treat diabetic wounds on legs, ankles, or feet with HBO. We have also found a reliable method to predict wound healing in ulcers and/or after an amputation and we think that we are able to determine the level of amputation in advance. The next step is to apply this in clinical practice and confirm the validity in a prospective trial.

CLINICAL TRIALS ON HBO

How to read and use publications on clinical trials?

Medical practice is constantly changing and clinicians are relatively helpless in deciding what new information to incorporate into their practice. All existing sources of information may be useful and helpful but have their own biases as well. Clinicians may choose to believe the most authoritative expert or the trusted colleague but it is difficult to exercise independent judgement. In 1981 the Department of Clinical Epidemiology and Biostatistics at McMaster University in Canada published a series of "Readers' Guides for busy clinicians to use when reading clinical articles about the diagnosis, prognosis, etiology, and therapy of their patients' illnesses" (20).

These Guides were received with great enthusiasm, were improved, and later published in the Journal of the American Medical Association (JAMA) between 1993 and 1995. They were then called "Users' Guides." These Guides have been inspired by the need to use the medical literature to solve real patient problems. They are designed to help provide our patients with care that is based on the best evidence currently available. We call this "evidence-based medicine."

Evidence-based medicine emphasizes the need to move beyond clinical experience and physiological principles to rigorous evaluations of the consequences of clinical actions.

Randomised clinical trials or therapeutic experiments are instruments with which expected therapeutic gain can be measured. These trials will also show something of the possible side effects. The trials must essentially serve the purpose of comparing two different treatment modalities: the new or "index treatment" and the control or "reference treatment."

When reading the literature on clinical trials the following questions are relevant and must be asked and answered

1. Was the assignment of patients to treatments randomised; was the randomisation list concealed? (major point).
2. Were all patients who entered the trial accounted for at its conclusion? (major point).
3. Were patients and clinicians kept "blind" to which treatment was being received?
4. Were the groups treated equally (aside from the experimental treatment)?
5. Were the groups similar at the start of the trial?

We will also have to look at the magnitude of the observed effect. Was the endpoint of the trial wound healing, improvement only, avoidance of amputation, etc? (31, 32, 33, 35, 53, 54, 59, 60).

Clinical trials on HBO in diabetic wounds

Anecdotal reports and retrospective studies have supported the finding that HBO is an effective adjunct in the (surgical) management of these wounds. Although the known pathophysiologic entity in diabetic wounds is tissue hypoxia, and we know that HBO is able to reverse this hypoxia, prospective randomised clinical trials are the next step to show the benefit of HBO. If all of what is said above is true, then that must not be too difficult. Unfortunately, very few, if any, of these trials have been done.

Some clinicians do not think that this is necessary. The argument for this is that the value of HBO is, at least in their opinion, based on the application of physical laws in a known pathophysiologic process. The indication then is the pathophysiology of local and/or focal hypoxia.

However, if we want to prove our point, that HBO is useful in selected patients in healing diabetic wounds, we need to perform these trials in a proper way, because this is today's standard.

With this in mind we will look systematically into publications in the literature on the use of HBO in patients with diabetic wounds.

"Anecdotal" and retrospective reports

The first publication was done by Hart et al. They reported on an open, retrospective, non randomised study in 11 patients with chronic, nonhealing diabetic wounds, all treated with HBO. The results were described as "a fair and good response"; 10 out of 11 patients, or 91%, healed (34).

We must remember that this was the standard way of reporting results in those days. Clearly, we shared the clinical experience of well-respected colleagues and we believed what they found.

It is equally clear that if we take the measure of "evidence-based medicine" and ask the above mentioned questions, that no one of them can be properly answered. In this respect we can not use this publication. Although the clinical experience and results are important, they are insufficient proof for efficacy of HBO in patients with diabetic wounds. This is sometimes difficult to accept for older clinicians, but the truth is that modern medicine can not be judged with standards formulated 30 or more years ago.

Paradoxically on the other hand, if a wound is not healing with all treatment modalities known for some time, say three months, and by adding HBO we get a complete different picture, healing in 60 or 70% of patients, this is, of course, an important experience. In these cases we like to say that the patients were their own control. Exactly this experience must, however, invite us to set up a proper randomised prospective trial in trying to end the discussion.

The same goes for the report of Matos, who described, retrospectively, treatment of non-healing wounds in 70 diabetic patients. He carefully formulates his conclusion, that where 60 % of his patients healed or showed significant improvement, this is suggestive for beneficial effects of HBO. In all patients there was ischemia, infection, and/or other neuropathic changes (46).

Pedesini reported good results in 88,6 % of his 26 patients (56).

Perrins and Barr found that of their 24 patients, 67% healed and in 18% amputation could be avoided; 1 patient only improved (57).

In a large clinical series of 168 patients with Wagner grade 3 and 4 diabetic foot lesions Davis reported a 70% success rate. The combined treatment protocol consisted of daily wound debridements, antibiotic therapy, aggressive wound care, metabolic control, and daily HBO for 30–60 days. Treatment failures were seen in older patients with occlusive vascular disease and absent pedal pulses (19).

Wattel et al. treated 20 patients during a twelve month period. In this group 11 patients had diabetic and 9 arteriosclerotic ulcers. They were treated with HBO twice a day. Complete healing was seen in 15 out of 20 patients. The value of $TcpO_2$ as a predictive factor for healing was confirmed (70).

In 1991, Wattel et al. reported about 59 patients treated over a two year period. It is not clear if the aforementioned group was a part of these patients. Of the 59 patients, 52 healed and in the other 7 patients amputation was necessary. Again one of the goals was to show the value of $TcpO_2$ in predicting outcome and not, for instance, percentage of healing after a predetermined number of treatments in a fixed time frame. A Wagner classification was not given and every patient referred for HBO with diabetic ulcers was enrolled. There was a significant difference between the $TcpO_2$ of the group that healed and the group of patients that failed to heal, measured in 2,5 ATA and 100 O_2 (p £ 0,005)(71).

Cianci et al. treated 41 patients of which 97 % had limb threatening infections. Fifty-five percent had undergone revascularisation procedures. Wagner grading was 4. Results were that 78% had their extremities salvaged (14).

Weisz reported on 14 patients with non-healing ulcers for at least three months. HBO was given at 2,5 ATA and 100 % O_2. Complete healing was achieved in 11 patients. $TcpO_2$ was highly predictive. All patients, however, had palpable pedal pulses (72).

In a review by Stone et al., it was noted that patients referred for HBO therapy had greater wound volumes, more wounds per patient, and a greater percentage recommended amputations. Despite this the limb-salvage rate was greater in the hyperbaric group (72 % vs 53 %; p £ 0,002) (64).

In a second review Stone and Scott concluded that the greatest healing rate was achieved in a group of patients treated with a combination of standard care, HBO, and growth factors (n = 49; 80 % healing) (65).

Finally, Lee et al. treated 31 patients. In 25 patients the foot was preserved. Their conclusion was that HBO seemed to be useful only when there was "a preserved circulation and a controlled infection." Again no controls or classification what makes one wonder about the indication for HBO. Risk factors for poor outcome were an elevated white blood cell count and a low ankle-brachial index (41).

There is one negative study by Ciaravino et al. This is also a retrospective study on a total number of 54 patients with a large variety of causes of non-healing wounds (including 17 diabetic patients). None of these patients healed completely. The number of complications of HBO therapy in their series is unheard of. All relevant data on the patients are lacking and comparison with any other study is impossible (16).

The conclusion from these retrospective reports, describing results in at least 464 patients, is that they all suggest a certain benefit of HBO. However, it is impossible to compare these studies. They have different patient selection, treatment schemes, outcomes, wound and/or ulcer grading, no controls, no randomisation, and all are retrospectively evaluated.

The questions suggested before to evaluate the evidence can not satisfactorily be answered.

A rather constant finding is that $TcpO_2$ measurements seem to be highly predictive for healing or non-healing and that older patients with occlusive vascular disease are the worst candidates for treatment.

It is, in fact, impossible to measure the effect of a treatment in a non-comparative study. Only one group of patients is treated and it is very tempting to take the observed effect as the effect caused by the therapy, but this is not true.

The observed disease course is a sum of the effect of the therapy, the natural course of the disease, non-specific factors like the placebo effect and others, and observers mistakes. We do need, besides the treated index group with all these factors, a reference group which is comparable, except for the fact that they do not get the specific treatment, and ideally, this must be the only difference between the two groups. In summary, a clinical trial is a comparison of two groups: the index group with the therapeutic intervention and the reference group without the therapeutic intervention.

The suggestion of benefit in the above mentioned studies, added to the theoretical and experimental rationale mentioned before, is a good reason or hypothesis that warrants a prospective study that is indeed very necessary. Let us see what has been done in this respect.

Prospective studies

Baroni et al. performed a prospective controlled study. He selected patients with grade 3 and 4 Wagner and all patients were hospitalized. The groups were matched for lesion size, subfascial involvement, and duration and severity of diabetes. Treatment was the same in both groups, the only difference being HBO treatment. The attending surgeons were blinded as to the different groups. The study (HBO) group consisted of 18 patients, with 16 patients in the control group. In the study group 16 patients healed and 2 underwent amputation and in the control group only 1 patient healed, 5 showed no change, and 4 had to be amputated (p £ 0,001). Since a review over the years 1979–1981 in the same center showed an amputation percentage of 40 % and in the present study group 11 % was found, they concluded that HBO was of benefit in the treatment of grade 3 and 4 Wagner diabetic wounds (4).

Remarks: Two things have to be noted on this study: firstly that the number of patients was not very large, which makes the statistical significance a little weak, and secondly that the patients were not randomized (which is a major point when judging evidence). Of the patients not treated with HBO, 10 out of the 16 refused because of psychological reasons.

The p-value is a test variable that can be positive (p £ 0,05) or negative (p≥ 0,05), of which the specificity is known and high (95% confidence interval), but where the sensitivity depends, among other things, on the size of the groups. The p-value has only value when the groups are large enough. The uncertainty about the relative risk (RR) can be quantified by determination of the 95% confidence interval (CI). The width of the interval is determined by the size of the treatment groups. The confidence interval in the above study is not mentioned.

Randomisation is meant to equalize the natural course of the disease and by blinding one tries to eliminate the observers mistakes. Randomisation was in fact not done in the study above. Some patients were excluded from the treatment because they refused HBO therapy.

Faglia et al. published a kind of follow up study on the above(?). The study group (HBO) consisted of 26 patients with 20 controls. Healing in the study group was observed in 24/26 and in 2/20 in the control group, whereas in the control group 8 patients had to be amputated. Unchanged in the control group were 10/20, in the HBO group 0/26 (Faglia et al. 1987).

The same remarks as above can be made here. We do not know if this is an extension of the same group as above (25).

Oriani et al. reported the effect of HBO in a group of 62 patients (different from the above?).

The matched control group consisted of 18 patients. There was no significant difference in age, severity, and duration of diabetes or its complications. Treatment was the same in both groups except for HBO. In the HBO group 96 % of patients healed and in the control group 66 %; 33 % of controls needed amputation (51).

Remarks: Again the same remarks as above. This seems to be an extension of the earlier study and patients were not randomised. The control group, which was considerably smaller, consisted of patients who refused treatment although they were selected for it. This is not randomisation.

This can be called a prospective controlled study. The study was not blinded. Again a suggestion of benefit from HBO, but not more than that.

Doctor et al. treated clinically 30 patients in 2 years: 15 with and 15 without HBO (?). Treatment scheme was 4 HBO treatments in 2 weeks (3 ATA and 100 % O_2). The number of amputations necessary in the control group was 43 % versus 10 % in the HBO group (p £ 0,05). A remarkable finding was that the number of positive wound cultures in the HBO group was reduced from 19 to 3 and in the non-HBO group from 16 to 12 (especially Pseudomonas and E. ccli) (21).

Remarks: We will follow the questions that can be found under "How to read and use publications on clinical trials?"

1. No details are given about how randomisation was done (major point).
2. The number of patients in each group is not sure. We suppose 15. Follow-up time is not mentioned.
3. Study was not blinded. Both patient and doctor knew who got HBO.
4. There is no detailed information if the groups were treated equally.
5. At the start of the study the groups seemed comparable (Table 1).

The amputation percentage is 13 % in the HBO group, versus 47 % in the controls, a RR of 0,33 (exact 95 % CI: 0,43–2,1) and an ARR (Absolute Risk Reduction) of 34 % (95 % CI: -66 % –5,9 %). NNT (Number Needed to Treat) would be 3; this means that for every three treated patients one major amputation is prevented.

This report has some typical potential shortcomings that can be found in other reports as well. There is a very brief description of the methods used; one can not judge if the study has been correctly done. It is a small study without a previously defined outcome and sample size calculation (two times 15 patients and a yes/no measurement). Normally this would be no study to start with; all relative risks less extreme than 0,1 can not be measured with confidence. An outcome percentage of 50 % must drop to under 5 % to give a reliable estimate. The p-value is just significant if we base ourselves on asymptotic p-values. This is not allowed with these small numbers. The real p-value is 0,0543, which is just not significant.

A second important point is that the doctors and the patients knew which treatment the patients had received. Since the outcome is in part subjective, "necessity of amputation," this can be a disadvantage, because knowledge of the therapy can influence the outcome. It is difficult to blind the patients, but the doctors who see and treat the patients besides the HBO can be.

In summary, not many very obvious mistakes, but a lot of things that could have been done better.

Oriani et al. reported in 1992 about 10 years experience. A lot has been published before (see above). In the HBO group there was 80% salvage versus 40% in the non-HBO group (52).

Remarks: This is in fact a retrospective report on a prospective study, but the continuation of the study after 1987 (4) can not be judged.

The largest prospective, randomized study so far is published by Faglia et al. A total of 70 patients with Wagner grades 2, 3 and 4 were treated, 35 with HBO and 33 without HBO.

Variables in patients did not differ significantly in any item of clinical characteristics. The presence of neuropathy and vasculopathy did not differ significantly in both groups.

As to the results, in the HBO group there were 3 major amputations (1 AKA and 2 BKA) which is 8,6 %, and in the non-HBO group 11 (4 AKA and 7 BKA) which is 33,3 %. This difference is statistically significant. The significance was highest in the group of patients with a Wagner classification of 4 (2/22 HBO, 11/20 non-HBO) (27).

Chantelau criticised the study. The low amputation rate in the HBO group, in his view, had to be attributed to more adequate vascular surgery that had been withheld in the non-HBO group because fewer patients in the non-HBO group had undergone angiography (13). Faglia et al. contradicted this however in a, in my view, convincing way (28).

Remarks:
1. No detailed information about the way of randomisation.
2. The data about the procedure are, incorrectly, far more extensive than those about the follow-up. There were 35 versus 33 patients. All patients are accounted for in Table 3.
3. The study was not blinded.
4. Whether the treatment was equal in both groups can not be concluded from the publication.
5. The groups were comparable at the start of the study.

The percentage was 33 in the control group versus 8,6% in the HBO group, a RR of 0,25 (95 % CI: 0,01 - 1,16), an ARR of 25 % (95 % CI 48 % - 1,4 %), or a NNT of 4. The statistical paragraph is far better than in any other study.

Zamboni et al. reported on a prospective, non-randomised trial of 10 patients. HBO was given in 5 patients and 5 were controls. The wound surface area (WSA) was measured and after 7 weeks of treatment the WSA in the HBO group was significantly smaller than in the non-HBO group (p £ 0,05). The wound size was measured and not the wound depth. Treatment was given at 2 ATA 100 % O_2 for 120 minutes in a monoplace chamber during 5 days per week for a total 30 treatments.

Follow up after 4–6 months showed that 80 % in the non-HBO group had not healed while 80 % in the HBO group had healed (78).

Remarks:
1. Non-randomised, selection possible.
2. 5 versus 5 is a very small study.
3. Not blinded.
4. Equal treatment supposed
5. ??

Faglia et al. published data about the change in amputation rate in their center for diabetic foot caring in the period from 1990–1993.

There were 115 patients hospitalized, and the amputation percentage in this group was compared with the amputation percentage in the years 1979–1981 and 1986–1989. Prognostic determinants of major amputation were Wagner grading, prior stroke, prior major amputation, $TcpO_2$ and ankle-brachial blood pressure index, while an independent protective role was attributed to hyperbaric oxygen treatment (29).

This was not a randomized study and it was not meant to be.

DISCUSSION AND CONCLUSIONS

Medicine is not a mathematical science. Doctors have to work with biological human material, so to speak, with many uncertainties, unexpected intervening factors, hypotheses but also a lot of biases in day to day practice. Many decisions made by physicians appear to be arbitrary, highly variable, and with no obvious explanation. Many decisions in medicine are undoubtedly correct, but also many are not. How to determine what is right and what is wrong?

Observers variation has been known for decades already in respect to the diagnostic process, physical examination interpreting laboratory results, and recommendations for treatment. Disagreement among observers looking at the same thing is possible in 10–50 % (22).

In looking at our studies, the controversy about the efficacy of hyperbaric oxygen in diabetic foot ulcers is not yet solved. There are strong indications for efficacy, but not yet convincing proof. No study is, compared with today's standards, without mistakes. No one is beyond criticism. On the other hand there is no reason to say that these studies are useless.

Major points of criticism are the randomisation procedure, blinding (at least of the observers, not so much of the treatment itself), numbers of patients that are too small, and study design (no definition of endpoint, no treatment schemes with a predetermined number of treatments followed by evaluation of results).

The question is, do we have to fulfill all this conditions? Do we have to satisfy all wishes from statisticians? I do not think that that must be our goal.

We must honour, however, their striving after improvement of our capacity to make better decisions. In this we can learn from them how to improve ourselves. These are healthy challenges that must appeal to us, because we strive continuously for quality improvement in our clinical work.

In hyperbaric medicine we are confronted with much opposition, and not always fair. Sometimes it seems that we have to prove our point with far more certainty than is asked for in any other therapy in medicine. We must not forget that less than 3% of what is done in medicine is "evidence-based" in the modern sense of the word. The rest is clinical experience or taken for granted because retrospectively we believe that it works. We must not defend that standpoint.

When we try to perform trials that are internally valid, we can generalise them externally as well. External validity is the measure in which the results can be translated to the clinic and generalized to future patients. Then, treatment can be called evidence-based.

A few last points beside what is said under "remarks."

1. The theoretical and experimental background to use HBO for diabetic ulcers in selected cases is sound.
2. Anecdotal and retrospective reports seem to support this finding.
3. Prospective trials lack in most cases a proper design and uniformity in various parameters. Choose clear endpoints: Wound healing, prevention of amputation, major or minor, or amputation? Is it the wound surface area or the depth of the wound?

Which patient selection criteria? Age, presence of large vessel occlusive disease (worst candidates!)? No patient without a full vascular investigation! Wagner grading 3, 4 and 5? Selection by outcome prediction with $TcpO_2$?

As to the treatment protocols, which pressure, how long for how many treatments per day and in total? Try to blind the observers and use a good randomisation procedure.

We have made a lot of progress these last years. Do not give up. One study is not enough. In a certain way we are almost there.

REFERENCES

1. Bakker DJ. The use of hyperbaric oxygen in the treatment of certain infectious diseases especially gas gangrene and acute dermal gangrene. Thesis, University of Amsterdam. Veen-man publ. Wageningen, 1984.
2. Bakker DJ. Clostridial myonecrosis. In: Davis JC, Hunt TK (eds). Problem wounds. The role of oxygen. Elsevier, New York, Amsterdam, 1984: 153-172.
3. Bakker DJ. Selected aerobic and anaerobic soft tissue infections. Diagnosis and the use of hyperbaric oxygen as an adjunct. In Kindwall EP (ed), Hyperbaric Medicine Practice. Best Publ. Flagstaff AZ, 1994: 395-417.
4. Baroni G, Porro T, Faglia E et al. Hyperbaric oxygen in diabetic gangrene treatment. Diab Care 1987; 10 (1): 81-86.
5. Bassett BE, Bennett PB. Introduction to the physical and physiological bases of hyperbaric therapy. In Davis JC, Hunt TK (eds) Hyperbaric Oxygen Therapy. Undersea Medical Soc. Inc. Bethesda MD, 1977: 11-24.
6. Boerema I, Meijne NG, Brummelkamp WH et al. Life without blood. Arch Chir Neerl 1959; 11: 70-84.
7. Boulton AJM. The diabetic foot. Med Clin N Am 1988; 72 (6): 1513-1530.
8. Brakora MJ, Sheffield PJ. Hyperbaric oxygen therapy for diabetic wounds. Clin Pod Med Surg 1995; 12 (1): 105-117.
9. Calhoun JH, Mader JT. Decision making in medicine. Infection in the diabetic foot. Hosp Pract, 1992; March 30: 81-104.
10. Campagnoli P, Oriani G et al. Prognostic value of TcpO2 during hyperbaric oxygen therapy. J Hyp Med 1992; 7: 223-228.
11. Carrico TJ, Mehrhof AI, Cohen IK. Biology of wound healing. Surg Clin N Am 1984; 64 (4): 721-733.
12. Centers for Disease control. Lower extremity amputations among persons with diabetes mellitus - Washington, 1988. MMWR 1991; 40:737-739.
13. Chantelau E. Hyperbaric oxygen therapy for diabetic foot ulcers. In: Letters to the editor. Diab Care 1997; 20 (7): 1207.
14. Cianci P, Petrone G, Green B. Adjunctive hyperbaric oxygen in the salvage of the diabetic foot. Undersea Biomed Res 1991; 18 (suppl): 108.
15. Cianci P. Adjunctive hyperbaric oxygen therapy in the treatment of the diabetic foot. J Am Pod Med Ass 1994; 84 (9): 448-455.
16. Ciaravino ME, Friedell ML, Kammerlocher TC. Is hyperbaric oxygen a useful adjunct in the management of problem lower extremity wounds? Ann Vasc Surg 1996; 10 (6): 558-562.
17. Consensus Meeting of the European Committee on Hyperbaric Medicine. Reports and recommendations of the jury. Centre Hospitalier regional Universitaire de Lille. Wattel FE, Mathieu D (eds). 1994: 62-63, 73-74.
18. Cruse PJE, Foord R. A prospective study of 23.649 surgical wounds. Arch Surg 1973; 107: 206-210.
19. Davis JC. The use of adjuvant hyperbaric oxygen in treatment of the diabetic foot. Clin Pod Med Surg 1987; 4 (2): 429-437.
20. Department of Clinical Epidemiology and Biostatistics, McMaster University. How to read clinical journals, I: Why to read them and how to start reading them critically. Can Med Ass J 1981; 124: 555-558.
21. Doctor N, Pandya S, Supe A. Hyperbaric oxygen therapy in diabetic foot. J Postgrad Med 1992; 38 (3): 112-114.
22. Eddy DM. Clinical decision making: From theory to practice. The challenge. JAMA 1990; 263 (2): 287-290.
23. Edmonds ME, Roberts VC, Watkins PJ. Blood flow in the diabetic neuropathic foot. Diabetologia 1982; 22: 9.
24. Edmonds ME. The neuropathic foot in diabetes. I. Blood flow. Diab Med 1986; 3: 111.
25. Faglia E, Baroni G, Favales F et al. Traitement de la gangrène diabétique par l'oxygène hyperbare. J de Diab de l'Hôtel Dieu Paris. Ed. Flammarion Medicine Sciences 1987: 209-216.
26. Faglia E, Favales F, Oriani G et al. Hyperbaric oxygen therapy in diabetic foot ulcer and gangrene. In: Oriani G, Marroni A, Wattel FE (eds). Handbook on Hyperbaric Medicine. Springer Verlag, Milano, Berlin, Heidelberg 1996: 542-568.
27. Faglia E, Favales F, Aldeghi A et al. Adjunctive systemic hyperbaric oxygen therapy in treatment of severe prevalently ischemic diabetic foot ulcers. A randomized study. Diab Care 1996; 19 (12): 1338-1343.
28. Faglia E, Favales F, Morabito A et al. In response to Chantelau E (1997). Diab Care 1997; 20 (7): 1207-1208.
29. Faglia E, Favales F, Aldeghi A et al. Change in major amputation rate in a center dedicated to diabetic foot care during the 1980s: Prognostic determinants for major amputation. J Diab Compl 1998; 12: 96-102.
30. Goodson WH III, Hunt TK. Wound healing and the diabetic patient. Surg Gynecol Obstetr 1979; 149: 600-608.
31. Guyatt GH, Rennie D. Users' guides to the medical literature; editorial. JAMA 1993; 270: 2096-2097.
32. Guyatt GH, Sackett DL, Cook DJ for the Evidence-based medicine working group. Users' guides to the medical literature. II How to use an article about therapy or prevention. A. Are the results of the study valid? JAMA 1993; 270: 2598-2601.
33. Guyatt GH, Sackett DL, Cook DJ for the Evidence-based medicine working group. Users' guides to the medical literature. II How to use an article about therapy or prevention. B. What were the results and will they help me in caring for my patients? JAMA 1994; 271: 59-63.
34. Hart GB, Strauss MD. Response of ischemic ulcerative conditions to OHP. In: Smith G (ed). Proceedings of the Sixth International Congress on Hyperbaric Medicine. Aberdeen. Aberdeen University Press 1979: 312-314.
35. Hayward RSA, Wilson MC, Tunis SR et al. for the Evidence-based medicine working group. Users' guides to the medical literature. VIII. How to use clinical practice guidelines. A. Are the recommendations valid? 570-574; B. What are the recommendations and will they help you in caring for your patients? 1630-1632. JAMA 1995; 274: 570-574, 1630-1632.
36. Hunt TK. Disorders of wound healing. World J Surg 1980; 4: 271-277.

37. Hunt TK. The physiology of wound healing. Ann Em Med 1988; 17: 1265-1273.
38. Kleij AJ vdr, Vink H, Bakker DJ et al. Red blood cell velocity in nailfold capillaries during hyperbaric oxygenation. Adv Exp Med Biol 1994; 345: 175-180.
39. Knighton DR. Mechanisms of wound healing. In: Kindwall EP (ed). Hyperbaric Medicine Practice, Best Publ. Flagstaff AZ. 1994: 119-140.
40. LaVan FB, Hunt TK. Oxygen and wound healing. Clin Plast Surg 1990; 17 (3): 463-472.
41. Lee SS, Chen CY, Chan YS et al. Hyperbaric oxygen in the treatment of diabetic foot infection. Chang Gung Med Journ 1997; 20 (1): 17-22.
42. Mader JT, Brown GL, Guckian JC et al. A mechanism for amelioration by hyperbaric oxygen of experimental staphylococcal osteomyelitis in rabbits. J Infect Dis 1980; 142: 915-922.
43. Mader JT, Adams KR, Wallace WR et al. Hyperbaric oxygen as adjunctive therapy for osteomyelitis. Infect Dis Clin N Am 1990;4: 433-440.
44. Mader JT. Phagocytic killing and hyperbaric oxygen: Antibacterial mechanisms. HBO Review 1981; 2: 37-49.
45. Mathieu D, Coget J, Vinckier L et al. Red blood cell deformability and hyperbaric oxygen. Med Sub Hyp 1984; 3: 100.
46. Matos LA. Preliminary report of the use of hyperbarics as adjunctive therapy in diabetics with chronic non-healing wounds. HBO Review 1983; 4 (2): 88-89.
47. Matos LA, Nuñez AA. Enhancement of healing in selected problem wounds. In: Kindwall EP (ed). Hyperbaric Medicine Practice, Best Publ. Flagstaff, Az, 1994: 589-612.
48. Morain WD, Colen LB. Wound healing in diabetes mellitus. Clin Plast Surg 1990; 17 (3): 493-501.
49. Nemiroff PM. Synergistic effects of pentoxifylline and hyperbaric oxygen on skinflaps. Arch Otolaryngol Head Neck Surg 1988; 114: 977.
50. Nylander G, Nordström H, Eriksson E. Effects of hyperbaric oxygen on edema formation after a scald burn. Burns 1984; 10 (3): 193-196.
51. Oriani G, Meazza D, Favales F et al. Hyperbaric oxygen in diabetic gangrene. J Hyperb Med 1990; 5(3): 171-175.
52. Oriani G, Sacchi C, Meazza D et al. Oxygen therapy and diabetic gangrene: a Review of 10 years' experience. In: Schmutz J, Wendling J (eds). Proceedings of the Joint Meeting on Diving and Hyperbaric Medicine. Foundation of Hyperbaric Medicine, Basel 1992: 178-181.
53. Oxman AD, Sackett DL, Guyatt GH for the Evidence-based medicine working group. Users' guides to the medical literature. I How to get started. JAMA 1993; 270: 2093-2095.
54. Oxman AD, Cook DJ, Guyatt GH for the Evidence-based medicine working group. Users' guides to the medical literature. VI. How to use an overview. JAMA 1994; 272: 1367-1371.
55. Pecoraro RE. The nonhealing diabetic ulcer: major cause for limb loss. Progr Biol Res 1991;365:27- 43.
56. Pedesini G, Oriani G, Barnini C et al. Hyperbaric oxygen therapy in the treatment of diabetic vasculopathies. In: Desola Ala J (ed): Proceedings of the IX Congress of the European Undersea Biomedical Society. Barcelona, EUBS, 1984: 207-212.
57. Perrins JD, Barr PO. Hyperbaric oxygenation and wound healing, In: Schmutz J (ed): Proceedings of the First Swiss Symposium on Hyperbaric Medicine. Basel, Foundation for Hyperbaric Medicine, 1986: 132-148.
58. Rabkin JM, Hunt TK. Infection and oxygen. In: Davis JC, Hunt TK (eds). Problem wounds: The role of oxygen. Elsevier, New York 1988: 1-16.
59. Richardson WS, Detsky AS for the Evidence-based medicine working group. Users' guides to the medical literature. VII. How to use a clinical decisions analysis. A.Are the results of the study valid? JAMA 1995; 273: 1292-1295.
60. Richardson WS, Detsky AS for the Evidence-based medicine working group. Users' guides to the medical literature. VII. How to use a clinical decision analysis. B. What are the results and will they help me in caring for my patients? JAMA 1995; 273: 1610-1613.
61. Robson MC, Stenburg BD, Heggers JP. Wound healing alterations caused by infection. Clin Plast Surg 1990; 17(3): 485-492.
62. Sheffield PJ. Tissue oxygen measurements. In: Davis JC, Hunt TK (eds), Problem wounds: The role of oxygen, Elsevier, New York, 1988.
63. Stewart RJ, Yamaguchi KT, Mason SW et al. Tissue ATP levels in burn injured skin treated with hyperbaric oxygen. Undersea Biomed Res (suppl) 1989; 16: 53.
64. Stone JA, Scott RG, Brill LR et al. The role of hyperbaric oxygen in the treatment of diabetic foot wounds. Diabetes Abstr Book, 55th Ann Meeting 1995; 71A: 44.
65. Stone JA, Scott RG. The role of hyperbaric oxygen and platelet derived growth factors in the treatment of the diabetic foot. Undersea Biomed Res 1995; 2: 78 (abstr).
66. Thom SR. Molecular mechanisms for the antagonism of lipid peroxidation by hyperbaric oxygen. Undersea Biomed Res (suppl) 1990; 17: 53-54.
67. Thom SR. Xanthine dehydrogenase conversion to oxidase and lipid peroxidation in brain after CO poisoning. J Appl Physiol 1992; 10: 413.
68. Visonà A, Lusiani L, Rusca F et al. Therapeutic, hemodynamic and metabolic effects of hyperbaric oxygenation in peripheral vascular disease. Angiology 1989; 40: 994.
69. Wagner FW jr. The dysvascular foot: A system for diagnosis and treatment. Foot Ankle 1981; 2: 64-122.
70. Wattel FE, Mathieu D, Coget JM et al. Hyperbaric oxygen therapy in chronic vascular wound management. Angiology 1990; 41: 59.
71. Wattel FE, Mathieu D, Fossati P et al. Hyperbaric oxygen in the treatment of diabetic foot lesions. J Hyp Med 1991; 6: 263-268.

72.   Weisz G, Ramon Y, Melamed Y. Treatment of the diabetic foot by hyperbaric oxygen. Harefuah 1993; 124 (11): 678-681, 740.

73.   White RA, Klein SR. Amputation level selection by transcutaneous oxygen pressure determination. In Moore WS, Malone JM (eds): Lower extremity amputation. W.B.Saunders, Philadelphia 1989: 44-49.

74.   Williams RL. Hyperbaric oxygen therapy and the diabetic foot. J Am Pod Med Ass 1997; 87 (6): 279-292.

75.   Williams RL, Armstrong DG. Wound healing. New modalities for a new millennium. Clin Pod Med Surg 1998: 15 (1): 117-128.

76.   Wyss CR, Robertson C, Love SJ et al. Relationship between transcutaneous oxygen tension, ankle block pressure, and clinical outcome of vascular surgery in diabetic and nondiabetic patients. Surgery 1987; 101: 56-62.

77.   Zamboni WA. The Microcirculation and Ischemia-Reperfusion: Basic Mechanisms of Hyperbaric Oxygen. In Kindwall EP (ed). Hyperbaric Medicine Practice, Best Publishing, Flagstaff Az, 1994.

78.   Zamboni WA, Wong HP, Stephenson LL et al. Evaluation of hyperbaric oxygen for diabetic wounds: a prospective study. Undersea and Hyperb Med 1997; 24 (3): 175-179.

NOTES

ADJUNCTIVE HYPERBARIC OXYGEN THERAPY IN THE TREATMENT OF FOOT LESION IN DIABETIC PATIENTS:
Selection of patients

Daniel Mathieu, Remi Neviere, Nicolas Bocquillon and Francis Wattel
Service de Réanimation Médicale et Médecine Hyperbare-Hôpital Calmette—
Lille, France

Diabetes is the most common underlying cause of lower-extremity amputations in Europe and North America. It is estimated that 50 to 80% of all lower extremity amputations are directly attributable to diabetes mellitus (1). Individuals with diabetes have a 15- to 30-fold greater risk of lower extremity amputation than those without diabetes (2). Treatement of a foot lesion accounts for up to one quarter of all diabetic patients who are admitted to hospitals (3–6). In October 1989, representatives of government health departments and patient organisations from all European countries met with diabetes experts under the aegis of the World Health Organisation and the International Diabetes Federation in St Vincent, Italy, and agreed on recommendations. One of those was to reduce by one-half the rate of limb amputations for diabetic gangrene (7). Despite the tremendous efforts and multiple actions launched by this declaration, 18 years after, the goal is not yet reached (8) even if promising pilot centers have opened the way.

Hyperbaric Oxygen Therapy (HBO) is a therapeutic measure in which the patient breathes oxygen at a pressure higher than atmospheric. Introduced in clinical practice in the early 1960s, HBO is actually used in decompression accident and air embolism, carbon monoxide poisoning, anaerobic infections, crush injuries, delayed wound healing, and tissue radiation damage (9). Pathophysiological bases for its use include increase in tissue oxygen delivery, redistribution of tissue blood flow toward ill perfused areas leading to correction of tissue hypoxia, direct killing effect on anaerobic bacteria, enhancement of microbicidal capabilities of polymorphonuclears, synergistic action with certain antibiotics, increase in fibroblast multiplication rate, and production of oxidized collagen (10). Based on these effects, HBO has been proposed as an adjunctive therapeutic measure in the treatment of foot lesion in diabetic patients (11–14). Recent randomized studies confirm HBO efficacy in diabetic foot lesions (15-16). However, considering the actual results of conventional treatment, not all patients have to be treated with HBO. Selection of patients is of major importance. In our view HBO is to be used in case of infected foot lesions or delayed healing despite correct conventional management (17).

WHICH PATIENTS REMAIN AT RISK OF AMPUTATION DESPITE APPROPRIATE CONVENTIONAL THERAPY?

The most common components in the causal pathway to loss of limb in patients with diabetes mellitus include peripheral neuropathy, peripheral vascular disease, structural deformity, ulceration, and infection (18–20). Evaluation of these parameters is essential to start an appropriate therapeutic program (21–22). Infection requires wound debridement and antibiotics. Treatment of ulceration due to neuropathy includes aggressive local wound care with removal of all necrotic tissue and callus, drainage of cavities, and reduction of weight bearing forces by appropriate chiropodic measures. An ischemic component due to vascular insufficiency must be identified by clinical evaluation and non-invasive vascular tests (pressure index, Doppler ultrasonography, transcutaneous oxygen measurement). If the ischemic part seems to be preeminent in the pathophysiology of the ulceration, peripheral artery angiography is mandatory to evaluate the possibility of revascularisation procedure: distal bypass or angioplasty.

However, despite efforts, depending on the combination of factors, failure to heal still happens in 10 to 40 percent of patients, leading to amputation. Many authors (6, 23–25) have studied the risk factors for amputation in diabetic patients. Patient education, glycemic control, careful daily foot hygiene, and appropriate foot wear have been recognized as preventable environmental factors, but prevention effort will act only in the long term. When analysing the reason why an amputation has been performed, non-healing ulceration, persisting ischemia, and infection are the 3 main indications (26, 27). Armstrong et al. showed that diabetic patients with a wound involving the bone are 11 times more likely to undergo an amputation, and patients with infection and ischemia are at a 90 times greater risk (28).

Severe lower limb ischemia is a critical factor leading to amputation. The 2nd European Consensus Conference has recommended a more precise description of the type and severity of chronic leg ischemia (29). Chronic Critical Leg Ischemia (CLI) was separated from other less severe forms of leg ischemia and defined in both diabetic and non-diabetic patients, by either of the following two criteria: persistent recurring ischemic rest pain requiring regular adequate analgesia for more than 2 weeks, with an ankle systolic pressure £ 50 mmHg and/or a toe systolic pressure of £ 30 mmHg, or ulceration or gangrene of the foot or toes, with an ankle systolic pressure of £ 50 mmHg or a toe systolic pressure of £ 30 mmHg. In addition to the above definition, the following information was said also desirable: arteriography to delineate the anatomy of the large vessel disease throughout the leg and foot, toe arterial pressure in all patients, and a technique for quantifying the local micro-circulation in the ischemic area (e.g., capillary microscopy, transcutaneous oxygen pressure [$TcpO_2$], or laser Doppler).

The interest of this definition is to separate two groups of patients with different outcomes. By assessment of previous reports, Wolfe and Wyatt showed that patients with CLI inevitably require amputation if treated conservatively, whereas more than 25% of those with subcritical leg ischemia retain the leg without intervention [30].

It was then recommended that all patients with CLI should be evaluated for revascularization and that a reconstructive procedure should be attempted if there is a 25% chance of saving a useful limb for the patient for at least 1 year. In spite of surgical efforts, patients with CLI have a high post-surgical mortality rate (15–25% at 1 year) and a 20–45% amputation rate (31). If an early graft failure nearly invariably leads to amputation, even graft patency may not be equivalent to limb salvage. Carsten et al. (32) have studied factors associated with limb amputation despite a patent infrainguinal bypass graft. In their series, 29 patients out of 158 (18%) have to be amputated. The most common primary causes of early limb loss (30 days from surgery) are overwhelming progression of soft tissue infection and insufficient run-off in the foot. In the late amputation group, amputation most often follows long treatment of a chronic proximal diabetic neuropathic foot ulcer with osteomyelitis.

In conclusion, despite complete evaluation and appropriate medical and surgical treatment, diabetic patients with foot lesion remain at high risk of major amputation if they present:

- A rapidly spreading soft tissue infection as gas gangrene or necrotizing fasciitis.
- A critical leg ischemia in case of unoperability or despite a revascularization procedure.
- A non healing ulcer with bone involvement or infection.

It is in these cases, where the commonly accepted treatment has failed, that the use of adjunctive HBO may be considered.

SELECTION OF PATIENTS FOR ADJUNCTIVE HBO

Soft tissue infection

Diabetic patients have long been recognized to be at high risk for anaerobic soft tissue infection (22).

a) Clostridial myonecrosis (gas gangrene) is a life-threating infection due to proliferation of Clostridia, releasing a large quantity of exotoxins in a area of low oxidation-reduction potential such an ischemic foot or leg in diabetic patient. Surgical excision of infected muscles associated to antibiotics and general intensive care is urgently needed, but mortality and major amputation rates remain high (33).

HBO exerts multiple anti-infectious actions. It has direct bacteriostatic and bactericidal effects on anaerobes. It stops alpha toxin production (32), it depletes the germs in reduced metabolites such as NADH and NADPH making those unavailable for protein and nucleic acid syntheses, and it induces an over-production of oxygen free radicals (OFR) which react and alter a variety of macromolecules in the bacteria (35). HBO also exerts an indirect effect in enhancing the microbicidal activity of polymorphonuclears (PMN). It has been shown that most of the microbicidal activity of PMN is oxygen-dependent acting through the generation of OFR inside the phagolysosomic vacuoles (36, 37). Hohn et al have shown that hypoxia suppresses this mechanism and allows germs to proliferate and destroy the PMN (38). Lastly, HBO potentiates the antimicrobial activity of certain antibiotics (39–41).

The beneficial effects of HBO in soft tissue infections has been demonstrated in animal models. In a model of Clostridial muscle infection in mice, Hill showed a considerable reduction in mortality using HBO (42, 43). In dogs, Demello showed the interest of the association antibiotics-surgery-HBO over the use of each of those alone or in other combination (44).

Since its introduction in clinical practice in the early 1960s [45], HBO has routinely been adjuncted to surgery and antibiotics in the treatment of patient with gas gangrene. Goulon in a large but uncontrolled study of 778 cases of all localizations reported a significant improvement in success rate when adjunctive HBO was used. From a review of the literature, Hart and Strauss also came to the conclusion that adjunctive HBO improves significantly the success rate (47).

Reporting on the large experience of the Amsterdam group, Bakker (48) emphasized the point that, when considering gas gangrene limited to foot or lower limb, the lifesaving capability of HBO may be considered as not so significant, but its tissue saving capacity is evident. In his series of cases of 173 lower limb gas gangrene, the overall amputation rate is 20%, with a difference according to the level of gas gangrene involvement: below the knee, amputation rate 12%, thigh and upper: 24%. This is to be compared to an amputation rate of about 50 % in series using only surgery and antibiotics. Jackson and Waddell also reported the same conclusion (49).

b) Other necrotizing soft tissue infections include necrotizing fasciitis and progressive bacterial gangrene. They are caused by a mixed aerobic and anaerobic bacterial flora and happen frequently in diabetics. If the mortality is lower than in gas gangrene, the infection process may have a fulminant extension and requires an immediate treatment associating surgery and antibiotics. Even in case of good outcome, morbidity remain high with multiple surgical procedures and prolonged hospitalization stay (50, 51).

The rationale to use adjunctive HBO is the same as that for gas gangrene. Several authors have reported beneficial clinical results (52). Riseman showed in a comparative but not randomized study a significant reduction in mortality and wound morbidity when using adjunctive HBO (53).

In conclusion, in soft tissue infections, the use of HBO in association with surgical debridement and appropriate antibiotic therapy is supported by a large body of evidence, although no randomized controlled clinical study is yet available. Diabetic patients have long been recognized as at a higher mortality risk in these infections and early use of HBO is recommended in these patients.

Critical Chronic Ischemia

Critical Chronic Leg Ischemia (CLI) is a clinical situation which has been individualized because of its high risk of amputation (29). Due to the lack of oxygen, the healing process is severely depressed (54,55) and the wound especially prone to infection (36,56). In this setting, to relieve hypoxia is mandatory and is best achieved by performing revascularization procedures such as surgical bypass or angioplasty. However, that may not be possible either because the patient is estimated "unoperable" or because no procedure can be performed after lower limb angiogram review. Moreover, distal hypoxia may persist after revascularization procedure because of severely narrowed distal arteries or in case of bypass thrombosis (57, 58). In those cases, the prognosis has been shown to be very poor and in case of patient survival, amputation has to be performed at a higher level than planned before the revascularisation attempt (59).

So, in case of CLI, when revascularization procedure has been ruled out or has failed, HBO may be used because of its effects on infection and healing processes.

The major problem, when faced with a foot lesion in a diabetic patient in CLI, is to determine if it is worth adding HBO to conventional treatment, and so to extend the treatment time for 3 to 6 weeks more, with a risk of failure and at the end amputation, or to amputate immediately in order shorten the hospitalization stay. To solve this problem, transcutaneous oxymetry has been shown to be an useful, non-invasive method for evaluation of residual perfusion and patient selection (60–64). This measurement is widely available and has a good predictive value (65–67). Patients with transcutaneous periwound value greater than 30–40 mmHg when breathing room air heal with conventional treatment most of the time. On the opposite, patients with less than 20 mmHg on room air have a poor prognosis (68-70). Unfortunately, in this last group, TcPO$_2$ in room air is not able to identify patients who will heal from patient who will need amputation (14). Measuring TcPO$_2$ under hyperbaric oxygen makes the difference between groups clearer (71, 72).

In a series of 59 diabetic patients with a periwound TcPO$_2$ lower than 40 mmHg in room air, HBO was added to conventional treatment. In 48 (81%), healing was achieved where as in 11 (19%) treatment failed leading to amputation. No difference could be seen between success and failure concerning age, sex, diabetes type or duration, diabetic complications, type of foot lesion. Transcutaneous oxygen pressures measured close to the wound show no difference between the success and the failure groups when patient breathes room air (26 +/- 17 vs 11 +/- 17 mmHg, NS) or 100% normobaric oxygen (102 +/- 80 vs 78 +/- 93 mmHg, NS). Conversely, a clear difference appears when measuring TcPO$_2$ in 2.5 ATA hyperbaric oxygen (786 +/- 258 vs 323 +/- 214 mmHg; p< 0.005) (Figure 1). The difference is even more impressive when considering the ratio between TcPO$_2$ at the wound site and at the subclavicular reference point (ambient air: 0.6 +/- 1 vs 0.3 +/- 0.5; NS - normobaric oxygen: 0.8 +/- 0.4 vs 0.7 +/- 1; NS - 2.5 ATA hyperbaric oxygen: 0.8 +/- 0.2 vs 0.3 +/- 0.2, p < 0.002).

Analysing data in terms of sensitivity and specificity, the threshold of 20 mmHg for periwound TcPO$_2$ in room air has a 83% sensitivity and a only 59% specificity to predict amputation when HBO is added to the conventional treatment. This low specificity is to be compared to the high specificity of this 20 mmHg threshold in series not using HBO, and means that some patients may keep their leg if HBO is added to conventional treatment. When considering ROC curves (Figure 2 and 3), no TcPO$_2$ level in room air appears to be a threshold value. In normobaric oxygen, TcPO$_2$ over 50 mmHg has a 79% sensitivity and 92% specificity for success. In 2.5 ATA hyperbaric oxygen, 2 critical levels appear with a very high specificity: a TcPO$_2$ under 200 mmHg predicts failure, leading to amputation with a 94% specificity; a TcPO$_2$ over 400 mmHg predicts success with HBO treatment with a 92% specificity.

Contrasting with the value of TcPO$_2$ measurements, we have been unable to find any predictive value of laser Doppler flowmetry in patients with CLI.

In summary, diabetic patients with foot lesion who present a chronic critical leg ischemia must be evaluated for revascularization. When no possibility exists or in case of healing failure after revascularization, HBO may be adjuncted to conventional treatment if periwound TcPO$_2$ in 2.5 ATA hyperbaric oxygen are over 200 mmHg. Periwound TcPO$_2$ over 400 mmHg in 2.5 ATA oxygen or over 50 mmHg in normobaric pure oxygen predict healing success with adjunctive HBO with a high accuracy. TcPO$_2$ in room air has no predictive value in this group, and TcPO$_2$ under 20 or 10 mmHg must not be considered as an imperative indication for immediate amputation.

Non healing ulcer with bone involvement or infection

Infection has long been recognized as a major factor involved in non-healing ulcers in diabetic patients. Diabetes mellitus adversely affects host defense against infection through 2 principal mechanisms (22, 73–75): local hypoxia due to vascular occlusive lesions and defective cellular and humoral immunity with a decrease in chemotadic response, and phagocytic activity of polymorphonuclears and abnormalities of lymphocyte functions.

Osteomyelitis of the foot is a common and serious complication and is frequently seen in neuropathic foot. Infection generally develops by spread of contiguous soft tissue infection to underlying bone. Osteomyelitis is recognized as a serious risk factor in delayed healing and subsequently amputation (76–78).

HBO has been proved beneficial in the treatment of osteomyelitis. It has a direct killing effect on anaerobes which have been found to be the most common organisms of clinical significance in diabetic foot infection and are present with Staphylococci in 75% of cases and Gram negative facultative anaerobes in 25% of cases (79).

It is able to elevate bone oxygen tension which is decreased in infected bone. As neutrophils require tissue oxygen tensions of 30–40 mmHg to kill bacteria by oxidative killing mechanisms, HBO is able to restore the bacterial killing activity at the infected focus (36-38). Lastly, HBO enhances antibacterial activity of some antibiotics such as aminoglycoside (39–41). This beneficial activity of adjunctive HBO has been also demonstrated in chronic S. Aureus and P. aeruginosa osteomyelitis rabbit model (80–82).

Beside this antimicrobial activity, HBO enhances fibroblast proliferation, collagen production, and capillary angiogenesis in hypoxic areas such as infected bone (83–85). Its also enhances osteoclastic activity and bone formation (86). Clinical studies reported in the literature confirmed animal data (87–89). Although no study specifically concerns osteomyelitis in diabetics, HBO may be used as an adjunct to debridement, wound care, and antibiotics as dictated by bone culture results (90).

CONCLUSION

Defective wound healing capability of foot lesions in diabetic patients is mainly due to infection and local hypoxia. Despite conventional treatment, including revascularization procedure when appropriate, three situations still lead frequently to amputation: soft tissue infection, persistent critical limb ischemia, and delayed wound healing with bone involvement. In these conditions, HBO may be adjuncted to conventional therapy and is associated with a better outcome. Transcutaneous oxygen measurement performed under HBO is a reliable tool to select patients who are the most likely to get benefit of adjunctive HBO.

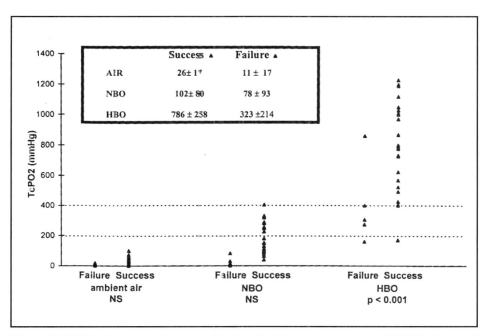

Figure 1. Relation between outcome and transcutaneous oxygen pressure (TcPO₂) at wound site in a series of 59 patients treated by HBO TcPO₂ are measured in three conditions : patient breathing room air at atmospheric pressure first, then normobaric oxygen, and finally 2.5 Ata hyperbaric oxygen. Note the 2 critical values of 200 mmHg for failure and 400 mmHg for success.

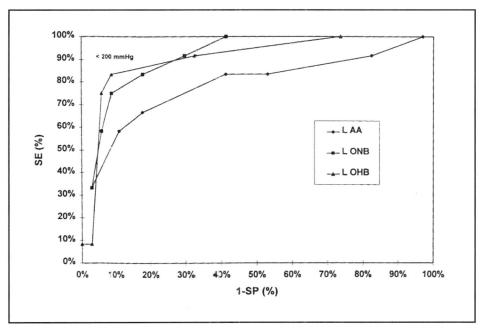

Figure 2. ROC curves of predictive value of TcPO₂ for failure. The best critical predictive value for failure is 200 mmHg in 2.5 Ata hyperbaric oxygen.

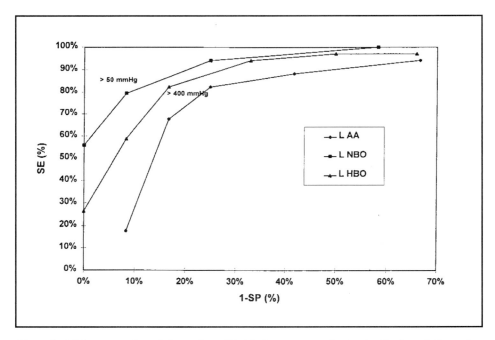

Figure 3. ROC curves of predictive value of TcPO$_2$ for success. The best critical predictive value for success is 400 mmHg in hyperbaric oxygen and 50 mmHg in normobaric oxygen.

REFERENCES

1. Lavery LA, Ashry HR, Van Houtom W, Pugh JA, Harkless LB, Basu S. Variation in the incidence and proportion of diabetes-related amputations in minorities. Diabetes Care ; 1996 ; 19 : 48-52.

2. Van Houtum WH, Lavery LA, Harkless LB. The impact of diabetes-related lower extremity amputations in the Netherlands. J. Diabetes Complications ; 1996, 10 : 325-330.

3. Levin M. Pathophysiology of diabetic foot lesions. In : Davidson JK, ed. Clinical Diabetes Mellitus : A Problem-Oriented Approach. Thieme-Stratton Inc, New York (USA) ; 1991 : 504-510.

4. Gibbons G, Eliopoulos GM. Infection of the diabetic foot. In : Kozak GP, Hoar CD, Rowbotham JL, eds. Management of Diabetic Foot Problems. WE Saunders Co, Philadelphia (USA) ; 1984 : 97-102.

5. Pliskin Ma, Todd WF, Edelson GW. Presentations of diabetic feet. Arch Fam Med ; 1994 ; 3 : 273-279.

6. Reiber GE, Pecoraro RE, Koepsell TD. Risk factors for amputation in patients with diabetes mellitus : a case control study. Ann Intern Med ; 1992 ; 117 : 97-105.

7. World Health Organization. Diabetes care and research in Europe : The Saint-Vincent declaration, World Health Organization, Regional office for Europe. Copenhagen (Denmark) ; 1990.

8. Stiegler H, Standl E, Frank S, Mendler G. Failure of reducing lower extremity amputations in diabetic patients : results of two subsequent population based surveys 1990 and 1995 in Germany. Vasa ; 1998 ; 27 : 10 - 14.

9. European Committee for Hyperbaric Medicine. Recommendations. In : Wattel F., Mathieu D. Eds : Proceedings of the First European Consensus Conference on Hyperbaric Oxygen Therapy, CRAM, Lille, (France), 1994.

10. Camporesi EM, Barker AC. Hyperbaric oxygen therapy. A critical review. UHMS, Bethesda (USA) 1991, 166.

11. Baroni G, Porro T, Faglia E et al. Hyperbaric oxygen treatment in diabetic gangrene. Diab Care ; 1987 ; 10 : 81-86.

12. Davis JC. The use of adjuvant hyperbaric oxygen in treatment of the diabetic foot. Clin Podiatr Med Surg. ; 1987 ; 4 : 429-437.

13. Oriani G, Meazza D, Favales F et al. Hyperbaric oxygen therapy in diabetic gangrene. J Hyperb Med; 1990; 5: 171-175.

14. Wattel F, Mathieu D, Coget JM et al. Hyperbaric oxygen therapy in chronic vascular wound management. Angiology ; 1990 ; 41 : 59-65.

15. Faglia E, Favales F, Aldeghi A et al. Adjunctive systemic hyperbaric oxygen therapy in treatment of severe prevalently ischemic diabetic foot ulcers. A randomized study. Diab Care ; 1996 ; 19 : 1338-1343.

16. Zamboni WA, Wong HP, Stephenson LL et al. Evaluation of hyperbaric oxygen for diabetic wounds : a prospective study. Undersea Hyperb Med ; 1997 ; 24 : 175-179.

17. Cianci P, Hunt TF. Adjunctive hyperbaric oxygen therapy in treatment of diabetic foot wounds. In: Levin ME, O'Neal LW, Bowler JH eds. The diabetic foot, 5th Edition, Mosby Year Book, St Louis (USA) ; 1993 : 305-319.

18. Pecoraro RE, Reiber GE, Burgess EM. Causal pathways to amputation : basis for prevention. Diabetes Care ; 1990 ; 13 : 513-521.

19. Kannel WB, McGee DL. Diabetes and glucose tolerance as risk factors for cardiovascular disease : the Framingham Study. Diabetes Care ; 1979 ; 2 : 120-126.

20. Frykberg R. Diabetic foot ulcerations. In : Frykberg R, ed. The High Risk Foot in Diabetes Mellitus. Churchill Livingstone Inc New York (USA) ; 1991 : 151-195.

21. American Diabetes Association. Foot care in patients with diabetes mellitus. Diabetes Care; 1995; 18 (suppl) : 26-27.

22. Caputo GM, Cavanagh PR, Ulbrecht JS, Gibbons GN, Karchmer AN. Assessment and management of foot disease in patients with diabetes. N Engl J Med ; 1994 ; 331 : 854-860.

23. Larsson J, Agardh CD, Apelqust J, Senstrom A. Clinical characteristics in relation to final amputation level in diabetic patients with foot ulcers : a prospective study of healing below or above the ankle in 187 patients. Foot Ankle int ; 1995 ; 16 : 69-74.

24. Moss SE, Klein R, Klein BE. Long term incidence of lower extremity amputations in a diabetic population. Arch Fam Med ; 1996 ; 5 : 391-398.

25. Flores Rivera AR. Risk factors for amputation in diabetic patients : a care control study. Arch Med Res ; 1998 ; 29 : 179 - 184.

26. Larsen K, Holstein P, Deckert T. Limb salvage in diabetic foot ulcers. Prosthet Ortho int ; 1989 ; 13 : 100-103.

27. Humphrey LL, Palumbo PJ, Butters MA et al. The contribution of non-insulin dependent diabetes to lower extremity amputation in the community. Arch Intern Med ; 1994 ; 154 : 885-892.

28. Armstrong DG, Lavery LA, Harkless LB. Validation of a diabetic wound classification system. The contribution of depth, infection and ischemia to risk of amputation. Diab Care ; 1998 ; 21 : 855-859.

29. European working group on Critical Leg ischemia. Second European Consensus Document on chronic critical leg ischemia. Circulation ; 1991 ; 84 : IV.1-IV.26.

30. Wolfe JHN, Wyatt MG. Critical and subcritical ischemia. Eur J Vasc Endovasc Surg ; 1997 ; 13 : 578-582.

31. Wolfe JHN. Defining the outcome of critical ischemia : A one year prospective study. Br J Surg ; 1986 ; 73 : 321-326.

32. Carsten CG, Taylor SM, Langan EM, Crane MM. Factors associated with limb loss despite a patent infrainguinal bypass graft. Am Surg ; 1998 ; 54 : 33-37.

33. Bartlett JG. Gas Gangrene. In Mandell GL, Douglas RG, Bennett JE Eds. Principles and practice of infections diseases. Churchill Livingstone, New York (USA) ; 1990 ; 1850-1860.

34. Van unnik AJM. Inhibition of toxin production in Clostridium perfringens in-vitro by hyperbaric oxygen. Antonie Leeuwenhoek J Microviol Seriol ; 1965 ; 31 : 181-186.

35.   Kaye D. Effect of hyperbaric oxygen on clostridia in vivo and in vitro. Proc Soc Exp Biol Med ; 1967 ; 124 : 360-366.

36.   Knighton DR, Halliday B, Hunt TK. Oxygen as an antibiotic : the effect of inspired oxygen on infection. Arch Surg ; 1984 ; 119 : 199-204.

37.   Park MK, Myers RA, Marzella L. Oxygen tensions and infections : Modulation of microbial growth, activity of antimicrobial agents, and immunologic responses. Clin Infect Dis ; 1992 ; 14 (3) : 720-740.

38.   Hohn DC, MacKay RD, Halliday B et al. The effect of O2 tension on the microbicidal function of leukocytes in wounds and in vitro. Surg Forum ; 1976 ; 27 : 18-20.

39.   Verkllin JR RM, Mandell GL. Alteration of effectiveness of antibiotics by anaerobiosis. J Lab Clin Med ; 1977 ; 89 : 65-71.

40.   Knighton DR, Halliday P, Hunt TK. Oxygen as an antibiotic. A comparison of the effects of inspired oxygen concentration and antibiotic administration on in vivo clearance. Arch Surg ; 1986 ; 121 : 191-195.

41.   Marzella L, Vezzani G. Effect of Hyperbaric Oxygen on Activity of Antibacterial Agents. In : Oriani G, Marroni A, Wattel F. eds. Handbook on Hyperbaric Medicine. Springer-Verlag ; Berlin (BRD) ; 1996 ; 699-713.

42.   Hill GB, Osterhout S. Experimental effects of hyperbaric Oxygen on selected Clostridial species. I. In-vitro studies. J Infect Dis ; 1972 ; 125 : 17-25.

43.   Hill GB, Osterhout S. Experimental effects of Hyperbaric oxygen on selected Clostridial species. II. In vivo-studies. J Infect Dis ; 1972 ; 125 : 26-35.

44.   Demello FJ, Haglin JJ, Hitchcock CR. Comparative study of experimental Clostridium perfringens infection in dogs treated with antibiotics, surgery, and hyperbaric oxygen. Surgery ; 1973 ; 73 : 936-941.

45.   Brummelkamp WH, Hogendijk J, Boerema I. Treatment of anaerobic infections (Clostridial myositis) by drenching the tissues with oxygen under high atmospheric pressure. Surgery ; 1961 ; 49 : 299-302.

46.   Goulon M. Gangrènes gazeuses : Etude multicentrique réunissant 778 cas. In : Les anaérobies : Microbiologie - Pathologie, Masson, Paris (France) ; 1981, 181-290.

47.   Hart GB, Strauss MB. Gas gangrene - Clostridial myonecrosis : a review. J Hyperbaric Med ; 1990 ; 5 : 125-144.

48.   Bakker DJ. The use of hyperbaric oxygen in the treatment of certain infectious diseases especially gas gangrene and acute dumal gangrene. monograph. Academisch Proefschrift, Drukkerij Veerman BV, Wageningen (NL) ; 1984 ; 118.

49.   Jackson RW, Waddell JP. Hyperbaric oxygen in the management of Clostridial myonecrosis (gas gangrene). Clin Orthop. 1973 ; 96 : 271-276.

50.   Mc Henry CR, Piotrowski JJ, Petrinic D, Malagoni DA. Determinant of mortality for necrotizing soft tissue infections. Am Surg. 1995 ; 221 : 558-563.

51.   Lille ST, Sato TT, Engrav LH, Foy H, Jurkovich GJ. Necrotizing soft tissue infections : obstacle in diagnosis. J Am Coll Surg ; 1996 ; 182 : 7-11.

52.   Bakker DJ. Necrotizing soft tissue infections. J Hyperbaric Med ; 1987 ; 2 : 161-168.

53.   Riseman JA, Zamboni WA, Curtis A et al. Hyperbaric oxygen therapy for necrotizing fasciitis reduces mortality and the need for debridements. Surgery ; 1990 ; 108 : 847-850.

54.   Hunt TK, Twomey P, Zederfeldt B et al. Respiratory gas tensions and pH in healing wounds. Am J Surg ; 1967 ; 114 : 302 - 308.

55.   Knighton D, Silver I, Hunt TK. Regulation of wound healing angiogenesis - Effect of oxygen gradients and inspired oxygen concentration. Surgery ; 1981 ; 90 : 262-270.

56.   Hunt TK, Linsey M, Grislis G et al. The effect of differing ambient oxygen tensions on wound infection. Ann Surg ; 1975 ; 181 : 35-39.

57.   Reifsnyder T, Grossman JP, Leers SA. Limb loss after lower extremity bypass. Am J Surg; 1997 ; 174 : 149-151.

58.   Yeager RA, Moneta GL, Edwards JM et al. Predictor of outcome of fore foot surgery for ulceration and gangrene. Am J Surg ; 1998 ; 175 : 388-390.

59.   Kazmers M, Satiani B, Evans WE. Amputation level following unsuccessful distal limb salvage operations. Surgery ; 1980 ; 87 : 683-687.

60.   Franzeck UK, Talke P, Bernstein EF, Golbranson FL, Fronek A. Transcutaneous PO2 measurements in health and peripheral arterial occlusive disease. Surgery ; 1982 ; 91: 156-163.

61.   White RA, Nolan L, Harley D, Shoemaker WC. Noninvasive evaluation of peripheral vascular disease using transcutaneous oxygen tension. Am J Surg ; 1982 ; 144 : 68 -75.

62.   Hauser CJ, Klein SR, Mehringer CM, Appel P, Shoemaker WC. Assessment of perfusion in the diabetic foot by regional transcutaneous oximetry. Diabetes ; 1984 ; 33 : 527-531.

63.   Wyss CR, Matsen FA III, Simmons CW, Burgess EM. Transcutaneous oxygen tension measurements on limbs of diabetic and nondiabetic patients with peripheral vascular disease. Surgery ; 1984 ; 95 : 339-345.

64.   Sheffield PJ. Tissue oxygen measurements. In : Davis JC, Hunt TK (eds). Problem wound, the role of oxygen. Elsevier, Amsterdam (NL) ; 1989 ; 17-51.

65.   Ratliff DA, Clyne Ca, Chant AD, Webster JH. Prediction of amputation wound healing : the role of transcutaneous PO2 assessment. Br J Surg ; 1984 ; 71 : 219-222.

66.   Bacharach JM, Rooke TW, Osmundson PJ, Gloviczki P. Predictive value of transcutaneous oxygen pressure and amputation success by use of supine and elevation measurements. J Vasc Surg; 1992 ; 15: 558-563.

67.   Prinzer MS, Sage R, Stuck R, Ketver L, Osterman H. Transcutaneous oxygen as predictor of wound healing in amputation of the foot and ankle. Foot ankle ; 1992 ; 13 : 271-272.

68.   Wyss CR, Robertson C, Love SJ, Harrington RM, Matsen FA. Relationship between transcutaneous oxygen tension, ankle blood pressure and clinical outcome of vascular surgery in diabetic and non diabetic patients. Surgery ; 1987 ; 101 : 56-62.

69. Ballard JL, Eke CC, Bunt TS, Killeer Jd. A prospective evaluation of transcutaneous oxygen measurements in the management of diabetic foot problems. J Vasc Surg. 1995; 22: 485-490.
70. Bunt TJ, Holloway GA. TcPO2 as an accurate predictor of therapy in limb salvage. Ann Vasc Surg ; 1996 ; 10 : 224-227.
71. Wattel F, Mathieu D, Fossati F, Neviere R, Coget JM. Hyperbaric oxygen in the treatment of diabetic foot. Undersea Biomed Res ; 1990 ; 17 (Suppl): 160-161.
72. Mathieu D, Nevière R, Wattel F. Transcutaneous oxymetry in hyperbaric medicine. In : Oriani G, Marroni A, Wattel F. Eds Handbook on hyperbaric medicine, Springer, Berlin (BDR) ; 1996 ; 686-698.
73. Goodson WH III, Hunt TK. Wound healing and the diabetic patient. Surg Gynecol Obst ; 1979 ; 149 : 600-608.
74. Morain WD and Colen LB. Wound healing in diabetes mellitus. Clinics in Plastic Surg ; 1990 ; 17 (3) : 493-501.
75. Levenson SM, Demetrion AA. Factors affecting tissue repair : Metabolic factors. In : Cohen IK, Diegelmann RF, Lindblad NJ. Eds Wound healing : Biochemical and clinical aspects. WB Saunders, Philadelphia (USA) ; 1992 ; 248-273.
76. Kaufman J, Breeding L, Rosenberg N. Anatomic location of acute diabetic foot infection. Its influence on the outcome of treatment. Ann Surg ; 1987 ; 53 : 109-112.
77. Balsells M, Viade J, Millau M et al. Prevalence of osteomyelitis in non healing diabetic foot ulcers : usefulness of radiologic and scintigraphic findings. Diabetes Res Clin Pract ; 1997 ; 38 : 123-127.
78. Eneroth M, Apelquist J, Stenstrom A. Clinical characteristics and outcome in 223 diabetic patients with deep foot infections. Foot ankle Int ; 1997 ; 18 : 716-722.
79. Klainer As, Bisaccia E. Clindamycin treatment of diabetic foot infections. Rev contemp Pharmaco ther ; 1992 ; 3 : 281-285.
80. Hamblin DL. Hyperbaric oxygenation : its effect on experimental staphylococcal osteomyelitis in rats. J. Bone Jt Surg ; 1968 ; 50 A : 1129-1141.
81. Mader JT, Guckian JC, Glass DL, Reinarz A. Therapy with hyperbaric oxygen for experimental osteomyelitis due to Staphylococcus aureus in rabbits. J Infect Dis ; 1978 ; 138 : 312-318.
82. Mader JT, Brown GL, Guckian JC, Wells CH, Reinarz JA. A mechanism for the amelioration by hyperbaric oxygen of experimental staphylococcal osteomyelitis in rabbits. J Infect Dis ; 1980 ; 142 : 915-922.
83. Yablon IG, Cruess RL. The effect of hyperbaric oxygen on fracture healing in rats. J. Trauma ; 1968 ; 8 : 186-201.
84. Niinikoski J, Penttinen R, Kulonen E. Effect of hyperbaric oxygenation on fracture healing in the rat : A biochemical study. Calcif Tissue Res ; 1970 ; 4 (suppl) : 115-116.
85. Penttinen R. Biochemical studies on fracture healing in the rat with special reference to the oxygen supply. Acta Chir Scand ; 1972 ; 432 (suppl) : 8-32.
86. Stedd DL. Enhancement of osteogenesis with hyperbaric oxygen therapy. A clinical study. J Dental Res ; 1982 ; 61A : 288.
87. Morrey BF, Dunn JM, Heimbach RD, Davis JC. Hyperbaric oxygen and chronic osteomyelitis. Clin Orthop ; 1979 ; 144 : 121-127.
88. Davis JC, Heckman JD, DeLee JC, Buckwold FJ. Chronic non-hematogenous osteomyelitis treated with adjuvant hyperbaric oxygen. J Bone Jt Surg ; 1986 ; 58A : 1210-1217.
89. Strauss MB. Refractory Osteomyelitis. J Hyperbaric Med ; 1987 ; 2 : 147-159.
90. Mathieu D, Wattel F. Intérêt de l'oxygénothérapie hyperbare dans le traitement des ostéites chroniques. In: Sutter B, Bianchi F, Fayada P et al eds. Les infections ostéoarticulaires à germes banals. Marson, Paris (France) ; 1998 ; 119-130.

NOTES

A COST-BENEFIT EVALUATION OF HYPERBARIC OXYGEN TREATMENT OF THE DIABETIC FOOT

Alessandro Marroni[1,3,4], Pasquale Longobardi[2,4] and Ramiro Cali-Corleo[1,3,4]

Diabetes is one of the most important and growing health care problems in Europe. It affects all age groups and generates a chronic illness with significant complications and is associated with premature death.

The diabetic foot is characteristically a late complication of diabetes. It is a multi-faceted syndrome, with several pathogenic mechanisms and a common denominator; diabetic foot lesions can lead to complications of such magnitude as to require the amputation of an entire lower limb. This clinical condition has a tremendous negative impact on the patient's quality of life and life expectancy (Chantelau, 1996; Diabetes Care and Research in Europe, 1994).

In the diabetic patient the risk of foot/limb amputation is 15 times higher than in the non-diabetic, furthermore this risk increases with age and with preceding amputations. Controlateral amputation becomes necessary in about 53 percent of the amputees within 4 years of the first amputation. Ipsilateral amputation becomes necessary in about 27 percent of the amputated patients (Cianci, 1990, 1991; Cignetti, 1991; Della Marchina, 1991; Vannini 1991).

Post-amputation hospitalisation is frequently longer than 60 days, with the associated possibility of a need for 20–50 days of intensive care and with a post-amputation mortality in excess of 31 percent. The cost of primary post-amputation rehabilitation in the USA is estimated to exceed US $30,000 (Cianci, 1990, 1991).

The Saint Vincent Declaration identified the diabetic foot as the most frequent current cause for lower limb amputation, stressed that such high amputation rates are not an unavoidable consequence of diabetic disease, but just a sign of inadequate treatment and prevention, and strongly recommended a reduction of the amputation rate to less than 50% (Diabetes Care and Research in Europe, 1994).

The use of Hyperbaric Oxygen Therapy in Diabetic Foot Syndrome has been reported to significantly help reduce the rate of major amputations in diabetics and to be related with limb salvage percentages in excess of 76%, with a mean hospital stay of 27 days and with 30–50 HBO sessions (Cianci, 1990, 1991).

The Italian experience is similar and the use of HBO in diabetic gangrene is associated with a reduction of the average hospital stay from 100 days to approximately 60 days, an increase of the treatment efficacy rate from 66.66% to 91.43%, and a reduction of major amputation rates from 33.33% to 8.57% (Baroni, 1987; Favales, 1989; Faglia, 1996).

1. Divers Alert Network Europe
2. Centro Iperbarico Ravenna, Italy
3. Division of Baromedicine, University of Malta
4. International School of Baromedicine, University of Belgrade

The "end point" which defined the outcome of the treatment was "limb conservation." An acceptable "limb conservation" includes minor amputation procedures of toes
or forefoot. Major amputation (BKA or AKA) was considered as a "treatment failure."
The group of HBO treated patients received an average number of 38 treatment
sessions (see Tables 1 and 2) (Faglia 1996).

The multivariate statistical analysis of the Faglia 1996 data seems to confirm a protective role of Hyperbaric Oxygen Therapy against the risk of major amputation in the
diabetic patient with ischemic ulcers of the foot (Wagner grade 3–4).

Table 1: Age and Gender Distribution - Faglia 1996 study			
	HBO group	Control group	Total
Total Patients	35	33	68
males	27	21	48
females	8	12	20
Mean Age	**61,7**	**65,6**	**63,6**

Table 2: Efficacy of Treatment - Faglia 1996 study		
	HBO group	Controls
Efficacy	91,43	66,66
no amputation	31,43	30,30
minor amputation	60,00	36,36
major amputation	8,57	33,33

COST-EFFECTIVENESS EVALUATION

The goal of an effective cost-benefit evaluation should be to evaluate the
convenience of a new form of treatment as compared to the "standard" alternative.
A correct evaluation should take into consideration not only the direct costs of the
clinical procedures involved, but other factors, such as the quality of life, long term
health care, and social costs, etc.

Such an evaluation should not be intended as a substitute to clinical evaluation and
judgement, but it should be used as an essential instrument for health management decision making (Diabetes Care and Research in Europe, 1994).

Marroni, Oriani, and Wattel (1996), based on an extensive literature review and on
original data obtained from the Regional Administration of Friuli Venezia Giulia in Italy
for the year 1989, estimated a potential Hyperbaric Oxygen Treatment cost of 6.000
European Currency Units (ECU) per diabetic patient and a possible saving of approximately 6.000 ECU per patient on hospital care costs for diabetic foot lesions.

The comparative analysis of the literature and the demographic data indicated that Hyperbaric Oxygen Treatment could significantly reduce the average duration of hospital stay, as well as the general and amputation-related morbidity and mortality rates in diabetic foot patients.

Based on the Faglia 1996 study, and on his previous 1995 data, Rychlik (1997) presented a model for the evaluation of the economic impact of Hyperbaric Oxygen Treatment for diabetic foot lesions, as compared to standard therapy.

The model also considered factors and elements which followed discharge from hospital and which included continuing social costs and the quality of life of these patients.

In particular, an estimate of the economic impact of the increase in social costs of a disabled patient until reaching his/her retirement age, instead of the absolute life expectancy data, has been preferred as an economic indicator, as only premature retirement, due to a significant disability after a major amputation, is likely to have a different economic impact when compared to the other possible treatment alternatives.

The decision making process to determine the economic efficacy of the treatment in the Rychlik's model considered both direct and strictly medical factors (no amputation, minor amputation, major amputation) as well as indirect cost-service factors (home care, prolonged hospitalization).

The direct costs involved in HBO treatment were generally higher when compared to the standard treatment approach of the individual patient (38.708 DM vs. 29.254 DM in the author's estimate), whereas the indirect costs were lower (2.565 DM vs. 5.171 DM).

The overall data reflecting the total treatment costs, if efficacy and final outcome are disregarded, seem to indicate that the choice of using HBO treatment for the diabetic foot may produce higher health care costs when compared to standard therapy, as is shown in Table 4.

However, when the cost of the two treatment alternatives is compared with the treatment's efficacy and final outcome, and when the factors affecting social costs and quality of life are taken into consideration, the situation is inverted and it appears that the use of HBO treatment may produce a saving of approximately 14%, per affected extremity, in the health care cost of the diabetic foot, as is shown in Table 5.

The saving results mainly from the significant reduction in the disability-related costs, due to an earlier healing, a shorter hospitalization time, and the fact that increased social costs due to premature retirement may be avoided or significantly reduced.

Rychlik (1997) concluded that adjunctive hyperbaric oxygen therapy in the treatment of the diabetic foot shows a better cost-benefit ratio when compared to a primary choice of major surgery and amputation.

Based on a study by Lapaucis et al. (1988), and using the data from the Faglia 1996 study, we evaluated the health economic indicator known as "Needed Number of Treatments (NNT)," which equals the ratio: <100/positive outcome percentage difference between two treatment modalities.

The NNT is considered a useful parameter when budgeting health care management and a tool in the decision making process of selecting the most appropriate form of treatment for a given condition. The NNT indicates the relative efficacy between two treatment modalities, and a low value shows an increased probability that a favorable event (i.e., healing) occurs. The NNT for HBO treatment of the diabetic foot is 4, which, according to the Lapaucis study (1988), can be considered a positive index of the efficacy of HBO treatment, when compared with primary surgical treatment.

Table 3: Economical indicators and HBO treatment of the Diabetic Foot - Marroni 1996					
	Mortality	Morbidity	Hospital stay	HBO Cost	Saving (ECU)
HBO	—%	< 5 % (amputation)	< 60 days	6.000	=
Non-HBO	>31% (amputation)	>30% (amputation)	> 100 days		> 6.000

Table 4: Clinical costs of HBO vs. Standard treatment - Rychlik 1997			
Treatment	Direct Costs	Indirect Costs	Total Cost
HBO	38.708 DM	2.565 DM	41.273 DM
Standard	29.254 DM	5.871 DM	34.925 DM

Table 5: Cost - Efficacy of HBO vs. standard treatment of the diabetic foot - Rychlik 1997			
Treatment	Direct Costs	Indirect Costs	Total Cost
HBO	42.336 DM	2.806 DM	45.141 DM
Standard	43.885 DM	8.507 DM	52.392 DM

ECONOMICAL EVALUATION

We evaluated economically the epidemiological and demographic 1995 data of the Italian Ministry of Health on ulcerated diabetic foot and diabetic foot lesions having an amputation risk (ISTAT coding: ICD-IX n. 2506- 25061- 25069, DRG 18), available through the Internet.

An estimated number of 7700 diabetic foot patients meeting the search criteria were found.

The need for HBO treatment was calculated using the formula elaborated by Persels (1987), on the basis of a previous paper by Workman (1984).

$$P5 = P1 \times M1 \times M2 \times M3$$

where:

P5 = total HBO sessions for a given patient population in one year

P1 = number of hospitalizations for a given diagnosis in one year

M1 = correction factor for outpatients affected by P1 condition

M2 = fraction of P1 diagnosed patients effectively responding to HBO treatment

M3 = mean number of HBO sessions required for the P1 diagnosed HBO indication

The "M" values for diabetic foot lesions as indicated by Persels are:

Diagnosis	P1	M1	M2	M3
Diabetic gangrene		2	0.4	30

Using Persels' formula on the number of diabetic foot patients discharged from Italian hospitals in 1995, shown above, a total of 6160 patients should/could have been treated with HBO for their condition, with a total number of hyperbaric oxygen treatment sessions of 184.800 nation-wide.

The average cost of a hyperbaric treatment session has been evaluated in Euro—at the value of 80 Euro per HBO session. The average cost of a hospital-day has been estimated in the range of 250 Euro per day, although it is understood that this cost may be somewhat underestimated, especially for severely ill patients, needing intensive medical and surgical care.

Table 6 shows the estimated number of HBO treatment sessions needed and their total cost.

Table 7 shows the potential saving if HBO treatment of the diabetic foot is adopted and the parameters considered by the studies we referred to are used in the calculation.

If all the 7.700 hospitalized patients are computed with an M2 multiplier of 1 (that is, if all of them were treated with HBO), the overall cost of treatment would obviously increase, but this would not significantly affect the end-point overall saving (see Table 8).

If the further saving, estimated according to the Rychlik model, is calculated, the potential saving produced, per diabetic patient's lifetime, according to Rychlik, is equal to 7251 DM, or 3.625 Euro per patient.

If this figure is applied to the estimated Italian diabetic foot patient population in 1995 (see above), this would result in a total saving (life-time) of (15.400 pts. x 3.625) = 55.825.000 Euro for the National Health Care system, for the considered patient population.

Our personal experience, as well as the available literature, indicates that the average age of the diabetic foot patient population ranges between 55 and 60 years. Considering the regular retirement age in Italy (65 years), this would mean a pre-retirement average period of approximately 8 years.

Table 6: Estimated number of annual HBO treatments and costs in Italy (1995 data). Costs expressed in Euro.				
Condition	Patients	Persels Formula	HBO Treatments	HBO cost
Diabetic Gangrene	7700	7700 x 2 x 0.4 x 30	= 184.800	14.784.000 Euro

Table 7: Estimated HBO absolute costs vs. resultant savings on hospitalization costs. Costs are expressed in Euro.			
Condition	HBO Costs	Hospital Costs Saving	Net Saving
Diabetic Gangrene	14.784.000 Euro	77.000.000 Euro	62.216.000 Euro

Table 8: Estimated HBO absolute costs vs. Resultant savings on hospitalization costs. Separate accounting for In-patients (M2 = 1) and out-patients (M2 = 0.4) Costs are expressed in Euro

Condition	HBO Costs	Hospital Costs Saving	Net Saving
Diabetic Gangrene In-pts. (7700 x 30 x 80)	18.480.000 Euro	77.000.000 Euro	62.216.000 Euro
Diabetic Gangrene Out-pts. (7700 x .4 x 30 x 80)	7.392.000	0	0
Totals	25.872.000	77.000.000	51.128.000

The consequent division of the lifetime saving estimated according to Rychlik, if the overall figures reported in Table 5 are evaluated on an annual basis instead of on a life-time period, would equal an overall annual saving rate of 6.978.125 Euro, which should be added to the previously computed Potential Net Saving (see Tables 7 and 8).

The final figures would therefore indicate a potential annual saving for the National Health Care system ranging between 58 and 69 million Euro, if Hyperbaric Oxygen Treatment would be included as a standard adjunctive treatment modality in the therapy of the diabetic foot.

CONCLUSIONS

Hyperbaric Oxygen treatment of diabetic foot lesions (Wagner grade 3–4) not only appears to be clinically effective, but it also seems likely to induce considerable savings in the general costs of a nation's health care and social systems and a better quality of life for the patients. Based on these data a prospective study on the economical impact of the use of HBO therapy, as an adjunctive treatment for diabetic foot lesions, is, in our opinion, highly recommend.

REFERENCES

1. Baroni G, et al. Hyperbaric Oxygen Therapy in Diabetic Gangrene treatment. Diabetes Care; 1987;10: 81.
2. Chantelau E., Spraul M., Berger M. Das Syndrom des diabetischen Fußes - Neue Aspekte. In: W. Hepp (a cura di): Der diabetische Fuß, Berlino Vienna; 1996.
3. Cianci P. Adjunctive Hyperbaric Oxygen in the salvage of the diabetic foot. Undersea Biomed Res; 1991; 18 (suppl): 108.
4. Cianci P, et al. Salvage of the difficult wound / potential amputation in the diabetic patient. Hyperbaric Medicine Proceedings. Foundation for Hyperbaric Medicine Basel; 1990; 4: 177.
5. Cignetti E., et al. Fattori di rischio del piede diabetico: studio su una popolazione in assistenza ambulatoriale. Atti VIII Congresso Nazionale AMD, Editoriale BIOS, Cosenza 1991: 171.
6. Della Marchina M., Trojani C. Piede diabetico dati epidemiologici e costi economici. Atti VIII Congresso Nazionale AMD, Editoriale BIOS, Cosenza, 1991: 197.
7. Diabetes Care and Research in Europe: The Saint Vincent Declaration. Diabetic Medicine; 1990, 7: 360.
8. Canadian Coordinating Office for Health Technology Assessment: Guidelines for Economic Evaluation of Pharmaceuticals. Canada, 1st Edition, Ottawa. 1994.
9. Faglia E., Favales F., Aldeghi A., Calia P. Quarantiello A., Oriani G., Michael M., Campagnoli P., Morabito A. Adjunctive systemic hyperbaric oxygen therapy in treatment of severe prevalently ischemic diabetic foot ulcer. Diabetes Care; 1996; 19 (12): 1338-1343
10. Favales F., et al. OTI e Diabete Mellito. In: Oriani G., Faglia E., Eds. Ossigeno Terapia Iperbarica, applicazioni cliniche. Edizioni SIO Milano; 1989, 111.
11. Laupaucis A., Sackett DL., Roberts RS. An assessment of clinically useful measures of the consequences of treatments. New Engl. J. Med; 1988; 318: 1728-1733.
12. Marroni A., Oriani G., Wattel F. Cost Benefit and Cost-Efficiency Evaluation of Hyperbaric Oxygen Therapy. In: Oriani G., Marroni A., Wattel F., (eds). Handbook on Hyperbaric Medicine. Springer-Verlag, 1996: 879-886.
13. Persels J. Developing the Hyperbaric Medicine Service. J. Hyper Med; 1987, 2: 97.
14. Rychlik R. in HBO Therapie - Kosten/Effektivitàts Analyse. Expertenforum: HBO im Gesundheitsweisen. Germany 14 May; 1997: 37-41.
15. Rychlik R. Stellenwert und Notwendigkeit der Pharmacoökonomie In: Die Pharmazeutische Industrie, 1995; 57: 274-277.
16. Vannini P., Ciavarella A. Criteri di prevenzione del piede diabetico. Atti VIII Congresso Nazionale AMD, Editoriale BIOS, Cosenza, 1991: 161.
17. Workman WT., et al. Medical Planning criteria for implementation of clinical hyperbaric facilities. Brooks Air Force Base, TX, USAF School of Aerospace Medicine, 1984.

NOTES

COST-EFFECTIVENESS—RELATION OF THE TREATMENT OF DIABETIC FOOT LESION WITH HYPERBARIC OXYGEN THERAPY VERSUS STANDARD THERAPY

Reinhard Rychlik

Institute of Empirical Health Economics—Am Ziegelfeld

28-D-51399 Burscheid, Germany

POSITION OF THE PROBLEM

Diabetes mellitus is a major and growing health problem at all ages and all countries. This incurable and lifelong metabolic disorder may lead to numerous complications in case of inadequate treatment. The diabetic foot lesion is a delaying complication typical of diabetes mellitus diagnosed 10 years before. Diabetic foot lesion is defined as a syndrome of various clinical pictures characterized by their different etiology and pathomechanisms. They all have in common that lesions of the feet of diabetes mellitus patients may result in complications at worst including amputation of all extremities. The clinical picture of diabetic food lesion has a major impact on quality of life and life expectancy, as well as prospects of all those affected.

Today, diabetic foot lesion is the most common cause of amputation of lower extremities. Such a high frequency of amputations by no means represents unavoidable late complication. Rather, they indicate the inadequacy of both prophylaxis and therapy. Consequently, the St. Vincent Declaration sets a target of the reduction of the frequency of amputation of 50%.

The therapy of diabetic foot lesion depends on the severity of the lesion based on the classification by Wagner 1984/Boulton 1988. As a rule normoglycemia must be guaranteed. At zero degree lesion prophylactic measures such as meticulous foot care, training of patients, and correction of foot deformities must be taken. At one degree local wound treatment with ablation of necrosis, local wound disinfection, wound drainage, and myocutanous transplantation would be necessary. Selective antibiotic treatment may rule out infections. The choice of antibiotics is based on recommendations by the Deutsche Gesellschaft für Chemotherapie for the treatment of soft tissue infections. Mainly bactericidal substances which have proven effective against Staphylococci and Streptococci must be considered, e.g., second generation cephalosporines. Moreover clindamycin is suitable due to its high bone resorption as well as its wide germicidal spectrum. Rheological measures (pentoxifylline, naftidrofuryl) and if necessary vascular surgical interventions (e.g., bypass) are intended to remedy the hyperfusion as well as the peripheral oxygen deficiency. Despite all measures taken it will often prove impossible to sufficiently provide even minor blood vessels with oxygen supply. Thus, patients will not be unable to escape amputation, resulting in being indicated for hyperbaric oxygen therapy.

The health economic cost-effectiveness analysis is an attempt to investigate the efficiency of the HBO therapy compared to standard therapy. Therefore advantages and disadvantages of both alternatives must be comprehensively considered. The health economical comparison will only be complete if all direct, indirect, as well as intangible costs will be taken into consideration.

The object of present analysis will be the introduction of adjuvant HBO therapy in the treatment of diabetic foot lesion. This analysis centered around the question of which of the alternative therapies—standard therapy plus hyperbaric oxygen therapy or standard therapy alone—incurs the best cost-effectiveness ratio. The comparison of costs and benefits was made on the basis of a cost-effectiveness analysis.

The perspective taken is that of the society.

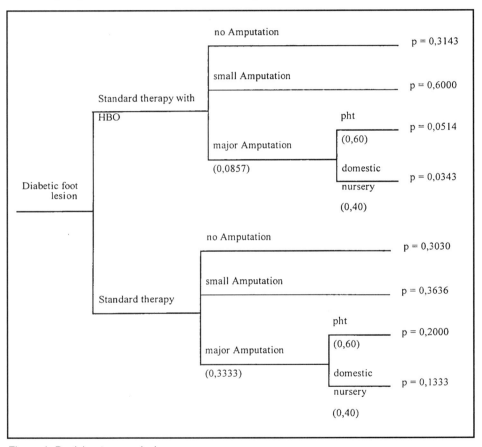

Figure 1. Decision tree analysis.

METHODS

This analysis based on a clinical trial from Faglia, E,. et al, 1996. The materials studied did not allow for a meta-analysis as the smallest common denominator of all study designs would neglect basic health/economical aspects. Moreover the result of a number of published studies would not be sufficient for present analysis. Also, patients hospitalized due to severe lesions received a randomized treatment of adjuvant HBO therapy. In addition the study comprises results differentiated according to no amputation, minor amputation, and major amputation which are essential from a health/economic perspective. The underlying clinical trial meets the guidelines as applicable for health/economical studies. The following populations have been evaluated as to the number of amputations (Table 1).

Whereas patients in the control group were exclusively treated according to the standard therapy protocol, the patients in the HBO group received an adjuvant HBO therapy. Accordingly the therapy was considered to have succeeded if the ulcer had been healed and only minor amputations had been necessary. Major amputations were judged to be therapy failure.

A decision tree with four endpoints was constructed:

1. successful therapy without amputations
2. small amputations
3. major amputations with post-hospital treatment
4. major amputation with domestic nursing

The effectiveness was defined as avoided major amputation.

Table 1: Populations compared in the clinical trial				
	HBO group	Control group	Total	
			absolute	relative (%)
Number of patients	35	33	68	100
Men	27	21	48	70.59
Women	8	12	20	29.41
Average age	61.7	65.6	63.6	-------

Table 2: Effectiveness of the alternative therapies				
	HBO group		Control group	
	absolute	relative (%)	absolute	relative (%)
Number of patients	35	33	68	100
no amputations	11	31.43	22	66.66
minor amputations	21	60	12	36.36
major amputations	3	8.57	11	33.33

Data regarding the number and severity of amputations underlying were taken from the underlying clinical study. Health care costs included in the model were all medical costs (hospitalization, surgical intervention, drug costs, etc.) and indirect costs (absence from workplace, retirement). The following effectiveness rates were revealed in the clinical study (shown in Table 2): population with adjunctive hyperbaric oxygen therapy (HBO) 0.9143, population only with standard therapy 0.6666.

Contrary to the clinical study cost relevant aspects after hospitalization are considered in the present model. Therefore the average patient resulting from the clinical trial has been looked at between hospitalization and retirement. This endpoint was preferred to death as—unlike an regular retirement—an early retirement will have an impact on the alternatives.

RESULTS

In order to assess the costs arising from the alternative therapies, each endpoint of the decision tree was consequently assigned measures incurring both direct and indirect costs. If the respective weighting resulting from the clinical trial is taken in consideration, both direct and indirect costs have been assessed.

All together, adjuvant HBO therapy is shown to entail higher costs than that with standard therapy. The results are presented in Table 3.

Table 3: Results				
Therapy	Direct Costs	Indirect Costs	Total Cost	Effectiveness adjusted cost
Therapy with HBO	DM 38,708 $21,504	DM 2,565 $1,425	DM 41,273 $22,929	DM 45,142 $25,079
Standard therapy	DM 29,253 $16,251	DM 5,670 $3,150	DM 34,925 $19,402	DM 52,398 $29,110

Standard therapy plus hyperbaric oxygen therapy resulted in total costs of DM 45,142 ($25,079) per successfully treated patient, Standard therapy incurred total costs of DM 52,398 ($29,110) per successfully treated patient.

Owing to the higher effectiveness of HBO therapy compared to standard therapy, HBO therapy incurs costs per avoided amputation may be decreased by approximately 14%.

In conclusion, both alternatives considered in the present model are seen to incur high direct costs there is, due to the introduction of treatment by HBO, a cost saving reduction of time off work, coinciding with a shortening of the healing process as well as avoidance of early retirement due to an incapacity to work resulting from an amputation. An adjuvant treatment of diabetic foot lesion with HBO therapy will lead to a more favorable cost-effectiveness ratio compared to standard therapy.

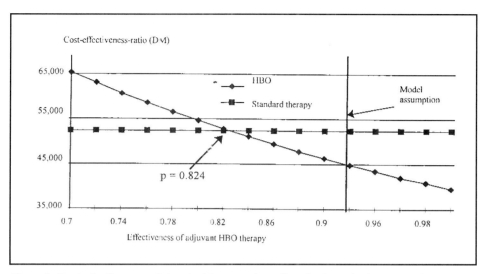

Figure 2. Cost-effectiveness of standard therapy plus adjunctive hyperbaric oxygen therapy.

SENSITIVITY ANALYSIS

To prove the robustness of the model a sensitivity analysis was performed to determine the influence of the efficacy on the incremental cost-effectiveness ratio.

This shows that the treatment of diabetic foot lesions with adjunctive hyperbaric oxygen therapy by a ratio of effectiveness of p = 0,824 would be equal in cost compared to standard therapy.

CONCLUSION

The outpatient treatment preceding hospitalization could not be included in the model due to a lack of data. This may be assumed to be the large potential of resources spent on the treatment of diabetic foot lesion as the treatment extends over a period of several years. Therefore the effectiveness of HBO therapy as proven in the clinical trial may indeed point to a potential for saving costs in the case of patients being hospitalized. This may be concluded from the reduction in long-term outpatient treatment with HBO. This hypothesis has to be proven in a prospective health economical study including quality of life.

REFERENCES

1. Chantelau, E., M. Spraul, M. Berger: Das Syndrom des diabetischen Fufles - Neue Aspekte; W. Hepp (Hrsg.): Der diabetische Fufl, Berlin Wien, 1996, S. 8.
2. Diabetes Care and Research in Europe: The Saint Vincent Declaration; Diabetic Medicine 1990, 7, S. 360.
3. Rychlik, R.: Stellenwert und Notwendigkeit der Pharmacoökonomie; die pharmazeutische industrie, 1995, 57, S. 247-277.
4. Faglia, E, F. Favales, A. Aldeghi, P. Calia, A. Quarantiello, G. Oriani, M. Micheal, P. Campagnoli, A. Morabito: Adjunctive Systemic Hyperbaric Oxygen Therapy in Treatment of Severe Prevalently Ischemic. Diabetic Foot Ulcer. Diabetes Care, 1996, 19 : 1338 - 1343.
5. Hannoveraner Konsensgruppe: Deutsche Empfehlungen zur gesundheitsökonomischen Evaluation. DMW, Thieme Verlag, 1996, 121. Jg., Nr. 51/52, A19-A 21.

EXPERIENCE OF A MULTIDISCIPLINARY UNIT

Pierre Fontaine
Diabetic Foot Unit—Clinque Marc Linquette—CHRU Lille, France

Chronic wounds of the lower extremity are common in diabetic patients (1). Foot ulcer incidence in France is estimated about 40 000 a year. These ulcers are the result of three pathogenic factors : arterial insufficiency, peripheral neuropathy, and infection (2,3) which are frequently associated. Foot ulcers are a grave complication of diabetes mellitus, but unfortunately, have received less attention than the other complications. The risk of lower extremity amputation is 10- to 14-fold higher in diabetic patients than in the non-diabetic population (4,5,6,7). Diabetes is the first cause of non-traumatic amputations in adult patients. Surgical complications and mortality are also increased in diabetic patients (7,8,9). Chronic wounds of lower extremities in diabetics are a public health problem in Europe and United States. The economic cost of treating these patients is extremely high (10).

In Europe, wound management is being influenced by the Saint Vincent declaration, the joint European World Health Organisation and International Diabetes Federation initiative, which emphasize prevention of diabetic complications (11). One of the principal goals was to reduce lower extremity amputation rate in diabetics by 50% in five years.

Traditional wound care practice was a fragmented approach without a coordinated diagnosis or treatment plan established between different specialists. Conversely, wound care clinics offer the advantage of a coordinated multidisciplinary care provided in a single setting.

THE DIABETIC FOOT AND THE ROLE OF A MULTIDISCIPLINARY CLINIC

Diabetic foot clinics offer many advantages over traditional approaches and contribute to achieving improvement in the quality of wound care practice. Reading many reports regarding multidisciplinary approaches, indicates that four specific points appear to be beneficial to patients with chronic wounds.

Multidisciplinary Team in a Single Setting

Treatment of a complex disease such as diabetic foot ulcers requires a multidisciplinary management with the close collaboration of a team for care.

The most important members of the team are the diabetologist as coordinator, the physical therapist, the podiatrist, the vascular surgeon, the orthopaedist, the pedorthist, and the nurse specialist in diabetes and wound care. Other members of the wound care team include the specialist of hyperbaric medicine, the radiologist, the plastic surgeon, the dermatologist and the bacteriologist.

The multidisciplinary setting is important factor of quality in care practice (12,13,14):

- access of patients to care is easy, allowing early intervention,
- presence of different specialists allow patients to benefit from rapid, coordinated care,
- patients are followed up by the same team until final outcome,
- care is improved by emphasizing compliance and continuity,
- multidisciplinary system is associated with relatively low cost,
- healing rate and duration are improved in multidisciplinary clinic over standard care.

Patient benefits are observed by all authors who have organised a multidisciplinary foot clinic (14,15,16).

Coordinated Wound Assessment and Wound Care Management

Wound management is a crucial aspect of patient care, but the effect of diabetes on wound healing is a very complex issue that continues to leave many unanswered questions.

The wound care team is often faced with the question of which approaches to provide an environment that supports healing and prevents complications? How different types of wounds should be dressed? What method of debridement to use? Whether dressing should be changed using sterile versus unsterile technique, and which adjunctive therapies to select under given circumstances (16,17,18,19,20)?

Multidisciplinary management allows coordinated process for different steps of assessment and care. Every member of the wound care clinic knows the comprehensive wound care program:

A. Patient evaluation by history, physical examination, and laboratory studies. Accurate assessment of neurologic, vascular, metabolic status is essential for addressing the etiologic factors involved.
B. Wound classification and measurement.
C. Wound care practice:

- Local surgical treatment of wound (wound debridement, incision and drainage of abscesses, bone resection for severe osteomyelitis, distal amputation for gangrene).
- Dressing to use in different types of wounds and in different stages of healing.
- Agents used to accelerate healing (topics, growth factors preparations, cultured cell preparations).
- Antibiotic therapy.

D. Measures to eliminate pressures and maintain weight bearing (insoles, protective shoes, custom footwear, total contact walking casts, or complete bed rest).
E. Limb salvage procedures in patient with ischemic ulcers (surgical by-pass or endoluminal procedure).
F. Skingrafts (free tissue transfer or pedicle flaps).

    G.   Use of adjuvant hyperbaric oxygen in treatment of severe ischemic foot ulcer or refractory infection.

    H.   Major amputation (above knee amputation).

Every out-patient or in-patient can be evaluated and treated under the same wound care program. This program is written in a background paper which is regularly updated.

All authors point to multispeciality integrated treatment protocol to produce the greatest success (14,15,21,22,23).

Prevention and Education Program

Diabetic patients and caregivers education (24,25,26,27,28)

- Prevention of primary and recurrent ulcers in diabetics can be increased through programs to educate patients and caregivers. Prevention program emphasizes education, regular follow-up, hygiene, and lifestyle modification; it is best implemented by a multidisciplinary team co-ordinated by the diabetologist. Such teams are variably composed and may include a nurse educator, a podiatrist, an orthotist, and the primary care physician.
- Foot screening can individualise specific foot problems and provide an understanding of risk factors to prevent complications. Diabetic patients with a high risk of foot ulceration are referred to the clinic for ongoing management to prevent complications and amputation. Education is an integral part of preventive program and of quality health care.
- Patients with foot ulcers are discharged from the acute care setting to the home care setting at a much earlier time in their recovery; wound care will be delivered by patients, family members, home healthcare providers rather than by the hospital nurse. Teaching regarding wound care, universal precautions, and prevention of wound complications have become a vital comportment of preparing the diabetic patients for optimal continuity of care at home.

Professional Education (29,30)

- Professional education strategies are developed in foot clinics. These strategies are aimed at all members of the comprehensive health-care team, especially primary-care practitioners, home care nurses, and podiatrists; professional education emphasizes appropriate management regarding assessment of clinical risk-status, regular foot examination, assurance of follow-up according the risk, treatment methods, and when to refer patients to multidisciplinary foot clinic. These programs increase coordination of care between foot clinic team and primary-care practitioners.
- Wound care clinics provide valuable experience for the training of physicians, student nurses, student podiatrists, and other health care personnel.

Evaluation Program

Multidisciplinary foot clinic allows the care team to develop three types of evaluation:

- Protocols to evaluate topically applied agents of wound healing or other medical or surgical therapies.
- Epidemiological evaluation of programs that seek to prevent low-extremity amputation in diabetic population.
- Economic analysis to evaluate cost of different wound care strategies.

Concerning economic analysis, treatment of diabetics patients with foot ulcers in a multidisciplinary clinic is associated with relatively low costs, because higher probability for primary healing in out-patients (31,32).

DIABETIC FOOT CLINIC—UNIVERSITY HOSPITAL OF LILLE: AN EXAMPLE OF MULTIDISCIPLINARY UNIT

The Foot Clinic

We organized a diabetic foot clinic in the university hospital of Lille in 1992. The clinic is under the direction of the department of diabetology, physical medicine, vascular surgery, and hyperbaric medicine with support of the departments of plastic surgery, orthopaedic surgery, vascular surgery, vascular radiology, infectious diseases and dermatology. The clinic have agreement with the school of podiatry. Podiatrist students and graduate assistants are present every day for care. Nurses are specialists in diabetes education and wound care.

The clinic is housed in a out patient unit of the department of diabetology. A suite of two examining rooms and two dressing rooms is available for patient evaluation and treatment. Diabetic out-patients are seen five afternoons each week. Rooms are used by nurses of the department of diabetology every morning for in-patients dressing.

In this clinic, we have developed a multidisciplinary approach with coordinated management.

Missions of the multidisciplinary team of the diabetic foot clinic are:

- assessment and care of out-patients with chronic wounds
- evaluation of new therapies
- prevention and education
- selection of high risk of wound diabetics
- professional education and training
- development of a computed database for epidemiological and economic analysis
- organisation of wound care in hospitals of the district around our clinic

Two hundred diabetic subjects were evaluated and treated in the clinic every year. Fifty percent were non-insulin dependent diabetic patients. The primary cause of ulcers was arterial insufficiency in 50% of cases and diabetic neuropathy in 50%. Infection was present in 25% of all cases.

Collaboration with hyperbaric department

In our clinic, hyperbaric oxygen therapy (HBO) is an adjunctive treatment for non-healing ulcers in association with surgery and local wound care. Collaboration with hyperbaric unit is then an important factor of success.

Adjunctive HBO therapy is proposed in treatment of severe ischemic foot ulcer, refractory infection, or skin grafting (33,34). In all cases, a coordinated care, especially with surgeon and hyperbaric medicine specialist, is very important. Rapid accessibility to the hyperbaric unit for treatment is a factor of success in wound healing.

HBO therapy initiated twice a day consists of pure oxygen a 2.5 ATA for 90 minutes. After 20 sessions, evaluation of healing is done by team for stop or continuation. During HBO therapy, dressing are done by nurses of hyperbaric unit with the same wound care protocol established in the clinic by care team.

Patients with ischemic ulcers have a rapid coordinated management for assessment and treatment with collaboration between foot clinic, vascular insufficiency, and hyperbaric unit. Vascular insufficiency is explored by Doppler, arteriography and transcutaneous oxygen pressure ($TcPO_2$) under different conditions. In all cases, possibility of revascularization is evaluated (35). In our experience, the distal $TcPO_2$ et 2.5 ATA pure oxygen is a reliable test to predict final outcome with ischemic wound healing when hyperbaric oxygen therapy is used (36).

CONCLUSION

Diabetic foot clinics with coordinated multidisciplinary care provided in a single setting appears to be a condition to achieve goals of Saint Vincent declaration concerning lower extremity amputation rate. The foot clinic is the base on which diabetic foot care can be organized in collaboration with primary-care practitioners. Diabetic foot clinics have to be developed for increased education, prevention, wound care, and for decreased economic cost. Accreditation processes engaged in western countries have to take account of these alternative experiences for wound care management.

REFERENCE

1. Bild DE, Selby JV, Sinnock P, Browner W, Braveman P, Showstack J. Lower extremity amputations in people with diabetes : epidemiology and prevention. Diabetes care, 1989 ; 12 : 24-31.
2. Edmonds ME. The diabetic foot : pathophysiology and treatment. Clin Endocrinol Metab, 1986 ; 15 : 889-916.
3. Mc Neely MJ, Boyko EJ, Ahroni JH, Stensl VL, Reiber GE, Smith DG, Pecoraro RE. The independent contributions of diabetic neuropathy and vasculopathy in foot ulceration : how great are the risks. Diabetes Care, 1995 ; 18 : 216-219.
4. Humphrey ARG, Thoma K, Dowse GK, Zimmet PZ. Diabetes and nontraumatic lower extremity amputations : incidence risk factors and prevention a 12 years follow-up study in Nauru. Diabetes care, 1996 ; 19, 7 : 710-714.
5. Edmonds M, Boulton A, Buckeman T, Every N, Foster A, Freeman D, Gadsby R, Gibby O, Knowles A, Pooke M, Tovey F, Unwin N, Wolfe J. Report of the Diabetic foot and amputation group. Diab Med, 1996 ; 13, 9: 527-542.
6. Most RS, Sinnock P. The epidemiology of lower extremity amputation in diabetic individuals. Diabetes Care, 1988 ; 6 : 87-91.
7. Siitonen OI, Siitonen J, Niskanen LK, Pyorala K, Laakso M. Lower-extremity amputations in diabetic and non diabetic patients. A population-based study in eastern Finland. Diabetes Care, 1993 ; 16,1 : 16-20.
8. Apelvist J, Larsson J, Agardh CD. Long-term prognosis for patients with foot ulcers. J Int Med, 1993, 233 : 485 - 491.
9. Donahue RP, Orchard TJ. Diabetes mellitus and macrovascular complications. An epidemiological perspective. Diabetes Care 1992, 15 : 1141-1155.
10. Halimi S, Benhamou PY, Charras H. Le coût du pied diabétique. Diabetes Metab, 1993 ; 19 : 518-522.
11. Piwernetz K, Home PD, Snorgaard O, Antsiferov M, Staehr-Johansen K, Krans M. Monitoring the targets of the St Vincent declaration and the implementation of quality management in diabetes care : the DIABCARE initiative. The DIABCARE Monitoring Group of the St Vincent Declaration Steering Committee. Diab Med 1993 ; 10,4 : 371-377.
12. Ghirlanda G, Mancini L, Castagneto M, Citterio F, Serra F, Cotroneo AR, Marano P. The foot clinic. Multidisciplinary management of the patient with diabetic foot. Rays, 1997, 22,4 : 638-643.
13. Knowlfs EA, Gem J, Boulton AJ. The diabetic foot and the role of a multidisciplinary clinic. J Wound Care, 1996 nov, 5, 10 : 452-454.
14. Steed DL, Edington H, Moosa HH, Webster MW. Organization and development of a university multidisciplinary wound care clinic. Surgery, 1993, 114,4 : 775-79.
15. Apelqvist J, Ragnarson-Tennvall G, Persson U, Larsson J. Diabetic foot ulcers in a multidisciplinary setting. An economic analysis of primary healing and healing with amputation. J Inter. Med. 1994, ; 235 : 463-471.
16. Edwards V. A multidisciplinary approach to foot care in diabetes. Community Nurse, 1998, 4,2 : 53-55.
17. Ennis WJ, Meneses P. Strategic planning for the wound care clinic in a managed care environment. Ostomy Wound Manage 1996 ; 42,3 : 54-56.
18. Maklebust J. Using wound care products to promote a healing environment. Crit Care Nurs Clin North Am, 1996 ; 8,2 : 141-158.
19. Meyers JS. Diabetes and wound healing. Crit Care Nurs Clin North Am, 1996 ; 8,2 : 195-201.
20. Hanft JR, Fisch SE, Fryberg R, Sage R, Sanders LJ. Wound management in the diabetic foot. J foot ankle surg 1997 ; 36,3 : 240-254.
21. Foster AV, Snowden S, Grenfell A, Watkins PJ, Edmons ME. Reduction of gangrene and amputations in diabetic renal transplant patients : the role of a special foot clinic. Diab et Med, 1995; 12,7 : 632-635.
22. Ciresi KF, Anthony JP, Hoffman WY, Bowersox JC, Reilly LM, Raapp JH. Limb salvage and wound coverage in patients with large ischemic ulcers : a multidisciplinary approach with revascularization and free tissue transfer. J Vasc Surg 1993 ; 18,4 : 648-653.
23. Faglia E, Oriani G, Favales F, Michael M, Aldeghi A, Calia P, Morabito A, Quarantiello A. Adjunctive systemic hyperbaric oxygen. Therapy in treatment of severe prevalently. Ischemic diabetic foot ulcer. Diabetes care, 1996 : 19,2 : 1338-1343.
24. Shenaq SM, Klebuc MJA, Vargo D. How to help diabetic patients avoid amputation : prevention and management of foot ulcers. Post Graduate Medicine, 1994 ; 96,5 : 177-191.
25. Litzelman DK, Slemenda CW, Langefeld CD, Hays LM, Welch MA, Bild DE, Ford ES, Vinicor F. Reduction of lower extremity clinical anomalities in patients with non-insulin dependant diabetes mellitus. Annals of internal medicine, 1993 ; 119,1 : 36-41.
26. Edmonds ME, Van acker K, Foster AV. Education and the diabetic foot. Diabet Med 1996 ; 13 suppl 1 : S61-S64.
27. MC Cabe CJ, Stevenson RC, Dolan AM. Evaluation of a diabetic foot screening and protection program. Diabet Med, 1998 ; 15,1 : 80-84.
28. Kravitz M. Out patient wound care. Crit Care Nurs Clin North Am, 1996 ; 8,2 : 217-233.
29. Barnett A. Prevention and treatment of the diabetic foot ulcer. Br J Nurs, 1992 ; 11,2 (1) : 7-10.
30. Doucette MM, Fylling C, Knighton DR. Amputation prevention in a high-risk population through comprehensive wound healing protocol. Arch Phys Med Rehabil, 1989 ; 70, 10 : 750-785.
31. Apelqvist J, Ragnarson-Tennvall G, Larson S, Persson U. Long-term costs for foot ulcers in diabetic patients in a multidisciplinary setting. Foot Ankle Ind 1995, 16,7 : 388-394.
32. Apelqvist J. Wound healing in diabetes - outcome and costs. Clin Podiatr Med Surg 1998 ; 15, 1 : 21-39.
33. Chantelau E. Hyperbaric oxygen therapy for diabetic foot ulcers. Diabetes care, 1997 jul ; 20, 7 : 1207-1208.
34. Uunger HD, Lucca M. The role of hyperbaric oxygen therapy in the treatment of diabetic foot ulcers and refractory osteomyelitis. Clin Podiatr Med Surg, 1990 ; 7, 3 : 483-492.
35. Chambon JP, Fontaine P, Vambergue A, Fournier A, Fossati P, Quandalle P. Results of sub-inguinal revascularization in the treatment of diabetic ischemic foot. Chirurgie 1996, 121 (6) : 401-405.
36. Wattel F, Mathieu D, Coget JM, Billard V. Hyperbaric oxygen therapy in chronic vascular wound management. Angiology, 1990 jan ; 41, 1 : 59-65.

SECTION II
ECHM WORKSHOPS

ECHM Workshop On

New Methods of Fire Fighting in Hyperbaric Chambers— Theory and Life Tests

Section II

May 21 and 22, 1999—Lübeck, Germany

ORGANIZED BY GERMANISCHER LLOYD, HYPER S.T. GKSS

CONTENTS

THE CONFERENCE IS SPONSORED BY

- Sechrist Industries Inc.
- Smith & Nephew Healthcare Ltd.
- Musgrave Systems Ltd.
- Environmental Tectonics Corporation
- Haux Life Support
- Hemocue
- Hytech Hyperbaric and Diving Systems
- Jane Saunders and Manning Ltd.
- Mara Engineering Ltd.
- Radiometer Ltd.
- RDG Medical
- Sat Medical
- Sayers Hyperbaric and Dicing Systems GmbH

THE USE OF SPRAYED WATER AS AN EXTINGUISHING AGENT INSIDE HYPERBARIC THERAPEUTIC CHAMBERS

Jean-Pierre Bargiarelli

There are two main ways to extinguish a fire:

- cool it down with water
- smother it by means of a neutral gas, foam, or blanket, etc.

Manually operated foam fire extinguishers have been used extensively in chambers for many years to effect. However, due to the specific nature of therapeutic chambers, a remotely-controlled system based on sprayed water and operated from the control console of the chamber would seem more appropriate.

We have carried out two kinds of tests to check capability of different nozzles, keeping in mind that we have to cover almost all the volume of the chamber:

FULL JET 1/2 GA
MISTEX 1AGTI
MISTEX 3YT8
FOGTEC 050031

1. SEE APPENDIX 1 AND VIDEO TAPE

1.1. To control at atmospheric pressure:
- flow rate versus supply pressure
- shape of the water spray

1.2. To control that the flow rate and the shape of the water spray are the same under pressure (3 ATA) and at atmospheric pressure
- This is confirmed by the figures in Appendix 1 and by the video cassette, provided that the over-pressure pushing the water remains the same.

2. SEE APPENDIX 2 AND VIDEO TAPE

These tests were carried out on a fire of one kilogram of paper, in a confined atmosphere but not under pressure. Two temperature sensors were installed:
- One located in the heart of the fire to indicate maximum fire activity and complete extinction.
- One located 60 cm from the fire to indicate temperature variations in the chamber.

Extinguishing means was 11 litres of water sprayed by means of air pressure. Graphics in Appendix 2 show duration of extinction.

DISCUSSION

As a result of these tests it was demonstrated that:

1. A significant fire inside a confined atmosphere can be extinguished using an appropriate sprayed water system.
2. Owing to the substantial volumes of smoke and vapour produced, survivability can only be guaranteed by breathing fresh air through the oral-nasal mask.
3. A series of fire tests must be conducted in a chamber under pressure to confirm ability of sprayed water under pressure.
4. We have also to develop an automatic fire detection system able to start automatically the water spraying system in hyperbaric conditions.

USE OF SPRAYED WATER EXTINGUISHERS FOR HYPERBARIC CHAMBER FIRE-FIGHTING RESULTS OF N° 1 NOZZLE TRIAL

	TRIAL N°	DEPTH	SUPPLY PRESS.	FLOW DURATION	FLOW
S.S.CO.50W :	1	Surface	5 Bar	20 Secondes	33 Litres/Min
	2	Surface	10 Bar	15 Secondes	44 Litres/Min
	3	Surface	15 Bar	12 Secondes	55 Litres/Min
	3*	Surface	20 Bar	10 Secondes	66 Litres/min
	4	20 Mètres	5 Bar	18 Secondes	33 Litres/Min
	5	20 Mètres	10 Bar	15 Secondes	44 Litres/Min
	6	20 Mètres	15 Bar	12 Secondes	55 Litres/Min
	6*	20 Mètres	20 Bar	10 Secondes	66 Litres/min
Mistex 1AGT1 :	7	Surface	5 Bar	60 Secondes	11 Litres/Min
	8	Surface	10 Bar	55 Secondes	14.5 Litres/Min
	9	Surface	15 Bar	35 Secondes	18.5 Litres/Min
	9*	Surface	20 Bar	30 Secondes	22 Litres/min
	10	20 Mètres	5 Bar	70 Secondes	9.5 Litres/Min
	11	20 Mètres	10 Bar	50 Secondes	13.5 Litres/Min
	12	20 Mètres	15 Bar	40 Secondes	16.5 Litres/Min
	12*	20 Mètres	20 Bar	30 Secondes	22 Litres/min
Mistex 3YT8 :	13	Surface	5 Bar	150 Secondes	4.5 Litres/Min
	14	Surface	10 Bar	90 Secondes	7.5 Litres/Min
	15	Surface	15 Bar	80 Secondes	8.5 Litres/Min
	15*	Surface	20 Bar	70 Secondes	9.5 Litres/min
	16	20 Mètres	5 Bar	150 Secondes	4.5 Litres/Min
	17	20 Mètres	10 Bar	95 Secondes	6.5 Litres/Min
	18	20 Mètres	15 Bar	80 Secondes	8.5 Litres/Min
	18*	20 Mètres	20 Bar	70 Secondes	9.5 Litres/min
Fogtec 050.031 :	19	Surface	20 Bar	200 Secondes	3.5 Litres/Min
	20	20 Mètres	20 Bar	195 Secondes	3.5 Litres/Min

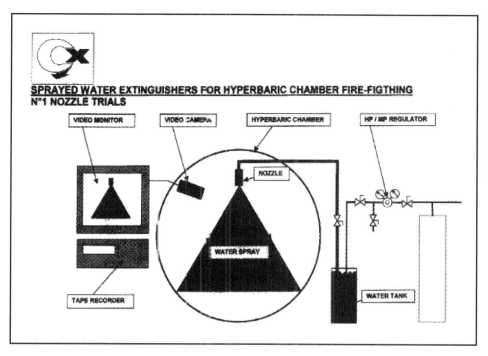

Figure 1. Sprayed water extinguishers for hyperbaric chamber fire-fighting N°1 nozzle trials.

USE OF SPRAYED WATER EXTINGUISHERS FOR HYPERBARIC CHAMBER FIRE-FIGHTING RESULTS OF N° 2 NOZZLE TRIAL

NOZZLE	SUPPLY PRESSURE	TIME TO LOWER TEMPERATURE FROM 500 TO 30°C
Fulljet S.S.CO.50W :	5 Bar	10 Secondes
	10 Bar	7 Secondes
	15 Bar	5 Secondes
	20 Bar	5 Secondes
Mistex 1AGT1 :	20 Bar	15 Secondes
Mistex 3YT8 :	20 Bar	3 Secondes*
	20 Bar	6 Secondes

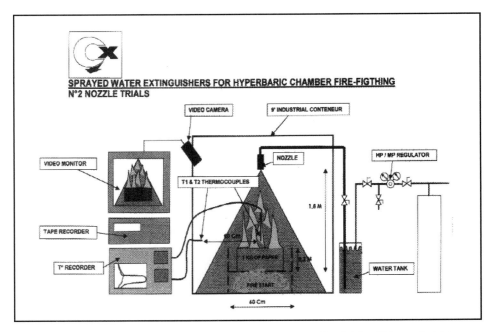

Figure 2. Sprayed water extinguishers for hyperbaric chamber fire-fighting N°2 nozzle trials.

FIRE SUPPRESSION IN HYPERBARIC CHAMBERS

William C. Gearhart
University of Pennsylvania Medical Center
Institute for Environmental Medicine

Fire Suppression in Hyperbaric Chambers is a review of the inspection, testing and maintenance procedures for fixed fire suppression equipment in the hyperbaric environment. The review was based on existing requirements presented by the National Fire Protection Association, National Oceanic and Atmospheric Administration, and the Undersea and Hyperbaric Medical Society.

OBJECTIVES

The objectives were two-fold. First, the various standards were presented to create familiarity with these references. Secondly, the importance of integrating the fire suppression system into the operational maintenance program was emphasized.

METHOD

An explanation of the importance for maintaining fire suppression systems was developed using data from the NFPA. The concept of "Scheduled" and "Emergency" impairments was explained along with their respective impacts on the operational capability of the hyperbaric chamber.

CONCLUSIONS

Fixed fire suppression systems are the first line of protection in the event of a chamber fire. Therefore, their reliability must be guaranteed, since the pressure boundary of the hyperbaric environment creates a situation where occupants cannot readily escape or seek refuge in another area. The potential for rapidly developing toxic gas fires in a confined space requires strict guideline adherence to prevent both loss of life and property damage. Fixed fire suppression systems are proven to be the most effective and cost efficient devices available for fire protection. Personnel involved in the operation of hyperbaric chambers should be knowledgeable regarding inspection, testing, and maintenance of fire suppression systems.

INSPECTION, TESTING & MAINTENANCE OF WATER BASED FIRE PROTECTION SYSTEMS IN CLINICAL HYPERBARIC CHAMBERS

The reliability and satisfactory performance for water based fire suppression systems in the hyperbaric environment (Class A) are contingent upon performing prescribed procedures as part of a scheduled program.

OBJECTIVES

Each participant should understand the purpose for inspection, testing & maintenance of the Fire Suppression System and be familiar with the supporting documents (codes & standards), system components, testing methods, testing schedules, and the importance of integrating the Fire Suppression System into the routine maintenance program of the facility.

LECTURE OUTLINE

I.   Purpose
    A. Ensure Reliability
      1. Operational
        a) Mechanical Systems
    B. Confidence
      1. No Second Chance
    C. Statutory and Regulatory Compliance
      1. National Fire Protection Association - NFPA 99, Chap 19-2.5
      2. UHMS - Guidelines for Clinical Multi-place Hyperbaric Facilities
      3. Standard Operating Procedures - SOP

II. Types of Tests
    A. Compliance Tests
    B. New Installations or Modifications to Existing Installations
      1. Acceptance Tests
        a) Design Criteria
          1) Supply Duration (NFPA 99, 19-2.5.2.4)
          2) Minimum Operating Time (NFPA 99, 19-2.5.2.5)
            a) 15 Seconds Operation by Stored Pressure
          3) Handline Pressure (NFPA 99, 19-2.5.3.4)
            a) 50 PSIG OBP

      2. Acceptance Test is the most comprehensive
        a) Should cover all facets of the design and performance criteria
      3. Documentation
        a) Pass/Fail
        b) Perform necessary adjustments / corrections
        c) Procure documentation for any waivers from authority having
          jurisdiction (AHJ), stating the rationale for providing the waiver
        d) Sign Off
          1) AHJ
        e) Benchmark for Routine Inspections & Testing
    C. Routine Inspections & Testing
      1. Operational Reliability
        a) Manual Activation Controls
        b) Automatic Activation Controls
      2. Initiation & Activation of Related Components & Systems (NFPA 99, 19-2.5.1.3)

          a) Visual & Aural Appliances

          b) Electrical Disconnect

          c) Emergency Lighting & Communication Systems

          d) Water Level Sensor to Prevent Sudden Pressurization of Chamber from Driving Air Source

    3. Annunciation to Building Fire Alarm System (NFPA 99, 19-2.5.1.4)

    4. Critical / Emergency Controls of Electrical System (NFPA 99, 19-2.5.1.6)

          a) Switch Gear

          b) Transfer Gear Test

          c) Load Test

    5. Operating Times

          a) Deluge Operation

             1) Water in 3 seconds or less (NFPA 99, 19-2.5.2.2)

    6. Pressure & Flow Test

          a) Handline Pressure Test (NFPA 99, 19-2.5.3.4)

             1) 50 psig OBP (residual)

             2) 5 GPM simultaneous any two hose lines

    7. Handline Hose Length

          a) Bilge Access (NFPA 99, 19-2.5.3)

  D. Test Schedule

    1. Hyperbaric Fire Suppression Systems are unique

    2. Several Guidelines exist for inspection frequency

    3. A composite of several guidelines has been used to create the attached guide

          a) Deluge Systems, functionally tested at least annually (NFPA 19-2.5.5)

          b) Handline Systems, functionally tested at least annually (NFPA 19-2.5.3.4)

          c) By-Pass tests performed monthly (UHMS Multi-place Guidelines)

III. Highlights

    1. Closed Valves—Valves not in Proper Baseline Position cause most problems

    2. Independent Hose & Deluge Water Sources

    3. By-Pass Test Valve Arrangement

    4. Water Quality - Potable Source

    5. No black iron pipe permitted

    6. Inspect pipe to ensure adequate brackets, hangers, and supports

IV. Integrate Fire Suppression System Maintenance into Routine Maintenance

    1. Don't create an Inspection, Testing & Maintenance nightmare

    2. Use Inspection & Testing Procedures as "Hands on Training" for all chamber personnel. Develop Emergency Preparedness Programs using Inspection & Testing Procedures as the simulator

    3. Document the test and the results

    4. Create a history

    5. Performing a proper test constitutes more than simply flowing water. All related electrical components such as alarms, sensors, and disconnects should also be tested

INSPECTION & TESTING

Schedule
Daily
1. Tank & System Pressure (measured directly in the piping system)
2. Tank & System Pressure (measured at the console)
3. Water Level in Tanks (preferably by sight glass or reliable instrument) (A malfunctioning pressure gauge will not indicate actual water level)
4. Control Valve Positions—All valves should be locked or supervised in their baseline position
5. Nozzle Obstructions—orifices checked visually and no impediments to discharge or shielding from other equipment in the chamber

Monthly
1. All daily inspections
2. Flow test using "By-Pass" Valve, Actuation by alternate switch*

Quarterly
1. All daily & monthly inspections
2. Flow test using "By-Pass" Valve, Actuation by alternate switch

Annual
1. All daily, monthly & quarterly inspections
2. Complete visual inspection: damaged, leaking pipe, hangers, brackets
3. Complete system discharge test using test hoses connected to internal chamber piping

Tri-Annual
1. Interior Water Tank Inspection (Pressure Tanks and Non-Pressurized Steel Tanks without corrosion protection
2. Other Tanks—Every Five Years

* Activate Deluge System using main panel, remote panel and internal chamber switches.

This document integrates information from NFPA 99, 25 and UHMS Multi-place Guidelines.

REFERENCES

1. Standard for Health Care Facilities, (NFPA 99, 1999 Edition) National Fire Protection Association, 1 Batterymarch Park PO Box 9101 Quincy, MA 02269-9904.
2. Standard for Inspection, Testing & Maintaining Water Based Fire Protection Systems, (NFPA 25, 1995 Edition) National Fire Protection Association, 1 Batterymarch Park PO Box 9101 Quincy, MA 02269-9904.
3. Fire Protection Handbook, (NFPA 17th Edition, 1991) National Fire Protection Association, 1 Batterymarch Park PO Box 9101 Quincy, MA 02269-9904.
4. Guidelines for Clinical Multi-place Hyperbaric Chambers, UHMS, Kensington, MD.
5. Safety Standard for Pressure Vessels for Human Occupancy, (PVHO-1 ASME) American Society of Mechanical Engineers, 1997 345 East 47th Street, New York, NY 10017.

NOTES

FIRE SAFETY STANDARDS, REGULATIONS AND SYSTEMS USED IN THE UNITED KINGDOM

Roly Gough-Allen

This lecture will describe the fire safety standards, regulations, and systems used in the United Kingdom. Fire safety is not just about one set of regulations. It is the whole facility approach to maintaining good staff education and a positive safety program.

OBJECTIVE

Attendees should have an overview of the British Hyperbaric Association (BHA) and the type of fire safety standards, regulations, and equipment presently used in the United Kingdom. Safety requires a team commitment to all aspects of safety.

THE SITUATION IN THE UNITED KINGDOM (UK) PRIOR TO 1990

The 1980s saw a significant increase in the use of hyperbaric oxygen (HBO) for the treatment of conditions other than diving.

In 1981 the Health and Safety Executive issued Diving at Work Regulations to improve the offshore oil industry diving safety record. These regulations covered all working divers and diving contractors. However, they were not suitable for clinical hyperbaric facilities, although many tried to apply them as nothing else existed. In 1997 these regulations were updated (1), but again, unless a facility registers as a diving contractor, they do not apply to clinical hyperbaric facilities.

THE BRITISH HYPERBARIC ASSOCIATION (BHA)

Due to the need for appropriate standards and a general lack of knowledge of hyperbaric oxygen therapy, the British Hyperbaric Association was formed in 1990.

The BHA is a professional group of medical, nursing, and technical practitioners and is working towards a co-ordinated approach for British facilities, in terms of clinical practice and management. It is hoped that consistency of service and quality can thus be achieved.

Membership is open to all hyperbaric facilities in the British Isles receiving emergency referrals. The membership consists of approximately 26 facilities and numerous individual associate members.

It is the chamber facilities which make up the primary membership, but within each facility all personnel, medical, nursing, and technicians are encouraged to participate and join as associate members for a nominal fee.

The aims are:

a) To promote the understanding and safe practice of hyperbaric medicine;
b) To provide a forum for discussion of hyperbaric therapy in the British Isles, with particular consideration to:
    - Clinical indications,
    - Therapeutic standards,
    - Audit and research,
    - Funding,
    - Management,
    - Safety Standards;
c) To foster friendship and communication between isolated doctors and recompression facility personnel;
d) To encourage exchange of information and treatment problems, a common database, the best use of resources available, and methods of closer unification;
e) To encourage a method by which peer group review is acceptable and current medical advances are disseminated;
f) To discuss methods of achieving long term financial support.

At present the BHA only produces guidelines and has no authority or desire to enforce standards.

In 1991 the BHA asked the Faculty of Occupational Medicine of the Royal College of Physicians of London to produce 'A Code of Good Working Practice for the Operation and Staffing of Hyperbaric Chambers for Therapeutic Purposes' (also known as the COX report)(2)

The code of practice was published in 1994 and went a long way to improve the UK situation. However it also highlighted additional needs and therefore the BHA formed working parties to publish guidelines on:

- Education and Training (3)
- Fire Safety Standards (4)
- Electrical Safety Standards (5)
- Health and Safety for Therapeutic Hyperbaric facilities. (6)

HYPERBARIC CHAMBERS CATEGORIES

Category 1 (ALS)

Multiplace chambers capable of supporting the treatment of patients who are critically ill from any cause and who may require hyperbaric intensive therapy; such facilities offer Advanced Life Support.

Category 2 (BLS)

Multiplace chambers capable of receiving elective or emergency referrals for any accepted application of hyperbaric oxygen therapy, but excluding patients who are critically ill at time of referral or who are likely to become so; such facilities offer Basic Life Support.

Category 3 (DIVERS)

Multiplace chambers specifically intended for the treatment of decompression illness; such facilities offer Basic Life Support.

Category 4 (MONOPLACE)

Monoplace chambers capable of receiving elective and emergency referrals in any diagnostic category, but who are unlikely to require emergency access during treatment; such facilities offer Basic Life Support and would normally be closely associated with a hospital.

GENERAL HEALTH AND SAFETY

The basis of UK health and safety law is 'The Health and Safety at Work Act 1974' (HASAWA)(7). The law states that employers have to look after everyone working for them or on their premises, and anyone affected by what they do. It covers all work premises. Employees also have a duty of care to look after themselves and their colleagues.

Health and Safety Regulations are law and further regulations are introduced from time to time, such as 'The Management of Health and Safety at Work Regulations 1992' (8). Both the above regulations give the employers the freedom to decide how to control risks. Some risks are so great that specific regulations are issued that set out explicit actions to be taken.

'Approved Codes of Practice' give practical advice on how to comply with the law. These or an alternative method may be used too but employers need to demonstrate that they have complied with the law.

Authorities can issue 'Guidance' (or professional bodies) and these provide information for best practice. They are not compulsory; they help people understand the problem.

'A Code of Practice' is a document drawn up by organisations with an interest in a particular field. A Code of Practice is not approved by the Health and Safety Commission and can not be used in court proceedings, unlike an Approved Code of Practice. Codes offer best practice at the date of issue. Health and Safety Legislation is administered by the Health and Safety Commission (HSC) and the Health and Safety Executive (HSE) The HSC develops health and safety policies and makes proposals. The HSE enforces the law and provides advice.

RISK ASSESSMENT

The HSE produces a free small leaflet called 'Five Steps to Risk Assessment (9)(8), and in this publication is a straight forward guide for every employer. All employers must conduct suitable and sufficient assessment of the risks to health and safety of its employees or others coming into the workplace. Risk assessment is a proactive process of assessing the risks associated with activities. This is an essential part of managing health, safety, and environmental issues within the organisation.

In carrying out a risk assessment, employers are required to assess the risks to workers and others that may be affected by their actions. Employers must document the assessments. Every hyperbaric facility must have a risk assessment generic to that site; this will identify the site hazards and decide who might be harmed and how, then evaluate the risks arising. The risks can then be either eliminated or reduced to as low as reasonably practical. This should be reviewed periodically and the risk assessment updated as necessary. The person who creates the risk owns, controls, and regulates it.

All significant risk assessments will then lead to the production of Standard Operating Procedures (SOPs) or Emergency Procedures (EPs). All therapeutic hyperbaric facilities must have buildings, plant, equipment and administration structures that are 'fit for purpose.' All SOPs and EPs should be in a manual accessible to all the hyperbaric team.

European legislation has had a significant impact on UK Health and Safety law. In recent years a set of regulations embodying the European directive on Health and Safety management were passed into UK law in 1992 (Management of Health and Safety at work Regulations) and Approved Codes of Practice (ACOPs). (4)

HEALTH AND SAFETY FOR THERAPEUTIC HYPERBARIC FACILITIES

In 1994 the BHA formed a Health and Safety working party with advice from the HSE and are due in 1999 to publish a document, 'Health and Safety for Therapeutic Hyperbaric Facilities: "A Code of Practice"(6).'

The code gives practical guidance on the safe operation of facilities to meet the requirements of existing health and safety legislation. The guidance in the code relates to the safety of personnel working in or adjacent to the hyperbaric facility and to others who may be affected by the operation of the facility.

The guidance advises specifically on the application of UK health and safety legislation to those providing hyperbaric treatment, whether it be to emergency or elective patients.

A therapeutic hyperbaric facility consists of the therapeutic chambers (multi- or monoplace) together with all associated plant and buildings, staff (technical and medical), and a specific administrative organisation led by the hyperbaric therapy provider.

The hyperbaric treatment team consists of all medical and technical personnel directly involved with the hyperbaric treatment of a patient.

The fundamental concept of this code is that the Hyperbaric Therapy Provider and the Supervising Chamber Operator have very defined responsibilities. Every facility shall have one person and one person only who is nominated as the Hyperbaric Therapy Provider, and who is in overall administrative control of the Facility.

The Hyperbaric Therapy Provider's general responsibilities are to ensure that:

a) Risk assessments have been carried out for all predictable technical or administrative aspects of the therapeutic hyperbaric facility operation;
b) There are sufficient personnel available in the hyperbaric treatment team to provide adequate patient safety and safe technical operation of the chamber during a hyperbaric treatment;
c) The personnel in the hyperbaric treatment team are competent;
d) Sufficient plant and equipment is provided for safe technical chamber operation and that it is fit for purpose, correctly certified, and maintained;
e) Medical equipment for use in the hyperbaric environment is sufficient, appropriately maintained, correctly certified, and fit for purpose, as advised by the medical director of the therapeutic hyperbaric facility;

f) Written Standard Operating Procedures (SOPs) and Emergency Procedures (EPs) are available, which include treatment protocols for guidance, and which include procedures for both medical and technical emergencies and contingency plans. The Standard Operating Procedures should be signed and dated by the hyperbaric therapy provider;

g) A Medical Director, Hyperbaric Facility Manager, and Supervising Chamber Operator are appointed in writing and the extent of their delegated responsibility is documented;

h) There is a clear reporting and responsibility structure laid out in writing;

i) There is appropriate occupational health provision for staff;

j) All other relevant legal requirements are complied with.

The Supervising Chamber Operator is responsible for:

a) Direct supervision of the pressure system;

b) The safety of the chamber and its occupants;

c) Minor maintenance;

d) Direction and supervision of other technical and maintenance personnel.

The Supervising Chamber Operator with responsibility for the hyperbaric treatment is the only person who can order the start of compression and must be in control of all technical aspects of the chamber operation. It is up to them to ensure staff are competent and the equipment suitable and 'fit for purpose.'

The guide also covers in detail all the other hyperbaric team members and their responsibilities in a similar fashion as the Royal College of Physicians document but in more detail. It discusses team sizes with a minimum of three for a multiplace chamber (Hyperbaric Duty Doctor, Supervising Chamber Operator, and Medical Attendant), and two for a monoplace (Hyperbaric Duty Doctor, Monoplace Attendant). The code of practice is essential reading for any UK clinical facility; it contains the comprehensive information needed to run a safe hyperbaric facility.

UK FIRE SAFETY STANDARDS

The basis of UK fire standards is 'The Fire Precautions Act 1971'(10) and 'The Fire Precautions, Work Place Regulations 1997' (11). Until 1996 no formalised or accepted standard of fire safety for hyperbaric therapeutic chambers was available. The working party 1991–93 produced 'Guide to Fire Safety Standards for Hyperbaric Treatment Centres' (4) and was published in 1996. The aim of this publication was to produce a safety standard to be achieved, rather than a set of measures to be rigidly applied in all circumstances. The guide can not take into account all circumstances and should not be used in isolation.

Where new hyperbaric facilities are being installed as part of a District General Hospital then the guidance issued by the Department of Health under the title of 'Health Technical Memorandum 81'(12) should be used. The facility should be treated as a life risk compartment and provided with the same fire separation and means of escape as an Intensive Care Unit or Operating Department.

Guidance for existing hospitals is contained in the Health Technical Memorandum 85 'Fire precautions in existing hospitals' (13), similarly, the Department providing

Hyperbaric Therapy facilities should have the same fire safety provisions as an Operating Theatre Department.

The document covers fire prevention, communications, alarms, escape, extinguishing fires, and emergency procedures. It must be remembered that the guide was written between 1991–93 and at the time they were goal setting, however sadly we have recently had horrific fires in Europe. At the time of writing, the BHA is considering updating the guidelines to reflect the latest 1999 NFPA-99 standards. New UK facilities would be wise to update their knowledge prior to building new facilities. The table that follows is a brief summary of the UK 'Fire risks and precautions within chambers used for hyperbaric therapies.'

The information listed covers fire risks, which may be experienced in clinical chambers with air environments between 1 and 6 bar. Precautionary measures are given though these are not detailed.

MATERIALS PROHIBITED IN THE CHAMBER

General

The following items comprise a reasonably comprehensive listing of items and materials that should not be allowed into the chamber. The letter(s) proceeding each item indicates the general reason for prohibiting it; the coding is shown below.

> C   possibility of damaging the fabric of the chamber.
> D   contamination of the environment.
> E   explosion risk.
> F   fire source or combustible substance.
> L   could be broken or damaged by pressure.
> M   will possibly cause a mess.
> P   affects the ability of the occupants.

Listing

> a   Adhesives (F)
> b   Aerosols (D,E,F)
> c   Aftershave, perfume, and cosmetics (D,F)
> d   Alcohol (D,E,P)
> e   Batteries with unprotected leads (F)
> f   Chemical cleaners, e.g., trichloroethylene, 'Freon', etc. (D,P)
> g   Cigarettes, cigars, tobacco of all kinds (F,M)
> h   Cleansing powder (C,F,P)
> i   Volatile Drugs (F,P)
> j   Electrical equipment including tape recorders, radios, etc. (F)
> k   Explosives/Ammunition
> l   Glass thermometers including batteries containing mercury (C,D,P)
> m   Ink pens (M)
> n   Lighters (F)
> o   Matches (F)
> p   Non-diving watches (L,M)
> q   Petroleum based lubricants, greases, fluids (F)

r   Sugar and fine powder and other flammable food stuffs (F,F)
s   Thermos flasks (L,P)
t   Non-fire-retardant bedding, including blankets, sheets, pillows, mattresses, etc., except 100% cotton or specialist hyperbaric material

Table taken from The BHA Guide to Fire Safety Standards for Hyperbaric Treatment Centres (4).

UK FIRE RISKS AND PRECAUTIONS WITHIN CHAMBERS USED FOR HYPERBARIC THERAPIES COMPRESSED ON AIR UP TO 6 BAR

Area of risk	Source	Precaution
1. Raised pressure	a. Fire risks in compressed air environments are greater than one atmosphere; e.g., ease of ignition and rate of burning is enhanced in compressed air atmosphere.	Systems should be so designed as to minimise the risk of fire and, in the event of such, procedures and hardware should exist to maintain life and minimise damage, e.g., fire extinguishing devices, BIBS, chamber fire procedures, chamber evacuation procedures.
	b. The physical features of the functional therapeutic chamber multiply the hazards of even a very small fire, by containing personnel and restricting escape. One of the most obvious actions to be taken in the event of a fire would be to evacuate the affected compartment, isolating personnel from the danger of fire and noxious gases. In many cases this will not be practical, or at least hampered by the condition of the patient.	Hyperbaric fire-fighting equipment should be fitted to all chamber compartments.
	c. Decompression obligations will negate, or at best delay, evacuation from the hazardous environment	
2. Raised oxygen percentage	a. BIBS leakage when administering oxygen and oxygen-enriched gases (>21%).	Correctly fitting oral nasal masks; provide adult and child sizes. Use BIBS and Hood Tents incorporating an 'overboard dump,' so exhausting expired oxygen-enriched gases from within the chamber. Regularly maintain system, check for leaks prior to use. A flexible extension tube from the internal chamber oxygen sampling line maybe used to discover systems leaks during operation.
	b. Atmosphere replenishment.	Oxygen replenishment systems should introduce gas into the chamber so as to facilitate mixing, e.g., oxygen could be bled into external regeneration return lines, onto internal scrubber fans, jetted at short bursts into the top of the chamber. Oxygen analysers should be fitted with 'high' and 'low' alarms.
	c. Patient ventilators.	Fit a scavenge line into ventilator exhausts so drawing off oxygen-enriched gases expired by the patient and dumping it outside the chamber.
		In all cases, chamber oxygen should be maintained below 24%; concentrations above this will require flushing through with air. (If ventilator is driven with oxygen then this will need drawing off to the overboard dumps.)

Area of risk	Source	Precaution
3. Flammable atmospheres	a. Dust in suspension in a dry atmosphere.	All gas lines should incorporate dust filters; chamber furnishing should be lint-free; chamber should be cleaned out daily.
	b. Volatile substances.	Spirit-based medical wipes should not be used in the chamber. Volatile drugs should be preloaded into syringes outside the chamber. Patients, their clothing and bedding, should be void of spirit based preparations, aftershaves, perfumes, hair spray, pens containing spirit based inks (See Appendix 2). All persons entering the chamber should be checked and relieved of these substances.
4. Flammable materials	a. Clothing: flammability and static arcing.	All chamber occupants should wear 100% cotton materials clean and free from oil and grease. Maintain Relative Humidity between 50%–70%.
	b. Bedding and chamber soft furnishing: flammability and static arcing.	Material of a standard acceptable to hospital use should be employed. Keep all bedding to minimum, as required for the therapy. (Ref. HTM 87).
	c. Foodstuffs: flammability low flashpoint.	Certain foods are inherently flammable and should not be introduced into the chamber in a raw state, e.g., sugar (should be pre-mixed into drinks), butter, etc. (pre-spread on bread).
	d. Lubricants: low flashpoint.	Only permitted lubricants should be used within the chamber, and on any equipment that may be introduced into it, e.g., ventilators, aspirators, stretchers, etc. All such equipment should be checked and authorised as safe prior to use. (Clearly label equipment that IS chamber compatible & if equipment is not labeled do NOT allow it into the chamber).
	e. Paints.	Chamber surfaces to be painted with special-to-purpose fire-retardant, non-toxic fuming materials, and of minimum thickness. Flaking paints should be feathered in and patched as soon as possible; thin sections will ignite readily.
	f. Electrical insulation.	Use fire-retardant, non-toxic fuming, insulated wiring. Electrical wiring feeding life-support and emergency systems should be protected from mechanical and heat damage.
	g. Medical supplies	Flammable materials, such as tissues, medical wipes, and bandages, should be kept to a minimum and may be stored in covered metal containers or drawers. Used materials should also be passed out of the chamber as soon as convenient.
	h. Paper products.	These should be kept to a minimum. Rubbish should be passed out of the chamber as soon as convenient.

Area of risk	Source	Precaution
4. Flammable materials...*cont.*	i. Imported items.	All personnel entering the chamber, regardless of whether it is to be pressurised or not, should declare all equipment they intend to take in with them so that it may be vetted by the chamber supervisor. If the chamber is to be pressurised then 4(a) applies. A notice containing the following or similar information should be prominently displayed over entry lock doors and medical lock doors. **WARNING: FIRE AND TOXICITY RISK** No flammable or toxic materials, such as lighters, matches, flammable liquids, oil containing articles or clothing, are to be taken into the chamber. Instruments containing mercury are never to be taken into the compression chamber. Remember the flammable and toxic danger from drugs, etc. Staff should be briefed prior to entering the chamber, the above restrictions being enforced.
5. Electrical/electronic systems.	a. Chamber fires may be caused by electrical defects.	Electrical equipment should be kept to the absolute minimum; that which is employed should comply with relevant regulations and standards (HSE, AODC, BS, and IEE). All systems should be protected by RCD's (ELCB's), trips being located in main control area. Wiring must be protected from mechanical damage. All systems should be regularly maintained and checked as part of the pre-therapy routine.
	b. Motors, e.g. scrubbers.	Should be encased in metal, brushless, and switched externally.
	c. Switches and connectors.	Power supplies should be located outside the chamber and initiated by external switching. Only intrinsically safe switches should be used inside the vessel. Batteries and connectors must not be connected / disconnected inside during pressure exposures, as this also is a source for arcing.
	d. Lighting.	Only hyperbaric compatible lighting should be used inside the chamber, e.g. monofilament fibre-optic light.
	e. Battery-powered equipment.	Medical equipment normally powered by internal batteries should be kept to a minimum. As a rule batteries should not be allowed in the chamber (though we know those of certain construction / materials can not contaminate the environment.)

ELECTRICAL SAFETY STANDARDS (5)

The use of electrically powered equipment in hyperbaric chambers has been hampered by:

a) Its perceived potential as a fire risk in oxygen enriched atmospheres;
b) By the need for electronic circuitry to be pressure resistant or pressure compatible;
c) By the possible requirement of it to be waterproof to protect it during fire suppression measures.

The low demand for equipment to meet these conditions has meant that a generally agreed manufacturing standard has not been developed. At the same time hyperbaric physicians are under an increasing obligation to use electronic equipment routinely available in the hospital ward when caring for patients under pressure. There is a need therefore for some guidelines to ensure safe practice.

Mains Free Supply (240 volts AC) (Recommended)

It is possible to reduce greatly the dangers of mains electricity by the use of an "earth free" mains supply. The system requires the addition of a 1:1 isolating transformer for every power output.

Fire Risk

The ignition temperature of paper is reduced by approximately 25% by compression to 6 atmosphere absolute in air and the rate at which paper burns is significantly increased. As oxygen concentration increases from 21%, ignition temperature falls and burn rate is further increased.

The risk of fire due to ignition from an electrical source in an oxygen-enriched atmosphere is the single most important factor, which limits the use of electrical equipment in pressure chambers. In order to avoid this risk, it is important to keep the level of electrical power used in the chamber to a minimum. Where high power utilisation is essential, such as in the use of a defibrillator, extra care and attention must be paid to avoiding the potential fire hazard.

In this context brief mention should be made of the power derived from batteries, although the voltage levels generated by batteries are generally low, the power produced can be high and 'shorting' across battery terminals can generate large sparks. Further, the lead acid type batteries which are incorporated into a number of medical electrical devices will generate hydrogen gas during recharging and care must be taken that this does not constitute an explosion hazard. More modern lead acid batteries are sealed and may avoid this risk.

Existing International Standards

The International Electrotechnical Commission (IEC) Publication 601:1988 (14) addresses the specification of medical electrical equipment connected to patients, however, does not explicitly deal with equipment to be used in a pressure chamber. The specification requires that equipment be designed for the following environment:

a) An ambient temperature of +10 ˚C to + 40 ˚C;
b) A relative humidity of between 30% to 75%;
c) An atmospheric pressure range of 70 to 106 kPa;
d) A temperature at the inlet of water-cooled equipment not higher than 25 ˚C.

Equipment to be used in a hyperbaric environment will be exposed to much higher pressures and may be intermittently exposed to a higher relative humidity.

As mentioned above, there are also no specifications with regard to oxygen enriched atmospheres.

Since currently accepted manufacturing 'norms' for medical electrical equipment do not make allowance for the hyperbaric environment in terms of humidity, pressure, or high oxygen content, it should be demonstrated that equipment for use in such an environment is 'fit for purpose.' Expert advice should be sought from manufacturers as to whether particular equipment is suitable for the environment.

All equipment should be designed and tested for hyperbaric conditions or be intrinsically safe with regard to them.

All electrical equipment and conductors used in a pressure chamber should be waterproof to a degree such that an electrical hazard is not generated in the event of activation of the fire-extinguishing sprinkler or deluge system.

OTHER RELEVANT POINTS

- Access to and from the chamber and site
- Fire alarms
- Noise levels on the chamber control and inside the chamber
- The regular testing at maximum chamber pressure of fire extinguishers (Empty the contents in to a large bucket)
- BA sets for the chamber control
- Nurse call systems
- Good communications
- Positive smoke extraction from the chamber room
- Location of liquid oxygen supply (distance from risk)
- Two hour plant room fire separation
- Chamber room fire separation from the rest of the building
- Electrical switch gear (RCD / ELCB's)
- Deluge / sprinkler / fogging systems
- Carbon dioxide flooding for plant rooms?
- New chemicals for fighting fires
- Other fire fighting equipment

SUMMARY

- Learn from others.
- Do not try to reinvent the wheel.
- Try not to look at things in isolation.
- Review the whole situation.
- Review all risk assessments regularly.

- Regularly test fire-fighting equipment for yourself at the pressure it needs to operate at.
- We must all maintain and continually update our knowledge and standards.
- The UK has already published many guidelines and more are due to be published soon.
- We must all push for realistic international standards and then regularly update these rather than all working in isolation.

REFERENCES

1. Diving Operations at Work Regulations 1997 HSE Books.
2. A Code of Good Working Practice for the Operation and Staffing of Hyperbaric Chambers for Therapeutic Purposes. The Faculty of Occupational Medicine of the Royal College of Physicians ISBN 1-873240-99-6 Published 1994.
3. Core Curriculum for the Training of Hyperbaric Unit Personnel. British Hyperbaric Association Due to be published 1999.
4. Guide to Fire Safety Standards for Hyperbaric Treatment Centres. British Hyperbaric Association ISBN 0-9527623-1-5 Published 1996.
5. Guide to Electrical Safety Standards for Hyperbaric Treatment Centres. British Hyperbaric Association ISBN 0-9527623-0-7 Published 1995.
6. Health and Safety for Therapeutic Hyperbaric facilities: 'A Code of Practice' British Hyperbaric Association Due to be published in 1999.
7. The Health and Safety at Work Act 1974 (Guidance L1). HSE Books ISBN 0-10-5437743.
8. Management of Health and Safety at Work Regulations 1992 (MHSAW) (SI 2051) (ACOP L21) HSE Books ISBN 0-11-886330-4.
9. Five Steps to Risk Assessment. HSE Books.
10. The Fire Precautions Act 1971 ISBN 010-544-071-X HMSO.
11. The Fire Precautions, Work Place Regulations 1997 (SI 1840) HMSO ISBN 011-064-7386.
12. Health Technical Memorandum 81. Fire Precautions in new hospitals HMSO.
13. Health Technical Memorandum 85. Fire precautions in existing hospitals HMSO.
14. The International Electrotechnical Commission (IEC) Publication 601:1988 Medical electrical equipment (BS 5724:1989) HMSO.

USEFUL ADDRESSES

HSE Publications and free leaflets can be obtained from:

HSE Books
PO Box 1999
Sudbury Suffolk
CO 10 6FS
www.open.gov.uk/hse/hsehome.htm

Dr. A. P. Colvin (Chairman)
British Hyperbaric Association
North Sea Medical Centre Ltd
3 Lowestoft Road
Gorleston On Sea
Great Yarmouth
Norfolk
NR31 6SG
Tel: 0149.341.4141
Fax: 0149.365.6253
Email: apcolvin@northseamedical.demon.co.uk

The Faculty of Occupational Medicine
of the Royal College of Physicians
6 St Andrew's Place
Regent's Park
London
NW 1 4LB
Tel: 0171.317.5890
Fax: 0171.317.5899

Her Majesty's Stationary Office (HMSO)
The Stationary Office
Publication House
Orders Department
PO Box 276
London
SW8 5DT
Tel: 0870.600.5522
Fax: 0870.600.5533
E-mail: book.enquires@theso.co.uk

Roly Gough-Allen
Supply and Demand
Three Point Cottages
Barton Road
Turnchapel
Plymouth
Devon
PL9 9RQ
Tel/Fax: 0044.1752.492490

NOTES

RECENT ACTIVITIES OF GERMANISCHER LLOYD IN THE FIELD OF FIRE PREVENTION AND FIRE FIGHTING IN HYPERBARIC CHAMBERS

Dr.-Ing. Harald Pauli and Germanischer Lloyd

ECHM WORKSHOP ON NEW METHODS OF FIRE FIGHTING IN HYPERBARIC CHAMBERS—THEORY AND LIFE TESTS

Since Germanischer Lloyd was founded in 1867 as a classification society, fire prevention and fire fighting have continuously played an important feature in the work for safety and quality control.

Following the concept of fire protection on board ships and submersibles, GL had put into force new rules for the special tasks of work and research activities in closed environments like diving systems, diving simulators, and hyperbaric treatment chambers in 1986. These rules showed their evidence during the activities of the GKSS underwater simulation system GUSI with manned dives down to 600m diving depth including research and welding procedures with a duration up to 6 weeks.

In the last years GL's point of view moved to fire prevention of equipment used in hyperbaric treatment chambers. So a lot of fire tests were performed in hyperbaric environments to get knowledge of the fire behaviour under real conditions. The results showed in many cases strong deviations from the fire behaviour under normal conditions. Another result showed the influence of positioning the equipment in combination with others and the importance of a sound construction demonstrated, e.g., with an intensive care ventilator.

After the Milan accident the German Government ordered the local authorities to verify the fire protection of the German Hyperbaric Treatment Centers. The criteria for these inspections were elaborated together with Germanischer Lloyd.

Recently GL tested new fire extinguishing systems for hyperbaric chambers utilizing water fog technology with performance nozzles. The results showed the suitability of these systems if especially designed for hyperbaric environment.

Due to national questions regarding fire extinguishing systems for pressure chambers and the worldwide lack of a rule or standard for these systems (except NFPA 99 for sprinkler systems), Germanischer Lloyd initiated a DIN subcommittee to develop requirements and testing standards with the aim to classify systems using different methods of extinguishing.

Place of performance and jurisdiction is Hamburg. The latest edition of the "General Terms and Conditions for Classification" and the "General Terms and Conditions for Classification" and the "General Terms and Conditions for Activities other than Classification" respectively are applicable. German law applies.

NOTES

HYPERBARIC MEDICINE— SAFE MEDICINE

Dr. K.-H. Kieft, Ch. Jung

Hyper S.T., Zentrum für hyperbare Sauerstofftherapie, Lübeck

Hyperbaric medicine covers a wide range, a combination of complicated technical equipment, and well trained people from different fields.

To achieve optimum safety for the patient the whole team should be aware of the interaction between technical and medical requirements and varying treatments.

Permanent training and hypothetical trouble shooting in emergency situations is a must. This should encompass fire fighting inside as well as outside the chamber and should be done in cooperation with local fire brigades and rescue teams. This way the whole team gains security.

An important point is to also include the staff which only works during weekends or employees who stay at the center for only a short period of time.

With regard to the human factor posing a risk in hyperbaric medicine, I will try to develop some ideas and theoretical aspects, which are based on the work and published data of Prof. Unger, who works in the field of security and sensomotoric science at the University of Bremen. He is interested in the behaviour and reactions of individuals in extreme situations, for example a parachutist who is in a situation of extreme stress and danger.

An incorrect action in the wrong moment can be dangerous, which could then result in a deadly accident. It is necessary to analyse and understand the conditions and reasons for these actions, and then develop rules and guidelines for education and training for behaviour in extreme situations. Stress can cause incorrect action. This will prove to be a main point of the following analyses, a result of which may be a better guideline for training and education.

Risk accidents happen in day to day life through wrong actions of people. Today only about 10% of all accidents happen for technical reasons; the other 90% of accidents are caused by human error, by perception or action mistakes. These mistakes happen at the work place, in street traffic, in air and shipping travel, and also during leisure time and last but not least in the field of HBO.

Over the last years risk and accident science has concentrated on the behaviour of individuals. Accident science is not merely quantitative; it analyses of the number of accidents, but also the risk and accident profiles, meaning the development of an accident and the progress thereof.

We were able to find special processing developments behind accidental mistakes. For example, in street traffic a stop sign is passed and a crash happens. This accident enters the statistical records as "stop sign passed." But why did the driver pass the sign; there could have been different reasons for him doing so. For example, the sign was not seen, the sign was recognized, but the decision to stop took too much time, or possibly the driver merely forgot to brake. This shows, that in the development of risk and accident profiles, the determining factor is the perception process of the person, his cerebral function, and his way of action.

Wrong or inappropriate human activity is determined by the sensomotoric operation of perception, cognition, and action. This is important for training and education; for safety processes the "drill" and educational training have to encompass perception, thinking, and action.

Now, I would like to say something about the reasons for stress and the work up of information. Stress is a multifactoral phenomenon. We can separate stress into eustress and distress. Eustress is perceived positively; we are able to work in a better manner (we are able to function better). Distress is recognized in a negative way; efficiency decreases. Distress induces negative feelings, eustress positive.

Distress incriminates our psychovegetative nervous system and decreases the work-up of information. Distress causes transpiration, increases the heart beat, and leads to psychic ill humor.

SPECIFIC REASONS FOR DISTRESS

Some years ago stress science and exploration searched for various single stress factors. The field became more and more complex and thus increasingly difficult to survey. The question unanswered was, does the human brain react specifically under distress caused by one "stressor," or are simple psychocerebral mechanisms a reason for distress reactions. The challenge was to find the common reasons for distress.

We know of three reasons for distress: (Abb./Figure 1)
- First: the excess of information
- Second: the lack of information
- Third: the work up of information

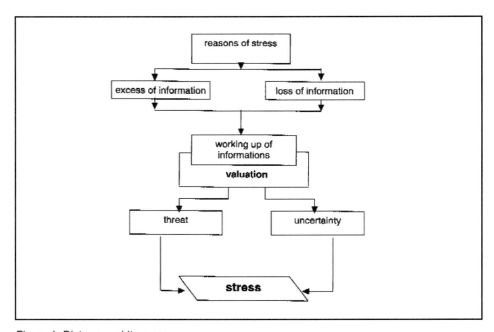

Figure 1. Distress and its reasons.

These are the basic factors which can vary. Excess of information appears when too many facts appear in short intervals of time. In such cases there might be a sudden overload of worked-up information; the person loses control.

Lack of information has not been known for long to be a cause of distress. The exploration of stress focused on excess of information. Thereby the influence of lack of information was neglected. Lack of information means that there is not enough data to find a solution in a specific situation; in case of the parachutist, he cannot find the pull ring, which moves like a pendulum. This situation means, for the skydiver, he does know what ought to be done, but something is missing.

The work up of information is dependent upon the psychocerebral actions in the brain. The main components of cerebral actions are illustrated on the following slide. (Abb./Figure 2)

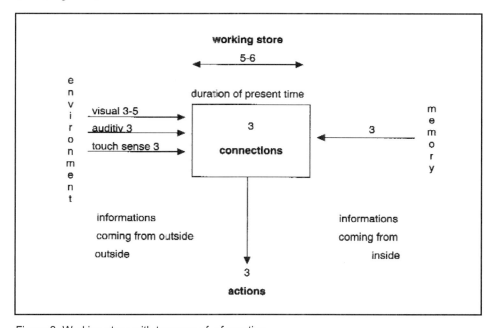

Figure 2. Working store with turnover of information.

First of all, we need to look at the work store of the brain. This is the region, where all information segments which are given are stored, recognized and processed. With known information, the information from the surrounding area is checked first, and then by calculation, weighting and deciding a solution for the problem at hand is found. This is a normal procedure.

Difficulties arise only in case of wrong information turnover, and this can occur under distress.

Information Turnover Becomes Deficient
1) The Incoming Information
We have to separate between vision and hearing. Visual information can constitute of up to 5 objects per second. Under distress this can be reduced. It is possible that only one information segment per second is recognized visually or even only one segement in two or three seconds. The hearing information also has its capacity borders. Per second we are able to recognize three words. Under distress this performance may decrease drastically. It can decrease to one word per second or one word in two seconds. The audible information itself can be the reason for the distress. If there are simultaneous influences for acting, viewing and hearing, the capacity limit is quickly reached.

2.1) The Velocity of Rememberance
In the brain the velocity of rememberance can be three facts per second. This may be words or physical movements. But it is not sufficient to merely achieve rememberance, it has to result in effective actions through transformation. And this cannot be achieved any faster than three words or grips per second. In an emergency case the velocity of rememberance is important. The brain should find the emergency rules quickly and transform it immediately into action. But often we find, after an accident has happened that there has been a significant lapse of time, for example, in street traffic, in case of an accident where there is no braking or delayed braking.

What were the reasons? In case of distress the rememberance velocity is reduced. Besides this there is a reduced velocity of information from the memory in the work store. The brain does not process three facts per second, but only one fact per second. In extreme situations we often need two or three seconds for finding the right action. There may also be a blockage. This is described as the well known black out, as for example happens during a test. This mechanism is also possible in the area of rememberance of learned actions.

Possible Reasons for Such Events
1.) The model (for example a word) was stored inaccurately. Inprecise educational instructions can cause such inaccurate storing. This is also possible when a new task is taught through learning by doing. The first solution may not be the right one. Learning by trial and error can prove to be fatal, for example for a skydiver. The brain stores the mistakes, which were then corrected by the trainer, but in case of an emergency (i.e., disfunctional stress) the mistakes will return.

2.) The training for behaviour in emergency situations used sentences which were too long. The instructions sentence should be short and exact. The storing of key words is preferable; they will reach the working store even in a case of stress. Training and education should emphasize the verb, which is the code for the task to be done. In the brain a verb is quicker activated than a substantive, adjective, or adverb. In case of emergency the brain works only with verb-substantive codes, as for example for the skydiver will. Such speech-fact combinations are called SOKOP units. These are products of sensomotoric combination action in the brain. To overrule disfunctional stress, they have to be strong and stable.

3.) The duration of present time. This is the time to recognize incoming information from the surrounding environment and from the memory and to keep it present in the working store. This takes about 5 seconds. That is normally enough time to recognize a given piece of information about a dangerous situation. We are able to activate the action schedules we have learned, transfer them into the working store and execute the required actions. Well trained actions need only a part of these 5 seconds, so there always exists a sufficient safety range and rest capacity in case of unexpected incidents. Under disfunctional stress the duration of present time can move towards zero. This means that, for example, the skydiver shows no reaction. The person cannot store any incoming information in his working store and has no possibility to use it for trouble shooting and finding a solution in this situation. He falls down without any reaction. He is not able to objectively analyse his situation.

Another example is a situation where individuals are in a burning multistory building and who then jump into the deep. They recognize the heat on one side of their body, while the other side is relatively cool. Their brain fluctuates between these simple decision rules. The long distance of the jump is not rightly realized. During this moment the duration of present time is not sufficient to calculate the jump nor its risks and following consequences; there is not enough capacity. The "heat" pushes for the "life saving" jump.

Comparing this with other emergency situations shows that it is of vital importance to have the resource capacity to visualise and check and play through the final results mentally. This requires precise learning and training and permanent optimation of these specific actions.

4.) The handling: For the brain to be able to realize certain actions to be the solution to a situation in a cognitive way, the actions need to have been followed through in reality. The brain is able to realize three actions (in the skydiver example three grips) per second. If the several actions are well trained they will need less time.

5.) The information store household. The information store household has a volume of 15 single information units, which can consist of words, grips or visual objects. It is important to know which unit dominates in case of an emergency. In case of disfunctional stress the information household is significantly reduced. A volume of less than 5 factors is possible. For the skydiver example: if 3 grips are necessary a volume of only two units remains. The simultaneous input of two words results in an end of the information household.

2.2.) Valuation of a Situation

Distress is caused not only by the dynamics of information work up (Abb./Figure 3).

A second reason may be the personal rating of a situation. A person can realize an excess of information as a threat, whereas thoughts such as, I will have no success, there is no solution for me, would be typical.

The lack of information is realized as uncertainty. Ideas and feelings are described as follows:

Something is missing. I can't get further on. This is shown in figure 4 (Abb. 4).

To be free of distress is merely an attitude of challenge. Threat and overtax result in extreme distress, and a mishap may occur.

The influence of excess of information but also lack of information can be minimised by training and education. The processing of information is improved by education and training in connection with perception, cognitive, and actional operations.

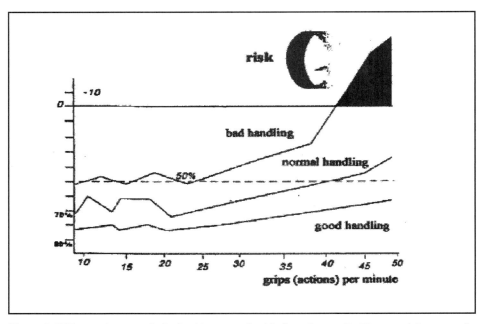

Figure 3. With growing speed of grips increases the binding of capacity. The remaining capacity decreases continuously.

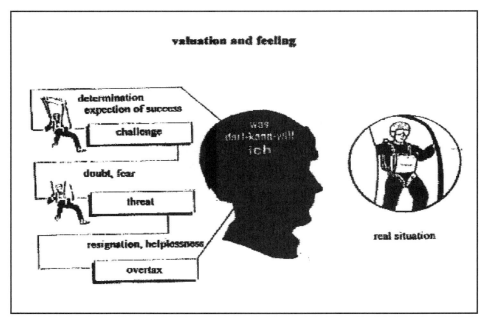

Figure 4. Different valuations of the same situation depending on individual mental attitude.

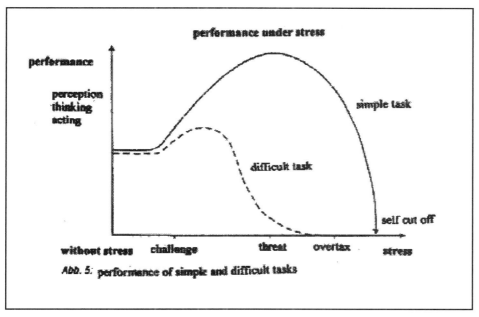

Figure 5. Performance of simple anc difficult tasks.

2.3.) If there is Distress the Performance Will Decrease in a Specific Way

First mistakes happen in tasks with difficult precise actions. "Basic actions" are done relatively well for quite a long time in distress situations (Abb./Figure 5).

Following these rules we can establish some guidelines for education and training. These guidelines could also be applicable for operators of hyperbaric chambers.

1. The teacher should have the necessary expertise in his line of work and be aware of all details and backgrounds.
2. All action and tasks should be well formulated in a correct and clear speaking mode.
3. During education and training there should be a happy mood/positive atmosphere. A bad mood/negative atmosphere during teaching is stored and in case of distress this can lower performance.
4. There should be no teaching and learning through trial and error. The brain stores mistakes made during training, and in an emergency case the brain returns to these mistakes.
5. A "trained" emergency procedure should not be changed.
6. Words which are used during training and education should be clear and precise.
7. All learned actions have to be drilled. We have to separate between training of perception, cognition, and action. All three have to be drilled for quick recognition, decision and quick action. Trained procedures are able to economise on unblocked rest capacity of the brain under stress.

8. Emergency situations cannot always be trained in real situations. They have to be simulated so as to create a mental scenery. The instructions with precise code words for the actions should be trained in a mental simulation; this achieves a high recognition velocity and a good mental support for emergency management.

I think a lot of these rules and thoughts are important also in the field of hyperbaric medicine.

REFERENCES

1. Prof. Dr. Unger: Fehlverhalten in Extremsituationen beim Fallschirmspringen; 1997; Verlag Peter Schäfer GmbH / Blue sky edition, D 34246 Vellmar.

QUALITY MANAGEMENT AND CERTIFICATION OF HYPERBARIC FACILITIES OF THE "VERBAND DEUTSCHER DRUCKKAMMERZENTREN (VDD) E.V." UNDER SPECIAL CONSIDERATION OF FIRE PROTECTION

D Peusch-Dreyer, K-H Dreyer

Center for Diving and Hyperbaric Medicine-ZETÜM-, D-28777 Bremen

Technical standards determined by the "Medizingeräteverordnung", the DIN norms, and the "Medizinproduktegesetz" as well as the supervision by independent experts, e.g., "Germanischer Lloyd" or TÜV, have been obligatory for the operation of a hyperbaric chamber for a long time.

Standards for the qualification of hyperbaric chamber staff and the certification of a complete hyperbaric facility, however, have been defined only recently.

It is the aim of such quality requirements for staff and facility to establish a checkable minimum standard which guarantees the safety of patients in a hyperbaric chamber, also with regard to sufficient fire protection.

In 1995 the German Society for Diving and Hyperbaric Medicine "GTÜM e.V." took a first step in this direction by publishing guidelines to qualify doctors in diving and hyperbaric medicine.

For the first time, the brochure "Qualitätsstandards Hyperbare Sauerstofftherapie —Richtlinien zur Qualitätssicherung in der hyperbaren Sauerstofftherapie" was issued in the fall of 1995 by the "GTÜM e.V." in cooperation with the "Bundesverband Deutscher Druckkammerzentren," the current "Verband Deutscher Druckkammerzentren (VDD) e.V.," and revised in June 1996.

The measures for quality management in hyperbaric medicine were further developed by the VDD e.V., which set up a quality management committee. Since August 1997 it is possible to certify not only physicians, but medical assistants and chamber operators of hyperbaric facilities as well.

The VDD e.V. has issued guidelines for education of the following occupational groups and carries out their certification:

- Nurse for Hyperbaric Medicine (VDD e.V)
- Medical Assistant for Hyperbaric and Diving Medicine (VDD e.V.)
- Hyperbaric Chamber Operator (VDD e.V.)

According to their educational level, Nurses for Hyperbaric Medicine (VDD e.V.) and Medical Assistants for Hyperbaric and Diving Medicine (VDD e.V.) are able to carry out the hyperbaric oxygen therapy on medical order and under medical supervision. They are responsible for the supply and care of patients during hyperbaric therapy and are competent contact persons with respect to the hyperbaric therapy.

After completion of training, the Hyperbaric Chamber Operator (VDD e.V.) carries out hyperbaric treatments according to medical requests. He masters the technical emergency management in the range of hyperbaric chamber engineering, and may accompany patients during hyperbaric treatment, provided that they are not dependent on medical or nursing assistance. Through his educational training, he is able to recognize problems and emergencies during the treatment and to inform the doctor immediately.

Beyond this, both occupational groups must also be certified in preventive fire protection and, if necessary, in sufficient fire fighting.

REQUIREMENTS FOR EACH SINGLE CERTIFICATION

1. Nurse for Hyperbaric Medicine (VDD e.V.)

The following references or documents have to be forwarded to obtain the certification as "Nurse for Hyperbaric Medicine (VDD e.V.)":

- Proof of position as a state-certified nurse
- A certificate showing a two-year training period / vocational experience in anaesthesiology / intensive care
- The certificate "Diving Physician Course A" (30 hours theoretic education) according to regulations of GTÜM
- The certificate "Hyperbaric Medicine Training Course," C, (40 hours education) according to regulations of GTÜM
- A two-week voluntary experience in a hyperbaric facility, working in compliance with VDD e.V. standards (80 hours education)
- A valid certificate proving fitness for diving as shown by regulations of professional trade organization (BG) G31/1.

2. Medical Assistant for Hyperbaric and Diving Medicine (VDD e.V.)

The following references or documents have to be forwarded to obtain the certification as "Medical Assistant for Hyperbaric and Diving Medicine (VDD e.V.)":

- Proof of position as a state-certified nurse, medical assistant of doctors, or paramedic
- Proof of participation in 40 lessons of theoretical / practical training in hyperbaric medicine according to curriculum "emergency management" VDD e.V.
- Proof of 40 hours work experience in an anaesthetic unit or intensive care unit
- The certificate "Diving Physician Course A" (30 hours theoretic education) according to regulations of GTÜM
- The certificate "Hyperbaric Medicine Training Course C" (40 hours education) according to regulations of GTÜM
- A two-weeks work voluntary experience in a hyperbaric facility working in compliance with VDD e.V. standards (80 hours education)
- A valid certificate proving fitness for diving as shown by regulations of professional trade organization (BG) G31/1

3. Hyperbaric Chamber Operator (VDD e.V.)

Following references or documents have to be forwarded to obtain the certification as "Hyperbaric Chamber Operator (VDD e.V.)":

- The certificate "Chamber Technician Course" according to regulation of VDD e.V. (40 hours education)
- A one-week voluntary experience in a hyperbaric facility working in compliance with VDD e.V. standards (40 hours education)
- A First-Aid-Course (minimum 16 hours) not older than one year
- A valid certificate proving fitness for diving as shown by regulations of professional trade organization (BG) G31/1, if accompanying patients during the lock operation or working in the hyperbaric chamber under pressure
- Minimum age 18 years

Since 1998, in context of the quality management, a certification of the hyperbaric facilities has become feasible.

The VDD e.V. has issued guidelines for this, too. The prerequisites for the certification of the facilities are checked by an association of independent experts, the "Germanischer Lloyd" (GL). The certificates are allocated by the VDD and the GL, jointly. The period of validity of such a certificate is one year. The extension of the validity by one year at a time is carried out on application and requires a further check of the facility.

The prerequisites for the certification of the facility are comparable in the main points to DIN ISO 9000. However, they have been raised through additional requirements in technical, therapeutic, and personnel standards.

Special value has been placed on the existence of sufficiently certified staff.

The medical head of a certified hyperbaric facility must fulfill the certification "Diving and Hyperbaric Medicine" according to the guidelines of GTÜM e.V. During regular treatment, the following staff members must be present permanently:

- 1 physician with the certificate "Diving Medicine (GTÜM e.V.)" and the certificate "Hyperbaric Medicine Training Course C," according to the guidelines of GTÜM e.V.
- 1 Medical Assistant for Hyperbaric and Diving Medicine (VDD e.V.) (alternatively a 2nd doctor with HBO certification or 1 Nurse for Hyperbaric Medicine)
- 1 Hyperbaric Chamber Operator (VDD e.V.)
- A valid certificate proving fitness for diving as shown by regulations of professional trade organization (BG) G31/1 is necessary for all staff if accompanying patients during the lock operation or working in the hyperbaric chamber under pressure.

After consultation with members of VDD e.V. and GL, the "Bundesinstitut für Arzneimittel und Medizinprodukte (BfArM)" in Berlin issued comments on preventive fire protection in 1998, which also receive consideration in the certification.

So patients are to be intensively instructed about behavior in case of fire and the handling of the fire fighting devices by the staff before beginning therapy. Adherence to the regulations has to be monitored by the staff at all times.

Only by sufficient quality management and strict certification regulations can an optimal cooperation of all components of a hyperbaric facility be achieved and therefore provide optimized benefits with minimized risks for our patients.

REFERENCES

1. Almeling, M., Welslau, W. (Hrsg.): Hyperbare Sauerstofftherapie - Qualitätsstandards. Archimedes-Verlag 1996.
2. Haux, G., Welslau, W.: Sicherheitsstandards, in: Grundlagen der hyperbaren Sauerstofftherapie, Hrsg. Almeling, M, Welslau, W., Archimedes-Verlag 1996, S. 109-110.
3. Peusch-Dreyer, D.: Richtlinien für die Erteilung des Zertifikats HBO-Therapieeinrichtung (VDD e.V.), Juni 1997, Verband Deutscher Druckkammerzentren.
4. Peusch-Dreyer, D.: Richtlinien und Anforderungen zur Personalqualifizierung durch den VDD e.V., September 1997, Verband Deutscher Druckkammerzentren.

WATER-BASED FIRE EXTINGUISHING

Sverre Lerdahl

GENERAL

Fire, what is a fire? It is important to learn the chemical mechanisms of fire in order to understand how fire can be suppressed and extinguished. As per definition, a fire is "A chemical chain reaction between oxygen and a combustible material under the development of heat, smoke, and gases."

The fire parameters are: Energy (heat) ultraviolet and infrared radiation, carbon monoxide, carbon dioxide and various nitrogen oxides.

Fire will start when a combustible material is heated to "flash point"—(evaporation temperature); oxygen is present and there is temperature and sufficient energy at ignition point of the released gasses.

At this moment the chain reaction is in progress and it will continue as long as there are oxygen and combustible material left, or till the fire is extinguished.

The methods of fire prevention or fire extinguishing are cooling, depletion of oxygen, using non-combustible material, or removing combustible material and chemical chain braking—inhibition.

The most common method is the use of water to cool down the environment and combustible material to a temperature below flash point. Different additives can be used with the water for special applications or fighting fires in materials where it is of importance to create a film on top of a liquid, to totally fill an area with high expansion foam, or to cover and seal an area to prevent re-ignition.

Secondly the use of carbon dioxide for oxygen depletion. Carbon dioxide however is a toxic gas, lethal in concentrations necessary for fire extinguishing, and is basically utilised in confined spaces where people are not present or must be evacuated before release and discharge.

Inert gases like Argonite and Inergen are currently used within the same areas as for carbon dioxide. These gases are nitrogen based and include a small percentage of argon and carbon dioxide.

These gases however will not create a lethal atmosphere in concentrations sufficient for fire extinguishing. Both carbon dioxide, Argonite and Inergen extinguish the fire by depletion of oxygen.

Dry chemical or powder is used mainly for portable fire extinguishers, but can also be utilised in fixed special applications. The powder extinguishes by cooling, prevention of fresh oxygen to reach the fire, and also by inhabitation. Most powders are non-toxic, but some special powders used for explosion suppression system are lethal at certain concentrations.

Halogenated hydrocarbons or "Halons" have been used since World War One when carbon tetrachloride (CCl4) was tested and found to be an excellent fire extinguishing agent however toxic and extremely dangerous even in small concentrations.

Halon 1301 (CF3Br) was approved and used for total flooding of confined spaces from the late sixties to 1986 when the Montreal Protocol was signed by most of the countries in the world. The Halons were banned due to global warming problems and depletion of ozone in the atmosphere

The Halon gases (1301)(1211)(2402)(1011) were all products with good fire extinguishing capabilities but with the two mentioned problems. These gases are all extinguishing fires by inhibiting the chemical chain reaction of the fire.

During the chain breaking process the halogenated hydrocarbons are generating toxic pyrolyse products as a function of the interaction with fire or heat. Some of these products are lethal even in low concentrations, like bromides, fluorides, bromine water, phosgene, chlorine water solution, etc. Halon 1301 however has the capacity to extinguish fires rapidly and at very low concentrations (4 to 6 %) by volume.

The production and generation of dangerous pyrolyse products are therefore at levels not dangerous to the human body.

Currently available with approvals in some countries are FM 200, NAF3, and Halotron.

These chemicals are all halogenated hydrocarbons that requires a much higher concentration by volume for successful fire extinguishing than Halon 1301, generate higher amounts of pyrolyse products, are more dangerous to the human body, but are environmentally friendly in the respect of global warming and ozone depletion in the atmosphere.

PREVIEW

Water as a fire extinguishing agent has been used since the beginning of time. Through the years water based systems have become more and more efficient when new ideas and knowledge have been developed into new technologies and equipment.

The distribution of the water into the fire was always a problem and from the days of the water bucket till today significant improvements have been taking place.

Spray nozzles and sprinkler systems, however, still with relatively low efficiency ratios, have been used for a long period of time. The systems extinguish most fires, but large amounts of water are necessary for successful fire extinguishing.

Secondary damages from the use of water have to be taken into consideration. Secondary damages and in particular water damage is a significant factor in the overall risk assessment, damage, and the aftermath of fire.

Systems using smaller and smaller amounts of water for successful fire extinguishing have the last 10 years been developed; the efficiency ratio is higher but still relatively large amounts of water are being used. Water damage as a function of fire extinguishing does still cause considerable claims and pay-outs from the insurance companies.

The Montreal protocol and the banning of halogenated hydrocarbons in 1986 and the fire and the catastrophe on the passenger vessel "Scandinavian Star," where 158 people were killed, resulted in the phase-out process of Halons together with new international rules and regulations for passenger ships carrying more than 36 passengers.

With this new situation for the fire protection industry, the engineers and the designers initiated the development of high performance water fog and water mist systems. A drop-in gas for halon was not likely to be approved world wide. Carbon dioxide, being toxic and dangerous to people, was not a good alternative, and weight and stability problems on older vessels opened the market for light weight high performance water based systems with high efficiency and little water usage. It was also likely to believe that water as such always would be world-wide approved as a fire extinguishing agent.

WATER AS A FIRE EXTINGUISHING AGENT

To improve the efficiency of water based fire extinguishing systems, basic investigations were performed to learn and understand the physical and chemical properties of water as such. The process of cooling, heat absorption, steam building ratios, expansion factors, and chemical decomposition temperatures are important parameters.

Water, one of the most basic elements on earth with the chemical formula H_2O, has two hydrogen and one oxygen atom in the molecule. Water is heavier than most flammable liquids.

Some liquids, however, are soluble in water under all circumstances, such as acetone, alcohol, and glycol. Some liquids are not soluble in water, but create a layer that floats on the water surface (ether) or sinks to the bottom (carbon sulphide).

Under normal atmospheric pressure water boils at 100 degrees C. At this temperature one litre of water converts to 1700 litres of water steam. If water is super heated to temperatures above 100 degrees C, small amounts are decomposed into hydrogen and oxygen. The result is a highly explosive mixture which could cause an explosion and rupture of the building construction.

The combination of high temperature and small water droplets will increase the decomposition process and the explosibility of the area. The hot contact surfaces are also important to the decomposition process, where plain surfaces are less dangerous than f.ex. metal chips or similar material with large surface areas.

Water has a large heat capacity or heat volume. At 100 degrees C, one litre of water has the capacity to heat absorb 2.253 Mjoul. It is a unique ability of water that large amounts of energy are necessary for the evaporation process. Water is therefore especially suitable as a cooling fire extinguishing agent.

With the right equipment used in a correct manner, water can absorb more heat from the fire than any other fire extinguishing agent.

When one litre of water evaporates to steam at 100 degrees C, 539,1 Kcal energy is released. One Kcal is equivalent to 426,9 kgm. One KW is equivalent to 101,98 kgm/sec. One Kcal/sec. is equivalent to 4,168 KW. One litre of water evaporated in one second requires 531,1 Kcal. One litre of water is capable of heat-absorbing 2,253 MW.

To increase the efficiency of the water, the discharge must be done in such a way that the evaporation process is as quick as possible. The larger the cooling surface area, the faster the evaporation process will take place, the more energy will be absorbed, and the faster the fire extinguishing.

If one droplet of water with the radius of one millimetre is devised into droplets with the radius of 0,001 millimetre, (one micron) the overall surface will be increased from 0,126 cm^2 to 126 cm^2 and the number of droplets will be 1.000.000.000.

Raindrops, as an example, have droplet sizes with a radius between 0,2 to 1 mm and fog from 0,004 to 0,04 mm. The immediate assumption would be that the most effective droplet for fire extinguishing would be the smallest possible. However, the smaller the droplets, the more difficult the transportation method will be.

Several factors will influence the effectiveness of transportation. The resistance in the air, wind, ventilation, and the pressure waves from the fire itself are factors that will have to be taken into consideration. A system capable of discharging a mass of water with small droplets and a large cooling surface area within a short period of time at high velocity and with high kinetic energy would be the most effective. One litre of water evaporated in one second has the capacity to heat-absorb 2,253 MW.

Fire extinguishing systems with these qualities however are difficult to design and there will always be a balance and compromise between the droplet size, the mass over time ratio, the velocity, and the price. The theory and technology must be adapted to real life situations.

Water is in most cases excellent as a fire extinguishing agent and can be used for most types of fires: A, B, C (E). However there are fires in materials where water should not be used, like reactive metals, metal oxides, metal amides, carbides, halides, sulphides, cyanides, or liquefied gases at cryogenic temperatures such as LNG (liquid natural gas) that will boil violently when heated by water.

WATER FOG / WATER MIST

Conventional sprinkler, deluge, and water spray nozzle systems produce relatively large water droplets with small cooling surface areas. In practice only a few percent of the water is evaporated and used for fire extinguishing. For this reason, large amounts of water are necessary to exceed the critical value. However, the transportation of water into the seat of the fire is relatively simple and easy, the momentum and penetration ability is high, and these systems will in most cases completely extinguish the fires. The spray patterns and cover areas can be well defined and, without considering the water usage and secondary damages, the fire extinguishing abilities are relatively good.

By utilising the water fog/water mist technology with small water droplets and large cooling surface area, the water usage is reduced by 60 to 90 percent compared to conventional sprinkler/deluge/spray nozzle systems.

One of the differences in performance between a conventional water deluge/sprinkler/water spray system is the water usage and the fact that small droplets can extinguish hidden fires better than the conventional technology. The water fog technology in general is utilising special nozzles to create droplet sizes between 20 to 200 microns.

The cooling surface area from one litre of water with droplet sizes of 50 microns is 120 m^2 while a 1 mm droplet size creates a cooling surface area of only 6 m^2.

To penetrate the fire ball and extinguish fires, nozzles of different types are available. It is important that the nozzle has the velocity to create sufficient momentum to penetrate the fireball and extinguish the fire.

The performance of the nozzle is important in order to extinguish within a short period of time with as little water usage as possible. If however the system does not extinguish and the fire is allowed to propagate and let the temperature rise, the phenomenon of water decomposition will occur and make the fire flare and in worst case a primary explosion could be the result.

The engineering methodology of water fog system is based upon results from a number of different test scenarios. The tests were executed to learn the overall efficiency of water fog as such, and the difference between nozzle constructions. In addition all the tests executed should present necessary scientific data to calculate water fog systems for different objects, areas, and applications.

Water fog as such is today recognised by authorities world wide as an equivalent to conventional sprinkler/deluge water spray technology using only small amounts of water for successful fire extinguishing.

WATER FOG IN HYPERBARIC CHAMBERS

Hyperbaric chambers are to be considered a high fire-risk installation where incidents in many cases are fatal.

The importance of fire prevention by means of using non-flammable materials, special clothing material, restrictions against devices that could cause a spark, devices with accumulated energy that could be released, and the use of intrinsically safe electronic equipment is of course very important.

However, it is not likely to believe that it is possible to totally eliminate the fire risk and therefore the incorporation of a fixed fire extinguishing system is important. In hyperbaric chambers under different hyperbaric conditions time is critical, and the system must be released immediately when a fire is discovered. In addition the system must have the capacity to extinguish the fire in less than 30 seconds.

Water deluge systems have been and can be used, however the performance in respect of time of extinguishing and the overall water usage is unsatisfactory. With the new water-fog fire extinguishing technology it is possible to extinguish fires under hyperbaric conditions within a short period of time using only small amounts of water. It is of importance that the release mechanism and the accessibility of the release units allow for immediate release when a fire is discovered or detected.

Under normal conditions, like atmospheric pressure in a confined space, a relatively low water fog concentration is sufficient to extinguish fires and to maintain an inerted atmosphere. Under hyperbaric conditions in a super pressurised atmosphere, the propagation of fire is significantly higher and requires higher water fog concentrations for successful fire extinguishing. Even with 1,5 bar over pressure and normal 20,9% oxygen, the fire is instant and the rate of temperature rise extreme. For successful fire extinguishing the space must be totally flooded with water fog in seconds.

First of all, the system must rapidly reduce the ambient temperature and then extinguish the fire. In a fire situation the system has one task only, to extinguish the fire rapidly and save human lives. If a fire is allowed to propagate under hyperbaric conditions, severe damage to people or death could be the result.

A typical system design should include the necessary number of high performance water-fog nozzles to totally flood the entire space within seconds. The nozzles must be located in such a way that the spray has optimal overlapping in order to maintain a homogenous water fog density. The transportation time of water in the piping should be kept to a minimum.

Tests must be carried out in order to prove the capacity and performance of the system. If the system is released manually, manual release stations must be located both inside and outside of the hyperbaric chamber. The accessibility of the release stations must be taken care of in order to release the system immediately when a fire is discovered.

FIRE DETECTION IN HYPERBARIC CHAMBERS

If the fire extinguishing system is designed with automatic release from an automatic fire detection system, the basic detection method should be a combination of IR and UV spark/flame detectors The early stage detection under hyperbaric conditions is important. Immediate release is the key word. Optical and ionisation smoke detectors are in this respect too slow, and the super sensitive aspiration detectors will not be suitable due to the over pressure. Traditional fixed and rate of temperature rise temperature detectors are also too slow and should not be used under hyperbaric conditions as triggers for a fire extinguishing system.

The fire detection system should consist of a fire detection panel with detector loops, manuel release station loops, valve release circuit, and alarm loops. The panel must be provided with batteries for at least 72 hours emergency power. The system should be configured with two detectors in coincidence (double knock) configuration, where both detectors detect the fire before release of the fire extinguishing system.

This system configuration will prevent false releases. The detectors are so quick that time delay is negligible. All electrical wires inside the hyperbaric chamber should be of flame proof and halogen-free type. Detectors should be of intrinsically safe type or be provided with EXd enclosure. If the detectors are of intrinsically safe type, the fines should be equipped with Zener barriers.

At all times, status of the system should be indicated on the fire detection panel. All loops and circuits should be monitored for failure (broken fine and short circuit). In addition it is wise to provide the system with monitoring facilities of the fire extinguishing hardware (water lever and pressure control).

In a fire situation the first detector will detect the fire, pre-alarm will illuminate and flash to alert the pilot. When the second detector detects the fire, the system will be released and the fire alarm bell will sound. The time between first and second alarm is dependent upon the propagation of the fire, but under hyperbaric conditions we know from experience and are estimating less than one second. If the system does not function, one of the manual release units must be activated. If the system still does not release, there must be a third means of release mechanism. The pilot must be able to manually activate the system from the water reservoir.

In many cases the detectors are faster and more reliable than the human eye and nose. A properly designed system with high quality components will provide extra safety to the installation as such. People do react differently and in many cases irrelevantly. Even well trained and educated people can have problems in a stressed situation. Fire detection and fire extinguishing installation must be provided with a daily/weekly/monthly control routine and an annual full control and service.

POSSIBILITIES FOR MINIMIZING FIRE RISK IN HYPERBARIC CHAMBER SYSTEMS

Dr.-Ing. Peter Szelagowski

GKSS Forschungszentrum Geesthacht GmbH

Max Planck Str., D 21502 Geesthacht

ABSTRACTS

Hyperbaric Therapy and Treatment chambers gain an increasing importance in medical treatment for the improvement of healing and curing of injuries.

The medical treatment is performed with an enriched oxygen or pure oxygen as a mask-breathing gas, which may influence the oxygen partial pressure or which raises the oxygen content of the compressed air chamber gas rapidly if leakage in the mask occurs. Higher oxygen contents and raised oxygen partial pressure increases material flammability or combustibility which results in increased fire risk for the chamber occupants. This situation requires extremely high attention to the chamber operation by the operating personal.

The paper will show different risk factors and describe the procedures and fire protection measurements in saturation diving and will provide recommendations for safety improvements for the chamber occupants living under compressed air and/or in oxygen enriched atmosphere.

INTRODUCTION

This paper covers experiences and results from research activities related to saturation diving several years ago. Problems which are related to safety of chamber occupants in hyperbaric therapy and treatment chambers today are similar to those in saturation diving and chamber operation about twenty years ago. Since that time quite some good improvements in this respect have been achieved and incidentally serious fatalities have been reduced remarkably.

In 1980 P. Rosengren stated, "the main danger for divers in chambers is fire. There have been 2,7 fatalities per event." This statement expressed all that had to be said at that time, getting across how important hyperbaric safety really is.

Intense experimental research was started already about thirty years ago to learn some lessons from heavy fire accidents in hyperbaric diving and treatment chambers. GKSS Research Ctr. Geesthacht was one of those research centers that performed some experimental research work in this respect to find out the flammability of materials and their hazardous standard in general to be found in hyperbaric chambers such as clothing of the occupants, the entertainment and recreation material (such as books, newspapers etc.) or the upholstery of the interior furniture respectively the furniture itself (1, 2).

The results have been accepted and have provided a base knowledge until today, extended and supplemented by additional experiments and experiences from application of new procedures, materials, and equipment.

The results and the experience achieved are reflected by numerous qualified and well-based standards, codes, and rules to improve fire safety in hyperbaric diving systems. Despite of the availability of these special standards, codes, and rules, which have to be carefully observed and obeyed during the operation of saturation diving chamber systems, some severe fire accidents have just been recently reported in hyperbaric treatment chambers, which initiated some new test activities in the check of fire fighting systems at GKSS Research Ctr, and which turned out to become the basis for the demonstrations at GKSS Research Ctr during this workshop. Before further details, possible procedures, and safety precautions can be discussed, related process behaviors and definitions behind the fire hazard in hyperbaric treatment and therapy chambers have to be discussed. This paper refers to those experiences, research activities, and achieved experimental results which have been procured mainly for saturation diving activities at GKSS Research Ctr. Geesthacht. As the interesting depth range is the same in saturation diving and hyperbaric therapy, this knowledge can be directly transferred to this special subject.

PARAMETERS AROUND THE COMBUSTION PROCESS

To start a combustion process an oxidant and an ignition source must be present and the fuel and the oxidant must be flammable.

Different parameters, such as temperature, pressure, oxidant- or fuel concentration and composition of gas mixtures, determine the individual flammability behavior of fuel-oxidant combinations.

Oxygen is the primary oxidant applied in diving technology as well in hyperbaric therapy and treatment and it is unavoidable in case the chambers are occupied by divers or patients.

Ignition sources contribute the thermal energy input, which is necessary to enable the combustion process to become self-sustaining. Independent from whether the fuel is a solid, a liquid, or a gas the flame reaction will be initiated in a gas or vapor phase. Possible sources of ignition may be:

- sparks (electrostatic, friction, impact)
- hot sources (heating, friction)
- hot gases (which will not in general occur in hyperbaric treatment or therapy chambers)

The flame propagation speed varies with temperature, pressure, and the presence of diluents (for oxygen these diluents in hyperbaric chambers can be nitrogen, helium, or hydrogen) At subsonic speed the combustion process is called deflagration; at supersonic speeds a detonation will occur. Both rapid reactions represent in common sense an explosion. The handling of diving gas mixtures, which could become explosive, has to be done with careful consideration of the flammability or the explosion limits and the full concentrated observation of the chamber operating personal.

Due to the depth range in which the treatment and therapy has to be performed, the patient has to stay in an environment with higher oxygen partial pressure.

This results at least in an atmosphere that does not reduce but increase the fire hazard to the occupants. This has to be aware to the occupants as well as to the chamber operating and medical staff of the center. Special precautions and procedures have to be available for emergencies.

The limits of flammability are generally defined as the limiting concentrations of fuel (lower/upper limit) necessary to sustain the combustion process at a given temperature and ambient pressure.

In special cases modified definitions are possible, e.g., flammability limits can refer to the concentrations of the oxidant due to the particular relevance in diving technology or in our case in therapy or treatment operations. Therefore attention should be paid to what is really meant.

Definitions of general interest are:
- Oxygen enriched atmosphere:
  An atmosphere which contains greater than 21-mole percent oxygen and/or contains a partial pressure of oxygen >0,21bar
- Atmosphere of increased burning rate:
  Oxygen enriched atmosphere with an increased fire hazard as related to the increased burning rate of material in the atmosphere (based upon a 1.2cm/sec. burning rate at 23,5% oxygen at 1 bar absolute)
- Flame retardant:
  Flame retardant refers to materials which do not continue to burn spontaneously in a compressed air atmosphere of at least 6 bar abs. (This is of special interest for the above mentioned subject)
- Lower/upper limit of explosion:
  Minimum/maximum concentration (vol.%) at which a mixture is inflammable.

The above mentioned have been determined in saturation diving. They can directly be transferred and applied to the actual situation in therapy and treatment chambers. All staff connected with the operation of the hyperbaric system and its handling as well as the related medical staff should be clearly aware of these definitions and what is meant behind them.

HAZARDS OF THE HYPERBARIC FIRE

Temperature increase, formation of toxic gases, pressure increase or pressure waves, and deoxidization are the main hazards in hyperbaric fire events, depending on the chamber dimensions, selection of adequate materials and outfit (e.g. furniture, bed sheets, blankets, clothing of occupants, books, and newspapers, etc.), and the gas composition with increased oxygen partial pressure or raised oxygen concentration inside the chamber. The seriously restricted and very limited escape possibilities complicate the situation extremely. Therefore primarily a well functioning and certified (by an independent certifying authority) fire extinguishing system should be compulsory equipment for each hyperbaric therapy and treatment chamber system.

Secondarily
- a well trained and very disciplined operational staff,
- well established operational and rescue (evacuation) procedures for the occupants,

• a well and comprehensive briefing of staff and chamber occupants on these procedures as well as:

an intensive check of the occupants and the materials they intend to take into the chamber will restrict the fire risk but cannot completely avoid it; the risk is omnipresent as demonstrated in the past serious fire accidents in diving systems, which lead to new standards, rules, and codes for these systems, and in the recently reported tragic fire accidents in hyperbaric treatment and therapy chambers.

It has to be considered that not only the fire itself and, in this respect the possibly related severe temperature and pressure rise, will seriously hurt or kill the occupants, but also the toxic combustion products and the hot gases will affect their health conditions seriously, as the respiratory tracks and the lungs will be severely affected by inhalation of these gaseous products.

Restriction in escape and rescue represent additional hazards in hyperbaric fire. A successful escape is a matter of structural boundary conditions as well as good training and briefing of the occupants and the housekeeping in the chamber.

All mentioned influencing factors cannot be regarded separately but only in total; they all act together more or less in composition but are unavoidable risk factors. These risk factors should be limited by very restricted system-related regulations.

CLASSIFICATION OF FIRE RESISTANT MATERIAL

In saturation diving it has become a compulsory operational regulation that in depth ranges with raised fire risk (due to increased oxygen partial pressure, which is similar to the operational depths in therapy and treatment chamber systems and which can additionally include raised oxygen content of the compressed chamber air due to leakage of individual breathing apparatuses), the chamber occupants have to be especially selected and are not permitted to take into the system inflammable material and have to wear fire-resistant clothing including underwear. Bed sheets, pillows, bed covers and blankets have to be from the same material. Paper material (such books, newspapers, booklets for their personal records, etc.) even have to be locked out in this special depth range.

Meanwhile the different materials have been classified according to their fire resistance, so that a purpose related selection can be performed. As an example the following classifications can be presented:

Mat. Cl. 0   Material burns in air at 1 bar (abs)
Mat. Cl. 1   Material requires a higher ignition temperature and burns at a lower rate at 1 bar (abs)
Mat. Cl. 2   Material that is non-flammable/self-extinguishing in air at 1 bar (abs)
Mat. Cl. 3   Material that is self-extinguishing/burns slowly in air at appr. 4 bar (abs)
Mat. Cl. 4   Material that is self-extinguishing/burns slowly in air at appr. 7 bar (abs)

Mat. Cl. 5   Material that is self-extinguishing/burns slowly in mixtures (25% O_2, 75% N_2) at 1 bar (abs)

Mat. Cl. 6   Material that is self-extinguishing/burns slowly in mixtures (30% O_2, 70% N_2) at 1 bar (abs)

Mat. Cl. 7   Material that is self-extinguishing/burns slowly in mixtures (40% O_2, 60% N_2) at 1 bar (abs)

Mat. Cl. 8   Material that is self-extinguishing/burns slowly in mixtures (50% O_2, 50% N_2) at 1 bar (abs)

Mat. Cl. 9   Material non-flammable in 100% O_2 at 1 bar (abs)

As shown in the table above the classification of materials of higher classes is based on experimental results achieved in atmospheres at 1 bar (abs). The behavior of such materials under elevated pressure in such gas mixtures is not known. Therefore it was necessary to start combustion tests in such gas mixtures under elevated pressure.

EXPERIMENTAL NEEDS

As stated above the main data available have been presented for 1 bar conditions only. It was felt necessary to establish in primarily experiments additional knowledge on the material's behavior in respect of influence of pressure on its ignition and flammability. Certain special test materials have been selected and tested in a hyperbaric chamber, 1993 at GKSS Research Ctr. to provide the required data for the safe performance of saturation dives in the GUSI-System. These results are of identical importance for the performance of treatment and therapy of patients under hyperbaric conditions with elevated oxygen content in the chamber atmosphere.

The experiments have been performed under the following conditions, as approved standard conditions were not available at that time:

- Size of specimen: (65–80) mm x 35 mm
- Ignition coil: coil with 4 turns of a dia of 12 mm, material: Cr(20%)-Ni (80%)-wire, 0,5 mm dia
- Distance between coil and rear side of specimen 2-3 mm
- Gas-atmosphere in pressure chamber: compressed air, synthetic mixed gases (He,N_2,O_2)
- Heating by adjustable transformer (up to 250 W max)
- Recording of ignition temperature at the rear side of specimen in a distance of 2–3 mm above the center of the ignition coil
- Test chamber facility: chamber can be pressurized up to 30 bar
- Temperature measurements: by thermal elements, located 3 mm above the ignition coil

EXPERIMENTAL RESULTS

Chamber-Atmosphere: Compressed Air

Premier tests were conducted to show the relation between ambient pressure in the chamber and heat transfer at the heating coil. The graph (Fig 1) shows the temperature relation to the heating time under different pressure levels with constant heating capacity of 60W. No specimens have been fixed above the ignition coil which guaranteed a non-obstructed heat transfer.

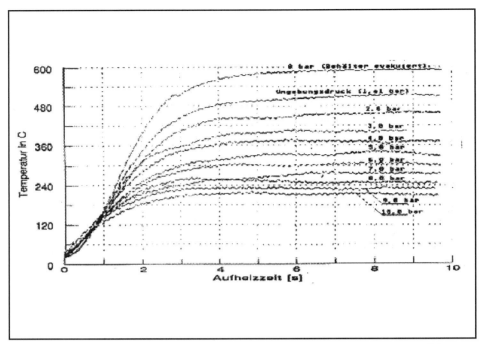

Figure 1. Heat transfer at the ignition coil in relation to the ambient chamber pressure [2].

It was found that raised pressure will increase the thermal flow based on the increased density, which is related to the increasing number of gas molecules.

Further results of a parameter study are presented in Figs. 2 and 3, which give an impression of influence of the surrounding pressure and the heating capacity at the ignition coil for compressed air (Fig. 2) and He-N_2-O_2-Atmospheres (Fig. 3). These experiments have been conducted with an asbestos plate with a rough surface fixed above the ignition coil to simulate a typical banked-up temperature below the specimen, resulting finally in fire ignition. The effective heating capacity has been calculated to 50–60% in the region of the ignition coil.

This paper will concentrate further only on the experiments in compressed air. First experiments on combustion behavior of materials under compressed air have been performed on paper, cotton, wood, and wool. The composition of the test specimens is shown below:

- paper: thick fabric high absorbent quality
- cotton: mixed fabrics 80% cotton fabrics, 20% polyester fabrics
- wool: mixed fabrics 60% woolen fabrics, 40% acrylic fabrics
- wood: veneer wood, pine and maple

Fig. 4 shows the achieved results of the ignition temperature values in relation to the atmospheric pressure (compressed air). It demonstrates the ranking of how the different materials have to be judged in their flammability. Especially in the depth ranges in which the therapy and treatment chambers are operated, paper shows the lowest ignition temperature, which demonstrates the high fire risk of this material. This risk increases

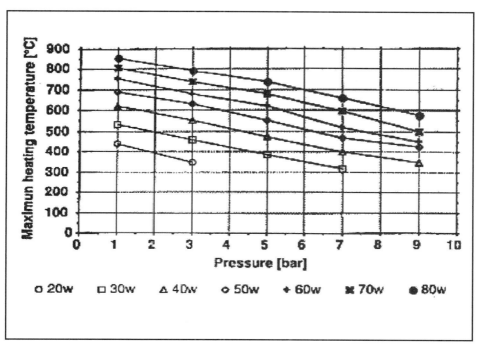

Figure 2. Relation between pressure atmosphere and max. heating temperature at the heating coil in compressed air atmosphere [2].

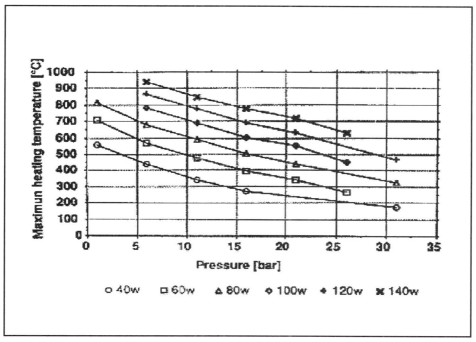

Figure 3. Relation between pressure atmosphere and max. heating temperature at the heating coil in He-N_2-O_2-atmosphere [2].

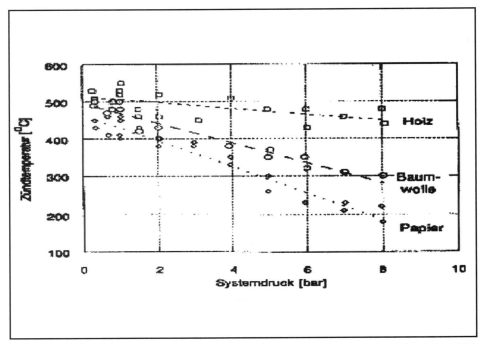

Figure 4. Ignition temperature of different materials in relation to the pressure of the system [2].

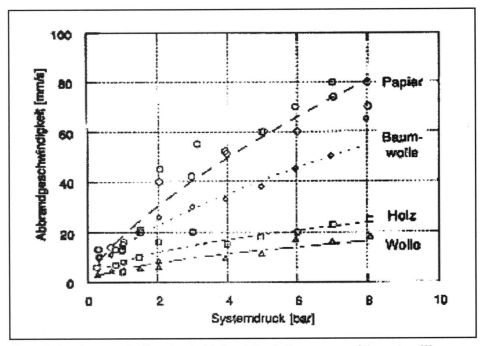

Figure 5. Burning rate of different materials in relation to the pressure of the system [2].

in higher oxygen concentrations which may occur due to leakage in the breathing apparatus with which oxygen treatment of the patient is performed. These results have been verified with the experimental demonstrations on the fire extinguishing system in the GUSI chamber on May 21,1999.

The conclusion out of this result should be such that for reduction of fire hazard in these treatment and therapy chambers no paper should be permitted during the treatment phase. Even the tested cotton mixture does not improve the safety of the chamber occupants very much so that it is strongly recommended to check even the clothing of the patients carefully before they are permitted to enter the system, and the material of the interior equipment, before releasing the chamber operation.

The burning rate of these investigated materials shows a similar behavior. Even here the highest flame propagation speed is found with paper fabrics as the highest one; the lowest speed could be evaluated for the tested woolen material.

It is common practice in saturation diving that the divers have to wear clothing manufactured from flame- or high temperature-resistant fabrics (as used by racing car drivers or astronauts), when living or working under fire hazardous conditions. Such materials have not yet been tested by GKSS Research Ctr so far but, from experience, this material will provide optimum safety conditions for the chamber occupants in the applied depth range.

Results of an additional test on the flammability behavior of a flexible tube under mixed gas conditions in relation to the oxygen concentration and the operational depth are shown in Fig. 6. Especially in the interesting depth range in which the treatment and therapy chambers are operated, a complete combustion of the material has been found for an oxygen concentration of appr. 14,5% at 20 m depth. This burning rate will

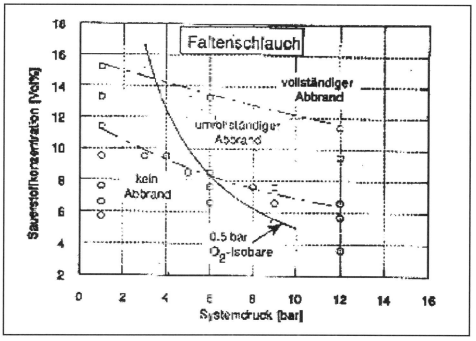

Figure 6. Combustion behavior of a flexible tube (not specially treated for flame resistance) tested under mixed gas conditions [2].

definitely increase when oxygen is supplied through such a tube as applied in a breathing system. The hazardous situation for the chamber occupant increases as he is applying the tube directly in the vicinity of his (in general) unprotected part of his body: his face. Fire on such a tube will in general lead to fatalities, and extreme special care should be applied on the selection of the tube material (if possible only fire resistant material to be selected) and on the positioning of such tube connections to the central breathing gas supply. It is strongly recommended to avoid as much as possible close contact to the face and to arrange the connections at the lower part of the chamber. In this case the tube should be led along the body and an around the waist, etc., but the arrangement of the connectors in head position should be avoided.

CONCLUSIONS AND RECOMMENDATIONS

First of all, in the application of hyperbaric treatment and therapy chamber systems on patients, there are some fixed facts that have to be accepted as they are in general unavoidable. These facts are:

- the chamber occupants live in a constraint-locked area with very limited possibilities for escape, especially in the case of elevated pressure.
- the chamber gas (in general compressed air) is applied in a depth range between 1 and 6 bar (abs).
- the partial pressure of oxygen is on an elevated level.
- leakage in the breathing apparatus can add oxygen to the chamber gas and can increase the concentration rapidly in a possibly uncontrolled manner.

As demonstrated in the previous fire extinguishing tests at GKSS Research Ctr on 22.05.1999, higher oxygen partial pressure and additional oxygen concentration in the chamber gas increase the fire risk for the occupants. The presented tests have shown that flammability and burning rate increases under these conditions remarkably and the fire extinguishing system will require more time to close down the fire. In some tests the fire could be stopped only by quick decompression and/or adding inert gas to the chamber gas.

A complete safe chamber system against fire hazards cannot be achieved or guaranteed. But special measurements in design, construction, operation, and management can reduce the risk for occupants and operators remarkably. Some of these measures will be listed as follows. The list does not apply for completeness and has to be added or reduced by related factors found and set for each special application and system.

As general requested measures the following should be observed

1. Chamber design and outfit of the system as well as operational procedure should meet standards, rules, and regulations set for the avoidance of fire risk in the chamber system (experience from saturation diving should be incorporated).
2. The built-in fire extinguishing system should be system tested and certified by an authorized body and routinely checked (Log-Book).
3. The chamber equipment should be fabricated from fire retardant or fire resistant material, incl. masks, supply tubes, etc.

4. An effective O_2-monitoring has to be installed and applied. The O_2-level in the chamber gas composition should never exceed the permitted level (23% max).
5. Approved operational and emergency procedures have to be available and the related staff trained with.
6. Clear conditions for restricted/permitted items introduced by the occupants into the chamber system has to be available. (Serious check of occupants before entering the system is essential.)
7. A serious briefing of the operational staff and the chamber occupants before entering the chamber system and starting the blow down should be essential.
8. A well trained and experienced chamber operation crew has to be available (preferably coming from previous saturation diving systems or offshore divers).
9. Responsibility should be clearly distinguished between medical and operational staff. No interference in between the responsibility areas (technical area, medical area) should be possible or permitted.
10. In case of different opinions in operation and possibly related hazards, this should be discussed and settled and fixed only by an "ethic" commission of the responsible staff members.
11. Exceptional wear of fire resistant clothing of the occupants, application of only fire resistant fabrics for bed sheets, bed covers, pillows, etc., for the time of chamber operation is generally to be observed.

The application of a quick or rapid decompression in chamber combustion can close down the burning fire in a chamber system, but the risk of achieving a fatal situation for the occupants increases with the treatment depth. This possibility of fire extinguishing should not be regarded as a serious arrangement to save the patients under such a condition.

REFERENCES

1. Schmidt,Klaus: Hyperbaric Fire Safety, GKSS Research Ctr. Geesthacht, GmbH, GKSS 90/E/47.
2. Schmidt,Klaus, H.Boie, A.Tiemann: Hyperbare Abbranduntersuchungen, GKSS Research Ctr. Geesthacht, GmbH, GKSS 93/E/80.

NATIONAL FIRE PROTECTION ASSOCIATION REQUIREMENTS FOR HYPERBARIC CHAMBER FIRE SUPPRESSION SYSTEMS IN THE UNITED STATES

W.T. Workman, MS, CHT
Chairman, Technical Committee on Hyperbaric and Hypobaric Facilities
National Fire Protection Association

HISTORY

The beginnings of using hyperbaric facilities for clinical purposes can be traced back to the late 1950s and early 1960s to the pioneering work of Dr. Boerema and his colleagues in Amsterdam, the Netherlands, where they validated the use of high pressure oxygen in the treatment of gas gangrene. Since then, there has been continued growth in the number of clinical hyperbaric medicine facilities throughout the world.

As with many developing technologies, there was an early interest in establishing the safety guidelines that would govern the administration of hyperbaric oxygen and for the equipment required to do so. In 1964, the National Fire Protection Association (NFPA), to address these concerns, created a Subcommittee on Hyperbaric and Hypobaric Facilities. Membership of this benchmark committee consisted of representatives from chamber and component manufacturers, chamber operators, fire service personnel, National Aeronautics and Space Administration (NASA), the military services, and others interested in hyperbaric safety Initially, work on developing this first standard was slow.

Unfortunately, there were two tragic events occurring within days of each other that served as the primary motivating factor to complete work on the standard. The first tragedy occurred on 27 January 1967 when the Apollo 1 Command Module erupted in fire, killing Astronauts Virgil I. Grissom, Edward H. White, and Roger B. Chaffee. Four days later, on 31 January 1967, two airmen were killed in a fire that occurred in a United States Air Force hypobaric test chamber that was pressurized with 100 percent oxygen at one-fifth of an atmosphere pressure (1). These two accidents resulted in completion of the first standard, which was adopted as a tentative standard, NFPA 56D, in 1968. Two years later, in 1970, NFPA 56D was transitioned to a permanent standard and remained largely unchanged until 1984. It was then extensively revised and integrated into NFPA 99, Health Care Facilities as a separate chapter devoted solely to hyperbaric facilities. The portion of the standard dealing with hypobaric facilities became a stand-alone standard, NFPA 99B, Hypobaric Facilities. The standard is revised every three years.

The major changes of the hyperbaric standard in the last few revision cycles of NFPA 99 were a direct result of the continual input from both military and civilian representatives on the Technical Committee (TC) on Hyperbaric and Hypobaric Facilities.

In preparation for the 1999 edition, membership of the TC was expanded to include representation from the Food and Drug Administration (FDA) and special expertise from the active fire research, fire sprinkler, and forensic communities. Their input proved invaluable to better understand the issues in support of the changes made to the 1999 edition. Of special note is that the most significant changes adopted for this edition were in the area of electrical requirements for Class A (multiplace) chambers. Support for these changes culminate many years of dedicated effort by committee members to update this portion of the standard and reflect an awareness of the technology now available to hyperbaric chamber designers that perhaps did not exist when the initial requirements were put into place. A better understanding of what constitutes an oxygen-enriched environment, the effects of hyperbaric conditions on the burning rate of materials, and the role that static electricity may play has also contributed to the ongoing revision process. It has been the committee's desire to reflect advances in technology and the ever-increasing understanding of the design and operation of hyperbaric facilities without compromising safety.

MISHAPS

It is unfortunate that the majority of the accidents involving hyperbaric facilities that have occurred within the last 10 to 15 years have been the result of human error. Two TC members, Dr. Paul Sheffield and David Desautels, recently reported information on 77 fatalities in 35 hyperbaric chamber fires from 1923 to 1996 (2). These mishaps occurred in Asia, Europe, and North America. Information on mishaps from other regions was not reported. Of the 77 fatalities cited, none occurred in North American clinical hyperbaric chambers. Prior to 1980, the primary cause of hyperbaric chamber fires was electrical; after 1980, the vast majority were attributed to either prohibited materials allowed in the chamber or operator error. Careful analysis of these data clearly points to the success of engineering and fire safety codes and standards as applied in North America to clinical hyperbaric medicine facilities. Because of recent tragic accidents in other countries, there is a growing recognition of the need for comprehensive fire safety standards in developing countries. Also, setting minimum training standards on the safe operation of hyperbaric systems will have a positive effect on maintaining hyperbaric safety standards throughout the world.

To my knowledge, there has only been one fire inside an occupied clinical hyperbaric chamber fire with no fatalities (2). In 1989, a multiplace chamber with four patients and two inside attendants was completing the HBO_2 treatment at 2.0 atms abs (33 fsw, 202 kPa) in a chamber atmosphere of about 21% oxygen. Responding to a request for a warm blanket for an infant patient, a cotton blanket was heated in the microwave for 2.5 minutes on the high setting. Upon removal from the microwave, a scorched odor was noted, but no fire was detected when the blanket was examined, so it was locked into the chamber. Upon removal from the medical lock into the chamber, the blanket ignited. The inside attendant successfully tried to reinsert the flaming blanket in the medical lock, but dropped it on the steel floor. The chamber operator activated the water deluge fire extinguishing system (FES) which rapidly extinguished the fire. Because of poor visibility and suspected continued smoldering, the FES was activated a second time. There were no injuries. The fact that the FES, as required by the standard, was an integral part of the system, and that it was fully functional, played a key role in the successful management of this potentially tragic event.

AREAS OF EMPHASIS

It is not the intent of this paper to replicate the contents of Chapter 19, Hyperbaric Facilities. Every hyperbaric facility should obtain a copy of the current standard for ready reference and application. However, for those readers not familiar with its contents, the general issues that are addressed in the standard are listed below (3).

- Purpose, scope and application of the standard
- Classification of chambers
- Nature of hazards
- Construction and equipment
    - Housing for hyperbaric chambers
    - Fabrication of hyperbaric chambers
    - Illumination
    - Chamber ventilation
    - Fire protection in Class A chambers
    - Fire protection in Class B and C chambers
    - Electrical systems
    - Communications and monitoring
    - Other equipment
- Administration and maintenance
    - Recognition of hazards
    - Responsibility
    - Rules and regulations
    - General requirements
    - Personnel
    - Equipment
    - Handling of gases
    - Maintenance logs
    - Electrical safeguards
    - Furniture
    - Conductive accessories
    - Fire protection equipment
    - Housekeeping

The general purpose of NFPA 99, Chapter 19, is to establish the minimum safeguards for the protection of patients, hyperbaric medical personnel, equipment, and surrounding facilities from the dangers of fire. It also provides guidance for rescue personnel who may not be familiar with the intricacies of hyperbaric chamber operation and their unique requirements.

The scope applies to hyperbaric chambers and related support systems used for medical and experimental purposes at pressures from 0 psig to 100 psig. It covers recognition of, and protection from, hazards associated with electrical, explosion, and implosion, as well as fire. It applies to both single and multiple patient occupancy chambers and to animal chambers whose size precludes human occupancy. It is only applied to new construction, new equipment added to new facilities, and new equipment added to existing facilities. It does not require the alteration or replacement of existing construction or equipment.

Chambers are generally classified according to occupancy. A Class A chamber is considered a multiple occupancy chamber; a Class B chamber is a single occupancy chamber, and a Class C chamber is animal occupancy only. Animal chambers that are equipped for human access are considered as Class A chambers by the standard.

The biggest distinction between building requirements for Class A chambers and Class B chambers is in the fire wall requirement. A Class A chamber requires 2 hour fire-resistive-rated construction and a B-label, 1 1/2 hour fire door rating. These requirements are not currently imposed on a Class B chamber installation. Other room requirements for both classes of chambers are exclusive use of the room for hyperbaric operations, floor support for the weight of the chamber, and room sprinkler protection.

As previously mentioned, all chambers used for clinical application are to be designed, fabricated, and installed in accordance with ASME-PVHO, Safety Standard for Pressure Vessels for Human Occupancy (4). Additionally, specific guidance is provided on flooring material, antistatic flooring properties, bilge installation, interior painting, viewports, access ports, electrical enclosures, illumination, environmental control, humidification, and minimum chamber ventilation rates. The need for individual breathing apparatus for each occupant is also cited in case the chamber environment becomes fouled for any reason. This apparatus must be immediately available and provide breathing gas independent from the chamber environment. Alternative breathing air sources for outside personnel of Class A chambers will also be available.

To help minimize the chance of contaminated chamber air, sources of air for the chamber atmosphere must be toxic free and flammability free. Compressor intakes are to be located in places to avoid air contamination from exhaust from vehicles, internal combustion engines, building exhaust outlets, etc. As a minimum, the air supplied to both Class A and B chambers currently shall meet the requirements of CGA Pamphlet G-7.1, Commodity Specification for Air[5], Grade D. Efforts are underway to bring the overall air quality requirements for hyperbaric operations into agreement with NFPA 99, Health Care Facilities, Chapter 4: Medical Gases. For bottled gases provided from a commercial source, periodic testing to insure gas quality is highly encouraged.

PATIENT HANDLING

NFPA 99, Chapter 19, does not prescribe a detailed procedure for patient handling. The majority of safeguards listed are aimed at minimizing the amount of hazardous materials that a patient can introduce into the chamber environment. One direct way of exercising control is to have the patient change from their street clothes into special clothing provided by the hyperbaric facility. Silk, wool, or synthetic materials are not allowed to be worn into either Class A or Class B chambers unless the fabric meets the flame resistance requirements as stated in NFPA 701, Standard Methods for Fire Tests for Flame-Resistant Textiles and Films (6). Therefore, personal clothing should never be allowed into the chamber. Only garments fabricated of 100 percent cotton, a special anti-static blend of cotton and polyester, or fire resistant garments made of materials such as Durette Gold, etc., should be used in any class of chamber. In addition to the requirement for textiles, the design of the garment shall be such that it is of the overall or jumpsuit type, completely covering as much of the skin as possible. Street shoes shall never be worn into the chamber because of the risk of sparking and introduction of hazardous hydrocarbons and solvents into the chamber from residue collected on the soles and heels of the shoes.

The use of flammable hair sprays, hair oils, and skin oils (cosmetics) are forbidden for all chamber occupants, patient and medical observer alike. Synthetic undergarments are also discouraged. Due to the length of treatment, patients are often allowed to bring into a Class A multiplace chamber a book or magazine to read during the course of treatment. Newspapers are never allowed due to the type of paper and inks used for printing. No reading material of any type is ever allowed to be used in a Class B chamber.

OPERATIONAL PROCEDURES

Although detailed operational procedures are not covered in the NFPA standard, general guidelines for administration and maintenance are. It is not enough to define how a hyperbaric system is to designed, fabricated, and installed. In order to create the safest environment possible for hyperbaric systems, careful attention must also be placed on how the facility is routinely operated and maintained. There are many good operational models available that provide representative pre- and post treatment checklists and outline solid maintenance programs that operators can follow. Many of these operational guides were developed by the US military and have been successfully used for many years. They are routinely adopted for general use.

One of the strongest cornerstones of any hyperbaric safety program is hazard recognition. Hazards can only be mitigated when all personnel involved, from the hospital administrator down to the most junior technician, clearly understand the nature of hazards that are possible in any hyperbaric facility. A partial description of these hazards is found in Appendix C-19 of the standard.

Even though the hazards and operational procedures are similar from one facility type to the next, it is highly recommended that all personnel (administrative, technical, and professional) jointly develop a series of operational procedures to follow for both routine and emergency situations. It is not enough just to develop the procedures; they must be practiced. Although proficiency can be achieved for routine procedures, emergency procedures must be practiced on a recurring basis to imprint the necessary steps that must be taken to appropriately deal with any emergency situation. In the case of fire, representative checklists are also included in Appendix C-19. Fire drills should be practiced frequently. These drills should also involve activation of the deluge fire suppression system at least annually.

Personnel Issues: Training, Staffing, Etc.

The one area that is less well defined is that of staffing and training. The standard is very clear that the ultimate responsibility for hyperbaric facility safety is placed on the governing board of the medical facility. It is incumbent on that body to insist that adequate rules and regulations are in place and that all personnel follow them. The standard also stipulates that a Safety Director be designated and responsible for all hyperbaric equipment. The Safety Director has the authority to restrict hazardous materials, supplies, or equipment from the interior of the chamber. There are no minimum staffing or training requirements mandated by the current standard.

Fire Protection in Class A (Multi-occupancy) Chambers
General Requirements (19-2.5.1)
A basic requirement for all Class A or multiplace hyperbaric chambers is that they must contain a fire suppression system (FSS) consisting of an independently supplied and operated handline and deluge system. The design of the FSS shall be such that the failure of any single component in either the handline or deluge system will not render the other system inoperable.

The system is further required to be designed so that activation of either the handline or the deluge system causes the following actions to occur:

- Visual and aural indication of activation shall occur at the chamber operator's console
- All ungrounded electrical leads for power and lighting circuits contained inside the chamber shall be disconnected. Intrinsically safe circuits, including sound-powered phones, are not required to be disconnected
- Emergency lighting and communications, where used, shall be activated

The standard also requires that a fire alarm signaling device be provided at the chamber operator's control console for signaling the telephone operator or suitable authority to activate the emergency fire/rescue network of the institution containing the hyperbaric facility. The use of fire blankets and portable carbon dioxide extinguishers are not permitted to be installed or used inside a multiplace hyperbaric chamber.

Booster pumps, control circuitry, and other electrical equipment involved in fire suppression system operations shall be powered from a critical branch of the emergency electrical system as specified elsewhere in the standard.

Deluge System Requirements (19-2.5.2)
A major requirement is for a fixed water deluge extinguishing system to be installed in all chamber compartments that are designed for manned operations. In those chambers that consist of more than one compartment or lock, the design of the deluge system shall ensure adequate operation when the chamber compartments are at different depths (pressures). The design shall also ensure the independent or simultaneous operation of the deluge systems.

There is one exception to this requirement. For a multiplace chamber that has a compartment or lock that is used strictly as a personnel transfer lock, and for no other purpose, no deluge fire suppression system is required in that compartment or lock.

Means of manual activation and deactivation of the deluge system controls shall be located at the operator's console and in each chamber compartment or lock containing a deluge system. These controls shall be designed to prevent unintentional activation. A new requirement for the 1999 edition is for water to be delivered from the sprinkler heads with 3 seconds of activation of any affiliated deluge control.

The number and positioning of the sprinkler heads shall be sufficient to provide reasonably uniform spray coverage with vertical and horizontal (or near horizontal) jets. An average spray density at floor level shall not be less than 2 gpm/ft² (81.5L/min/m²) with no floor area larger than 1 m² receiving less than 1 gpm/ft² (40.75 L/min/m²).

There shall be sufficient water available in the deluge system to maintain the flow specified above simultaneously in each chamber compartment or lock containing the deluge system for one minute. The limit on maximum extinguishment duration shall be governed by the chamber capacity (bilge capacity also, if so equipped) and/or its drainage system. The deluge system shall have stored pressure to operate for at least 15 seconds with electrical branch power.

Handline System Requirements (19-2.5.3)

In addition to a deluge FSS, each chamber compartment or lock shall contain a hand line system as well. At least two handlines shall be strategically located in the treatment compartments or locks. At least one handline shall be located in each personnel transfer compartment or lock. If any chamber compartment or lock is equipped with a bilge access panel, at least one handline shall be of sufficient length to allow the use of the handline for fire suppression in the bilge area.

All handlines shall have a 1/2 inch minimal internal diameter and shall have a rated working pressure greater than the highest supply pressure of the supply system. Each handline shall be activated by a manual, quick-opening, quarter-turn valve located within the compartment or lock. Hand-operated, spring-return to close valves at the discharge end of the handline shall be permitted. Handlines shall be equipped with override valves placed in easily accessible locations outside the chamber.

The water supply for the handline system shall be designed to ensure a 50 psi (345 kPa) minimum water pressure above the maximum chamber pressure. The system shall be capable of supplying a minimum of 5 gpm (18.8 L/min) simultaneously to each of any two of the handlines at the maximum pressure.

Automatic Detection System Requirements (19-2.5.4)

Automatic fire detection systems are optional. Whether installed and used in an alarm function or in an automatic deluge activation function, they shall meet the following requirements. Surveillance fire detectors responsive to the radiation from flame shall be employed. Type and arrangement of the detectors shall be such as to respond within 1 second of flame origination. The number of detectors employed and their location shall be dependent on the sensitivity of each detector and the configuration of the spaces to be protected.

The system shall be powered from the critical branch of the emergency electrical system or shall have automatic battery backup. If used to automatically activate the deluge system, the requirements for manual activation/deactivation and response time shall still apply. The system shall include self-monitoring functions for fault detection and appropriate fault alarms and indications.

Testing Requirements (19-2.5.5)

The deluge and handline systems shall be functionally tested at least annually. This test must be performed to verify the respective system performance criteria listed above. If a bypass system is used, it shall not remain in the test mode after completion of the test.

During initial construction, or whenever changes are made to the installed system, testing of spray coverage as cited above shall be performed at surface pressure, and at maximum operating pressure. The performance requirements above shall be satisfied under both conditions. A detailed record of the test results shall be supplied to the authority having jurisdiction and the hyperbaric facility safety director.

Fire Protection in Class B (Single-occupancy) Chambers

There are currently no internal fire deluge system requirements for Class B, single-occupancy hyperbaric chambers.

Regulatory Issues

Presently, the standards as contained in NFPA 99, Health Care Facilities are mandated by the local government or municipality authorities having jurisdiction (AHJ). Typically, AHJs are local Fire Marshals, but can be local building code inspectors or others. It can vary from one location to another. A major obstacle in the United States is that NFPA 99 only applies to designated health care facilities. Even though the document is very clear on what constitutes a health care facility, it is not always interpreted by the AHJs in that manner. There are many free-standing facilities, not affiliated with a "health care facility," that are not required to comply with the standard. To further complicate the issue, not all governments have adopted the current version of the code for enforcement. It is not uncommon for a city to have adopted a version that is several editions old. Major educational efforts are underway to ensure that these deficiencies are addressed to improve overall hyperbaric facility safety in the United States.

What Does the Future Hold?

The NFPA can be very proud of its contributions to hyperbaric facility safety. Since creation of the tentative standard in 1968, there has not been a single fatality in a clinical hyperbaric chamber in North American due to fire and only two documented fire mishaps (2). However, when first developed, the standard was so restrictive that many facilities simply ignored it. Over the years, dedicated committee members worked very hard to revise the standard to make it more realistic without compromising safety. This devotion is even more evident today, with members willing to position the committee to be more proactive. Instead of focusing its efforts only on evaluating and integrating changes into the standard, the committee is now expanding its interest into safety education, research, and hyperbaric community involvement.

The committee is actively promoting safety education efforts in a variety of different venues. Special panel discussions at meetings such as the annual scientific meeting of the Undersea and Hyperbaric Medical Society, awareness presentations at the annual meeting of the National Board of Pressure Vessel Inspectors, and seminars in conjunction with international NFPA affiliated activities are just a few examples of these efforts. One of their biggest undertakings is to advocate an international fire safety standard for hyperbaric facilities. Recent fire accidents in hyperbaric facilities throughout the world have raised the awareness level of the need for comprehensive safety standards. Work is progressing on that effort.

Fire monitoring and suppression technology has made dramatic advances since the early hyperbaric application research sponsored by the United States Navy and Air Force in the late 1960s and early 1970s. Improvements in monitoring for environmental contaminants that can serve as fuel sources, advanced flame and heat detection, enhanced nozzle design, and alternative suppressant agents such as water mist and non-toxic chemical agents all support renewal of research efforts to determine their applicability to the hyperbaric environment.

The committee supports pursuit of these research opportunities to integrate proven new technology into the standard to reduce the mishap risks and to minimize the cost of these life saving systems.

While organizations such as the NFPA, ASME, FDA, etc., have done a superb job in ensuring that hyperbaric pressure vessels and related systems are safely designed, manufactured and installed, it is up to the operator to ensure that the equipment is properly used and maintained. All personnel involved in hyperbaric medicine need to have a complete understanding of the safety requirements in this and other standards. There must be an active, ongoing safety awareness and training program that involves the entire hyperbaric staff and local fire personnel. Prevention and training are key elements to any effective safety program. There is much work needed to ensure that all jurisdictional agencies fully understand how hyperbaric facilities are currently used, appreciate their rate of growth, and exercise their enforcement role as it exists today. Standards need to be uniformly applied across all venues to ensure that we continue to enjoy our superb safety record.

REFERENCES

1. Health Care Facilities Handbook, 5th Edition, Burton R. Klein, Ed., National Fire Protection Association, Quincy, Massachusetts, 1996.
2. Sheffield, P.J. and D.A. Desautels. Hyperbaric and Hypobaric Chamber Fires: a 73-Year Analysis. Undersea & Hyperbaric Medicine, 1997; 24(3): 153-164.
3. Standard for Health Care Facilities, NFPA 99, 1996 Edition, National Fire Protection Association, Quincy, Massachusetts, pp. 108-119.
4. ANSI/ASME PVHO-1-1997, Safety Standard for Pressure Vessels for Human Occupancy, American Society of Mechanical Engineers, New York, 1997.
5. GCA Pamphlet G-7.1-1989, Commodity Specification for Air, Compressed Gas Association, Inc., Arlington, Virginia, 1989.
6. NFPA 701, Standard Method of Fire Tests for Flame-Resistant Textiles and Films, 1996 Edition, National Fire Protection Association, Quincy, Massachusetts, 1996.

HBO—CHAMBER SAFETY

Jörg Zimmermann

WAYS AND MEANS OF FIRE PREVENTION IN HBO CHAMBERS

Fire outbreaks in pressure chambers, in relation to frequency of missions, occurred relatively seldom. But once broken out, fires astonishingly always rapidly evolved, with fatal effects on chamber occupants in cases where the content of oxygen exceeded 21% (1).

Fires in hyperbaric atmospheres are difficult to control, due to

- increased oxygen partial pressure in the chamber atmosphere
- high temperatures and thereon resulting pressure increase
- short period for irreversible damages to occur
- limited effectiveness of applicable fire extinguishing means

The disastrous fire in the Milan HBO chamber led to an intensified awareness of danger by some of the users as well as manufacturers, with different results and solutions.

A positive point is the acceptance of the demand for stationary fire extinguishing systems for multiplace chambers in the DIN 13256, part 2.

Manufacturer, classification association, and user are dealing intensively with the problems of fire and fire extinguishing, respectively, the development of fire fighting systems.

- New chambers are only supplied if equipped with fire extinguishing systems.
- Some users have clearly shown their readiness to have their chambers modified.
- Some users have improved their preventive measures.

But also continued carelessness can be found. As for instance smuggling of forbidden items into the chamber is not yet consequently under control in most places. There are chambers in which school bags or ladies' handbags are an absolutely normal thing.

- An effective fire extinguishing system is of importance.
- Fire prevention as a whole of all means is of greater importance.
- The one who has to activate a fire extinguishing system has already committed errors before.

The installation of fire extinguishing systems must permanently be accompanied by a high sense of awareness to prevent an outbreak of fire.

To be more precise:

- a highly effective fire extinguishing system
- stock of fire fighting means lasting for several minutes
- even an automatic release system cannot look into the various bags being carried by chamber occupants.

It must always be pointed out distinctively that activating the fire extinguishing system can only be the last instance to perhaps finally rule out a catastrophe.

An attentively working, competent staff cannot be substituted by anything else. Wanting to save funds at this very end can easily have negative consequences.

Unqualified chamber operators cannot be compensated by additional demand upon any technical advances.

OXYGEN LOAD AND OXYGEN DISTRIBUTION IN MULTIPLACE CHAMBERS

In all multiplace chambers used in Germany the therapy pressure is built-up with breathing air.

The exhaled oxygen is discharged from the chamber (overboard dump).

All this because each increase of the oxygen proportion considerably raises the ignition and fire risk, essentially promotes burning, or causes rapid or total burning. (Figure 1).

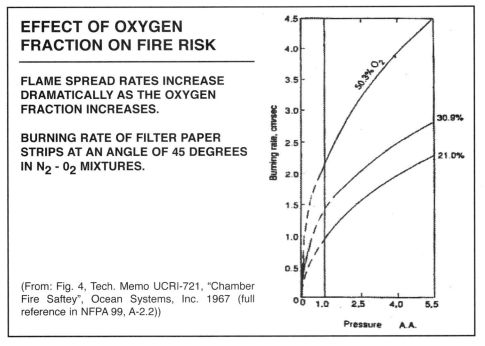

Figure 1. Burning velocity of filter paper strips in a oxygen nitrogen atmosphere.

The chamber atmosphere's oxygen content is under control permanently. Exceeding 23%, alarm is released and oxygen supply to the chamber disconnected. In many systems an automatic change-over from oxygen to air is found.

Normally for this control continued gas samples are taken at random in the chamber to measure its oxygen content (Figure 2).

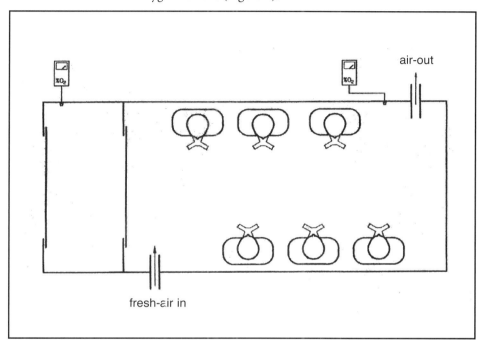

Figure 2. Gas samples are taken to measure oxygen content in the chamber.

Under normal working conditions the oxygen content of the chamber atmosphere raises unnotedly. A brief O_2 increase of approximately 0,1% occurs after masks are taken off.

As long as the value remains below 23% minimum reaction is an increase of fresh air ventilation.

It could also be that at times this measure follows after the alarm signal.

It was reported of cases describing switching off of alarm and continuation of oxygen supply, I quote: "but there is only 23% and we are operators from the fire-brigade."

An increased oxygen concentration is mainly caused by leaking breathing masks, that is to say, escape of oxygen between face and mask. Technically fit systems are a precondition.

Such leakages are mainly caused in cases in which shape and size of the mask do not fit shape and size of the user's face or if fitting of mask and adjustment of harness was not done properly.

Individual selection and adjustment of the mask for each patient and exercising of how to put on and tighten the mask is of utmost importance. (Something also an extinguishing system cannot do.)

If masks are tightened by an assistant a much better tightness is possible (3).

Many chamber occupants are not able to recognize a leaking mask; even a flow of gas between face and mask is not found worthy to be announced. Inconveniences resulting from improper fitting of the mask are also often tolerated.

As a result of a leaking breathing mask, oxygen clouds with at times a high concentration can build up (Figure 3).

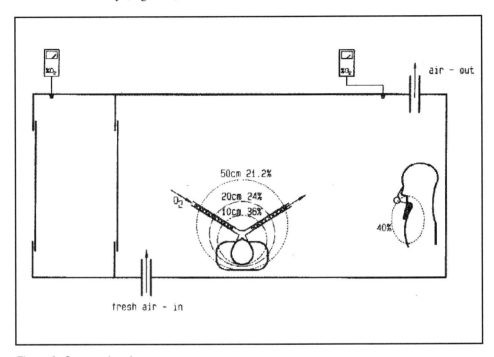

Figure 3. Oxygen drag-in.

They are not, or only with a delay, registered by the central control of oxygen content.

With a measuring result below 23% oxygen in the chamber atmosphere in general a concentration of more than 40% in the face areas and upper part of the body was found on patients with non-fitting mask or those bearded. In such cases only the slightest ignition energy could lead to fire out-break.

EXAMPLES

10-Person Chamber Occupied with 6 Persons, Ventilation Air Set for 6 Persons

- Patient with small beard, oxygen content at the side below the chin within 5 cm distance 36%, within 15 cm 24%, within 50 cm 21,2%.
- Patient with oversized mask, leaky in the nasal dorsum-corner of the eye area, within a 10 cm distance 36% O_2.
- No increased oxygen values detectable at the rest of the chamber occupants. Central control of oxygen content in the chamber indicates 21,5%.

10-Person Chamber, Occupied with 9 Persons. Ventilation Air Set for 10 Persons:

- Patient with oversized mask, leaky in nasal dorsum-corner of the eye area, within a 10 cm distance 33% O_2
- Patient with visually firm mask, 10 cm beside the face 27,2% O_2
- Patient, first time in chamber (leakage each time exhaling can clearly be seen), within a distance of 10 cm 35% O_2 and still 25% O_2 30 cm beside the face.

These Examples Demonstrate:

- Isolated oxygen clouds in the chamber cannot be detected by the central control of oxygen content.
- Already with only a slightly increased indication oxygen clouds could develop at one or the other chamber occupant and clothing could be saturated with oxygen.
- It would need only a minimum of ignition energy, possibly also through an electrostatic discharge in clothing, to initiate a fire outbreak.
- Only in cases in which absolutely no increase of O_2 content is evident a sufficiently high grade of security can be assumed.

Visual control of mask fitting brings to light bad mask fitting in nine out of ten cases if only the responsible assistants are alert enough.

Improvement Can Be Reached:

- By an improved air ventilation in the chamber
- and objective control of mask tightness by an oxygen measuring device suitable for use in a chamber (Figure 4)

The safest way is the control of discharge gas of each patient. This way the oxygen content of exhaled gas is individually measured by a suitable sensor (Figure 5).

Slightest mask leakages, that means oxygen transportation into the chamber, becomes clear without delay (Figure 7).

For patients not needing further monitoring this control can simultaneously serve as quality proof for the therapy.

This technology has proved successful in quite a number of our chambers for more than a year.

The chamber computer or the patient's monitoring can be used for the evaluation. A good example is the "HBO-Report" (Figure 8). The programme shows the oxygen partial pressure actually possible in percent.

If below 80% for more than 3 minutes, alarm is released with a remark in the patient's protocol.

For the development of extinguishing systems a test chamber has been in use at HAUX- LIFE -SUPPORT for some time. Starting with the examination of how the different sprinkling nozzles are reacting under different pressures, the test series were followed by designing stationary extinguishing systems for new chambers and the ones to be modified.

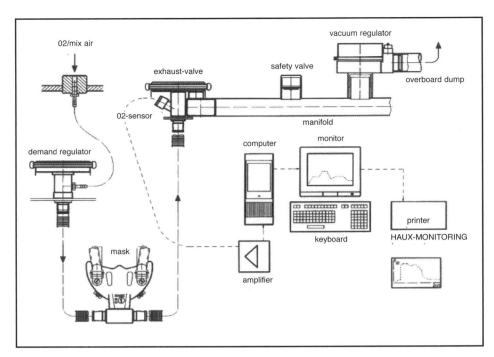

Figure 4. 0_2 Breathing System.

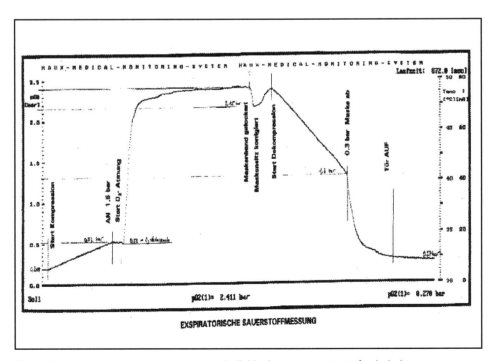

Figure 5. An appropriate sensor measures individual oxygen content of exhaled gas.

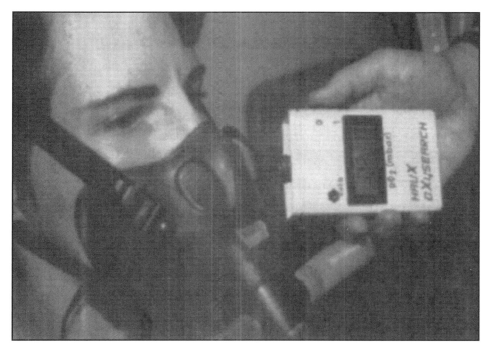

Figure 6. The oxygen administered to this patient is being monitored.

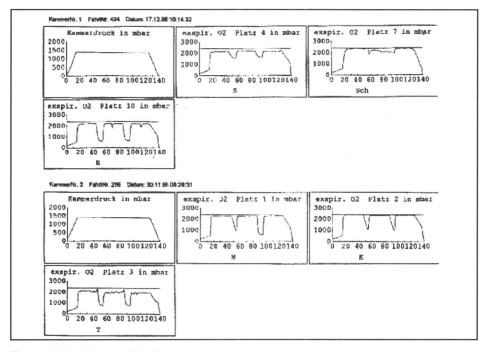

Figure 7. Monitoring mask leakages.

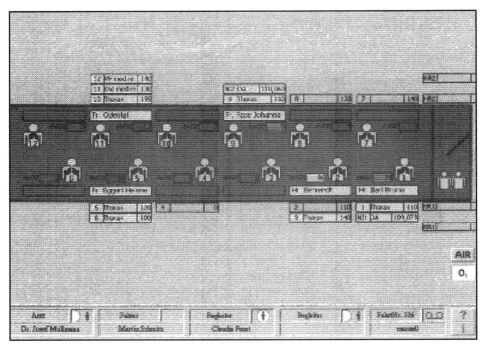

Figure 8. HBO Report.

Practice Teaches Us That
- with a sufficiently high oxygen content in the chamber atmosphere (>30%),
- with a sufficient delay of activation of the extinguishing system (> 15 seconds) a fire cannot be extinguished by the extinguishing system only. It dies once the combustible material is burned off. Temperature and pressure rise considerably (Figures 9a & 9b). Even silicone cables are burnt to ashes.

Sufficient Extinguishing Effect is Reached if
- system is activated immediately after the ignition occurred
- enough water
- the necessary energy is used on the seat of fire
    - and at least a reduction of the oxygen partial pressure is reached by a pressure reduction.

A system according to DIN 13256 is ready for operation. A second version which is also specially suited for modification will be available in about 4 weeks.

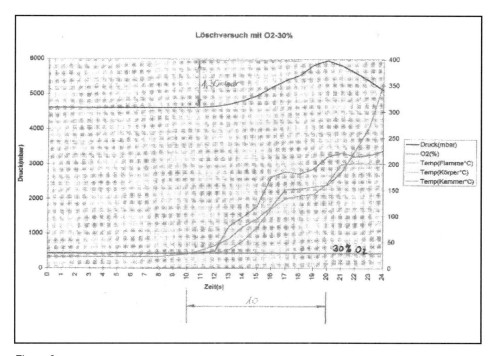

Figure 9a.

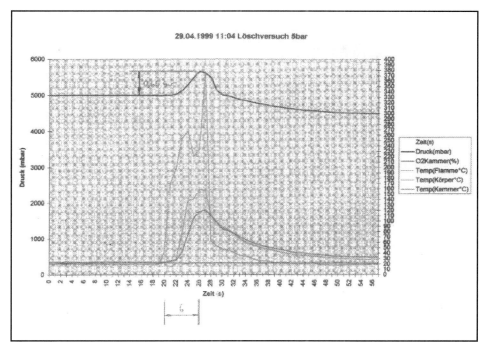

Figure 9b.

Figures 9a and 9b demonstrate rises in temperature and pressure.

REFERENCES

1. SHEFFIELD, DESAUTELS; Hyperbaric and hypobaric chamber fires: a 73-year analysis; UHMS, 1997.
2. REIMERS; Technical aspects of hyperbaric chamber safety; 1997, zit. acc. Chamber Fire Safety, Ocean Systems Inc. 1967.
3. STEPHENSON, MACKENZIE, WATT, ROSS; Measurement of oxygen concentration in delivery systems used for hyperbaric oxygen therapy; UHMS 1996.

SECTION III
ECHM REPORTS

Training Standards for Diving and Hyperbaric Medicine

Section III

PREPARED BY THE JOINT MEDICAL SUBCOMMITTEE OF ECHM AND EDTC

CONTENTS

INTRODUCTION

These training standards are the result of some years of international discussion which began prior the 1st European Consensus Conference on Hyperbaric Medicine, Lille, in September 1994 where one session was devoted to "Personnel education and training policies." A comprehensive paper by J. Desola, MD, and the subsequent debate defined the 5 different personnel categories ideally involved in the staff of a Centre of Hyperbaric Medicine:

- the medical doctors (including the Medical Director),
- the nurses,
- the attendants,
- the chamber operators, and
- the technicians.

The definition, functions, background, academic requirements, dedication, and the continuous education of each category were agreed upon. (This full document is reproduced in Appendix 1.) A working group is being formed to define the requirements for medical doctors in the fields of diving and hyperbaric medicine. An important feature of this project was the collaboration between the European Committee for Hyperbaric Medicine (ECHM), which is primarily a medical committee, and the European Diving Technology Committee (EDTC), which is a 15-nation committee with not only government, industry, and trades union representatives but also with a doctor nominated from each member country. The Goal-setting Principles for Harmonised Diving Standards in Europe was published by the EDTC in 1997 and includes a section on the "Qualifications, education and training of medical doctors" (Appendix 2).

The work presented here has been done by the Joint Medical Subcommittee of these two main committees and, from time to time, reports by this Subcommittee have been submitted to and approved by each of the two parent bodies.

It is the purpose of this paper to summarise what has been accomplished and to look at the future tasks of a Joint Medical Subcommittee of the ECHM & EDTC.

DEFINITION OF JOBS

Before any consideration of a training programme, the training objectives of each job need to be defined in relation to the competencies that are expected from the incumbent. A number of the jobs in diving and hyperbaric medicine have tasks and objectives in common, and so it is possible to optimise the efficiency of the educational program and avoid too much overlap by adopting a modular structure. Thus the first task was to prepare the job definitions which are compatible with EDTC and ECHM:

I. "Medical examiner of divers"
- Competent to perform the periodic "Fitness to dive assessments" of working and recreational divers and compressed air workers, except the initial assessment of novice professional divers.

CONTENTS OF MODULES

Modules of Formation and Subjects

		Jobs:	I	IIa	IIb	III
1		**Physiology & pathology of diving and hyperbaric exposure:** Hyperbaric physics				
	1	Diving related physiology I (functional anatomy, respiration, hearing	b	c	c	c
	2	and equilibrium control, thermo regulation) Hyperbaric pathophysiology (Immersion effect, blackout mechanism	b	c	b	c
	3	incl. apnea, psychology, working performance/endurance under water) Hyperbaric pathophysiology (decompression theories, bubbles)	b	c	a	c
	4	Acute Dysbaric disorders, DCI (Barotrauma, DCS) Chronic Dysbaric disorders (Long term effects)	b	c	b	c
	5	HBO-Basics (effects of hyperbaric oxygen)	b	c	b	c
	6	O_2 Intoxication	b	c	a	b/c
	7	Inert gas-effects (Narcosis/HPNS)	-	b	c	c
	8	Medicaments under pressure	a	c	c	c
	9	Non-dysbaric diving pathologies (Hypothermia, near drowning, fauna	a	c	a	c
	10	& flora effects, injuries and accidents in water, the sick diver)	b	c	c	c
	11	Diving fatalities	a	c	-	c
		Diving technology and safety:				
	12	Diving procedures (Bell diving) Diving procedures (SCUBA, surface supplied, bell, TUP, SURD, 02-	a	a	-	b/c
2		Deco, mixed gas diving				
	1	Divers (Recreational SCUBA diving, technical and deep diving,	b[1]	b[1]	-	a/c
	2	Apnea-diving, professional diving: offshore, inshore, scientific, media, recreational diving instructor, caissonwork, astronauts)	b	c	a	a/c
	3	Diving gear (SCUBA, SSUBA, mixed gas, rebreathers, monitoring equipment, working tools, suits) Diving tables and computers (incl altitude and interval) Regulations and standards for diving	b	b	a	a/c
	4	Safety planning / management (monitoring)	b	b	a	a/c
	5	**Fitness to dive:**	b	b	b	a/c
	6	Fitness to dive criteria and contraindications (for divers, tunnel workers	b	b	-	a/c
	7	and HBOT patients and chamber personnel) Fitness to dive assessment (diagnostics)	b	b	-	a/c
3						
	1	Fitness to dive standards and regulations (prof. and recreational d.)	c	c	c	c
	2		c	c	c	c
	3		c	c	b	c

[1] as required

	Jobs:	I	IIa	IIb	III
4	**Diving accidents:**				
1	Diving accidents / incidents (assessment and preclinical treatment incl. ORL, barotraumas, CPR)	a	c	a	c
2	Diving accident management clinical (Diagnostics, patient care, follow-up)	-	c	c	c
3	Diving accident management: Differential diagnosis	a	c	c	c
4	HBO-T for diving accidents (Tables and strategies)	a	c	c	c
5	Rehabilitation of disabled divers	-	a	a	b/c
5	**Clinical HBO:**				
1	Chamber technique (multiplace, monoplace, transport chambers, wet recompression)	-	b	c	c
2	HBO: Mandatory Indications	-	a	c	c
3	HBO: Recommended Indications	-	-	c	c
4	HBO: experimental and anecdotal Indications	-	-	b	c
5	Data collection / statistics / evaluation	-	b	b	c
6	General basic treatment (nursing)	-	b	c	c
7	Diagnostic, monitoring and therapeutic devices in chambers	-	c	c	c
8	Risk assessment, incidents monitoring and safety plan in HBO-Chambers	-	b	c	c
9	Safety regulations	-	c	c	c
6	**Diverse:**				
1	Research standards	-	a	a	c
2	Paramedics teaching program	-	b	a	c
3	Management /Organisation of HBO facility	-	a	a	c
7	**Practical training:**				
1	Fitness for chamber-dive test (of the course participants)	-	+	+	+
2	CPR	-	+	+	+
3	Practice in field first aid (diving accidents)	-	+	-	+
4	Practical training FTD exam (skills)	+	+	+	+
5	Demo : professional diving	+	+	-	+
6	Demo : HBO-T	-	+	+	+
7	Introduction to (wet)-Diving	(+)[2]	+[4]	-	+
8	Practice in HBO-T (including pressure test)	-	+	+	+
9	Practice in paramedics teaching	-	+[3]	-	+

[2] recommended

[3] as required

[4] exceptions possible, if important reasons of unfitness to dive

IIa. "Diving medicine physician"

- Competent to perform the initial and all other assessments of working and recreational divers or compressed air workers.
- Can manage diving accidents and advise diving contractors and others on diving medicine and physiology* (with the back-up of a hyperbaric expert or consultant).
- Should have knowledge in relevant aspects of occupational health. (He or she does not need to be certified specialist in occupational medicine to be in accordance with the standards).

IIb. "Hyperbaric oxygen physician"

- Responsible for HBO sessions at the treatment site (with backup of a hyperbaric expert or consultant).
- Should have appropriate experience in anaesthesia and intensive care in order to manage the HBO patients (he or she does not need to be certified specialist in anaesthesia to be in accordance with the standards).
- Competent to assess and manage clinical patients for HBO treatment.

III. "Hyperbaric expert or consultant (hyperbaric and diving medicine)"

- Competent as chief of a hyperbaric facility (HBO centre) and/or to manage the medical and physiological aspects of complex diving activities*.
- Competent to manage research programs.
- Competent to supervise his team (HBO doctors and personnel, health professionals, and others).
- Competent to teach relevant aspects of hyperbaric medicine and physiology to all members of staff.

IV. "Associated specialists"

- This title is not a job qualification, but rather a function. It covers experts, consultants, and specialists of other clinical specialities who can be nominated as competent to advise within their own speciality upon specific problems in the diving and hyperbaric field.

*optional additional qualification for bell diving (saturation, mostly off-shore)

STANDARDS FOR COURSE ORGANISATION AND CERTIFICATION

Teaching Courses

In order to comply with this EDTC/ECHM standard the person responsible for the professional contents of the course must be a hyperbaric medical expert or consultant (job type III):

1. The course curriculum should be declared as being "in conformity with the ECHM/EDTC standards" and the educational objective (jobs I and IIa, IIb) stated.
2. The course organisers are invited to send a copy of the curriculum to the joint medical subcommittee of ECHM/EDTC (through the national co-ordinator).
3. The final tests for individual evaluation are mandatory, and should cover all the taught subjects (see list) at the level of competence required for each subject.

The standards do not prescribe the status of the teaching institution but it is strongly recommended that courses are university based, are approved for such training courses by national health authorities, speciality training boards, or are under the auspices of the national scientific society for diving medicine and/or hyperbaric medicine.

How a course is to be organised is not prescribed in these standards. Evenings, weekends, or full weeks are possible For clinical teaching, an internship or residency may be appropriate. The acknowledgement of a high teaching standard is based on a credible final test of the candidates.

Modules and Course Organisation

The actual organisation and conduct of the modules will be influenced by local factors and so it is proposed that these details can be decided on a national basis and probably left to the individual course directors. The following proposal indicates the

I	Medical examiner of divers	25 lecture hours + 3 hours practical
IIa	Diving medicine physician	The above + 30 additional lectures + 10 hours practical
IIb	Hyperbaric medicine physician	60 hours + a practical phase (5 different types of clinical cases with different indications for treatment)
III	Diving and hyperbaric medicine expert or consultant	This needs further review (see below)

total teaching hours considered necessary to achieve appropriate competencies in the following jobs.

The proposal serves as a guideline and is not mandatory. When one of these teaching programmes includes topics covered elsewhere a reduction in the number of lecture hours may be justifiable.

Recognition of an expert

The experience needed to become an expert cannot be learned from a course. The essentials have already been described in general terms. The candidate should already be an accredited specialist or equivalent.

Except in those countries where some equivalent or higher standards already exist, those who wish to be acknowledged as experts or consultants in the fields of diving and hyperbaric medicine should send their curriculum to their national co-ordinator (representing the Joint Medical Subcommittee, or to that subcommittee itself if that nation has no co-ordinator) who may decide on the basis of the agreed standards. The Joint Medical Subcommittee will be informed by the national co-ordinator and can issue a list of experts if required. In the future the verification of achieved qualifications will be done by a national health authority or a scientific body (EU legislation). The aim is to achieve a recognition of the standards by those so that they automatically could take over the role of the national co-ordinator.

CONTINUOUS EDUCATION (QUALITY CONTROL AND COMPETENCY)

In most countries, the conditions for maintaining the active status of an individual are defined by some system of continuous medical education credit points (CME, as introduced in the USA some time ago). The ECHM & EDTC need to define the minimum requirement for this in a flexible way that provides enough freedom for the national bodies to establish a more detailed system. It is expected that these national requirements will be compatible with our guidance.

Our proposals are the following:

- **Job I:** A minimal activity of 10 medical assessments of diver's fitness per year is needed plus attendance at one refresher course (usually 2-days) in two years. Reactivation after a lapse needs participation in two 2-day refresher courses or a repeat of the full basic course.
- **Job IIa:** Continuing experience in the field of professional diving (e.g., advising a professional diving contractor or some equivalent activity) and participation in a course or congress previously approved by the national coordinator. Reactivation after a lapse should be on the basis of a specifically approved course. Where this cannot be achieved, the candidate should submit an alternative training programme to the national co-ordinator for approval.
- **Job IIb:** Active employment in an HBO facility (or equivalent activity) and attendance at one national and/or international congress on hyperbaric medicine per year. Reactivation after a lapse needs a 10 working days in a HBO facility and attendance at two congresses in two years.
- **Job III:** Will rely on the decision of the national co-ordinator.

The refresher seminars can serve to update the participants in order to confirm their active status and to reactivate those who temporarily have not maintained their required activity. They can also serve as an introduction to doctors of other specialities, who may also gain CME credits in their own specialities. This not only can help the financing of a course but can be a chance for promoting HBO to those who would not attend the HBO scientific congresses.

THE JOINT MEDICAL SUBCOMMITTEE OF ECHM AND EDTC

This committee will operate on the basis of the tasks outlined above. The members are the two chairmen of the education and training subcommittee of the ECHM and of the medical subcommittee of the EDTC respectively. Further, two to three members are nominated by the chairmen on the basis of their special competence and experience in one of the relevant topics. As the chairmen, each represents a specific subcommittee; any major changes or decisions must be discussed within these subcommittees before going to the meetings of the EDTC or ECHM respectively.

Each country interested in educational courses recognised by EDTC/ECHM should be represented by a member who has been acknowledged by the national hyperbaric medicine authority (or of all such authorities if there are more than one such authority in a country). Normally this would be either the national member of ECHM or the national medical representative on the EDTC. If not the same individual, both could attend if appropriate.

The EDTC and ECHM representatives of each country should nominate a national co-ordinator of teaching programmes, who could be the joint subcommittee member himself or who could delegate for that purpose (for instance to the national health and safety authority or any representative scientific body covering all aspects of hyperbaric medicine). The national co-ordinator will have the duty to supervise the national programs, the certification procedures, and the status of the course directors.

In order to enhance credibility of certification and to help those who do not yet have the experience necessary to establish a good validation system, the Joint Medical Subcommittee will create a pool of multiple choice questions with an evaluation grid, in the main European languages. This will be available for all members. Evaluation of the answers should be done by an international group nominated by the Joint Medical Subcommittee. This Subcommittee may also certify a national teaching syllabus or educational course if desired by its organisers, thus helping the national societies or other authorities in getting accepted by their governmental health and safety department or by their speciality boards.

For the Joint Medical Subcommittee of ECHM and EDTC:
J. Desola, D. Elliot, P. Longobardi/P. Pelaia, F. Wattel, J. Wendling

NOTES

ECHM RECOMMENDATIONS FOR SAFETY IN MULTIPLACE MEDICAL HYPERBARIC CHAMBERS

D. Mathieu, Coordinator, and J.C. Lejechon, Consultant

1-PRINCIPLES

1.1 - Scope of work

The purpose of this document is NOT to produce a new set of rules, standards, or regulations for the safety of HBOT. These rules, standards, and regulations exist and are available in various forms and countries. A list of the major international ones is given below for reference.

This document is intended to be guidelines for the manager or any responsible person in an HBO operation to help him making sure that all necessary safety precautions are taken care of properly.

1.2 - Risk assessment

To make sure safety precautions are adapted to the situation, a risk assessment is necessary; this is depending on the type of hyperbaric installation, the patients, and the indications, as well as the number of exposures carried out on a regular basis in the hyperbaric facility.

This document will not provide answers to all questions; it is only guidelines. An adapted response to eliminate the risks and to reduce the unavoidable ones to an acceptable level must be established under the manager control for each particular Hyperbaric Centre.

1.3 - List of reference documents

European Directives:

CEN Medical devices:	93/42/CE	dated 14 June 1993
CEN Pressure vessels:	97/23/CE	dated 29 May 1997
CEN Noise at work:	86/188/CE	dated 12 May 1986
CEN Chemical agents:	98/24/CE	dated 07 April 1998
CEN Electric devices / explosive atmospheres	94/9/CE	dated 23 March 1994
CEN Electric devices / electrocution	73/23/CE	dated 19 February 1993

Standards:
> Air quality standard (medical air, breathable air, etc.)
> ASME PVHO   1998
> NFPA   1996
> UHMS (Monoplace 1991
>   and Multiplace 1994 - HBO
>   Chamber Safety)
> ECHM (Training standard)   1997

Other documents:
Many independent control organs have produced rules or certification policies for hyperbaric and diving systems which may be used for conformity assessment of pressure vessels for human occupancy of HBO chambers (Bureau Vèritas, Germanischer Lloyd, Lloyds, DNV, etc.).

1.4 - Major points to be considered
Establishing and controlling a safety policy, at work for the attendants as well as in medical practice for the patients, is one of the duties of the manager of the hyperbaric facility. Sub-delegation of responsibilities should be clearly set and made known to the personnel.

The equipment used for HBO treatment is susceptible to generate risks both to the personnel and to the patients, therefore some construction and maintenance standards should be referred to for the equipment control and for the monitoring of the maintenance and in case of any modification carried out on that equipment. This topic includes fire protection and fire extinguishing systems.

Operational procedures needs to be specified, posted, and logged.

2 - MANAGEMENT AND ORGANIZATION

2.1 - Responsible persons
It is the duty of manager of the Hyperbaric Center to organize safety in the facility and he should designate in writing who is in charge of:

- Equipment, its maintenance and control (from compressed gases supplies to the chambers, the controls panel, and the exhaust of gases and fire fighting equipment outside and inside the chambers),
- Running the sessions and monitoring the operation,
- Informing the patients, controlling their personal items and objects eventually carried inside the chamber.

2.2 - Supporting documentation
Safety Manual
The safety manual is prepared and signed by the manager of the facility; it should include all information necessary to carry out the hyperbaric sessions safely, including the description of duties of the personnel involved. The content of this Safety Manual should be known by all and specific information should be given to new comers to make sure they are perfectly aware of its content.

Hyperbaric Equipment Construction Data Book (As built)

A technical document should contain all information concerning the plant, as-built drawings, all certificates with a list and dates of validity for easy check, basic operational procedures, maintenance program recommended by the manufacturer, and logging of all modifications carried out on the equipment.

Maintenance Register

Based on the manufacturer recommendations, a register of maintenance should be opened to log all actions of the maintenance team, in particular formal inspections, re-certifications, and spare parts changes. Near missed or break down should also be entered for further actions.

Compression and Decompression Procedure Manual

All pressure profiles used in the treatment should be categorized and identified with proper description. This includes decompression procedures applicable to the exposed personnel on the occasion of the attendance of the patients.

Any emergency compression (access), decompression (evacuation), or recompression (in case of DCI symptoms) procedures to be used for the attendants should also be in that document.

Day to Day Logging of Personnel Pressure Exposures

A register of exposure should receive information about individual staff exposures, and the same data should be logged in a personal log-book supplied by the employer to each person qualified to be exposed to pressure.

2.3 - Personnel training / medical fitness

Any person exposed to pressure should be fit to do so. This is based on occupation medical fitness to undergo pressurization. A specific assessment is needed on a yearly basis. A certificate of fitness should be issued, and eventually entered in the personal log-books.

The content of medical examination may be under national rules. If not, it should be defined and agreed with the concerned occupational doctor.

2.4 - Relationship with external emergency services

A joint visit of the plant with the Fire Brigade in charge of the place is highly recommended and the conclusion should be a jointly-defined contingency plan for fire outside the chamber and help in case of fire inside.

2.5 - Safety posters on site

Throughout the plant, where specific safety information is needed, proper posters should remind the patients and personnel of the applicable safety rules (non-smoking area, items not to be taken in the chamber, maximum value for oxygen monitoring, and action in case of high alarm signal, etc.).

At the lock attendant position, information on panel operation should be clearly displayed (valve function, positions, piping diagrams, emergency items, etc.).

3 - EQUIPMENT

3.1 - Construction of hyperbaric chamber
Pressure Vessel

Specific construction and inspection rules apply to pressure vessels according to various national rules. After 2002, European pressure vessels regulation will have been harmonized under the Directive: CEN Pressure Vessels, 97/23CE, dated 29 May 1997.

Architecture

Basically the number of chambers in an installation should be such that in case of emergency it should be possible to enter the treatment chamber and provide assistance inside. The minimum is a 2 compartment installation, one chamber being kept at atmospheric pressure to give access. It is generally considered acceptable to carry out decompression of personnel in that access chamber provided a procedure is prepared to free that chamber quickly to face the need to enter the main chamber.

Patient access to the treatment chamber is of primary importance for the personnel and all effort should be made to provide mechanical help for handling beds and stretchers when the entrance doors are not with easy and wide access. Many chambers derived from diving chamber engineering are very poorly designed in this respect. In addition this is a serious hazard in case of emergency evacuation.

Electric devices

Electricity may cause two types of hazards: Electrocution and Fire.

Electrocution prevention

Any electrical medical device in contact with the patients should be protected against the hazards of electrocution of the patients in accordance with medical rules applicable to such medical devices.

Any electrical device used in the chamber as tools or equipment should be protected against electrocution as a tool or equipment used in a conductive environment (CEN Electric devices, electrocution, 73/23/CE, dated 19 February 1993).

Fire precautions

Fire may be triggered in the chamber either by conductors overheating (short circuit) or by sparks. Due to the high partial pressure of oxygen always present in compressed air, fire will develop extremely fast if material burning in compressed air is present at the place of fire trigger, therefore:

- All power wires should be selected in the category M2.
- All equipment should be built in such a way that no spark may start a fire.
- Any equipment not specifically designed for use in compressed air should be validated by a competent person who will assess the risk of bursting a fire during normal use and in case of breakdown (fail safe).

A simple way to prevent dangerous sparks is to select electrical equipment with CE marks showing it is acceptable for use in flammable or explosive atmosphere (CEN Electric devices, explosive atmospheres, 94/9/CE, dated 23 March 1994).

Plumbing

Regular piping should be in agreement with pressure vessel systems rules.

Oxygen and gases with high oxygen concentration ($FO_2 > 0.25$) circuits, require special precautions (reduce pressure as much as practicable in all distribution lines, all equipment must be oxygen compatible and internally cleaned by a competent person on installation). No ball valve should be used to operate oxygen circuits. All gas storage areas should be properly ventilated or equipped with a leakage alarm (high oxygen content).

Connecting oxygen cylinders to the circuit should be made only by qualified personnel.

Measurements, analysis, recorders

Calibration of meters (gauges) is part of the maintenance program. It should be done at regular intervals and logged into the maintenance register.

Pressure profiles and oxygen content of the atmosphere should be recorded.

Fire fighting systems

Internal fire fighting system includes: A manual extinguishing system operable by the attendant, a sprinkler type water deluge triggered independently from inside or outside. Override valves (inside and outside) should be available to prevent flooding when fire is eventually under control.

It is part of fire prevention to be able to decompress quickly the chamber for evacuation and at the same to cool efficiently the burning material and reduce immediately the partial pressure of oxygen closer to 0.2 bar. A fast decompression valve operable from outside at the attendant position, eventually sealed with a safety breakable thread, is a strong recommendation.

Breathing masks

In case of fire it is extremely important that any extra oxygen input in the atmosphere should be stopped, and that breathing masks be available for all. Shifting HBO masks to air will cover the need for the patients; extra masks should be available, one for each attendant eventually present in the chamber.

Very little can be done to protect hoses delivering gases to the masks; they should be built of heat and fire resistant material. The deluge system is intended to protect them until evacuation can be carried out.

Lock attendant station

Special care should be given by the manufacturer of the system to make the control of the chambers easy and fool proof. Proper markings are needed showing gas circuits and functions of valves as well as their position. When video screen are used, their location and brightness should be controlled. The communications system should have a back-up arrangement, and the quality of microphones and speakers in the chambers should be high; a permanent listening capability for the lock attendant is needed. A telephone line in connection with the telephone control panel of the building should be available at the position of the lock attendant.

Noise level due to decompression of gases should be removed from the place by proper piping and silencers.

3.2 - Construction of buildings

Patients access

In addition to the access to the chamber some care should be given in the room available for patient preparation, inspection and handling around the installation in particular when intensive care patients are concerned.

Connection with hospital

Many of the indications of HBOT are for intensive care patients which require special equipment and transport from the hospital, a close connection with the hospital is a must for hyperbaric centers accepting intensive care indications. This includes laboratories and medical analysis capabilities.

Fire precautions

The hazard of fire in the hyperbaric facility are related to gas storage, oxygen circuits, pressure vessels, and the fact that for some indications decompression of patients for evacuation may be fatal to the patient (arterial embolism, DCI, some CO poisoning cases). And it also may be dangerous for the attendant involved in such cases.

A contingency plan should be prepared with the fire brigade to take into account those specific hazards and organize fire fighting procedure accordingly.

All markings in relation with fire fighting and evacuation must be displayed.

Gas storage, compressors room, distribution plumbing, etc.

It is of primary importance that, in all situations, pressure could be maintained in the chamber and that ventilation should not be interrupted for more than a few minutes. The gas supply system should be so arranged that in case of failure (compressor, electricity, cooling water, piping breaks, etc.) a back up system becomes operational at once to match the gas requirements for the treatment and the possible required decompression of personnel. This can be achieved via gas storage, emergency compressors, emergency electric supply, etc. A document should demonstrate the risk assessment which leads to the choice of an adapted solution. The corresponding emergency procedure should be in writing and should be part of the training of the personnel in charge.

Equipment authorized for use under pressure

The equipment permanently used in the chamber and designated for use under pressure should be devoted to that activity and be clearly identified. It should have been evaluated for suitability of the purpose either by the initial manufacturer of the chamber or jointly by the user and the manufacturer of the equipment.

A list of those equipment items should be part of the safety manual. Example: hospital wheel chairs should be greased with non-burning grease, Private wheel chairs have to be left outside.

Any new item to be entered into the chamber should be controlled by a competent person who will sign an authorisation to use under pressure, eventually in association with special recommendations or safety rules when applicable and after questioning the manufacturer.

3.3 - Maintenance program

Schedule for maintenance operations
In the instruction manual provided by the manufacturer of the installation, there should be proper guidelines for the maintenance schedule. The manager of the installation will formalize the maintenance program in the safety manual.

In particular, only products and spare parts recommended by the manufacturer should be used (oxygen compatible lubricants for example).

Air quality controls.
The frequency of air quality controls is depending of the type of compressors used, the type of filtering units, and the activity of the center. This should be defined in agreement with the guidelines given by the manufacturer(s) of the gas production plant and incorporated into the safety manual.

Maintenance logging
All maintenance operations carried out by technicians should be logged in the maintenance register and signed by the technician in charge.

Entries should be left open for the personnel to report on day to day breakdowns and remedial actions taken.

Emergency drills
The manager of the installation should recommend safety drills, mostly oriented towards fire prevention and fire fighting; all personnel should participate to those safety drills, which should also be logged in the operation log-book.

4 - OPERATIONS

4.1 - Staffing
Number and role of persons
During any treatment the functions involved are:

- Supervision of the treatment (medical aspect and safety of operations)
- Operation of the chambers
- Attendance of patients under pressure
- Emergency assistance under pressure if needed

Depending on the type of center and the number of simultaneous pressure chamber operations, the minimum team size is variable. There should be a minimum of three qualified persons outside (supervision lock attendant, and emergency help).

Any staff member accepted for compression should be medically fit to undergo pressurization.

Under pressure patients attending policy
It is presently a common practice in several hyperbaric units not to attend walk-in patients for the whole session, the attendant being locked out after compression or even not being compressed at all when patients have experience of the exposure.

The policy on patient attending under pressure should also be clearly defined in the safety manual. Instructions to unattended patients should be sufficient for them to face minor problems under pressure and to control properly oxygen mask leakage (both ways).

4.2 - Patient preparation / control
Information to the patients

The content and the procedure of information to the patients should be clearly established, eventually with a specific leaflet or document to be given to the patients, on the occasion of exposures. Who is in charge of this information and copies of the documents are to be included in the safety manual.

Medical preparation

Before entering the chamber, all patients should be controlled to assess their medical situation, in particular when they are connected to medical devices or when they wear dressings on wounds.

Practical preparation

Policy concerning patients clothing, bedding equipment, inspection of personal items is needed. A recommendation should be that patients keep a minimum of personal clothes and receive at least a blouse covering the remaining clothes, that blouse being made out of low flammability material (cotton). Consequently a personal items storage locker should be made available for each patient.

5 - CONCLUSION

Basically there are few construction problems left when the manufacturer of the HBO facility is safety conscious and the buyer ready to invest in a safe system. Most of the safety problems in HBOT are related to the procedures used and the precautions enforced during the day to day work.

These precautions are directly under the control of the personnel. The personnel should be well aware of the center safety policy, he (she) should have received the initial training, a copy of the safety manual, and be given a clear definition of his (her) responsibilities during the sessions.

The management, after establishing that policy in a safety manual, should also make sure it is properly applied. This needs personal involvement and frequent controls.